Reach for the Stars!
The Complete Guide to

Successful NURSING ASSISTANT Care

Diana L. Dugan, RN

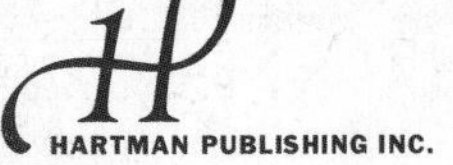

HARTMAN PUBLISHING INC.

hartmanonline.com

Credits

MANAGING EDITOR
Susan Alvare

COPY EDITOR
Celia McIntire

COVER AND INTERIOR DESIGNER
Kirsten Browne

ILLUSTRATORS
Thaddeus Castillo/Robert Christopher

PAGE LAYOUT
Thaddeus Castillo/Susan Alvare

PHOTOGRAPHY
Art Clifton/Dick Ruddy

PROOFREADER
Suzanne Wegner

SALES/MARKETING
Gailynn Garberding/Debbie Rinker

CUSTOMER SERVICE
Yvonne Gillam/Kim Williams

Copyright Information

8529-A Indian School Road, NE
Albuquerque, New Mexico 87112
(505) 291-1274
web: www.**hartman**online.com
e-mail: orders@hartmanonline.com

ISBN 1-888343-50-8

NOTICE TO READERS
Though the guidelines and procedures contained in this text are based on consultations with healthcare professionals, they should not be considered absolute recommendations. The instructor and readers should follow employer, local, state, and federal guidelines concerning healthcare practices. These guidelines change, and it is the reader's responsibility to be aware of these changes and of the policies and procedures of her or his healthcare facility.

The Publisher, author, editors, and reviewers cannot accept any responsibility for errors or omissions or for any consequences from application of the information in this book and make no warranty, expressed or implied, with respect to the contents of the book. The Publisher does not warrant or guarantee any of the products described herein or perform any analysis in connection with any of the product information contained herein.

GENDER USAGE
This textbook utilizes the pronouns he, his, she, and hers interchangeably to denote healthcare team members and residents.

Special Thanks

A sincere thanks to all of our knowledgeable and insightful reviewers:

Marianna Kern Grachek, MSN, CNHA, CALA
Elmhurst, IL

Lyla Berry, EdD, MA, RN
Brea, CA

Cheryl Dilbeck, MN, RN, PHN
Fresno, CA

Genevieve Gipson, RN, MEd
Norton, OH

Rita Krummen, BSN, RNC
Columbus, OH

Jill Holmes Long, RN, BS, BSN, MA
Peachtree City, GA

Karen Walborn, PhD, RNCS
McLean, VA

Joan Wolff
Scottsdale, AZ

Ileen F. Sullivan, RN, BSN
Salem, NH

Regina St. George, RN, MEd
Atlanta, GA

Bernard A. Brown
Tucson, AZ

Paula S. Ayers, RN, BSN, MS
Grand Junction, CO

Glenda Stapf, RN, MSN
Union City, CA

Karen A. Hergert, RN, MS
Waltham, MA

Beatrice L. Nyback, RN
Salem, MO

Paula L. Windler, RN, BS, MS, CLNC
Chandler, AZ

Ellen A. Latour, RN
Holyoke, MA

Nancy O'Keefe, RN
Pittsburgh, PA

Lorraine H. Mulligan, MSN, RN

Kathleen M. Litz, RN

We are especially grateful for Judith Clinco, Cynthia McAndrew and everybody at Catalina In-Home Services for helping us find Rachel, Gus, and Myriam for our photo shoot.

Thanks to Dr. George W. King for being such an agreeable and informative model. And thanks to his grandson, Alex Berger, for fulfilling the demanding roles of photographer's assistant and part-time model.

Permissions

To the Teacher

"It's a funny thing about life; if you refuse to accept anything but the best, you very often get it."

—**W. SOMERSET MAUGHAM, 1874-1965**

Background

Imagine a textbook fashioned step-by-step with the student's success in mind. Imagine a text inspired by years of students' suggestions, comments and constructive criticism. During my teaching career (my first year teaching nursing assistants was 1978), I started imagining just that. In 1988, while teaching for a community college, the first flicker of my own book actually started to glow. Over the past 11 years, that flicker has turned into a virtual inferno due to the overwhelming insistence of my students, family and friends that I had to write my very own textbook.

So, I finally asked myself, "How would I write a better textbook?" I'm originally a graduate of one of the old diploma nursing programs, the one that used to be at Northwestern Memorial Hospital in Chicago. The structure of that phenomenal school was quite instrumental in my success as a registered nurse and a nurse educator. I soon realized that if the basic structure of our diploma program worked for us, then a similar structure could work for nursing assistants.

I have taught in a variety of settings, from very short to extended courses, and I have found that no matter how hard I searched, a textbook was not available that suited me and my students. There are many fine textbooks out there; however, each one is missing vital information. I often wished that I could find a book that would set me free from the task of compiling endless additional information. Finally, I decided I would have to create one myself.

Then I asked myself, "How could I make a text more interesting?" Again, it dawned on me that there was no special trick to this; I simply must write the textbook using exactly the same methods I use to teach my successful nursing assistant course. I must package all of the interesting and entertaining aspects of my course into this new textbook.

It is my fervent desire to make this textbook the only one that you will ever need in order to effectively teach your own special nursing assistant course. I welcome all of your comments and suggestions.

With admiration for your dedication to teaching,

Diana Dugan, RN

To the "Star" Student

"A professor can never better distinguish himself in his work than by encouraging a clever pupil, for the true discoverers are among them, as comets amongst the stars."

—**CARL LINNAEUS, 1707-1778**

Reach for the stars!

Today is the first day of the rest of your life! I say that to each group of students on the very first day of class. You have chosen to take that first step and enter the exciting field of health care. Look around you at the other eager, uncertain faces. They each took a risk and chose to begin a new day by entering a new profession. So, whether you are young or not-so-young, male or female, let me congratulate you for being here. I'm proud of each one of you! You have chosen an honorable profession, a caring one that will be of service to your community.

I must tell you that I am as fascinated with the world of medicine today as I was when I first entered this field many years ago. I worked as a nursing assistant while I was in nursing school, and those memories are very dear to me. When you actually start your new profession, you will remember your firsts: your first resident to turn 100 years old, your first resident who survives a stroke and actually returns home, and the first family member who tells you that a loved one could not get through a day without your excellent care.

Countless students have sat in front of me over the years. Each one has been a very unique and special person. That is part of what will make your class interesting: the different faces and backgrounds of your peers. You may develop close friendships with your fellow students that will last a lifetime.

My students always ask me what led me into teaching. I teach so that I can train hundreds of nursing assistants in the same philosophy: "Your resident always comes first!" This textbook is the result of constant encouragement from my students over the years. They have made it clear that I could, should, and must write a better textbook, and they have never accepted any excuses. Thus, I have tried to create a textbook made just for you. I hope you will find this text easy to use and interesting, yet also one that will consistently challenge you to learn more about your residents and the care they require. In closing, I leave you with this recipe for success:

The Nursing Assistant "Recipe for Success"

MIX TOGETHER:
Motivation: Work hard every single day.
Interest: Keep learning forever.
Steadfastness: Never take shortcuts in resident care.
Safety: Remember to always think, "Safety first."
Imagination: Be resourceful p.r.n. (when necessary).
Objectivity: Do not judge staff, residents, or visitors.
Nobility: Always expect nothing but the best from yourself and others!

Your **mission** is to study hard, graduate, and go forward to help us change health care! Each and every day, I challenge you to strive to make resident care a little better than it was the day before. Together, we can make it happen!

Diana Dugan, RN

For All My Stars

This book is dedicated to my dearest loving husband John, the biggest star in our family, the quintessential soulmate, and a truly extraordinary husband and father. Words cannot express the appreciation I have for your love and devotion, help and support these many years. You are truly "my rock." With the greatest respect and admiration for your love, patience, dedication and your expertise on behalf of our families and our friends, your patients and your staff.

To our very own best and brightest stars, our dearest son Mark and our dearest daughter Marissa—computer wizards, copy editors, and technical advisors extraordinaire. Your love, hugs, and your enthusiasm regarding this book have helped me push ever forward and reach for the stars!

To my dearest Mom and Dad, Robert and Margaret, my dearest brother Paul and his wonderful family, Paula, Matthew, and Leah, my dear mother-in-law and father-in-law, Thomas and Mary Alice and John's big, wonderful family, my loving Gramma and Grampa and Granny, and all of our good friends, for your great love, encouragement, and tremendous support. To my dear puppies Snowball and Cassandra, for keeping me company.

To special colleagues, dear friends, and associates: Richard L. Luebke, Sr., Jo Ann Luebke, Richard L. Luebke, Jr., Stan Bodzioney, Robin Sipos, Concetta Tynan, Judith Clinco, Cynthia McAndrew, Judith T. Kautz, J. C. Martin, George E. Barrett, Phil Higdon, Marsha Hidgon, Mark Ogram, Angie Kaelberer, Kimberly Graber, Mary Kay Kerbel, Barry Kerbel, Kathryn Kiernicki, Roy Kiernicki, Lorri Ostruszka, Paul Ostruszka, Elizabeth Hayward, Robert Hayward, Rochelle Pozner, Jeanne M. Sierka, Bernard A. Brown, Barbara J. Ramutkowski, Ruth Darling, Barbara R. Rockwell, Judy E. Bodzioney, Marguerite Roop, Irene C. Suchodolski, Joyce A. Chace, Devona Dee Manning, Mike and Jeanne, Chuck and Dana, David and Marita, Michael DeMuch, Yvonne Buckley, Grace Middlebrook, Zona Pinto, Jeanna Skinner, Susan M. Sacharski and Northwestern Memorial Hospital.

To Mark Hartman, my publisher, for his vision and faithful support from the very beginning. Your quiet encouragement, creative talent, commitment to the integrity of the text, wisdom, and editorial expertise, along with your terrific sense of humor helped me "stay the course" to success!

To Susan Alvare, my editor, for her incredible dedication and determination, unlimited energy, enthusiasm, organizational skills, and enormous attention to detail, along with her sharp editorial judgment, flexibility, and constant availability. It has truly been a joy working with you! My heartfelt thanks for your incredible efforts on behalf of this book.

To everyone who helped at Hartman Publishing—Thaddeus, Celia, Gailynn, and Yvonne. To our book designer Kirsten Browne and our photographer Art Clifton, thank you both for your patience, creativity, and expertise. To all of our wonderful and photogenic models for your patience and help; you were a joy to work with!

To all of my very own STAR students over the many, many years. . .

Finally, to Mrs. McDonald, who wanted me to become a doctor; I decided to aim slightly higher and become a nurse, an educator, an author, and most importantly, a wife and a mom.

Diana L. Dugan, December, 2001

Table of Contents

10 Your Facility: The Place Your Residents Call Home 152

11 Quality Infection Control: Breaking the Chain of Infection 164

12 Your Safety Review: Preventing Accidents and Injuries 184

13 Your Introduction: Emergency Care, Disasters, and First Aid 202

37 Your Position: The Star Employee 512

Table of Principal Steps, Practical Procedures & Star K.A.R.E.

Practical Procedures

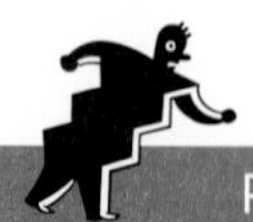

Principal Steps

Star K.A.R.E.

Using your textbook

Color Tabs:

Because you also use your book as a reference, each chapter has been assigned a color tab which is visible at the top of each page, making it easier to find what you need.

Learning Objectives:

e.g. 5 Describe twelve tools provided in this textbook to help you succeed.

Everything you will learn in this book is organized around each chapter's numbered learning objectives. A learning objective is a specific piece of knowledge or a very specific skill. For clarity, this book and the accompanying workbook are referenced to these learning objectives.

Key Terms:

e.g. 1 Spell and define all **STAR** words

The first learning objective of each chapter reviews key terms you should know to better understand the chapter. They are in **bold** and are repeated in **bold** wherever they are used within the chapter.

Procedures:

e.g. Procedure title

All care procedures are highlighted by the same background color for easy recognition.

Principal Steps:

e.g. 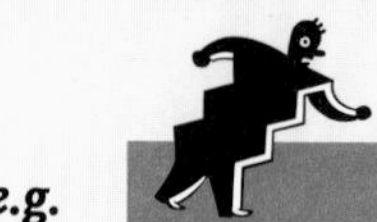 Principal Steps

Principal Steps include general instructions for using equipment, guidelines for caring for residents with particular illnesses, and helpful techniques with which you should become familiar.

Star K.A.R.E.:

e.g. 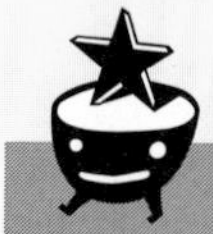 Star K.A.R.E.

Star K.A.R.E. teaches how to observe, report, and promote independence for each disorder.

Anti-Abuse

Important information teaches about abuse and neglect and ways to recognize and prevent both.

Voice of Experience

Experienced nursing assistants share their advice with you whenever you see this icon.

Tips and Trivia

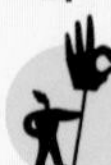

We know that the majority of nursing assistant students are adults, many of whom are managing households, raising children, and leading busy lives. These icons call out interesting and educational tidbits that you can use inside and outside of work.

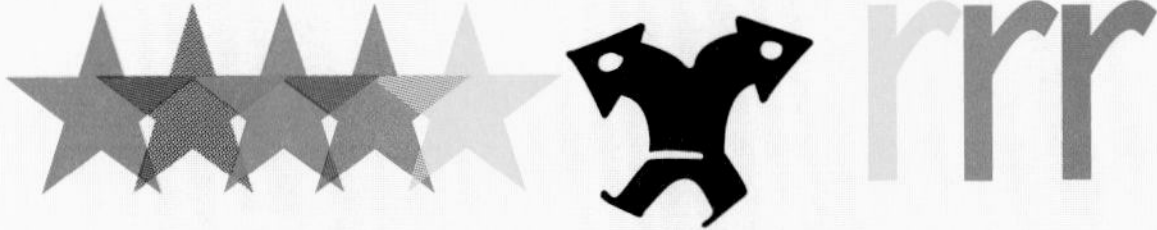

The "5 Stars" icon in each procedure reminds you to follow the five important steps when beginning or ending care.

Beginning Steps

★ RESPECT
Knock first, ask and receive permission to enter a resident's room.

★ INFECTION CONTROL
Wash hands.

★ COMMUNICATION
Greet and identify the resident. Identify yourself. Explain the procedure, encouraging the resident to be as independent as possible throughout.

★ BED SAFETY
Lock bed wheels. Raise bed to safe working height. Lower one side rail if required.

★ PRIVACY
Provide for privacy by closing the door and covering the resident appropriately.

Ending Steps

★ RESIDENT SAFETY AND COMFORT
Secure the resident, lowering the bed, and raising the side rails if ordered. Check that the resident is comfortable and properly aligned.

★ PRIVACY
Remove any added privacy measures, such as a drape or a privacy screen.

★ ESSENTIALS
Place the call light, fresh beverage, and other items within reach.

★ COURTESY
Ask the resident if he or she needs anything else. Say thank you and goodbye.

★ INFECTION CONTROL
Wash hands.

The "3Rs" is a tool listed at the end of each procedure to help you learn and remember to: Report, Record, and Recheck!

r **Report** your care and any important observations to the nurse.

r **Record** your care and any important information/observations such as vital signs in the appropriate place.

r **Recheck** your resident for any changes as directed by the nurse!

The Finish Line:

e.g. 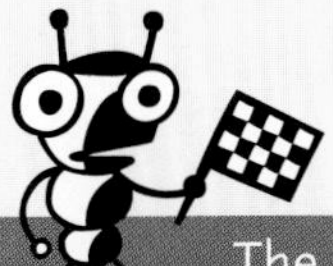 The Finish Line

When you reach The Finish Line at the end of each chapter, it's time to evaluate which learning objectives you know and which need more review. Each Finish Line includes the following review tools:

What's Wrong With This Picture?

This section helps students sharpen their observation skills by making them amateur detectives.

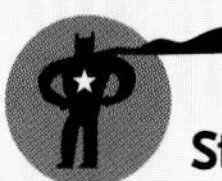

Star Student Central

This material helps mold students into quality employees.

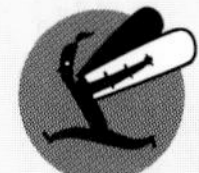

You Can Do It Corner!

This challenges students to remember and practice what they have learned.

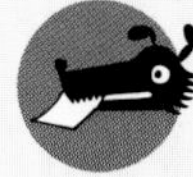

Star Student's Chapter Checklist

The last part in every chapter reminds students to complete all of the necessary study tasks.

Quintessential Quotes and Time Capsules

Carefully-chosen quotes begin each chapter and may be used for discussion. Time Capsules highlight how health care has changed over the years by detailing interesting events in medicine from the past.

for

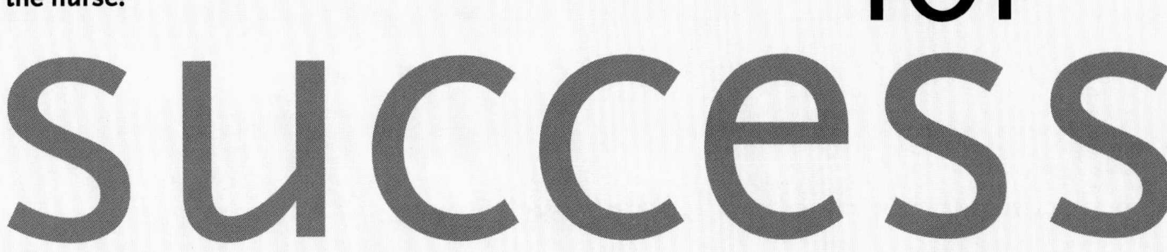

1

Your Guide: Becoming a Star Student

Look Like a Star!

Look at the Learning Objectives **and** The Finish Line **before you begin reading this chapter.**

Look at your pocket calendar.
With your pencil, put a bracket ( ) around a study period every single day.

Look at your homework for this chapter.
Plug each piece of homework into a certain time slot.

Look at the Star Student's Chapter Checklist **at the end of this chapter. Check off each item as it is completed.**

"If one advances confidently in the direction of his dreams, and endeavors to live the life which he has imagined, he will meet with a success unexpected in common hours."

Henry David Thoreau, 1817-1862 from *Walden*

"Chiefly the mould of a man's fortune is in his own hands."

Francis Bacon, 1561-1626

Learning Objectives

1. **Spell and define all STAR words.**
2. **Discuss the importance of professional behavior and goal-setting.**
3. **Define seven terms in the Grammar Connection.**
4. **Describe five punctuation marks in the Punctuation Corner.**
5. **Explain ten capitalization rules in Capital Row.**
6. **Identify the seven steps to improve your reading skills.**
7. **Name three methods of note-taking.**
8. **Identify the two "Secrets of the Stars" memory tips.**
9. **List nine tips to improve your organizational skills.**
10. **List seven materials needed for expert studying.**
11. **Discuss three ways to study effectively around children.**
12. **Describe three ways to prepare physically before an exam.**
13. **Describe six common mistakes to avoid while taking a test.**
14. **Demonstrate skill in four basic types of mathematics.**
15. **Explain how to convert decimals, fractions, and percentages.**
16. **List three different kinds of graphs.**

Nurses' Aides: Helping Hands During WWII

One of the early times nurses' aides were used in America was during wartime. The United States trained nurses' aides in 1941 to help deal with a shortage of nurses due to the World War. Employers in the United States expected nurses' aides to volunteer during this time. The country set a goal of training 100,000 nurses' aides to assist nurses in the care of patients. These individuals toiled each day without being paid. Imagine being hired today as a nursing assistant and being expected to do the job without receiving any pay!

1 Spell and define all **STAR** words.

decimal: a fraction whose denominator is a power of ten. Example: 0.5

fraction: an amount less than the whole.

goal: an aim or objective.

grammar: the rules of a language.

learning objective: aim or goal of acquiring specific knowledge or skill after completion of area of learning; goals must be specific and measurable to help achieve desired outcome.

nursing assistant: an important member of the healthcare team who assists the nurse with the care of the sick and disabled.

peers: individuals with equal standing in age, class or rank.

percentage: a fraction with 100 understood as the denominator. Example: 50%

procedure: a particular method of doing a task.

professionalism: the act of displaying appropriate behavior for a certain job.

punctuation: the use of marks in writing to separate words and ideas.

resident: a person who lives in a long-term care or assisted living facility.

2 Discuss the importance of professional behavior and goal-setting.

Professional behavior is a vital part of today's workplace. **Professionalism** has to do with the way we present ourselves to other people in the community. People may have more respect for those who behave professionally. When someone acts in an unprofessional manner, other people may respond negatively. A healthcare facility is a place where people expect the very best in professional behavior.

As we move through the early chapters of this textbook, professional behavior in the healthcare field will be an ongoing focus. You must first consider what professional behavior means to you. The growth process toward the goal of professional behavior begins here and now. You are on your way to becoming an important part of a professional healthcare team—a skilled **nursing assistant**.

Professional Behavior	*Unprofessional Behavior*
Keeping resident information private	Telling a friend or family member about Mrs. Olsen's illness
Leaving personal problems at home	Telling Mr. Crawford, "I'm in a bad mood because my boyfriend and I got into a fight."
Never gossiping or talking badly about your co-workers	Whispering to another nursing assistant that you think your supervisor is having an affair
Speaking politely to a visitor at the front desk	Telling a visitor, "I'm on the phone; you'll have to wait."

To become a *star* employee in the healthcare field, you must communicate well with many different types of people. Doctors, nurses, family members, and other visitors may ask you for information about your residents. **Residents** will want an explanation of the **procedures** you perform each day. Sometimes nursing assistants need to be able to answer the telephone and exchange accurate information about residents or peers. Your **peers** are your co-workers or people who have an equal standing in age, class, or rank. In short, you are a part of a team of caring people, and you will make a great difference in the lives of your residents.

Learning to speak in front of a small group of people can make you feel more at ease in your everyday work. In class, raise your hand often and ask questions in front of your new peers (Fig. 1-1). It can take a while to feel comfortable doing this, but it will make you feel more confident. It will also become much easier to speak up when you begin your job search.

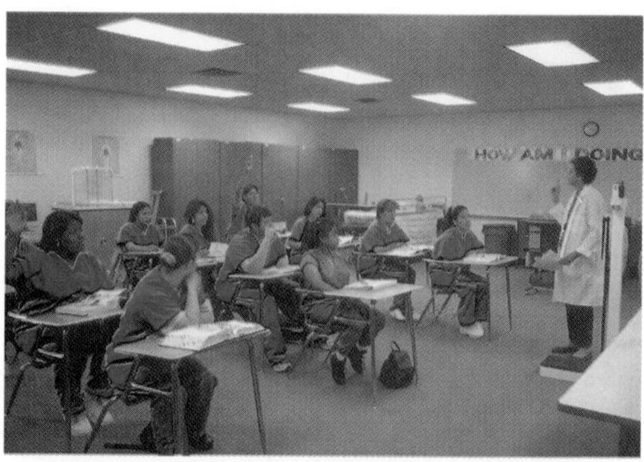

Figure 1-1. Raising your hand in class may make you feel more confident.

The best way to start participating in a class is to begin *right now*. One helpful exercise at the start of a new class is for each student to set personal goals. Goal-setting is an important part of everyday life. As you read this textbook, you are setting **goals**, possibly without realizing it. This textbook is organized around **learning objectives**—goals of acquiring specific knowledge or skills after completing an area of learning. After reading each learning objective, you should have accomplished the goal of being able to *do* what that learning objective describes.

A new student can set many goals, both short-term and long-term goals. A short-term goal may be something that you would like to accomplish in the near future, perhaps within the next month or the next year. A long-term goal is a goal that you might want to complete in five years or more.

Goals can help people focus on their dreams. Some people dream of being successful parents and raising terrific children. Others have grand career goals. Setting financial goals for the future is common in many families. No matter what your dreams are, goals can help you reach them.

Setting goals within a group can be a way to identify one or more of your dreams in front of other people. When you say a goal out loud, you may be more likely to succeed in reaching that goal. You are making a kind of promise or vow to yourself and to others. Others now know your dreams. They may encourage you and help you make your dreams come true.

You may feel a bit "rusty" in this process at first. To help polish your communication skills and help you feel more comfortable speaking in front of others, we need to first learn the basics.

3 Define seven terms in the Grammar Connection.

Speaking well and using **grammar** correctly says something about a person. If you went to a doctor's office and the receptionist said, "Ain't it a great day? You here to see the Doc?" her lack of professionalism might surprise you. It is important for everyone to look closely at the way they present themselves to others. The Grammar Connection reviews some important basic grammar terms.

The Grammar Connection

1. **Noun:** Person, place, or thing. Examples: *car, home, lipstick, school.*
2. **Adjective:** A word that describes a noun. Examples: *blonde* hair, *grey* sweater.
3. **Pronoun:** A word that takes the place of a noun. Examples: *I, he, him, she, them, we.*
4. **Verb:** A word that expresses an action or the condition of a person. Examples: *jumps, drives, lifts.*
5. **Adverb:** A word that describes a verb, adjective, or adverb. Examples: He smiled *happily*. She skated *quickly*.
6. **Conjunction:** A connecting word. Examples: *and, but, neither, nor, or.*
7. **Sentence:** A group of words with a subject and verb. It makes a complete thought. Example: *The fireman rescued the cat from the tree.*

4 Describe five punctuation marks in the Punctuation Corner.

Punctuation is the use of marks in writing to separate words and ideas. If you did not use punctuation, you might not know where one sentence ends and another begins. The Punctuation Corner reviews some important terms.

Punctuation Corner

1. **Comma:** Separates thoughts or items in a list (for example, in a list of adjectives). Example: The hospital sat on top of a tall, grassy hill.
2. **Semicolon:** Connects two sentences with closely related ideas. Example: John has great patience; we appreciate him.
3. **Colon:** Introduces a list or indicates that an addition is coming. Example: Kelley picked up these items: a comb, a razor, and soap. There was only one thing they needed to make their family complete: a pet.
4. **Apostrophe:** Shows possession (ownership) and indicates where letters are missing in contractions. Examples to show possession: That is Doug's house. Susan took Sarah's toy. Examples of use in contractions: wasn't (contraction of *was not*), didn't (contraction of *did not*).
5. **Quotation Marks:** Show you are copying what someone has said or written. Example: The resident said, "I am having pain in my shoulder."

5 Explain ten capitalization rules in Capital Row.

Capital Row

Capitalize the following:

1. The first word of a sentence, question, or quote. Example: The gate is open.
2. Proper names and titles. Example: "Hello, Mr. Dickens. How are you and Margaret today?"
3. Races or names of peoples. Example: Asian
4. Names of religious groups and of sacred texts. Examples: Catholics, the Koran (Muslim holy text), the Bible
5. Names of countries, states, cities, or areas. Examples: Italy, Massachusetts, Tucson, the Pacific Northwest
6. Names of streets or roads. Example: Thatcher Road
7. Names of buildings, organizations, colleges, schools. Examples: Yale University, the United Nations, Roosevelt High School, the White House
8. Holidays, historical and special events, and holy days. Examples: Labor Day, Passover, the Civil War
9. Days of the week and months of the year. Examples: Tuesday, May
10. Trade names. Examples: Arby's, Target, Nike

6 Identify the seven steps to improve your reading skills.

Reading well is an art. If you enjoy reading for pleasure, you know how much fun it can be. Sometimes we read to our children, family members or friends. When you are in the healthcare field, you must be able to read assignments, menus, activity schedules, and many other things. Brushing up on your overall reading skills can assist you in these situations. It will also help you do your homework and study for your tests. Make sure you choose a place to read where you can concentrate. For some people, that is in a room with loud music. Others must have absolute quiet in order to concentrate. When you read any textbook, the best way to begin is to follow "The Seven Steps to Star Reading."

1. Know yourself. Choose the site where you can read best.
2. Use glasses or contact lenses if you need them.
3. Have enough light to read.
4. Sit comfortably so that you do not hurt your back or neck.
5. Practice saying words you are unsure of.
6. Do not be too embarrassed to ask for help pronouncing a word.
7. Use your dictionary wisely. Do not miss a chance to increase your vocabulary. In fact, set a goal to look up one new word each day!

7 Name three methods of note-taking.

We take notes all the time. Everyone is different; some people write tiny notes and post them on their refrigerator. Taking notes while reading a textbook or listening to a teacher in class can be hard if you have not chosen a plan. There are many fine note-taking methods out there; here are three for you to consider using in class.

1. **Outline Method:** Write down the subject, and then put all sentences about that subject under it in outline form. (See Box 1-1) Use a highlighting marker to highlight the subjects and important words or points you need to remember.
2. **Index Card Method:** Write down all of your notes neatly on large index cards instead of in a spiral notebook. Use one card for each small subject. Use rubber bands to keep them together. Or punch a hole in the left-hand corner of the cards. Buy a ring at a discount store to hold them together (one ring for every chapter).
3. **Rewrite Method:** If you are using plain notebook paper, rewrite your notes in a neat, orderly fashion in a spiral notebook to keep them together. As you rewrite them, you will "write to learn" the material and actually remember some things because you wrote them down a second time.

Taking Notes - Outline Method Box 1-1

I. First Topic

A. Key Term 1
B. Key Term 2

II. Second Topic

A. Key Term 1
  a. Secondary Information
  b. Secondary Information
B. Key Term 2

III. Third Topic

A. Key Term 1
  a Secondary Information
  b. Secondary Information
B. Key Term 2

8 Identify the two "Secrets of the Stars" memory tips.

Remembering things can be difficult for some people. If you can learn to improve your memory, it will help you take better, safer care of your residents. These two memory tips can assist you in remembering things when you are unable to write them down.

Memory Tip 1: Use the first letter of each item you need to remember to create a sentence or phrase that is easy to remember. For example, if you are trying to remember to get syrup, oatmeal, and sandwiches, pull out the "S", the "O", and the "S." Then give each item a name: for example, "Sally, Oscar, and Sam." Or you can create a sentence or a phrase. For example, "Same Old Stuff." To cement this in your memory, say it out loud or whisper it at least five times.

Memory Tip 2: Use the first letter of each item to spell an easy-to-remember word or abbreviation. For example, syrup, oatmeal, and sandwiches can spell the abbreviation "SOS."

As you practice memory techniques, you will be able to choose those that work best for you. You can actually come up with new memory techniques of your own!

9 List nine tips to improve your organizational skills.

It is very important to be organized as a nursing assistant. Organization does not come naturally to some people. If you are not an organized person, there are ways to improve your organizational skills. A few simple steps can make the difference between feeling overwhelmed and feeling ready for each new day. One way is to "compartmentalize," or put each thing on your list into a box. This allows you to do one thing at a time, check it off, and then go on to the next item.

To get started, look at the following tips. These tips will be at the beginning of each chapter in this book. Following these tips can help you get through each day feeling like you have accomplished a great deal!

Look Like a Star!

1. Look at the Learning Objectives and "The Finish Line" before you begin reading this chapter.
2. Look at your pocket calendar. With your pencil, put a bracket ( ) around a study period every single day.
3. Look at your homework for this chapter. Plug each piece of homework into a time slot.
4. Look at the "Star Student's Chapter Checklist" at the end of each chapter. Mark off each item as you complete it.

Now that we have discussed methods of organizing your study time, let us discuss improving your life organizational skills. Review the following hints:

1. Buy and use sticky notepads. Keep them all over your house with pens.
2. Buy an inexpensive daily planner. Make sure it is divided into hours of the day. See Figure 1-2.

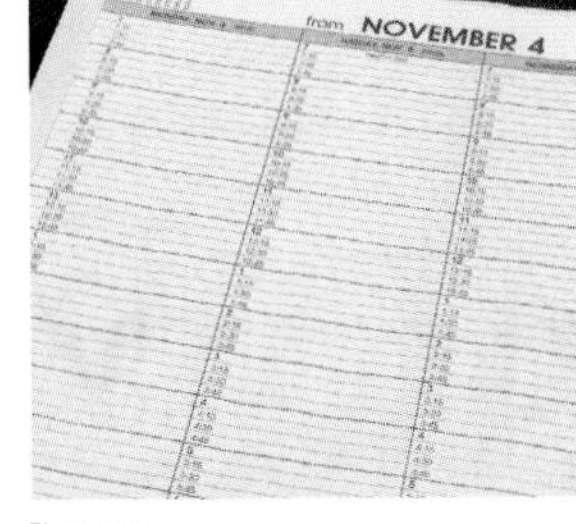

Figure 1-2.

3. At the end of every month, write in everything you must do in the next month. This includes school, work, birthdays, holidays, appointments, games, etc.
4. At the beginning of each week, review the week ahead so that you can be prepared.
5. Use a magnetic refrigerator notepad to remind family members of important things. Make it clear that all telephone messages will be written on this magnetic pad and that each member of the household should check it each time they

come home. Some families choose to use an electronic message machine.

10 List seven materials needed for expert studying.

It is not enough to just sit down and start studying. Students must have the right tools to make the most of their study time. Make sure you have gathered the following items before you set out to study for the first time:

- A large pad of paper for writing a list of questions.
- Regular pens and highlighting pens. Highlight all important words and main subjects.
- A cassette-tape player to record your thoughts and ideas about each chapter. We may remember things better when we hear them out loud. We will call this your "tutor tape." Some people replay their thoughts while resting.
- A timer. Set your timer for one hour from the time you start studying. When it rings, get a drink, use the bathroom, or run around the yard with your pets. It is best to take frequent breaks. Reset it for the next hour when you return.
- A regular dictionary.
- A medical dictionary. This may be supplied by your school. If it is not supplied, please consider buying one. Swap meets or used bookstores often have terrific sales on these books.
- A "Pocketful of Terms" personal notebook. Purchase a small spiral notebook so that you may write down any unfamiliar terms from your lectures or textbook. Look each term up once in one of your dictionaries, and write the meaning in your notebook. Simply pull this out to study for each test or quiz.

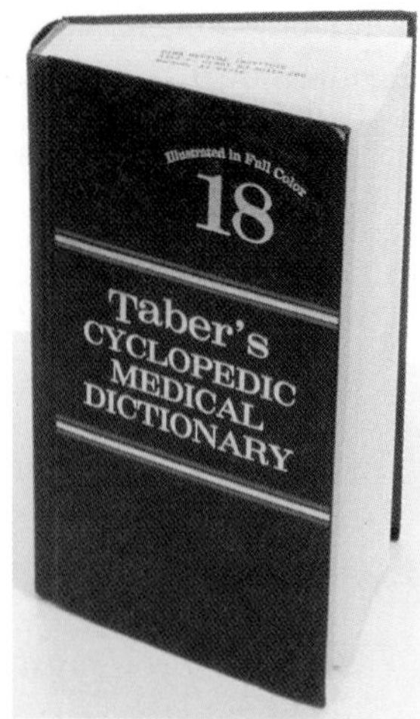

Figure 1-3.

11 Discuss three ways to study effectively around children.

Children are certainly one of the world's greatest blessings. They can brighten our lives and make our days worthwhile. Studying with children underfoot, however, can be something of a challenge. Here are some helpful ideas to make it easier.

1. If you are working on the computer and you have a problem, ask your children to help you fix it. Many children have advanced computer skills and are flattered when you ask them for help.
2. Ask your children to quiz you for your exam. If they can read, they can quiz you. Children as young as five or seven can help parents study medical terms. By the time the studying is done, the children may also have memorized the terms!
3. Ask your children to help around the house while you study if they are old enough to do a task. This keeps them busy and makes them feel like they are needed. Reward them later with a special treat.

12 Describe three ways to prepare physically before an exam.

Students sometimes put so much effort into the book preparation for a test, they may forget to prepare their body as well. When you take a test, you use all of your mental energy. Your brain needs food, too! Please remember to do the following things before an exam:

1. Do not stay up past your regular bedtime. If you are overtired the day of the test, you may score lower, so get a good night's sleep.
2. Eat before the test. Students often skip meals when they are in a hurry. Feed your brain so it can do its best during the test! Eat things that will "stick" like breads, cereals, juices, and proteins. Try to stay away from simple sugars like candy, doughnuts, or soda. If you eat these items, you may notice a sudden drop in energy mid-morning or -afternoon when the sugar level in your blood goes back down.
3. Decrease your overall stress level before an exam. Fill up the car with gas or get cor-

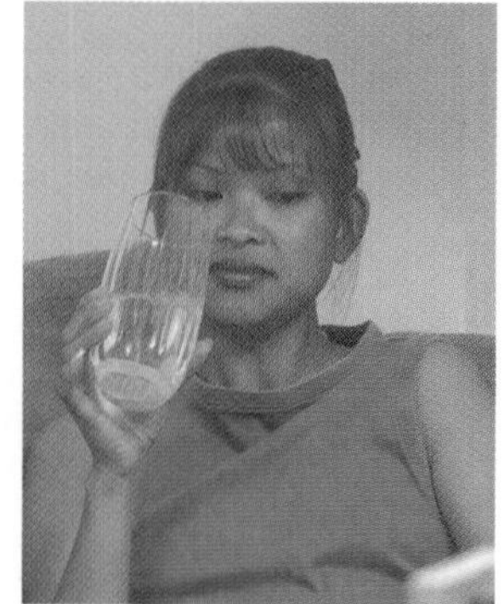
Figure 1-4. **Avoid drinking soda; drink water instead.**

rect bus fare the day before. Make everyone's lunch the night before. In short, do not allow yourself to get stressed the morning of an exam. Stress may negatively affect your grade.

Relaxation Breathing — Box 1-2

When people are stressed, they will sometimes hold their breath or take very shallow breaths. This can cause their bodies to tighten up further and can increase their overall stress level. Whenever you feel stressed, try following the simple steps listed below:

1. Sit up straight (or lie in bed) with your hands on your abdomen.
2. Take a breath (inhale) through your nose, forcing the air into your abdomen instead of your chest. This will cause your hands to move upward.
3. Let the breath out (exhale) through your lips. Purse your lips or bring them close together when you exhale.
4. Try this two different ways–with your eyes open and with your eyes closed. Which method do you like better?
5. Breathe in this way until you feel your body begin to relax.
6. With each breath, focus on relaxing one part of your body. Start at the top of your body with your jaw and neck and move downward. Finish at your toes and feet.
7. Do not let yourself fall asleep (unless you are in bed)! This type of breathing can really help a person relax.

13 Describe six common mistakes to avoid while taking a test.

Sometimes there are only a few points between one letter grade and the next one above or below it. In other words, you may need each and every point you can get. Here are some tips on how to prevent mistakes that will cost you unnecessary points.

1. When you are done with a quiz or a test, stop and go over the entire answer sheet. Check to make sure you have circled an answer for each question.
2. Hold a ruler or a piece of colored paper under each line on your answer form to make sure you answer the right question on the right number.
3. Read the entire question at least two times before you choose or write an answer. Read every word carefully. If you miss one word, you might pick the wrong answer.
4. Does the question ask for more than one answer? Double-check that you have included a second or even a third answer if requested.
5. Cover your answer sheet. The person next to you may not have studied as hard as you did last night. Do not put yourself in a position where you get into trouble because someone copied off your paper. *Teachers can usually tell when a student has been cheating.*
6. If English is your second language, check to see if a translator aid is allowed, or if you are allowed to take the test in your first language.

Math: The Old-Fashioned Way

The study of math started a very long time ago. Five thousand years ago the people living in Egypt and Mesopotamia used some of the earliest written numbers. The word "calculate" comes from the Latin word for pebble, "calculus." Figure 1-5 shows some of the different ways to write the same numbers using numerals from many lands

Arabic	Egyptian	Babylonian	Roman	Greek	Mayan
1	I	V	I	A	•
2	II	VV	II	B	••
3	III	VVV	III	Γ	•••
4	IIII	VVVV	IV	Δ	••••
5	III II	VVV VV	V	E	—
6	III III	VVV VVV	VI	F	• —
7	IIII III	VVVV VVV	VII	Z	•• —
8	IIII IIII	VVVV VVVV	VIII	H	••• —
9	III III III	VVVVV VVVV	IX	Θ	•••• —
10	∩	<	X	I	=
20	∩∩	<<	XX	K	[illegible]
50	∩∩∩ ∩∩	<<< <<	L	N	[illegible]

Figure 1-5. **Different kinds of numerals. (Reprinted with permission from *Let's Investigate Numbers* by Marion Smoothey.)**

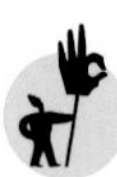

Little Letters, Big Meanings

Have you ever wondered what the following little abbreviations mean?

et al. (Latin et alia): means "and other things." Only "al" has a period at the end.

i.e. (Latin id est): means "that is." Both letters have a period.

e.g. (Latin exempli gratia): means "for example." Both letters have a period.

14 Demonstrate skill in four basic types of mathematics.

Sometimes students have been out of school for a while. Many people overuse calculators and begin to rely on them too much. If you are in this situation, do not despair. This section includes a basic math review that may help bring you up-to-date in a subject many people find very challenging.

Addition

Remember to carry over:

3,457	11,999
+ 398	+ 7,657
3,855	19,656

Subtraction

Do not forget to borrow!

27,785	179,746
- 9,358	- 37,437
18,427	142,309

Multiplication

3,754	92
x 129	x 37
33,786	644
75,080	+2,760
+ 375,400	3,404
484,266	

Division

49	33
26 | 1,274	16 | 528
-104	-48
234	48
-234	-48
0	0

15 Explain how to convert decimals, fractions, and percentages.

Many people leave school without learning that decimals, fractions, and percentages are all related. A **decimal** is a **fraction** whose denominator is a power of 10. A **percentage** represents a fraction where the assumed denominator is 100. To express one-half (1/2) as a decimal, we would say 0.50. To express one-half (1/2) as a percentage, we would say 50% or 50/100. Here are some examples for you to review:

Problem 1: ½=0.5=50%

To get the decimal 0.5 from ½, divide the denominator (2) into the numerator (1).

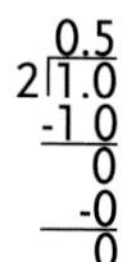

To change 0.5 into a percent, move the decimal sign two places to the right and add the percent sign. Drop the decimal sign if there are no numbers to the right of the decimal sign.

0.5 = 50%

Problem 2: ¼ = 0.25 = 25%

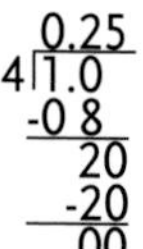

To change 0.25 into a percent, move the decimal sign two places to the right and add the percent sign. Drop the decimal sign if there are no numbers to the right of the decimal sign.

0.25 = 25%

Problem 3: ¾ = .75 = 75%

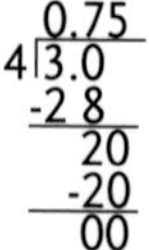

To change 0.75 into a percent, move the decimal sign two places to the right and add the percent sign. Drop the decimal sign if there are no numbers to the right of the decimal sign.

0.75 = 75%

16 List three different kinds of graphs.

We see graphs used regularly in the community. You may see graphs on the side of a bus or on a news program. In the healthcare field, graphing may be required in order to complete some of your duties, such as graphing a temperature reading for a resident. Figure 1-6 shows some examples of the different kinds of graphs you may use.

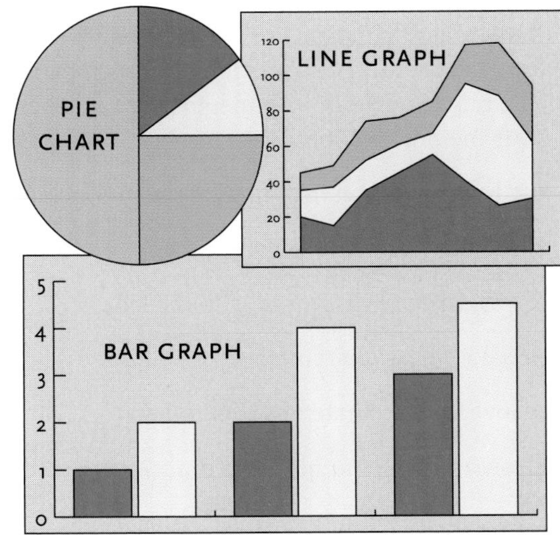

Figure 1-6. **Different types of graphs**

Useful Information

Conversions

1 kilometer (km) = 1,000 meters (m)

1 liter (l) = 1,000 milliliters (ml)

1 gram (g) = 1,000 milligrams (mg)

Meters	Yards	Inches
1.000	1.093	39.37
0.914	1.000	36.00

Centimeters	Inches	Feet
1.00	0.394	0.0328
2.54	1.000	1/12
30.48	12.000	1.000

Kilometers	Miles
1.000	0.621
1.609	1.000

Grams	Ounces	Pounds
1.00	0.035	0.002
28.35	1.000	1/16
453.59	16.000	1.000

Kilograms	Ounces	Pounds
1.000	35.274	2.205

Liters	Pints	Quarts	Gallons
1.000	2.113	1.057	0.264
0.473	1.000	½	1/8
0.946	2.000	1.000	1/4
3.785	8.000	4.000	1.000

60 seconds = 1 minute
60 minutes = 1 hour
24 hours = 1 day
7 days = 1 week
30 days = 1 calendar month
12 months = 1 year
365 days = 1 common year
100 years = 1 century
2 pints = 1 quart (qt.)
4 quarts = 1 gallon (gal.)
12 inches = 1 foot
3 feet = 1 yard
12 units = 1 dozen
12 doz. = 1 gross
1 hand = 4 inches
1 knot = 6,086 feet
2,000 pounds = 1 ton (T.)

Multiplication Table

1	2	3	4	5	6	7	8	9	10	11	12
2	4	6	8	10	12	14	16	18	20	22	24
3	6	9	12	15	18	21	24	27	30	33	36
4	8	12	16	20	24	28	32	36	40	44	48
5	10	15	20	25	30	35	40	45	50	55	60
6	12	18	24	30	36	42	48	54	60	66	72
7	14	21	28	35	42	49	56	63	70	77	84
8	16	24	32	40	48	56	64	72	80	88	96
9	18	27	36	45	54	63	72	81	90	99	108
10	20	30	40	50	60	70	80	90	100	110	120
11	22	33	44	55	66	77	88	99	110	121	132
12	24	36	48	60	72	84	96	108	120	132	144

Summary

In order to be a "STAR" nursing assistant student, you must have a solid understanding of the basic skills necessary to succeed. This chapter has outlined many of the skills you will need. In life, we should continue trying to improve ourselves each and every day. Do not stop here! Always be on the lookout for new ideas and ways to improve yourself. Strive to learn something new every day!

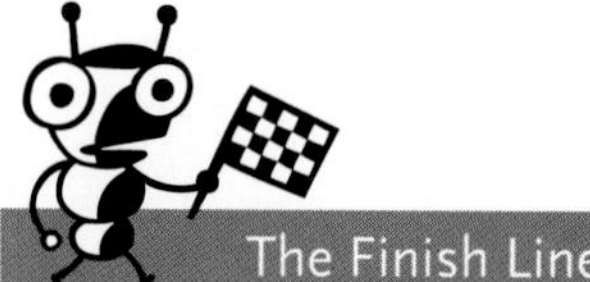

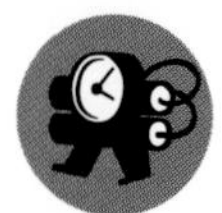

What's Wrong With This Picture?

1. Look at the paragraph below and find all of the errors in grammar and punctuation.

   "The resident were going to the bathroom, She fall down and hurted her head on the hard floor? When the nurse comed to visit, he wrote down his notes about the fall. Then we listened to the nurses talk at the nurses station. Afterward, the resident got in the bed and lied down."

2. Read through the paragraph and try to find the incomplete sentences.

   "We went to the care conference and saw people we had not seen for a long time. When we left the care conference. Our supervisor handed out bonus checks to each of us for working so hard. The checks to the bank at the corner. We couldn't wait to spend our bonus checks!

3. Review the paragraph and find all of the mistakes in capitalization.

   The windsong Nursing Home is set high on a hill in some beautiful woods far up north in New hampshire. The director of the Facility is named john Holland. When you look out the window of his office, You can see a beautiful view of the Atlantic ocean.

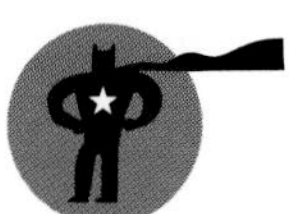

Star Student Central

Complete the following exercises:

1. Write out two short-term goals and two long-term goals.

2. Outlining Skills

   Look at your notes from Chapter 1. Practice writing your notes in simple outline form.

   Use the sample outline in Chapter 1 along with this section as a guide.

3. Practicing Memory Techniques

   Remember that these tips can be used when you are not able to write something down on paper. The more you work with memory tips, the better your memory will become.

Choose four items you may need at the grocery store.

1. Write down the first letter of each item.
2. Try to develop a fun word with the letters.
3. See if it helps you remember the items.

Write down two separate phone numbers.

1. Say each phone number five times in a row.
2. Set a timer for 10 to 15 minutes.
3. When the timer goes off, quickly try to remember the numbers.

Make a list of three names of family members using their last names. (Mr. Holmes, Mrs. Watson, Mr. Chan)

1. Create a phrase that has meaning. For example, "Holmes, Watson and Chan solved a case!"
2. Practicing this memory technique may help you remember things, for example, removing three treatments from three residents in a very short period of time.

3. Time Management Exercises

   Make a chart of everything you do in one day. You may fit study time into any open time slots. These slots could be time periods spent watching television or doing something else that could wait until after your course has ended.

   Try making a to-do list for the next day every night before you go to bed. This way, you will feel extremely organized every night before you fall asleep and when you wake up in the morning. You will be ready to take on the day!

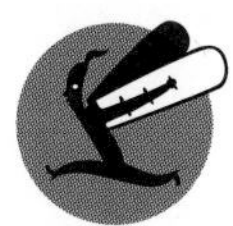

You Can Do It Corner!

1. Complete the following math problems. (LO 14)

A. Addition Practice

```
  672          8,256
+ 349         +9,744
```

B. Subtraction Practice

```
  9,397       10,735
 -4,868      - 6,973
```

C. Multiplication Practice

```
  62           43
 x 57         x 32
```

D. Division Practice

12,936 ÷ 24 496 ÷ 16

2. Complete the chart by filling in the blanks. (LO 15)

Decimal	Fraction	Percentage
	4/5	80%
0.15	3/20	
0.75		75%
0.10		10%

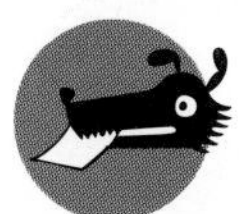

Star Student's Chapter Checklist

1. I have read my textbook chapter.
2. I have reviewed my own "Pocketful of Terms."
3. I have listened to my tutor tape.
4. I have reviewed and highlighted my class notes.
5. I have read and completed any handouts from this chapter.
6. I have completed "The Finish Line."
7. Star Time! Choose your reward!

Your Title: The Star Nursing Assistant

Look Like a Star!

Look at the Learning Objectives and The Finish Line before you begin reading this chapter.

Look at your pocket calendar.
With your pencil, put a bracket ( ) around a study period every single day.

Look at your homework for this chapter.
Plug each piece of homework into a certain time slot.

Look at the Star Student's Chapter Checklist at the end of this chapter. Check off each item as it is completed.

"The best of healers is good cheer."

Pindar, 522-422 B.C.

"Never promise more than you can perform."

Maxim 45

Learning Objectives

1. **Spell and define all STAR words.**
2. **List seven qualities of a STAR employee.**
3. **Discuss seven grooming skills of a STAR employee.**
4. **Describe six hairstyle, makeup, and nail care guidelines.**
5. **State two reasons team members must not use any scented materials, such as perfumes and aftershaves.**
6. **Explain five ways jewelry can pose a problem in resident care.**
7. **Discuss two factors about appropriate footwear in long-term care.**
8. **Explain two reasons to wear an identification badge and the importance of leaving personal valuables at home.**
9. **Describe necessary organizational skills and ten sample nursing assistant tasks.**
10. **Describe the residents for whom you will care.**
11. **Demonstrate the ability to convert regular time to military time.**
12. **Discuss three common types of time clocks.**

What Life was Really Like in Nursing School...

The early nursing schools in the 1800s and early 1900s maintained very strict rules for their students. The classes at that time were made up entirely of women, and they normally lived together in a building. The schools usually had women who acted as "housemothers" for the students. Rigid curfews, rules restricting smoking, drinking and foul language, strict dress codes, and strict separation of the sexes were common. The students were normally not allowed to date or marry. Women who broke the rules suffered severe punishment.

The nursing students were expected to work long hours and, in addition to caring for patients, had to wash and wax floors and do chores that today are completed by other health team members.

1 Spell and define all **STAR** words.

assignment: the responsibility of care for a group of residents.

accountable: answerable for one's actions.

conscientious: guided by morals; principled.

courteous: polite, kind, considerate.

empathetic: able to enter into the feelings of others.

facility: an agency that provides health care.

first impression: a way of classifying or categorizing people at the first meeting.

halitosis: bad-smelling breath.

obligations: responsibilities.

policy: planned course of action.

prioritize: to place things in order of importance.

responsible: answerable for one's actions.

resident: a person living in a long-term care or assisted living facility.

trustworthy: deserving the trust of others.

2 List seven qualities of a STAR employee.

A "STAR" employee is a one-of-a-kind, irreplaceable person. Some qualities of the "STAR" employee are listed below. As you read through this list, ask yourself whether or not you have these qualities.

1. **Patient and understanding.** Do you have a low "boiling point"? Do you let people finish their sentences? Are you calm most of the time? Are you slow to anger?
2. **Honest and trustworthy.** Can you keep a secret? Do people trust you with their homes? their children? their money? their secrets? Do people consider you a **conscientious** person? Can you stay away from gossip? Can you keep confidential information private?
3. **Enthusiastic.** Do you see the glass as half-empty or half-full? Do others say you have a P.M.A. (positive mental attitude)?
4. **Courteous and respectful.** Do other people describe you as polite? Do you respect other beliefs even if they are different from yours?
5. **Empathetic and skilled at listening.** Can you imagine what it would be like to be "in your resident's shoes"? Do your family members and friends come to you for guidance and support?
6. **Dependable and responsible.** Are you always on time? Do you pay your bills on time? Are you there for others? Do you always try to follow policies and procedures?
7. **Humble and open to growth.** Are you willing to admit when you're wrong? Can you accept your limitations? Are you able to ask others for help? Do you hold yourself **accountable** when you make a mistake? Can you say the words, "I made a mistake"? Can you say the words, "I am sorry"?

3 Discuss seven grooming skills of a STAR employee.

A "STAR" has to look sharp. Other people take notice of this person. **First impressions** can make the difference between getting a job, getting another date, or even getting good service in a store. When you visit your barber or hairstylist, if he or she looks smart, you feel comfortable allowing that person to touch your hair. On the other hand, an unkempt barber with dirty teeth and messy hair may make you turn around, run out the door, and never look back. **Residents** living in facilities are no different than you. If a nursing assistant walked into a resident's room with hands covered in black grease, the resident may ask the nursing assistant to leave the room! Below is a listing of some common uniform rules. As you review this list, think about how you prepare to go out and meet the world each day.

Which nursing assistant would you choose?

The "STAR" in Uniform	Someone Else
Pressed uniform	Wrinkles
Fresh breath	**Halitosis**
Clean body	Body odor
No perfumes	Strong cologne
Clean teeth	Stained teeth
Short nails	Very long nails
Clean shoes	Dirty shoes

4 Describe six hairstyle, makeup, and nail care guidelines.

There are guidelines for keeping the look of a star nursing assistant. Some of these guidelines have to do with hairstyles, which can be vivid statements of the impression people want to give to others. If your hair is messy all the time, others may develop a negative impression of you. If you have long hair, keep it neatly tied back and away from your face. Long hair that is not tied back can block your vision and even fall into your residents' faces as you give them care.

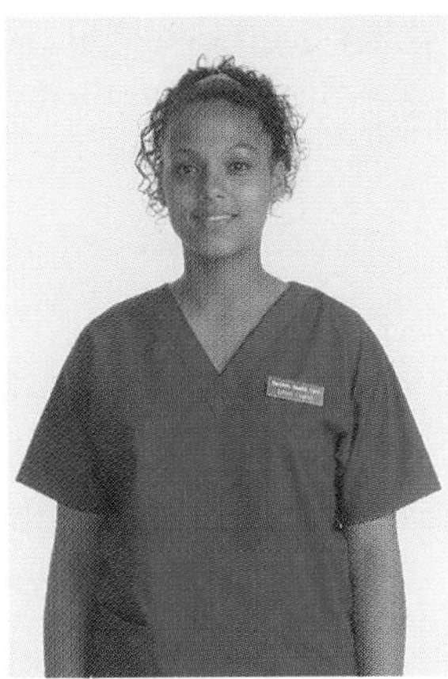

Figure 2-1. **If you have long hair, keep it tied neatly back, away from your face.**

For men, beards can also pose a problem for residents if they are long and messy. It is best to keep beards trimmed neatly. In addition to the way a messy beard looks, a beard can hide bacteria that could harm the resident.

A nursing assistant must be careful not to wear too much makeup. Makeup should be applied skillfully and sparingly. A professional-looking nursing assistant must learn how to apply makeup so that the beauty of the face shows through. The first thing other people should see when they look at you is your beautiful face, not your makeup.

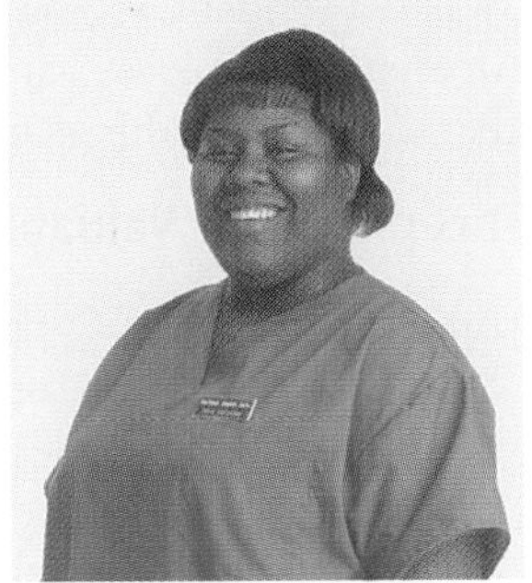

Figure 2-2. **Apply makeup lightly.**

Fingernails can be a potential problem in health care. We all scratch ourselves from time to time. Imagine scratching an elderly resident and tearing the fragile skin on his arm. For safety's sake, all healthcare team members must keep fingernails short and clean.

In addition, false nails of any kind must not be used. No matter how well hands are washed, dangerous bacteria can hide within false nails. The bacteria in false nails can also be transferred to your residents.

Nail polish is another risk factor in health care. Some facilities allow pastel or clear nail polish to be worn during resident care. Other facilities have a **policy** against wearing any nail polish. Nail polish hides bacteria, especially if it has chipped. Follow your facility policy regarding wearing nail polish.

5 State two reasons team members must not use any scented materials, such as perfumes and aftershaves.

Allergies are on the increase in our society. In recent years, stores have begun to stock more unscented items like facial and toilet tissue and laundry detergents. You may know many people with serious allergies. Every day a person with scent allergies must spend time trying to avoid scents that will trigger an allergy attack. Some people hesitate to attend functions like weddings where others will be wearing heavy cologne or perfume. It's very important for healthcare workers to always show respect for residents. One way to accomplish this goal is by smelling fresh and unscented at all times. Choose unscented deodorants and hair care products and avoid colognes, perfume, and aftershaves.

Residents may also be acutely aware of scents around them simply because they may not feel very good. Consider the way you feel when you are sick, especially with a cold. Scents tend to become exaggerated during illness, and even a bouquet of fresh flowers may affect a person negatively. If a resident does not feel well, you may be asked to remove any bothersome items, such as flowers or sachet. If you are wearing a lot of perfume one shift, a resident may ask for a different nursing assistant for that day. You need to understand that this is part of the process of making a resident comfortable, and nursing assistants must always respond cheerfully to this type of request.

Kill the scent!

Wearing colognes and perfumes when you know a resident has serious allergies may be considered abuse. We must always try to meet the needs of our residents in every way, and that means respecting their individual problems and putting the residents' comfort first!

NAs: In demand in 1945

Nursing assistants, it seems, have been in demand for many years. This list of "unfilled positions" in hospitals at that time appeared late in 1945:

- *Registered Nurses 65,000*
- *Non-nursing personnel 90,000*
- *Nurses' Aides 90,000*
- *Untrained volunteers 45,000*

6 Explain five ways jewelry can pose a problem in resident care.

Jewelry can be a major problem in the healthcare industry. It may scratch residents, other staff, or even you. Precious stones can fall out while making a bed or reaching for equipment. Residents can pull on earrings, injure you, and damage your expensive jewelry. Jewelry can pass infection from one resident to another. You may also bring this infection home to your own family. Jewelry presents a problem for nursing assistants and residents alike, so remember the following:

1. Wear only perfectly smooth rings without openings or holes that might transfer dangerous germs.
2. Leave rings with stones at home. Stones may scratch others or fall out of settings.
3. Leave necklaces at home. Residents may pull on necklaces and break them, or pull hard enough so that you could be hurt.
4. Wear small earrings that will not snag on things and that residents cannot grab and pull out of your ears.
5. Do not wear bracelets. They interfere with wearing gloves and can collect bacteria.

The main exception to the jewelry rule is to wear a simple, waterproof watch. You will use a watch when you take a resident's pulse and respirations (covered in Chapter 16), as well as for recording events.

7 Discuss two factors about appropriate footwear in long-term care.

Shoes can make or break your workday. You cannot afford to have your feet hurt every day or night when you get home from work. Purchase one quality pair of shoes that you will be able to wear for many hours and that will never cause your feet to hurt. Change your laces when they become stained or soiled, and keep your shoes clean. Never buy shoes with open toes or without backs, like clogs, for your position as a nursing assistant. Many facilities have a standing policy that forbids this style of shoe because it can cause falls and on-the-job injuries.

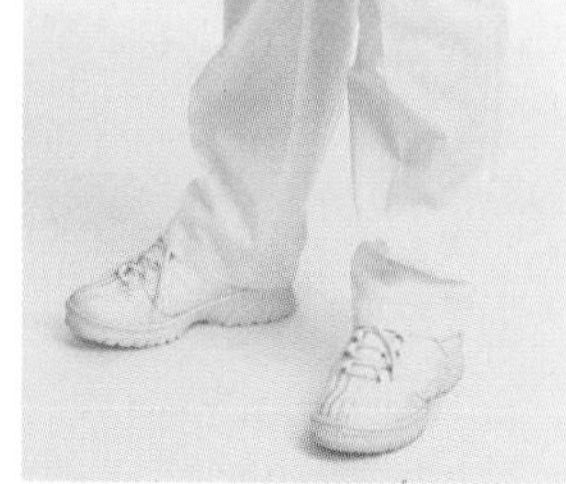

Figure 2-3. Wear the proper shoes for the job.

8 Explain two reasons to wear an identification badge and the importance of leaving personal valuables at home.

An identification badge is vital to the healthcare worker. You may need this name badge or card to enter a **facility**. You may be asked to insert it into a device or machine that will open an entrance door to a facility. In other facilities, a guard may check each person's identification badge or card. A new nursing assistant must quickly get used to wearing a name badge at all times. Residents and family members rely on name badges to identify staff members. Searching a uniform for a name badge can be frustrating to visitors and staff alike. When a resident, visitor, or another employee can easily identify a staff member, it can make things easier and less frustrating.

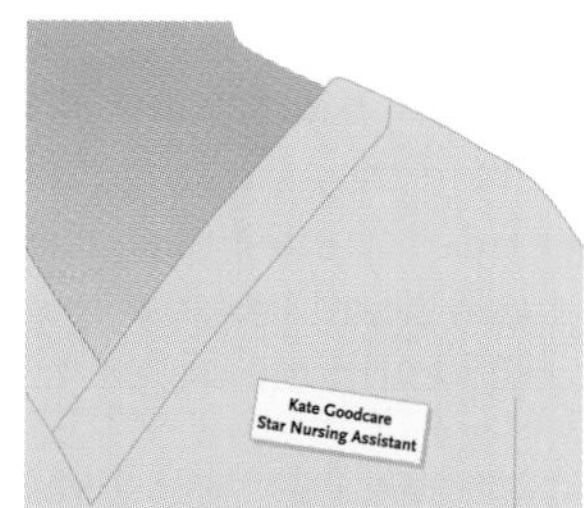

Figure 2-4. Always wear your name badge.

Keeping Your Valuables Safe

A healthcare facility is open to the public, and that means anyone may be able to wander onto a floor. It is wise to leave valuables, like purses, at home. Some facilities are not equipped with lockers for personal belongings. In some places, staff will choose to keep purses and valuables in a cabinet under the front desk. This is unwise because anyone could find out about this practice and take advantage of the situation by stealing the purses and other valuables. Also, personal belongings should never be stored in service areas or where care is provided. Only bring to work things that you must have to get through your day. Leave everything else at home.

9 Describe necessary organizational skills and ten sample nursing assistant tasks.

Organized people can meet most of their **obligations** each day. A disorganized person may be the individual who forgets to pick up a child from school or the person who always forgets items at the grocery store. Imagine a long-term care facility running out of milk or bread! Think about what would happen if a shuttle bus took a resident for an appointment and then forgot to pick him up. The world would simply not run well without organized people to keep things moving along properly.

When you take care of residents, it is important for you to organize and **prioritize** your work every day. At home, you may do the following regularly: make meals, pay bills, keep up with correspondence like letters and cards, wash laundry, clean house, water plants, and feed pets. If you are able to balance your life and meet all of those responsibilities, then you may be described as a well-organized person. In the healthcare field, there are certain **assignments** you will complete each day for your residents. Brushing teeth, bathing, serving meals, cleaning rooms, and helping residents read their mail are some of the duties of a nursing assistant. If you can successfully complete your duties at home, then there is every reason to believe you will become a well-organized nursing assistant. As each month passes, you will feel more and more organized in your new role.

What kinds of assistance will you provide for your residents? You will help them in many ways. Residents learn to depend upon nursing assistants to make their days more comfortable and more pleasant. A list of some sample resident requests and nursing assistant tasks follows:

Nursing Assistant Task List

Serving trays and feeding residents
"I can't wait until dinner! I hear we are having turkey with stuffing tonight. Oh, my favorite!"

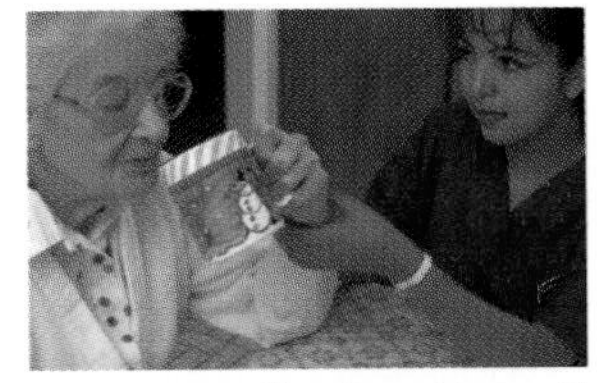

Figure 2-5. **You will assist residents with eating and drinking.**

Soaking a resident's tired feet
"My feet hurt. I walked a lot today on our trip to the botanical gardens!"

Dressing a resident for a son she has not seen for six months
"My son, his wife, and two children are coming! I am so excited!"

Bathing residents and bedmaking
"I am really sorry; I didn't make it to the bathroom in time. Can you please help me get cleaned up?"

Shampooing hair
"My head is scratchy! I think I need a shampoo. Can you please help me wash my hair this morning?"

Shaving residents
"I want to look nice for my card game. My beard needs a shave today. Can you help me find my razor and shaving cream?"

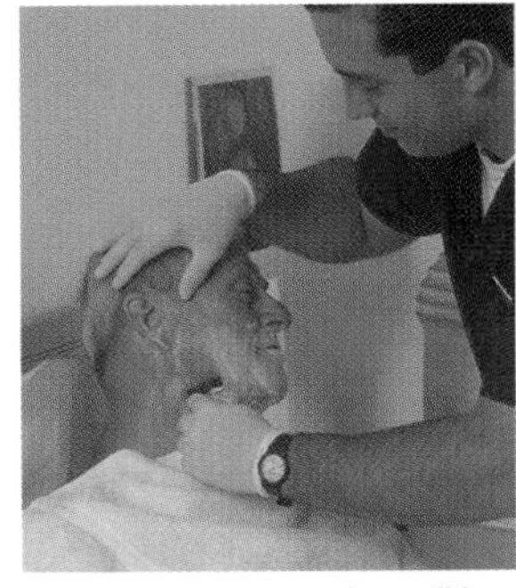

Figure 2-6. **Shaving a resident will be one of your tasks.**

Applying ice bag (with a doctor's order)
"I fell during shuffleboard; my ankle hurts badly and is turning black and blue."

Taking the vital signs of residents, including temperature, pulse, respiration, and blood pressure
"I suddenly feel very dizzy; I have to lie down."

Giving back massages
"My neck feels achy this morning! I think I slept on it wrong last night."

Reporting constipation or other complaints to the nurse
"I haven't been to the bathroom for two days. Can you please help me get something that will make me more comfortable?"

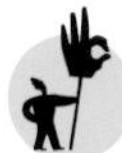

Organizing Your Work

Do you use sticky notes to remind yourself to do things at home? Many nursing assistants and other healthcare team members use a similar method to organize their work. A small notebook stored in your pocket can make the difference between feeling organized and feeling overwhelmed each workday.

10 Describe the residents for whom you will care.

There are some general statements that can be made about the population of residents in nursing homes across the country. However, more important than understanding the entire population, is understanding the individuals for whom you will care. Always make sure you know how to provide care for your resident based on his or her needs, illnesses, frailties, and desires.

Almost 91 percent of residents are over age 65. This means that only nine percent are younger than 65 and are admitted for a variety of disabilities or disorders. Almost 72 percent of residents are female. More than 85 percent are Caucasian, a much larger percentage than the population as a whole. Approximately one-third of residents come from a private residence; over 50 percent come from a hospital or another facility.

Almost one-half of residents admitted will remain for six months or more. These residents need enough assistance with their activities of daily living that 24-hour care is required. Often, they did not have caregivers available to provide enough care to allow them to live in the community. The groups with the longest "average stay" are the mentally retarded and developmentally disabled, who are often younger than 65.

The "other half" of residents remain for a period shorter than six months. This group generally falls into two categories. The first category is residents admitted for terminal care who will die in the facility. The second category is residents admitted for rehabilitation or illness who will recover and leave to live in a community setting. As you can imagine, care of these residents may be very different.

Various studies estimate the number of nursing home residents who suffer from dementia to be between 50 and 90 percent. Dementia is defined as the loss of mental abilities, such as thinking, remembering, reasoning, and communicating. To be certain, dementia and other mental disorders are major causes of nursing home admissions. While many residents are admitted with other disorders, the disorders themselves are often not the reason they are being admitted. Rather, it is most often the lack of ability to care for oneself and the lack of a support system to assist with care that leads people into a facility.

To illustrate how important a support system is in allowing the elderly to live outside a facility, consider this fact: for every elderly person living in a long-term care facility, there are at least two people living in the community with the same disorders and disabilities.

You may notice this lack of outside support among your residents. It is another reason you will care for the "whole person," instead of focusing only on the illness or disease. Residents have many needs beyond their activities of daily living that go unmet if staff do not work to meet them.

11 Demonstrate the ability to convert regular time to military time.

The healthcare industry sometimes uses the 24-hour clock, or military time, to record data in facilities. This way of keeping track of time is very simple to learn. Figure 2-7 shows the divisions in the 24-hour clock and the corresponding military time. Examples of the way the numbers are written are listed below:

Example One: Regular to Military
11:00 = 1100 (eleven-hundred hours)

Example Two: Military to Regular
1115 = 11:15

To change the regular hours between 1:00 p.m. to 11:59 p.m. to military time, 12 must be added to the regular time. These steps are followed:

Step One: Change 4:00 p.m. and 10:00 p.m. to military time.

Step Two:

4:00 p.m.	10:00 p.m.
+ 12	+ 12
1600 hours	2200 hours

To change back from military time to standard time, you must subtract 12 from military time. These steps are followed:

Step One: Change 1600 hours and 2200 hours to standard time.

Step Two:

1600	2200
- 12	- 12
4:00 p.m.	10:00 p.m.

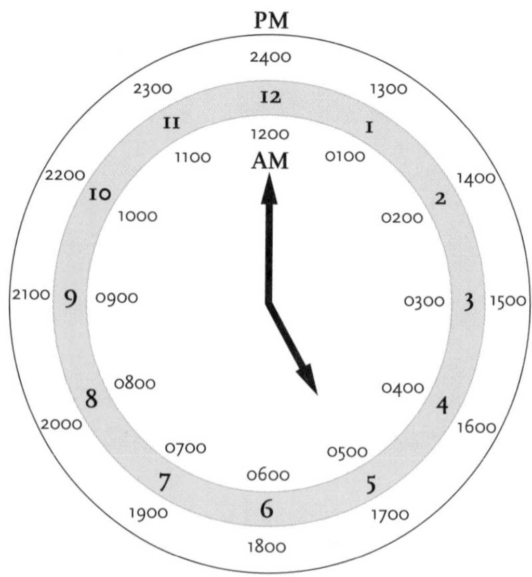

Figure 2-7. **Divisions in the 24-hour clock.**

12 Discuss three common types of time clocks.

Learning how to keep track of the hours you work in a healthcare facility can take time. It is not unusual to forget to punch in once in a while when you first start your new position. When you use a time clock in a responsible manner, you will help to make sure that you get paid correctly. Paychecks are very important to most people, so you must remember to complete your time card each pay period. That way, you will always receive a paycheck. Some facilities have one-week pay periods, while others use a schedule with two-week pay periods.

There are many types of time clocks. Some companies use a manual system. The employee simply writes in the time of arrival and departure from the facility. Others use an automated system. This type of system requires employees to punch a time card when arriving and leaving each workday. Another type of time clock is one that requires each staff member to swipe a card through the time clock. This registers employee hours automatically. Some tips to remember regarding time clocks are:

1. Make sure you write on or punch your own card. When you're in a hurry, it is easy to grab someone else's time card.
2. Add up your hours carefully. If you are asked to add up your hours, do this when you are not in a hurry. Make a note in a small notebook of the hours you worked this pay period. If you add the numbers wrong, you could lose pay. Fixing a problem like this takes time because your supervisor must research the situation. Also, some employers do not pay people who forget to add up their hours on their time card.
3. Write in, swipe your card, or punch in for hours allowed. When you come in for a special meeting, make sure you ask your supervisor if you should punch your card that day.

Summary

Becoming a "STAR" employee is a desirable and attainable goal. A nursing assistant must always try to look good, wear a minimum of makeup, and have a hairstyle that suits the position. A name badge must be worn at all times while on duty so residents and family members or visitors are able to recognize your position. It's important that you take care of your feet and always wear comfortable shoes. You must follow the rules of time clocks and time cards so that paychecks come on time. The nursing assistant who follows the rules outlined in this chapter will become a valued employee.

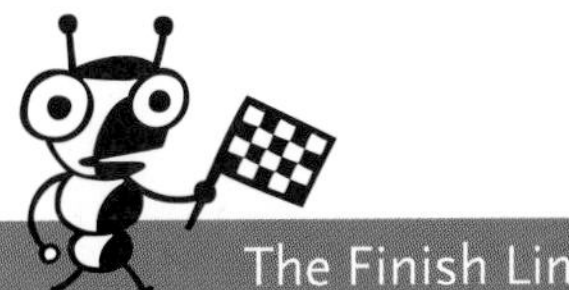

The Finish Line

What's Wrong With This Picture?

Look at each of the drawings. Find the errors in dress code in each of the following pictures:

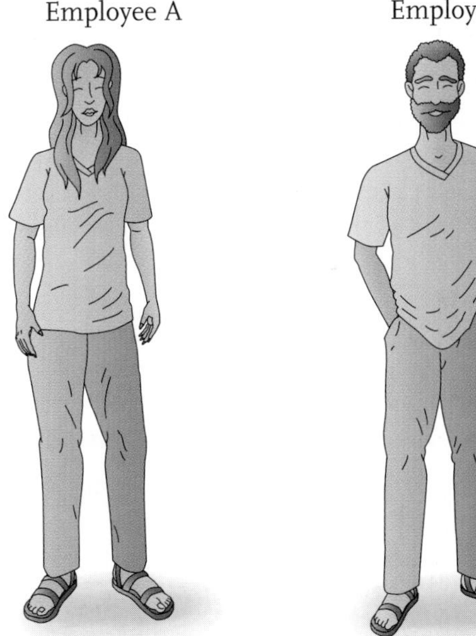

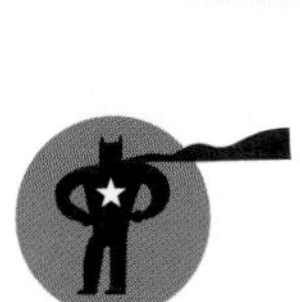

Star Student Central

Improving your appearance is an ongoing process. Everyone can improve aspects of their appearance. Try the following suggestions to update and improve your appearance:

1. Schedule a free skin care consultation. It should be held at a trusted place with high standards using disposable, one-time-use supplies.

2. Go to a public library and check out a "dress for success" book. Find one book that suits you and follow its advice. Other tips include:
   - Acetone is an inexpensive liquid that can keep white shoes cleaner.
   - Keep the jewelry that is acceptable for work separate from your other jewelry.
   - A simple, professional hairstyle may take less time to style before work.
   - Keep your badge, watch, and other work necessities together to make getting ready simpler.

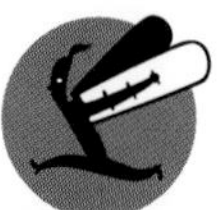

You Can Do It Corner!

True or False. Circle a "T" for true or an "F" for false for each of the following statements.

1. Perfume, aftershaves, and colognes often help severe allergies. (LO 5) T F
2. Being dependable means people can rely on you. (LO 2) T F
3. Long or false nails can hide bacteria. (LO 4) T F
4. Shoes that have open backs, like clogs, should be worn if you work in health care. (LO 7) T F
5. A pressed uniform is a sign of a well-groomed nursing assistant. (LO 3) T F
6. Helping a resident eat is one of the tasks nursing assistants can expect to perform. (LO 9) T F
7. After a nursing assistant enters her facility, she can remove her name badge. (LO 8) T F
8. A watch is an acceptable form of jewelry for a nursing assistant to wear. (LO 6) T F
9. Being respectful means a nursing assistant can make fun of a resident's religion. (LO 2) T F
10. Organization is an important skill for a nursing assistant to have. (LO 9) T F
11. Fill the correct time for each blank entry listed.

Regular Time	Military Time
__________ p.m.	1400
3:00 p.m.	__________
10:45 p.m.	__________
__________ p.m.	2315
6:00 p.m.	__________
__________ p.m.	1730
midnight	__________
11:15 a.m.	__________
__________ a.m.	0915

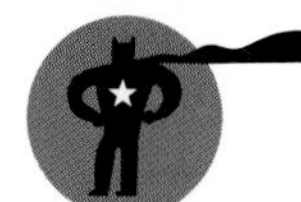

Star Student's Chapter Checklist

1. I have read my textbook chapter.
2. I have reviewed my own "Pocketful of Terms."
3. I have listened to my tutor tape.
4. I have reviewed and highlighted my class notes.
5. I have read and completed any handouts from this chapter.
6. I have completed "The Finish Line."
7. Star Time! Choose your reward!

Your Guidelines: Living by a Code of Ethics and Understanding the Law

Look Like a Star!

Look at the Learning Objectives and The Finish Line before you begin reading this chapter.

Look at your pocket calendar.
With your pencil, put a bracket (   ) around a study period every single day.

Look at your homework for this chapter.
Plug each piece of homework into a certain time slot.

Look at the Star Student's Chapter Checklist at the end of this chapter. Check off each item as it is completed.

"Wherever there is a human being, I see God-given rights inherent in that being, whatever may be the sex or complexion."

William Lloyd Garrison, 1805-1879

"Three may keep a secret, if two of them are dead."

Benjamin Franklin, 1706-1790

Learning Objectives

1. **Spell and define all STAR words.**
2. **List the three branches of the United States government.**
3. **Identify different courts in the United States judicial system.**
4. **Name and define the terms used to identify the people involved in the court system.**
5. **Define, discuss, and compare the terms "law," "ethics," "moral values," and "etiquette."**
6. **Identify two different types of laws.**
7. **Name the "Standards Three" relating to legal and ethical issues in the nursing assistant profession.**
8. **Explain the nine components of professional and ethical behavior as described in the acronym "CATCH ME UP."**
9. **Describe a nursing assistant code of ethics.**
10. **Identify nine specific components of the Residents' Rights.**
11. **Explain the importance of the OBRA Act of 1987.**
12. **Describe six legal issues relating to the nursing assistant.**
13. **Summarize negligence and what it means to the nursing assistant.**
14. **Recognize the importance of obtaining liability insurance.**
15. **Discuss the Good Samaritan Act and how it relates to nursing assistants.**
16. **Explain seven types of resident abuse and describe signs of abuse.**
17. **Explain methods of reporting resident abuse when following the chain of command.**
18. **Discuss the ombudsman's role in preventing resident abuse.**

The First Code of Ethics

An English physician named Thomas Percival wrote a code of ethics called "Percival's Medical Ethics" in 1803. This was used in 1847 to help develop the American Medical Association's first code of ethics. The American Medical Association Principles is still the code of ethics that physicians use today. Here is a sample from that first code of ethics: "A physician ought not to abandon a patient because the case is deemed incurable, for his attendance may continue to be highly useful to the patient, and comforting to the relatives around him . . ."

1 Spell and define all STAR words.

Activities of Daily Living (ADLs): all of the activities people do for themselves each day, like brushing teeth, bathing, dressing, toileting, and eating.

assault: an attempt to threaten or harm another person.

battery: the actual touching of another person without the person's consent.

chain of command: the order of authority in a facility.

civil law: private law; law between persons.

criminal law: public law; related to committing a crime against the community.

defamation of character: to attack the reputation of another.

defendant: person accused of a crime.

domestic abuse: abuse related to the family or family situations.

elder abuse: the seven types of abuse of the elderly include psychological or verbal abuse, physical abuse and neglect, sexual abuse, domestic abuse, involuntary seclusion, financial abuse, and exploitation.

ethics: standards or guide of conduct.

executive branch: the branch of the government administering the laws of the nation.

exploitation: to make unethical use of a person for one's own profit.

false imprisonment: unlawfully keeping a person away from others.

financial abuse: stealing from or deceiving a person into giving away money or assets.

fraud: deceiving or tricking another person.

Good Samaritan Act: a law in many states that protects persons who assist others in an emergency situation from possible lawsuits.

invasion of privacy: a violation of the right to be left alone and the right to control personal information.

involuntary seclusion: confinement or separation from others in a certain area; done without consent or against one's will.

judicial branch: the branch of the government dealing with the courts and judges.

legislative branch: the branch of the government having the power to make laws.

liability insurance: insurance that can protect an individual in case of a lawsuit.

libel: defamation or lies in writing or in print that injure the reputation of another person.

malpractice: negligence by a professional such as a doctor, nurse, pharmacist, or attorney.

neglect: lack of proper care.

negligence: carelessness; failing to do the proper thing.

no call, no show: when a person does not show up for work and does not call the facility.

OBRA: Omnibus Budget Reconciliation Act; law originally passed in 1987 which standardized requirements for facilities that accept Medicare residents.

ombudsman: a person who investigates and tries to settle complaints; may be a government official.

physical abuse: harming or injuring a person's body in some way.

plaintiff: the person who files and brings a lawsuit into court.

psychological abuse: emotional or verbal abuse of another person.

Residents' Rights: numerous rights identified by the OBRA law for the residents in long-term care facilities or nursing homes; purpose is to inform residents and others of their rights within these facilities and to provide an ethical code of conduct for healthcare workers.

sexual abuse: forcing another person to perform sex acts against his or her will.

slander: a spoken falsehood (lie) that damages the reputation of another person.

substandard: below the standard (something established as a rule); poor.

tort: wrongful act for which a civil action may be brought.

verbal abuse: oral or written statements threatening or insulting a resident in some way.

2 List the three branches of the United States government.

Laws exist everywhere. Understanding the law and how it affects you in your new position can help you provide better care. Before we discuss legal and ethical issues specifically related to you and other members of the healthcare team, let us review the overall legal system of the United States. The three branches of government are the legislative, the executive, and the judicial branches. The legislative branch of the government consists of the House of Representatives and the Senate. The House of Representatives is currently made up of 435 members, each of whom is elected from one of the 50 states in the union. If the population increases or decreases in a state, the number of representatives elected from that state changes, too. The Senate is made up of 100 members, with two members elected from each state. The Vice President serves as the President of the Senate. The **legislative branch** makes the laws.

The President and the members of the President's cabinet make up the **executive branch** of our government. The executive branch enforces the laws.

The **judicial branch** is made up of the court systems. The judicial branch interprets the laws. Figure 3-1 outlines the branches of government.

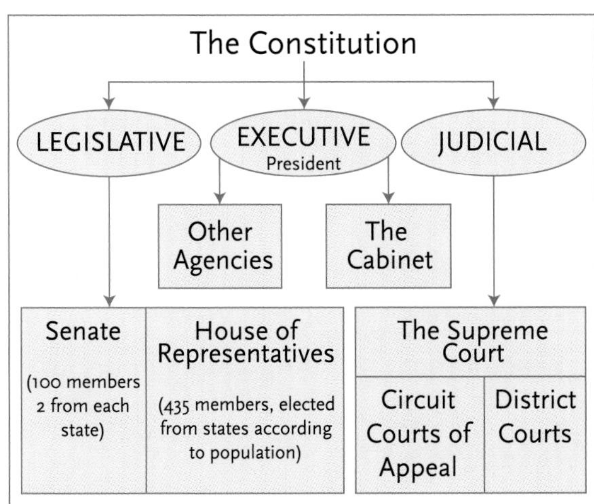

Figure 3-1. **Branches of the United States government.**

3 Identify different courts in the United States judicial system.

The judicial branch consists of the court systems. Our court system is composed of federal courts and state courts. Figure 3-2 outlines the federal court system. Some of the federal courts are the Supreme Court, the U.S. Tax Court, and the District Court. The Supreme Court is the most famous court in the United States. This court hears appeals from other federal courts and from state courts. State courts include criminal and civil courts, as well as state supreme courts.

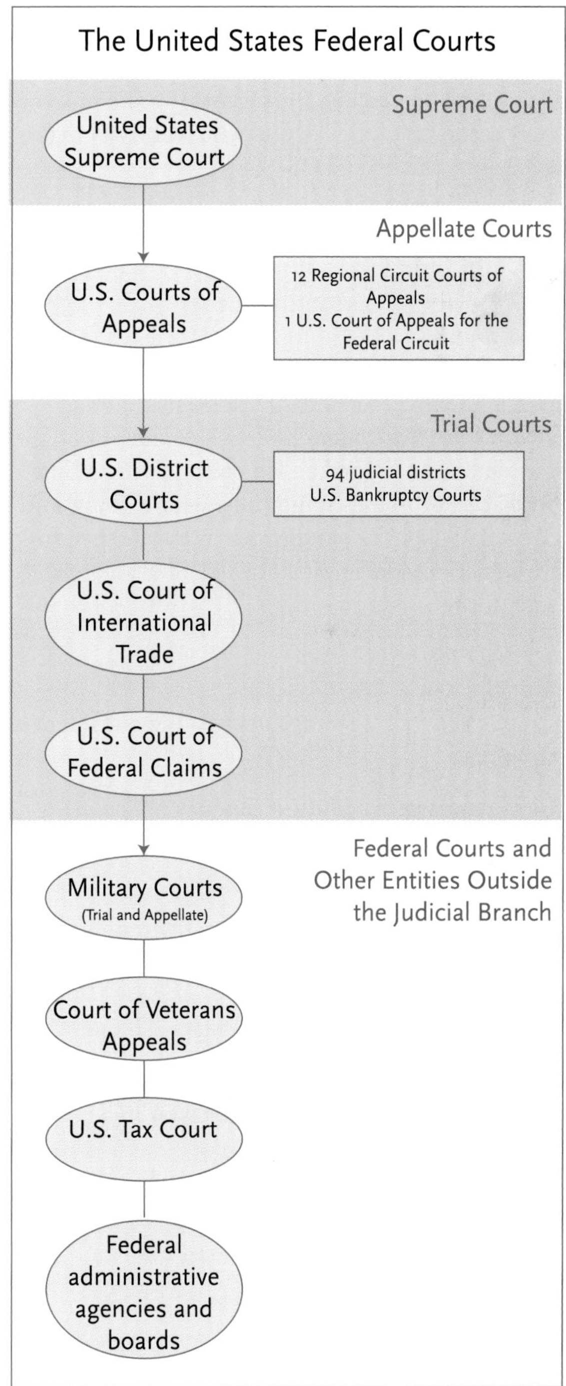

Figure 3-2. **The United States judicial system.**

4 Name and define the terms used to identify the people involved in the court system.

There are many people who play an important role in the court system. Some positions people may hold in the court system are defendant, plaintiff, judge, lawyer, bailiff, court reporter, the jury, and clerk. The **plaintiff** is the person in court who has filed a complaint of some kind against another party. The **defendant** is the person who has been charged with the complaint. The defense is composed of the lawyers who will defend the defendant. The prosecution is made up of the lawyers who will try to make a case against the defendant.

5 Define, discuss, and compare the terms "law," "ethics," "moral values," and "etiquette."

There are many legal and ethical terms that relate to resident care. **Ethics** and morals help determine the many decisions we make each day at home, in our workplaces, or in the community. Before going into more detail about law and ethics, it may be helpful to have a solid understanding of what all of the related terms mean.

Law: rules set to protect the public; may be civil or criminal.
Example: There is a law against stealing a resident's belongings.

Ethics: standards or guide of conduct.
Example: Keeping a resident's information confidential is ethical behavior.

Moral values: beliefs about right and wrong that help guide one's life; influenced by family, religion, and culture.
Example: A resident believes all people should wait to have sex until they are married.

Etiquette: proper manners and behavior in a certain setting.
Example: Asking "How may I help you?" when you answer the phone at your facility is proper telephone etiquette.

6 Identify two different types of laws.

Two well-known types of laws are criminal and civil law. **Criminal laws** are written in order to protect society from people or organizations that try to do them harm. This type of law protects the public; it is also called public law. **Civil law** refers to disputes between individuals. Problems with landlords, conflicts with neighbors, and divorce and custody issues are examples of areas covered by civil law. Civil law is sometimes referred to as private law.

Criminal law includes the following categories of offenses (crimes):

Misdemeanor. Assaulting someone or disturbing the peace are examples of misdemeanors. A misdemeanor is not as serious an offense as a felony.
Felony. Homicide (murder) and bribery are examples of felonies. A felony is much more serious than a misdemeanor.

Criminal law cases will often have jury trials, while civil cases may have a judge make a decision.

7 Name the "Standards Three" relating to legal and ethical issues in the nursing assistant profession.

We will divide legal and ethical issues as they relate to nursing assistants into three different standards, called the "Standards Three." The first is "Standards of Behavior." This identifies a set of desired professional and ethical behaviors for nursing assistants and other healthcare team members. The second is "Standards of Care," outlining the formal rights identified to keep patients and residents safe in healthcare facilities. The third and final is "Standards of Training," reviewing the OBRA law (Omnibus Budget Reconciliation Act of 1987) and its overall importance to the nursing assistant profession and to residents and their families.

8 Explain the nine components of professional and ethical behavior as described in the acronym "CATCH ME UP."

A nursing assistant's personal ethics and value system can be the most important reasons for becoming a successful healthcare team member. The understanding of right and wrong behavior starts soon after birth. Parents start to say the dreaded word "No!" to their infants during the first year. An infant usually does not like to hear a parent speak firmly in this way, and may try to change his behavior to make the parent happy again.

From the moment children are born, they start growing into adults and learning to make choices each day. These choices often revolve around what is right and wrong. Consider the following decisions you may need to make in a given day:

- Should I call my elderly relative, or am I too busy?
- Should I return the $10.00 the grocery clerk accidentally overpaid me with my change?
- Should I leave a job without giving appropriate notice?

These types of decisions will multiply thousands of times as the weeks and years pass. Ethical behavior often affects everything people do. Other people may develop an impression of you because of the ethical decisions you make.

Professional and ethical behavior in a healthcare facility is vital to the safety and well-being of the residents. An easy way to remember these guidelines for success is to use the first letter of each guideline to create the acronym "CATCH ME UP." This acronym sums up many important behaviors that may affect a healthcare team.

CATCH ME UP

Communication skills and **C**ommon sense.

Attitude of a STAR!

Tact in dealing with others.

Confidentiality with resident and staff information.

Honesty and trustworthiness.

Managing mistakes responsibly.

Empathy for resident and staff problems.

Understanding and respect for everyone.

Patience.

ON THE STAR PATH TO SUCCESS!

Effective communication is essential to the success of any team. When common sense teams up with excellent communication skills, staff members are more efficient. Recall someone you know who seems to have a lack of common sense. Ask yourself what that means. Does this person frequently do things that accidentally cause harm to herself or to others? Does she make poor decisions that affect others negatively? As a nursing assistant, you must always think before acting, especially with your residents.

Attitude is everything! You may have heard potential employers say they would hire someone with a great attitude before a person who has a problem getting along with others. As a nursing assistant, you will deal with a large number of people every day. A good attitude is a valuable asset. Cheerful, enthusiastic people cheer up everyone around them! Residents deserve people who will try to make their days as pleasant as possible. A person with a professional, positive attitude is someone people like to be around!

Tact is the ability to understand what is proper and appropriate when dealing with others. It is the ability to speak and act without offending others. Team members need to consider consequences before they say or do anything. By limiting negative comments and actions, you will nurture self-esteem in your residents. It is important to treat residents with respect and maintain their self-esteem.

Keeping resident information confidential is one of the residents' rights covered later in this chapter. All team members must keep all resident information confidential. Keeping staff information confidential means that you must not share private information about your coworkers at home or anywhere else.

The ability to trust other people is very important in long-term care facilities. Trust issues can keep groups of people together or tear them apart. Within a facility, the residents must be able to trust the entire staff. Employers must be able to trust their employees. And employees need to have trust in their supervisors. For employers, trusting an employee means knowing that the employee will come to work each day on time. When an employee is frequently a "**no call, no show**" (does not show up for work and does not call), the boss cannot trust that employee to come to work each day. Employers also trust that employees will come to them first if they have a problem. This is called following the **chain of command**.

Making a mistake in your daily life may or may not affect others negatively. Making a mistake in the healthcare field can have serious consequences. It is important to report all mistakes promptly to prevent any further problems from happening. Reporting mistakes promotes the safety and well-being of all residents.

Empathy means being able to put yourself in the shoes of your resident and imagine what it is like to *be* that resident. Being able to do this can bring you to a whole new level of understanding.

An understanding person feels and shows sympathy for others. Sympathy means sharing in the feelings and difficulties of others. Respect means allowing others to believe or act as they judge best. So an understanding person would be sympathetic towards someone who is ill and would also respect the ill person's actions or beliefs regarding the illness, despite his or her own personal feelings.

Having patience means a person has the ability to deal with a resident's pain, troubles, difficulties, and hardships without complaining or becoming angry or frustrated. **Activities of Daily Living** (ADLs), such as eating, dressing, brushing teeth, bathing, and toileting may take longer. Whether the resident has great pain, difficulty moving, or is a slow eater, a nursing assistant should allow the resident to do the task at his own pace. The more patient you are, the better care you will provide.

9 Describe a nursing assistant code of ethics.

Many facilities have adopted a formal Code of Ethics to help their employees deal with issues related to right and wrong conduct. Codes of ethics differ, but all revolve around the idea that a resident is a valuable human being who deserves ethical care. A sample code of ethics, written specifically for nursing assistants, is shown below:

1. I will strive to provide and maintain the highest quality of care for my residents, fully recognizing and following all of the Residents' Rights.
2. I will communicate effectively, serve on committees, read all material as provided and required by my employer, attend educational in-services, and join organizations relevant to nursing assistant care.
3. I will display a positive attitude toward my residents, staff, family members, and other visitors.
4. I will always provide privacy for my residents and maintain confidentiality of resident, staff, and visitor information.
5. I will be trustworthy and honest in all dealings with residents, staff, and visitors.
6. I will strive to preserve resident safety and will report mistakes I make, along with any situation that I deem dangerous, promptly to the appropriate person(s).
7. I will have empathy for the difficulties of my residents, the staff, and all visitors, providing support and encouragement whenever necessary.
8. I will have respect for all people, without regard to the person's age, sex, ethnicity, religion, economic situation, sexual orientation, or diagnosis.
9. I will strive to have the utmost patience with all people I have dealings with at my facility.

10 Identify nine specific components of the Residents' Rights.

In 1987, the **OBRA** law was passed by the federal government. This law identified numerous rights for the people who were placed in long-term care facilities or nursing homes—the residents.

The purpose of **residents' rights** is to inform residents of their rights within long-term care facilities and to provide an ethical code of conduct for healthcare workers. You also need to become familiar with residents' rights. Residents' rights are very detailed.

Overview of Residents' Rights — Box 3-1

Quality of Life
Each nursing home is required to care for its residents in such a manner and in such an environment as will promote maintenance or enhancement of the quality of life of each resident. This statement highlights an emphasis on dignity, choice, and self-determination for nursing home residents.

Providing Services and Activities
Each nursing home is required to provide services and activities to attain or maintain the highest practicable physical, mental, and psychosocial well-being of each resident in accordance with a written plan of care which . . . is initially prepared, with participation to the extent practicable of the resident, the resident's family, or legal representative. This means that a resident should not decline as a direct result of the nursing facility's care.

Nursing home residents are also granted these specific rights:

The Right to Be Fully Informed, including:
The right to be informed of all services available as well as the charge for each service;
The right to have a copy of the nursing home's rules and regulations, including a written copy of their rights;
The right to be informed of the address and telephone number of the State Ombudsman, State licensure office, and other advocacy groups;
The right to see the State survey reports of the nursing home and the home's plan of correction;
The right to be notified in advance of any plans to change their room or roommate;
The right to daily communication in their language;

The right to assistance if they have a sensory impairment.

The Right to Participate in Their Own Care, including:
The right to receive adequate or appropriate care;
The right to be informed of changes in their medical condition;
The right to participate in planning their treatment, care, and discharge;
The right to refuse medication and treatment;
The right to refuse chemical and physical restraints;
The right to review their medical record.

The Right to Make Independent Choices, including:
The right to make independent personal decisions, such as what to wear and how to spend free time;
The right to reasonable accommodation of their needs and preferences by the nursing home;
The right to choose their own physician;
The right to participate in community activities, both inside and outside the nursing home;
The right to organize and participate in a Resident Council.

The Right to Privacy and Confidentiality, including:
The right to private and unrestricted communication with any person of their choice;
The right to privacy in treatment and in the care of their personal needs;
The right to confidentiality regarding their medical, personal, or financial affairs;

The Right to Dignity, Respect, and Freedom, including:
The right to be treated with the fullest measure of consideration, respect, and dignity;
The right to be free from mental and physical abuse, corporal punishment, involuntary seclusion, and physical and chemical restraints;
The right to self-determination.

The Right to Security of Possessions, including:
The right to manage their own financial affairs;
The right to file a complaint with the State survey and certification agency for abuse, neglect, or misappropriation of their property if the nursing home is handling their financial affairs;
The right to be free from charge for services covered by Medicaid or Medicare.

Rights During Transfers and Discharges, including:
The right to remain in the nursing facility unless a transfer or discharge:

- is necessary to meet the resident's welfare
- is appropriate because the resident's health has improved and the resident no longer requires nursing home care
- is needed to protect the health and safety of other residents or staff
- is required because the resident has failed, after reasonable notice, to pay the facility charge for an item or service provided at the resident's request

The right to receive notice of transfer or discharge. A thirty-day notice is required. The notice must include the reason for transfer or discharge, the effective date, the location to which the resident is transferred or discharged, a statement of the right to appeal, and the name, address, and telephone number of the state long-term care ombudsman;
The right to a safe transfer or discharge through sufficient preparation by the nursing home.

The Right to Complain, including:
The right to present grievances to the staff of the nursing home, or to any other person, without fear of reprisal;
The right to prompt efforts by the nursing home to resolve grievances.

The Right to Visits, including:
The right to immediate access by a resident's personal physician and representatives from the health department and ombudsman programs;
The right to immediate access by their relatives and for others subject to reasonable restriction with the resident's permission;
The right to reasonable visits by organizations or individuals providing health, social, legal, or other services.

11 Explain the importance of the OBRA Act of 1987.

The OBRA Law of 1987, updated several times since, was drafted in large part as a response to numerous reports of abuse and **substandard** (poor) care within the nursing home industry. Reports were common during that time period of the horrendous conditions of some elderly people living in nursing homes. Congress stepped in and set minimum standards of care, including standardizing the training of the most common caregiver, the nursing assistant. The OBRA law requires that states set minimum standards for the type and length of nursing assistant training, develop a nursing assistant competency evaluation (testing program) consisting of a written and manual examination, and set up and keep track of annual continuing educational requirements for nursing assistants. OBRA also requires that states maintain a current list of nursing assistants in a state registry. In addition, OBRA identified certain standards the instructors must meet to qualify as a formal nursing assistant trainer.

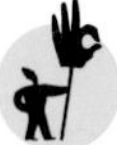

What is the State Board of Nursing?

In your state, this agency might have a different name; however, the responsibilities will be similar. Many State Boards of Nursing are in charge of the licensing of nurses and the testing or certification of nursing assistants. It is wise to keep the telephone number and address of your state board readily available. This agency may also handle issues and problems that occur with nurses and nursing assistants.

What is reciprocity?

When you have completed an approved nursing assistant course, you may be eligible for nursing assistant certification. When you move to another state, your nursing assistant certification may sometimes transfer to the new state. This is called reciprocity. Before moving to another state, it is wise to contact the agency in the new state that handles nursing assistant issues. Then you can find out if you qualify for reciprocity. If necessary, you can gather any important paperwork from your original state before you leave. Obtaining a new certificate in your new state is your responsibility.

12 Describe six legal issues relating to the nursing assistant.

A **tort**, or civil wrong, falls within the category of civil, or private, law. Torts may be intentional (the person did it on purpose) or unintentional (the person accidentally committed a wrong). We will define and discuss six torts. These are assault, battery, invasion of privacy, false imprisonment, fraud, and defamation of character.

1. **Assault** means that a person has threatened to touch or harm another person. A person has to prove that he was afraid harm would be done to him. Many lawsuits that include assault also will include battery.
2. **Battery** means a person has touched another person without permission. Example: Battery can be charged against a caregiver in a healthcare facility if an alert resident specifically refused a procedure and the healthcare team member performed the procedure anyway. If any resident refuses to allow you to perform a procedure, check with the nurse before you make any further decisions.
3. **Invasion of privacy** is defined as the violation of a person's right to be left alone or to have personal space. This can include a situation where private facts have been released without consent, such as medical records being shared without the patient's consent. Example: Invasion of privacy could be charged against a caregiver if that caregiver released medical information about a recently-admitted resident to a newspaper.
4. **False imprisonment** happens when a person restrains or confines another person against her will. The type of restraint may be physical (tie-down restraints), chemical (drugs), or emotional (threatening with something). Example: False imprisonment can be charged if a resident is restrained without the approval of the doctor and family members.
5. **Fraud** is when a person behaves in a deceitful (dishonest) manner. The elderly are more frequently becoming the targets of "scam" artists—untrustworthy people trying to gain money or something else from them. In addition, physicians' offices and nursing facilities can be charged with fraud. An audit may uncover services billed and not actually delivered. Example: A nursing assistant documents specific care that she never really performed.
6. **Defamation of character** is identified as a type of written or oral communication that is not true. This communication must injure the reputation of another person and/or cause damage to the person's ability to make a living.
   a. **Libel** is defamation in written form. Example: A nursing assistant may be charged with libel if he drew a negative cartoon about a well-known resident and published it.
   b. **Slander** is defamation in oral form. Example: A nursing assistant may be charged with slander if she supplied negative or private information to a tabloid newspaper.

13 Summarize negligence and what it means to the nursing assistant.

Negligence can be defined as an unintentional tort (wrong). **Negligence** may be charged when a person performed, or failed to perform, an act that a reasonable person would or would not have done in similar circumstances. Example: A nursing assistant leaves the side rail down on a resident's bed. The resident has a doctor's order for side rails. The resident falls out of bed and breaks her hip. Nursing assistants must be very careful to double-check resident rooms for safety before leaving them. Later in the textbook, a method for remembering the steps to take when entering and leaving a resident room will be outlined. The steps are called the "**5 Stars** and **3 Rs.**"

14 Recognize the importance of obtaining liability insurance.

The number of lawsuits against healthcare providers is increasing every year. Many lawsuits name everyone at fault, from the administrator and vice-president of patient care services, to the managers and nurses on the units. The best insurance against a lawsuit is to be careful in everything that you say and do while working. However, even though you might make every effort to provide good care, sometimes lawsuits occur. Insurance can then be a life-saver. Professionals like doctors and nurses must consider buying malpractice insurance as their form of **liability insurance**.

Some facilities will cover employees who are charged with negligence. **Malpractice** differs from negligence in that it is "incorrect or negligent treatment performed by a professional such as a physician, dentist, or a nurse."

You may also purchase additional liability insurance to have in case of a lawsuit. Many healthcare providers choose to purchase their own insurance so that they know there is someone who will look out for their best interests. That is what your insurance company should do—look out for you! The facility insurance will be busy looking out for everyone. The safest route is to gather information about personal liability insurance. Liability insurance for the nursing assistant is usually available at a low cost.

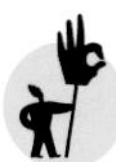

Never call yourself a nurse!

Nursing assistants must never identify themselves as nurses. If you do this, you may put yourself at serious risk of being named in a lawsuit (being sued). A nurse's responsibilities are different from a nursing assistant's, and people generally have higher expectations of a nurse. It is possible that you could also face a charge of "illegally posing as a nurse," in addition to the risk of being sued by others. So never use the term "nurse" lightly; always identify yourself as a nursing assistant.

15 Discuss the Good Samaritan Act and how it relates to nursing assistants.

Many states have passed laws that protect people who attempt to assist others in an emergency from being sued. These laws are called **Good Samaritan Acts**. These acts differ from state to state. The name comes from the Bible story of someone who gave aid to a stranger who had been beaten up. It normally covers people who accept no payment and are trying to provide emergency care within their scope of practice to help people at the scene of an accident.

In some states, the protection is limited to doctors while in others, all healthcare providers and even laymen (people without formal medical training) are also protected. A Good Samaritan Act usually does not apply when a person is being paid for services.

If you would like additional information about the Good Samaritan Act in your state, contact a local legal aid society. You can also contact your state's bar association, an ombudsman, or your local nurse's association.

16 Explain seven types of resident abuse and describe signs of abuse.

Elder abuse can occur both in private homes and within the walls of any facility, from adult daycare centers to nursing homes. Figure 3-3 identifies percentages of some of the types of elder abuse. Types of elder abuse include the following:

1. Psychological or verbal abuse
2. Physical abuse and neglect
3. Sexual abuse
4. Domestic abuse
5. Involuntary seclusion
6. Financial abuse
7. Exploitation

Psychological abuse includes emotional, mental, or verbal abuse of a resident. Emotional abuse happens when a resident is humiliated, harassed in any way,

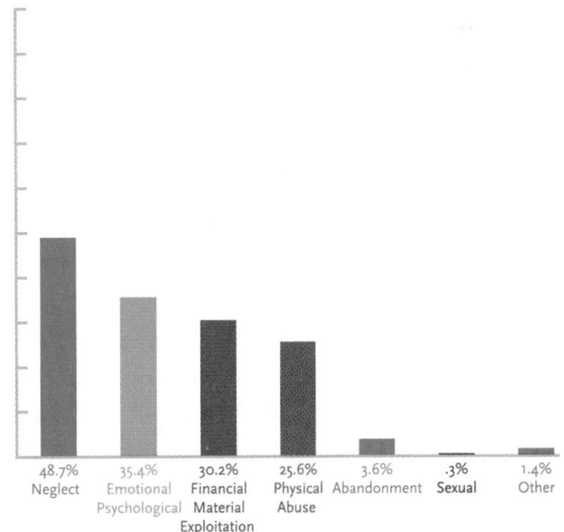

Figure 3-3. **Types of resident abuse.**

or feels threatened. **Verbal abuse** is defined as oral statements, written statements or pictures, or gestures that are threatening, embarrassing, or insulting to a resident. Team members must never use foul language or tease residents. Team members must also be sensitive to residents' cultures and backgrounds. Using insulting names that refer to a person's race, culture, religion, or sexual orientation can be devastating to a resident and can put your job at risk. Threatening to punish a resident in any way is not permitted.

Examples:

a. A team member insults a resident's race.

b. A team member threatens to harm a resident if he tells another team member about some problem that has occurred.

c. A team member loudly announces that a new resident wet the bed last night in front of other residents in a dayroom.

Physical abuse of residents is defined as causing physical harm or neglecting residents. A resident can be harmed physically if he is treated in a rough manner during personal care. Physical abuse also occurs when someone hits, kicks, pushes, or touches a resident in any way that causes pain, discomfort, and/or injury.

Examples:

a. A team member pushes a resident when she does not move fast enough toward a dayroom.

b. A resident is hit by a team member during personal care when he, the resident, tries to stop the care for some reason.

c. A team member pinches a resident when she tries to tell someone something the team member wants kept a secret.

Neglect means that a team member fails to follow through and give the correct care or treatments ordered for the resident. Neglect can be charged if anyone fails to provide personal care of any kind and this failure causes the resident discomfort or injury. Failure to provide adequate food and fluids for a resident is also neglect. *Not responding to a resident's call light is considered neglect.*

Examples:

a. A resident has wet the bed, and a team member places a pad under the resident instead of changing his sheets.

b. A resident who is unable to feed himself has a dinner tray placed in the room on the overbed table. The tray is left there, but the resident is never actually fed.

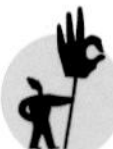

They are ALL our residents!

Remember, all of the residents within your area or unit are your residents. Even though you may be assigned a certain number of residents, you are still expected to respond to any resident in need. You should never say, "He/she is not my resident."

Sexual abuse occurs when residents are forced to perform or participate in sexual acts against their will. This would also include introducing sexual literature of any kind to a resident. In addition, sexual harassment of any resident falls under the definition of sexual abuse. Harassment is any kind of improper sexual advances or comments causing the resident to become fearful and feel threatened sexually.

Examples:

a. A resident is forced to perform sexual acts when no other staff are nearby.

b. A team member forces a resident to look at obscene literature.

c. During personal care, a team member rubs up against a resident inappropriately.

Domestic abuse is sometimes difficult to spot in the elderly population. This type of abuse may have existed within the home for some time. When a couple is moved from a home into a facility, the abuse may continue. If this type of abuse is suspected, you must immediately report it to your supervisor. Your supervisor will then make the appropriate decisions regarding this difficult and complex situation.

Examples:

a. A woman recently admitted to a double room with her husband has unexplained bruises on her arms.

b. A male resident was observed being hit by his wife because he could not understand what she was trying to tell him.

Involuntary seclusion happens when a resident is confined to his room or one particular area and separated from the rest of the facility without consent or against his will.

Examples:

a. A team member does not place the call light within easy reach of a resident.

b. A resident is made to stay in her room with the door closed during the dinner hour.

Financial abuse of a resident can occur both in the home and within a facility.

Examples:

a. A team member offers a resident "extra-special" care if the resident or a family member will give the team member a certain amount of money.

b. A team member requests that a resident give financial help to the team member's friend.

Witnessing a Will

Many facilities have a rule that staff members should never witness a will of any kind. It is not appropriate to witness a will for one of your residents. Witnessing a will is a serious legal responsibility and can involve family and friends who may not get along well with each other. To avoid potential legal problems in the future, it is simply the safest route to never witness a will. Make sure you know your facility's policy about witnessing any legal documents.

Exploitation is a type of financial abuse. The elderly can be quite vulnerable and defenseless against people known as "scam artists."

Examples:

a. An elderly person is asked to withdraw money from an account to invest in a "sure thing."

b. A team member attempts to convince an elderly male to name her in his will.

Abuse can be suspected when certain signs are identified. All healthcare team members must be watchful for these signs and follow the rules of reporting them in their particular state. Many of the signs of abuse are listed below.

Signs of Abuse (Box 3-2)

Signs of Physical Abuse
- Unexplained broken bones
- Similar injuries that occur over and over, such as an injury shaped like a belt buckle
- Burns shaped in certain ways, like a cigarette burn or a burn caused by an iron
- Bite marks
- Unexplained weight loss, extremely dry and cracked skin, or signs of dehydration
- Blood in underwear
- Bruising in the genital area
- Sexually transmitted infections

Signs of Emotional Abuse
- Mood swings
- Fear and anxiety, especially when a caregiver is present
- Lack of appetite
- Flinching when a certain person is near

Other Signs of Abuse:
- Missed doctor's appointments
- Changing doctors frequently
- Wearing makeup or sunglasses to hide injuries
- Family concern that abuse is occurring
- Person does not seem to be taking his medication
- Caregiver does not allow anyone to be alone with the resident

17 Explain methods of reporting resident abuse when following the chain of command.

In 1987, elder abuse, along with neglect and exploitation, was defined in amendments to the Older Americans Act passed by the federal government. The government gave the responsibility of enforcement to the individual states. Many of the 50 states have passed laws identifying methods of reporting elder abuse.

Be familiar with the laws in your state regarding the reporting of elder abuse. If you would like more information about the laws concerning elder abuse in your state, contact your state or local ombudsman or the state agency on aging. If you suspect abuse, you are legally required to report it. Follow the chain of command at your facility.

1. You must document any complaints of abuse told to you by residents or other staff, and anything you may have witnessed yourself.
2. Report this situation to your supervisor.
3. If action of some kind is not taken, continue reporting up the chain of command until action is taken.
4. If no appropriate action is taken at the facility level, contact the state abuse hotline. Usually this is an anonymous telephone call. If no abuse hotline exists in your state or town, a state agency must be contacted to report the abuse.

Hopefully, facility management will work to correct the problem. If they do not solve the problem, report directly to the ombudsman or another advocate. This can be done in a way that protects you and does not identify you. They are then required to investigate.

Never retaliate against a resident making a complaint of abuse. If you witness another member of the healthcare team retaliating against a resident who made a complaint, you must again follow the proper chain of command and report it.

If residents want to make a complaint of abuse themselves, you must assist in every possible way. This includes informing them of the process and their rights, and letting them know about the ombudsman program.

18 Discuss the ombudsman's role in preventing resident abuse.

The word "ombudsman" originally came from Scandinavia. In parts of Scandinavia, an ombudsman is an official of the government who investigates complaints of the citizens. In the United States, we have adopted the ombudsman approach for the reporting of elder abuse. In nursing homes, an **ombudsman** is established by law as the legal advocate for the resident. Ombudsmen visit the facility, listen to the residents, and decide what course of action to take if there is a problem. They provide an ongoing presence in long-term care facilities, monitoring care and conditions.

In some states, a group of specially-selected people on a watchdog committee may investigate all reports of abuse that occur in healthcare facilities. Citizens who are interested in quality care of the elderly may serve on this committee. For more information about the role of a long-term care ombudsman, contact the department in your state that handles elder care or your legal aid society.

Summary

The law can be complicated. Legal issues related to healthcare facilities are sometimes difficult to understand. When all healthcare workers have a basic understanding of the law, it can make a facility safer and more secure for everyone. The purpose of the Resident's Rights is to inform residents of their rights, as well as to provide an ethical code for nursing assistants and the rest of the healthcare team. Understanding Residents' Rights is one of the best ways to provide quality care for your residents.

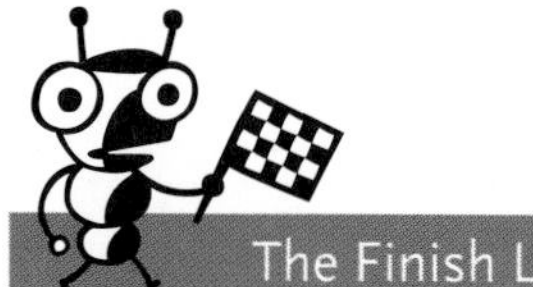

The Finish Line

What's Wrong With This Picture?

Each of the following scenarios describes a violation of one of the Residents' Rights. Following the scenario, identify the right violated and your course of action.

1. One morning, resident Alexandra Rietz asks her new nursing assistant for her name and position. The nursing assistant identifies herself and says she just started work that morning. Ms. Rietz then states that she would rather not have a new nursing assistant care for her. The nursing assistant tells Ms. Rietz she did not have a choice in the matter.

Right Violated:
Your Actions:

2. Mrs.Twila Montgomery is 97 and has just been admitted to the Geneva Ridge Facility with her husband. The couple has approximately the same ability to care for themselves and perform their daily activities. Mrs. Montgomery is not happy because she has been placed in Room 24 and her husband has been placed in Room 27.

Right Violated:
Your Actions:

3. Mr. Sky Jones is at Orion Care Facility for his 12th year. He is unhappy because the new administrator has said that Sky may not continue painting. Sky has been painting for 12 years. The doctor has approved this activity.

Right Violated:
Your Actions:

4. Minnie Mercado is the oldest resident at Harvest House, the largest care facility in town. The family has asked to have a small party with a few relatives and friends for her 100th birthday. The Harvest House management has refused, stating that not enough advance time was given to the facility.

Right Violated:
Your Actions:

5. Ms. Sun Ho is a new resident. She is a Buddhist and has placed religious items around her bed. A staff member makes insulting remarks about her religious items.

Right Violated:
Your Actions:

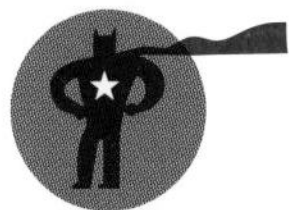

Star Student Central

1. Choose one topic listed below and gather further information that is specific to your state. Choose from: The Good Samaritan Act, the state or area hotline for reporting elder abuse, and the local ombudsman. This information can then be shared with your class.
2. Write down a problem you have had in the past with a neighbor or friend. Did you ever reach a point when you considered asking someone for help? Now think about residents in a long-term care facility. Consider this situation: a resident plays her radio too loudly in the same room as another resident. What could be done by the staff to solve the situation?

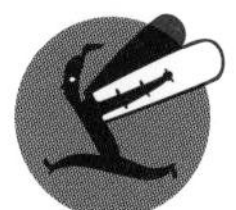

You Can Do It Corner!

1. Using the Standards of Behavior acronym "CATCH ME UP," write down as many of the professional and ethical behaviors as you can. (LO 8)
2. List the steps to follow in the chain of command when reporting resident abuse. (LO 17)
3. What are nine specific components of Residents' Rights? (LO 10)
4. List each branch of the United States government and what it does. (LO 2)
5. Give an example of negligence. (LO 13)
6. List how the protections of criminal and civil law differ. (LO 6)
7. List seven different kinds of elder abuse and give one example of each. (LO 16)
8. List ten possible signs of abuse that you might see in residents. (LO 16)
9. Name one reason why personal liability insurance might be a good idea for a nursing assistant. (LO 14)
10. Give one example of each of the following: upholding a law, demonstrating ethical behavior, and using proper telephone etiquette. (LO 5)
11. Name three federal courts in the United States. (LO 3)
12. Describe what the OBRA law covers. (LO 11)
13. List who the Good Samaritan Act normally covers. (LO 15)
14. Describe some of the ways an ombudsman advocates for a resident. (LO 18)
15. Give examples of each of the following: assault, battery, invasion of privacy, false imprisonment, fraud, and defamation of character. (LO 12)
16. List each of the "Standards Three" and how they relate to legal issues. (LO 7)
17. Describe five points of a typical nursing assistant code of ethics. (LO 9)
18. List the roles of plantiffs and defendants in legal disputes. (LO 4)

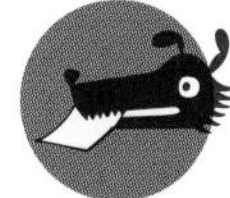

Star Student's Chapter Checklist

1. I have read my textbook chapter.
2. I have reviewed my own "Pocketful of Terms."
3. I have listened to my tutor tape.
4. I have reviewed and highlighted my class notes.
5. I have read and completed any handouts from this chapter.
6. I have completed "The Finish Line."
7. Star Time! Choose your reward!

4

Your Guide: Celebrating Diversity and Religious Differences

Look Like a Star!

Look at the Learning Objectives **and** The Finish Line **before you begin reading this chapter.**

Look at your pocket calendar.
With your pencil, put a bracket ( ) around a study period every single day.

Look at your homework for this chapter.
Plug each piece of homework into a certain time slot.

Look at the Star Student's Chapter Checklist **at the end of this chapter. Check off each item as it is completed.**

"The great law of culture is:
Let each become all that he was
created capable of being."

Thomas Carlyle, 1795-1881

"Religion is a great force - the only real motive force in the world: but what you fellows don't understand is that you must get at a man through his own religion and not through yours."

George Bernard Shaw, 1856-1950

Learning Objectives

1. **Spell and define all STAR words.**
2. **Define nine common terms related to diversity.**
3. **Define "immigrate" and "emigrate" and list two reasons people may move to the United States.**
4. **Explain four ways to promote cultural competence as described in the acronym "DOOR."**
5. **Name five ways residents may want health information communicated.**
6. **Discuss different methods of seeking health care.**
7. **Describe two ways to deal with a language barrier.**
8. **Describe eight responses to pain and why it is important for nursing assistants to understand residents' views of pain.**
9. **Describe ways cultural and ethnic practices relating to food and nutrition impact health care.**
10. **Define "spirituality" and "religion" and discuss the ways religion should be accommodated in health care.**
11. **Identify the ways religious beliefs can affect death practices.**
12. **Explain why the behavior of nursing assistants serves as a role model for their residents.**

The Black Death: The Plague That Didn't Discriminate

60 MILLION PEOPLE DEAD. In the 14th century, the Black Death, also known as the Bubonic Plague, first reared its ugly head. The name "Black Death" came from the black areas on the skin commonly seen in plague patients. It is thought to have developed in the Far East. This plague moved across Asia and into North Africa, slipping into Europe by way of Italy. Italian merchants at the time traveled to Asia searching for beautiful wares to sell. When they set sail for home, they carried the specter of the Black Death with them to Italy without realizing it. The plague spread over Italy and then over England. An estimated 60 million people died of the plague from 1340 to 1350. The plague killed people from many cultures and ethnic groups. Disease strikes everyone from every age group. It truly does not discriminate!

1 Spell and define all STAR words.

barriers: obstacles preventing an advance or access; things that may slow down or hold up progress.

bias: a preference based on prejudice.

culture: a set of beliefs and customs of a group of people.

cultural competence: taking into account a person's culture when giving care to maintain or restore health and wellness.

cultural diversity: many cultures living and working together; the state of being culturally different.

customs: generally accepted behavior or practices of a particular group of people or a social group; fixed traditions of a society.

emigrate: to leave one's country to live in another country.

ethnic group: a group sharing a common social and cultural background, usually having the same language and customs.

healthcare provider: healthcare professionals, such as doctors and nurses, who provide care to residents in order to promote wellness or to restore health.

immigrate: to enter a country in which one is not a native to live there permanently.

interpreter: a person who can translate words from another language and interpret the meaning and message of the words.

persecution: causing others to suffer or harassing others, esp. regarding religion or politics.

race: a distinct group of people with members who share and transmit to their children the same inherited physical characteristics, such as skin color and hair type.

religion: organized system of beliefs, rituals, and practices, esp. regarding marriage and death.

rituals: traditional religious ceremonies that are consistent and common to a certain religion.

spirituality: all behaviors that give meaning to life and provide strength to the individual.

stereotype: a biased and preconceived opinion about an ethnic or religious group.

taboo: prohibition of certain things on religious or social grounds.

traditions: continuation of a culture by transmitting beliefs, principles, behavior, and customs.

traits: distinguishing physical characteristics or features of a person like skin color, hair color, height, size, and facial features.

2 Define nine common terms related to diversity.

The term **culture** refers to a people's set of beliefs and customs. The world is full of many different groups of people. Each group has its own unique way of looking at the world. As nursing assistants on the front lines of health care, you will have the opportunity to take care of people from many cultures. Having a better understanding of other cultures will help you give better care to your residents. Your own culture influences you in many ways.

Cultural diversity has to do with the wide variety of people living and working together throughout the world. Cultural diversity is about acceptance and knowledge, rather than **bias**, or prejudice. Each culture may have different lifestyles, religions, customs, and behaviors. All of these things have a great impact on our daily lives.

Customs are the fixed traditions of a society. These **traditions** may be made into laws in some countries. An individual's culture and background often have an impact on overall behavior during times of illness. In order to provide the best health care and be the best caregivers we can be, we must try to understand other cultures and the different ways they may deal with health and disease. You need to be sensitive to and respect people who are different from you. Becoming familiar with many different cultures is a wonderful experience you will have in your position as a nursing assistant.

Race is defined as a way to categorize a group of people who have common physical traits. **Traits** are distinguishing characteristics or features about a person. Traits are things like skin color, hair color and type, overall height and size, and facial features. An **ethnic group** is a group of people who usually have the same language and customs. The same race may be made up of different ethnic groups. Examples of ethnic groups are the Japanese, the Spanish, and the Irish.

A **stereotype** is an oversimplified thought, opinion, or image about an ethnic or religious group. People who belong to one ethnic group are not all the same.

Do not assume a group is a certain way because of what you have read, heard, or seen on television or at the movies. Instead of assuming, ask questions in a friendly manner. Some people are happy to talk about their backgrounds and educate others about where they are from.

It is inappropriate and unprofessional to make fun of, tease, or concentrate negatively on people who look and act differently than you do. Try celebrating differences instead. It would be very boring if all people looked and acted the same way.

When nursing assistants are sensitive to cultural differences during daily care, residents benefit from it. When people accept and do not judge the beliefs or ways of life of others, there are more opportunities to learn about others and create lasting relationships. Residents will feel comfortable with you and your care and look forward to seeing you each day.

You are an important part of the nursing team for many reasons. One of the reasons you are so valuable is that you will offer detailed observations to the nurses. The most professional way to communicate with the staff is to gather your observations and report them to the nurses without being judgmental in any way about your residents. These observations may then be used by the nurses to help them plan and provide the best nursing care possible.

By Tanya Looney, CNA

As NAs caring for your residents, remember to always be considerate of their beliefs, despite the fact that they may be different from yours. Race, customs, religions, and preferences differ greatly in many ways. All of these things factor into the choices your residents make, from hair care to diets. Take it upon yourself to know that your resident in room 201 does not eat pork because he is Muslim, or that your African American resident in room 104 washes her hair once every two weeks because excessive washing causes it to become dry and brittle. Understand that all residents have different backgrounds. For example, one resident in your care grew up listening to country music. Another resident prefers gospel or R&B. Be sensitive to each of your residents' differences. Take time to learn about your residents' beliefs or customs by talking to them and their families. You can learn so much!

3 Define "immigrate" and "emigrate" and list two reasons people may move to the United States.

The United States began as a nation of immigrants looking for a better life across the sea. Many of these people came here because of religious persecution.

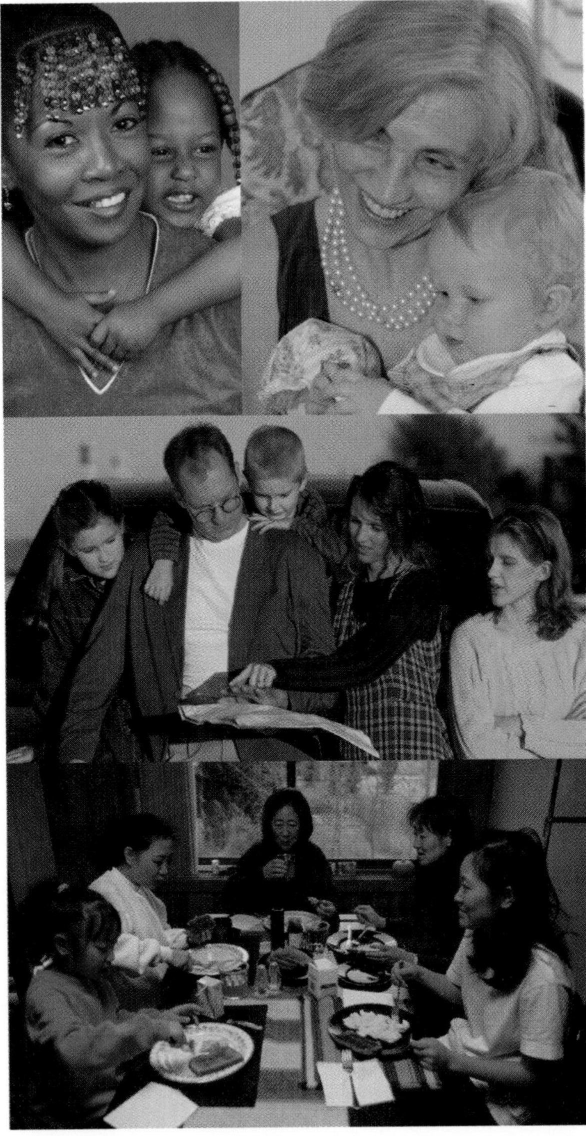

Figure 4-1. Families come in many shapes and sizes.

Persecution means being made to suffer or being harassed by others. Others came looking for "riches beyond compare."

We now have people immigrating here from all over the world. To **immigrate** means to move into a country in which one was not born, in order to live there permanently. To **emigrate** means to leave your home or country and settle in another.

Today, immigrants primarily come to the United States to find a better way of life. There are also other, more specific reasons for immigrating, depending on the culture. For example, some people come to this country because they do not have religious freedom within their home country. Others move here to be able to participate in a free style of government and have the right to vote for the candidates of their choice.

These immigrants are of different races and come from various ethnic groups. They may have a variety of cultural backgrounds, religions, and ways of dealing with illness that will greatly affect your ability to care for them. Some cultures may be unfamiliar with the "western model" of health care. It can be an interesting challenge for the staff to blend the healthcare practices of this nation with a resident's special individual beliefs.

4 Explain four ways to promote cultural competence as described in the acronym "DOOR."

Cultural competence—taking into account a person's culture when giving care—is of prime importance to the delivery of quality health care. When caregivers better understand the needs of people of different cultures, the quality of care improves.

Developing cultural competence can be a process. Four important aspects in the development of cultural competence include avoiding judging people, promptly securing the services of an **interpreter** or translator, making careful observations of all residents to learn from them, and respecting all people, regardless of culture. These four aspects are outlined in the acronym "DOOR."

When you try to follow these steps, you are delivering quality care to your residents.

DOOR

Do not judge anyone you meet.

Obtain the services of an interpreter as soon as possible, if necessary.

Observe all residents carefully to look for changes in condition and to learn from them about their culture and customs.

Respect all people.

5 Name five ways residents may want health information communicated.

Communication is a key to quality health care. Residents from various cultures may have certain customs they follow when dealing with others, especially medical professionals. Your residents may fall into one of these categories:

1. Resident would like information given directly to him- or herself.
2. Resident wishes information to be given to family members first.
3. Resident is unable to accept and understand information due to some physical problem or medication.
4. Family member or friend asks that information be withheld from the resident.
5. Resident may ask that family and/or friends not receive any health information for a certain period of time.

Staff members should be aware of personal preferences and differences regarding the way residents may want their health information to be handled. Honoring the wishes of each resident to the best of your ability is a part of quality care.

6 Discuss different methods of seeking health care.

Different cultures and ethnic groups have unique ways of dealing with health and illness. **Healthcare providers** need to be sensitive to differences between groups in order to offer the best care.

You will see many different methods of seeking health care. Certain people may seek help from a family member before making an appointment for a visit to a clinic or an office. Some people may delay making appointments due to fear, shyness, or embarrassment. Other people may not like to deal with professional caregivers, and may feel more comfortable working with people from their own ethnic groups or culture. They may feel intimidated by medical professionals. Some people may first ask special members of their culture who take care of the sick to treat the ill person.

Different ethnic groups may treat health and illness quite differently. Having a basic understanding of the healthcare practices and behaviors of the most common ethnic groups in your area may assist you in your goal of providing sensitive, quality care to all of your residents.

Ask, acknowledge, and accept!

Focus on compassionate, respectful, and sensitive care. Always treat your residents as they wish to be treated, NOT how you want to treat them. Your cultural background and experiences have shaped the way you think; other people come from different cultures and life experiences that have shaped the way they think. Something you may want or need from another person may be much different from what your resident wants or needs. Always remember to ask questions to find out what is appropriate. Never try to make your residents change their beliefs in any way.

7 Describe two ways to deal with a language barrier.

Language **barriers** can present unique problems that prevent the healthcare team from adequately communicating with a resident. One method of dealing with a language barrier is to obtain an interpreter to exchange information. Sometimes very slight changes in pronunciation will totally change the meaning of a word or group of words. An interpreter will make sure that your resident can fully understand the information you are giving him. The interpreter translates the words along with explaining the meaning and message in the words.

When the nurse is unable to arrange for an interpreter, another method of dealing with a language barrier is to learn some common medical phrases in other languages. Box 4-1 shows common phrases in Spanish that may be useful when caring for your Spanish-speaking residents. The box contains just a few examples; for a more complete list of medical phrases in other languages, use resources recommended by staff, residents, and their families.

Speak so they can understand.

Abuse comes in many forms. When you care for your residents, always speak in a language they can understand or find an interpreter (someone who speaks their language). Do not hold conversations with other staff members in a different language in front of residents. Residents might think you are saying something bad about them, and it is disrespectful.

Common Medical Phrases in Spanish Box 4-1

You are okay.	Está bien.
Lift your head.	Levante la cabeza.
I am hot	Tengo calor.
I am cold	Tengo frío.
Are you nauseous?	¿Tiene nausea?
Are you allergic?	¿Tiene Usted alergias?
Shot/injection	Inyección
Sit in the chair.	Siéntese en la silla.
Move your legs.	Mueva sus piernas.
Be calm.	Esté Usted tranquilo.
We are going to your room.	Vamos a su cuarto.
Toilet	Cuarto de baño.
Urinal	Orinal
Bedpan	La chata
Breathe.	Respire Usted.
Squeeze my hand.	Apriéteme la mano.

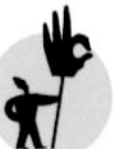

¡Un poco de Español!

When a resident speaks a different language, you might try to learn a few words in the resident's native language. This could be done by working with an interpreter or translator or perhaps a family member or friend of the resident. Flash cards or picture cards can assist with communication. Books may also help you accomplish this goal. Being able to speak a few words in residents' native languages helps provide a bit of comfort to them in a world that sometimes can be lonely and frightening.

8 Describe eight responses to pain and why it is important for nursing assistants to understand residents' views of pain.

Ethnic groups may deal quite differently with the concept of pain. When people are open and speak freely about pain, healthcare providers may find it easier to plan and provide care. However, when people do not communicate that they are in pain, this makes it more difficult for family, friends, and healthcare providers to see that they receive the best care. Understanding the way your residents view pain can make you watch for more subtle "messages" that they may be in pain. For example, if a resident does not often complain of pain, he may show other symptoms, such as squeezing his eyes shut, tightening his jaw, or sweating.

The following outlines some of the possible ways people may handle or respond to pain:

- high pain tolerance
- low pain tolerance
- loud verbal response to pain
- quiet response to pain
- belief that pain comes from God or that pain is good
- belief that pain is a curse or that pain is evil
- belief that pain must be tolerated
- being too embarrassed to report pain

Regardless of your resident's culture, it is important for you to recognize and respond to pain. When nursing assistants are observant regarding pain and communicate their observations promptly to the nurses, residents' pain may be kept under better control. No member of the healthcare team wants a resident to suffer needlessly.

9 Describe ways cultural and ethnic practices relating to food and nutrition impact health care.

Food can be one of the most important components in a culture, or food may be something a culture views as simply an element of survival. When we are ill, the importance of food may increase. We must get enough nutrition to get well as soon as possible. Some cultures serve food that is not healthy for an ill person. Adjustments have to be made to the diet, at least on a temporary basis and perhaps permanently, in order for the person to return to good health.

Your observations of residents, as they relate to diet and nutrition, are crucial in the delivery of quality health care. Many times you will be the only person who will notice a resident accepting food brought in by a family member or friend. The food may or may not be on the resident's diet, and the nurse should be made aware of the situation. You must always notify the nurse when a situation like this occurs in order to protect the resident.

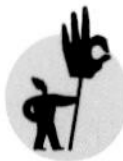

Start a "Recipe of the Month Club!"

Think about the favorite recipes that you hold dear in your family. Some of your residents may also have many recipes that they treasure. Consider having a favorite recipe day each month. A resident's or staff member's recipe could be chosen by a committee, and the dietary department might be able to make it (or a variation of it). Some residents may not be able to share certain foods because of a special diet, but these details can always be worked out.

Culture, ethnicity, income, education, religion, and even geography can affect attitudes about nutrition. Residents may miss ethnic or favorite dishes; their appetites may decline, causing unnecessary weight loss. Some residents will have specific dietary rules as a part of their religion.

Nursing assistants may see some of these habits affect food choices and behaviors within the long-term care setting. You should be familiar with the diet orders of all of your residents. This ultimately protects your residents from harm.

10 Define "spirituality" and "religion" and discuss the ways religion should be accommodated in health care.

Spirituality can be defined as all that concerns the life of the soul. Spirituality may also be thought of as simply believing in a higher power. **Religion** can be defined as an organized system of beliefs and practices related to the sacred. Each religion may have certain practices that include **rituals** (traditional religious ceremonies that are consistent and common to a certain religion). Some people who belong to a particular religious group do not abide by all the customs or rules of that religion. Some people consider themselves spiritual, but do not subscribe to any religion. Spiritual and religious beliefs can have a tremendous impact on healthcare habits.

The word **"taboo"** refers to things that are prohibited. For example, some religions do not allow their members to eat certain foods. Some kinds of meat may be taboo; coffee or tea may not be allowed, or milk and other dairy products may not be able to be paired with certain foods. These are just a few examples. If a resident shows reluctance to eat and drink certain things at particular times, it may be related to a religious practice.

Certain religions require members to treat days, weeks, or even months as holy periods. Always try to honor any special requests your residents have during these times.

Religious icons, symbols, statues, and literature should be handled carefully, according to the resident's wishes. Team members must immediately refer a resident to a member of the clergy whenever the request is made.

Healthcare team members need to be aware of the differences in residents' spiritual and religious beliefs. This is important, not only so that you can honor residents' requests, but also because by knowing your residents more fully, you are able to provide better care. Never judge or make fun of any beliefs or practices. Remember, your role is to care for the residents. They have a right to practice, or not practice, the religion of their choice. You do not have the right to impose your beliefs on them or to try to change their beliefs in any way.

11 Identify the ways religious beliefs can affect death practices.

The way people handle death and dying can vary considerably from one religion, culture, or ethnic group to another. No one group handles death and dying in a "right" or "wrong" fashion. All differences must be respected.

Some ethnic groups do not perform any special rituals to the body of the deceased. Others have certain ceremonies that are performed; sometimes they include the use of certain oils or special materials on or around the body.

After a person dies, some cultures have long, serious ceremonies that involve many people. Others have special kinds of joyous gatherings when a person dies. Some may talk very little about the person's death, while others may use talking about and remembering the person who has died as a way of comforting family and friends.

It is important that you do not judge any person's healthcare practices, regardless of what they are or whether you agree with them or not.

Being familiar with the individual practices of your residents may allow you to give better care during the dying process. More information on death and dying can be found in Chapter 36.

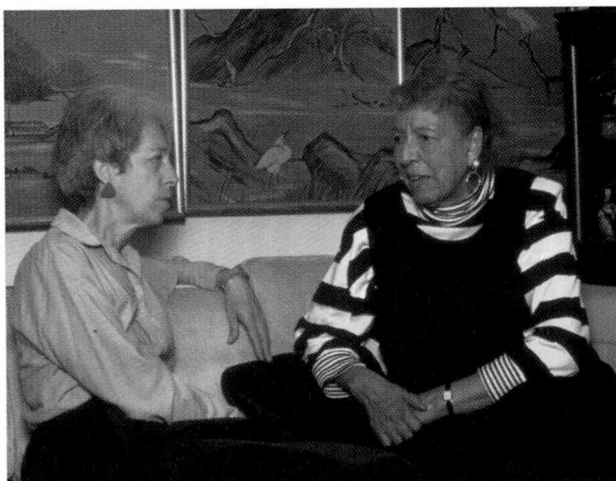

Figure 4-2. **Cultural practices affect the way people deal with death.**

12 Explain why the behavior of nursing assistants serves as a role model for their residents.

In many facilities, people of all ethnic and religious backgrounds may come together to live and work. In a diverse environment, there is potential for conflict among residents, families, and even staff. By respecting and accommodating the wonderful differences among people, you become an example for others.

Take advantage of the diversity around you. Learn as much as you can about people who are different from you. Take great care in your attitudes and behaviors toward each of your residents. If it seems hard, remember: people are watching you. Be a good example.

Summary

The ethnic and cultural makeup of the United States changes constantly. Diversity can be a wonderful thing for a country; it can make a country infinitely more interesting and enjoyable. As different cultures move to the United States, healthcare providers and the entire healthcare team must adjust to allow for specific cultural, religious, and healthcare practices. Nursing assistants need to become familiar with the cultural differences of their residents in order to provide the best care. They must be sensitive to the differences in the various ethnic groups they will care for and never form judgments about residents. Each and every person needs to work hard to encourage acceptance. It is important for healthcare workers to treat all residents with the same respect and courtesy. Nursing assistants should always exhibit professional behavior when caring for a culturally-diverse group of people. Celebrate diversity!

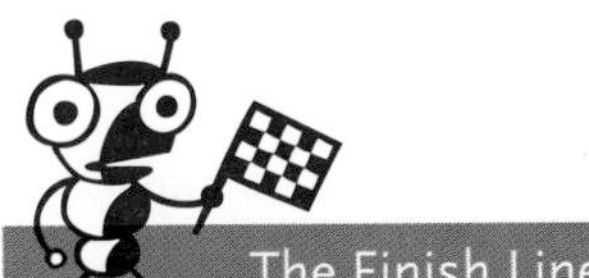

The Finish Line

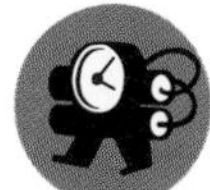

What's Wrong With This Picture?

Read the following scenario. List some possible ways you can promote respect and show support.

> Scenario: You are a nursing assistant on the afternoon shift, and today the Baptist minister is coming to do a service. You go into Mr. O'Brien's room to invite him to attend and he responds, "I wish you would leave me alone about these Baptist services! I am an Episcopalian."

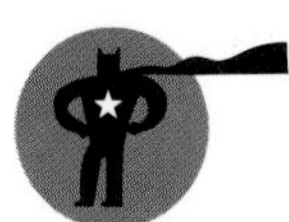

Star Student Central

1. Each student should choose one religion or denomination within a religion. Students should search the Internet or the local library for additional information about the religion and present it to the class. Each presentation may be about two to three minutes in length.
2. Each student should choose one country, being sure to include countries from which local immigrants arrived. Students can search the Internet or the local library to locate information about the group that could impact the life of a resident. Ideas include: diet, language, attitudes about illness or death, and traditions.

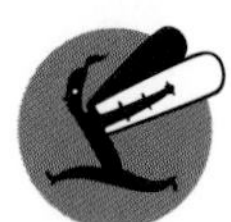

You Can Do It Corner!

True or False. Circle a "T" for true or an "F" for false for each of the following statements.

1. You should observe for signs of pain even if a resident has told you he is not in pain. (LO 8) T F
2. Most people have long funeral services after family members die. (LO 11) T F
3. Sometimes immigrants come to the United States to find religious freedom. (LO 3) T F
4. A person's income level does not affect her nutritional intake. (LO 9) T F
5. A healthcare team member can talk to a resident about his religion if he feels the resident needs spiritual guidance. (LO 10) T F
6. Cultural competence means taking into account a person's culture when giving care. (LO 4) T F
7. Spirituality and religion are the same. (LO 10) T F
8. Learning about other cultures and preferences can actually improve care. (LO 10) T F
9. Most residents will not want to be told about their health information. (LO 5) T F
10. All residents from the South like fried food, such as fried chicken and fried okra. (LO 9) T F
11. If a resident does not speak English, it is okay for you to tell him to learn it. (LO 7) T F

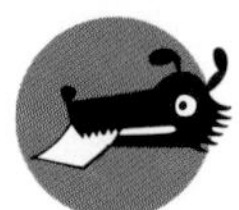

Star Student's Chapter Checklist

1. I have read my textbook chapter.
2. I have reviewed my own "Pocketful of Terms."
3. I have listened to my tutor tape.
4. I have reviewed and highlighted my class notes.
5. I have read and completed any handouts from this chapter.
6. I have completed "The Finish Line."
7. Star Time! Choose your reward!

5

Your Guide:
The Language of Medicine

Look Like a Star!

Look at the Learning Objectives and The Finish Line before you begin reading this chapter.

Look at your pocket calendar.
With your pencil, put a bracket ( ) around a study period every single day.

Look at your homework for this chapter.
Plug each piece of homework into a certain time slot.

Look at the Star Student's Chapter Checklist at the end of this chapter. Check off each item as it is completed.

"A good book is the precious lifeblood of a master spirit . . . treasured up on purpose to a life beyond life."

John Milton, 1608-1674

"Books are the carriers of civilization."

Barbara Tuchman, 1912-1989

Learning Objectives

1. **Spell and define all STAR words.**
2. **Summarize the use of roots, prefixes, suffixes, and abbreviations in medicine.**
3. **Recognize, pronounce, define, and spell some common prefixes.**
4. **Recognize, pronounce, define, and spell some common roots.**
5. **Recognize, pronounce, define, and spell some common suffixes.**
6. **Recognize, pronounce, define, and spell some common abbreviations.**
7. **Recognize some common symbols used in the medical field.**

Hippocrates: The "Father" of the Language of Medicine

Hippocrates, known as the "Father of Medicine," formed some of the earliest medical words in his writings. He lived during the time period of about 400 B.C.

Beginning with the period of about 100 A.D., the early Romans developed the basis for the medical language of today. They started keeping records of the new words they developed because of all of their experiences with wounded soldiers in the battlefield. This impressive record-keeping by the Romans ultimately laid the groundwork for Greek and Latin to become the two primary languages of medicine.

1 Spell and define all STAR words.

abbreviation: a shortened word.

examination: inspection or a testing of knowledge.

Greek: one of the languages from which medical terms are formed.

inflammation: a tissue reaction to injury, causing pain, redness, swelling, and heat.

instrument: a special tool for doing something, such as recording and measuring.

Latin: one of the languages from which medical terms are formed.

medical specialty: a branch of medicine in which a physician specializes.

prefix: a word part added to the beginning of a word.

root: the main part of a word.

suffix: a word part placed at the end of a word.

symbol: a sign representing something.

2 Summarize the use of roots, prefixes, suffixes, and abbreviations in medicine.

Medical language is really quite fascinating. Many people who have worked in medicine for some time truly love the language of medicine. Medical people may keep medical dictionaries close by and use these books often.

In order to "speak" this special language, we must first look at the different word parts. Very soon, you will be able to look at many of these word parts and recognize them immediately.

Defining Medical Words — Box 5-1

There are three basic steps for defining medical words.
First, define the suffix, or last part of the word.
Second, define the prefix, or first part of the word.
Last, define the middle of the word.
Here is an example.

gastr/o	enter/	itis
stomach	intestine	**inflammation**
(2)	(3)	(1)

Read as follows:
1. Inflammation (of) [suffix]
2. Stomach (and) [first part of the word]
3. Intestine [middle]

The definition of gastr/o/enter/itis is "inflammation (of) stomach and intestine."

(Reprinted with the permission of F.A. Davis from *Medical Terminology: A Systems Approach* by Barbara A. Gylys and Mary Ellen Wedding.)

Pronunciation Guidelines — Box 5-2

Although medical words usually follow the rules that govern the pronunciation of English words, they may be difficult to pronounce when you first encounter them. Here are some general rules you will find helpful:

For ae and oe, only the second vowel is pronounced.
Examples: bursae, pleurae, roentgen

c and g are given the soft sounds of s and j, respectively, before e, i, and y in words of both Greek and Latin origins.
Examples: cerebrum, cycle, gel, giant

c and g have a hard sound before other letters.
Examples: cardiac, cast, gastric, gonad

e and es, when forming the final letter or letters of a word, are often pronounced as separate syllables.
Examples: syncope, systole, nares

ch is sometimes pronounced like k.
Examples: cholesterol, cholera

i at the end of a word (to form a plural) is pronounced "eye."
Examples: bronchi, fungi, nuclei

pn at the beginning of a word is pronounced with only the n sound.
Example: pneumonia

pn in the middle of a word is pronounced with a hard p and a hard n.
Examples: orthopnea, hyperpnea

ps is pronounced like s.
Examples: psychology, psychosis

All other vowels and consonants have ordinary English sounds.

(Reprinted with the permission of F.A. Davis from *Medical Terminology: A Systems Approach* by Barbara A. Gylys and Mary Ellen Wedding.)

The Rich Root

Roots are rich in the history of the medical language. They come mostly from the **Greek** or **Latin** words we talked about in this chapter's "Time Capsule." A **root** is the part of a word that gives the word its meaning. Here is an example of a root and a medical term with a root:

The root "scope" means an **instrument** to look inside. The prefix "oto" means ear. An otoscope is an instrument used to examine the ear.

The Powerful Prefix

The **prefix** always comes at the front of the word. It works with a word root to make a new term. Here is an example of a prefix.

The prefix "brady" means slow. The root "cardia" means heart. "Bradycardia" means slow heart rate or pulse.

The Super Suffix

Suffixes are a sort of "super" word part found at the end of a word. A suffix by itself does not form a full word. When you add a prefix or a root, the "Super Suffix" turns this new term into a working medical term. Here is an example of a suffix and the working word it can become:

The suffix "meter" means measuring instrument. The prefix "thermo" means heat. A thermometer is an instrument that measures body temperature.

Putting Some "Word Buddies" Together

When you combine a prefix and root, or a prefix and suffix, a new term is formed. For example:

Prefix+Root = new term

tachy+cardia = tachycardia

fast or rapid+heart = rapid heartbeat

Prefix+Suffix = new term

poly+uria = polyuria

many or much+urine = a lot of urine

One of the most common suffixes is "-logy," which means the study of something. You will mostly see it when it refers to a **medical specialty**, such as cardiology. Cardiology is the study of the heart.

The Amazing Abbreviation

Abbreviations are amazing—they make our lives much simpler. Imagine if a doctor or nurse had to write out every word completely all of the time about every resident. How time-consuming that would be! Instead, they use shortened versions of words to save their valuable time. A couple of examples of this are:

b.i.d. means two times a day

t.i.d. means three times a day

Take this b.i.d and call me in the morning!

When using abbreviations like b.i.d., t.i.d., and q.i.d., remember they are formed from the Latin words.

B = 2 (L. bis) (Think bi or two)

T = 3 (L. ter) (Think tri or three)

Q = 4 (L. quarter) (Think quad or four)

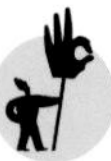

I am not an oxymoron!

The terms "metaphor," "simile," and "oxymoron" are frequently confusing. Review their definitions and then look at an example.

1. *A metaphor is a figure of speech which describes one thing as something else, even though it is not exact. Example: "nerves of steel"*
2. *A simile is a figure of speech that compares one thing to another using the words "like" or "as." Example: "clear as crystal"*
3. *An oxymoron is a figure of speech using terms that are contradictory. Example: "cruel to be kind"*

3 Recognize, pronounce, define, and spell some common prefixes.

Powerful Prefixes
prefix: meaning
medical term = definition

a, an: without, not, lack of
analgesic = without pain

ante: before, in front of
antepartum = before delivery

bi: two, twice, double
bifocal = two lenses

brady: slow
bradycardia = slow pulse, heartbeat

contra: against
contraceptive = prevents pregnancy

dis: apart, free from
disinfected = free from microorganisms

dys: bad, painful
dysuria = painful urination

endo: inner
endoscope = instrument for examining the inside of an organ

epi: on, upon, over
epidermis = outer layer of skin

erythro: red
erythrocyte = red blood cell

ex: out, away from
exhale = to breathe out

hemi: half
hemisphere = one of two parts of the brain

hyper: too much, high
hypertension = high blood pressure

hypo: below, under
hypotension = low blood pressure

inter: between, within
interdisciplinary = between disciplines

leuk: white
leukocyte = white blood cell

mal: bad, illness, disorder
malformed = badly made

micro: small
microscopic = too small for the eye to see

olig: small, scant
oliguria = small amount of urine

patho: disease, suffering
pathology = study of disease

per: by, through
perforate = to make a hole through

peri: around
pericardium = sac around the heart

poly: many, much
polyuria = much urine

post: after, behind
postmortem = period after death

pre: before, in front of
prenatal = period before birth

sub: under, beneath
subcutaneous = beneath the skin

supra: above, over
suprapelvic = located above the pelvis

tachy: swift, fast, rapid
tachycardia = rapid heartbeat

4 Recognize, pronounce, define, and spell some common roots.

Rich Roots

root: meaning
medical term = definition

abdomin (o): abdomen
abdominal = pertaining to the abdomen

aden (o): gland
adenitis = inflammation of a gland

angi (o): vessel
angioplasty = surgical repair of a vessel using a balloon

arterio: artery
arteriosclerosis = hardening of artery walls

arthr (o): joint
arthrotomy = cut into a joint

brachi (o): arm
brachial = pertaining to the arm

bronchi, bronch (o): bronchus
bronchopneumonia = inflammation of lungs

card, cardi (o): heart
cardiology = study of the heart

cerebr (o): cerebrum
cerebrospinal = pertaining to the brain and spinal cord

cephal (o): head
cephalagia = headache

chole, chol (o): bile
cholecystitis = inflammation of the gall bladder

colo: colon
colonoscopy = **examination** of the large intestine or colon with a scope

cost (o): rib
costochondral = pertaining to a rib

crani (o): skull
craniotomy = cutting into the skull

cyan (o): blue
cyanosis = blue, gray, or purple tinge to the skin due to lack of oxygen in the blood

cyst (o): bladder, cyst
cystitis = inflammation of the bladder

derm, derma: skin
dermatitis = inflammation of the skin

duoden (o): duodenum
duodenal = pertaining to the duodenum, the first part of the small intestine

encephal (o): brain
encephalitis = inflammation of the brain

gaster (o), gastro: stomach
gastritis = inflammation of the stomach

geron: aged
gerontology = study of the aged

gluco: sweet
glucometer = device used to measure blood glucose

glyco, glyc: sweet
glycosuria = glucose (sugar) in the urine

gyneco, gyno: woman
gynecology = study of diseases of the female reproductive organs

hema, hemato, hemo: blood
hematuria = blood in the urine

hepato: liver
hepatomegaly = enlargement of the liver

hyster (o): uterus
hysterectomy = surgical removal of the uterus

ile (o), ili(o): ileum
ileorrhaphy = surgical repair of the ileum

laryng (o): larynx
laryngectomy = excision of the larynx

lymph (o): lymph
lymphocyte = type of white blood cell

mamm (o): breast
mammogram = x-ray of the breast

mast (o): breast
mastectomy = excision of the breast

melan (o): black
melanoma = mole or tumor, may be cancerous

mening (o): meninges; membranes covering the spinal cord and brain
meningitis = inflammation of the membranes of the spinal cord or brain

necro: death
necrotic = dead tissue

nephr (o): kidney
nephrectomy = removal of a kidney

neur (o): nerve
neuritis = inflammation of a nerve

onc (o): tumor
oncology = study of tumors

ophthalm (o): eye
ophthalmologist = eye doctor

oste (o): bone
osteoarthritis = disease of the joints

ot (o): ear
otology = science of the ear

pharyng (o): pharynx
pharyngitis = inflammation of the throat, sore throat

phleb (o): vein
phlebitis = inflammation of a vein

pneo (a): breathing
tachypnea = rapid breathing

pneum: air, gas, respiration
pneumonia = inflammation of the lung

pod (o): foot
podiatrist = foot doctor

proct (o): anus, rectum
proctology = study of the rectum

pulm (o): lung
pulmonary = relating to the lungs

splen (o): spleen
splenomegaly = enlarged spleen

stomat (o): mouth
stomatitis = inflammation of mouth

therm (o): hot, heat
thermoplegia = heatstroke

thorac (o): chest
thoracotomy = incision into chest wall

thromb (o): blood clot
thrombus = blood clot blocking a vessel

toxic (o), tox (o): poison
toxicology = study of poisons

trache (o): trachea, windpipe
tracheostomy = incision to make an artificial airway

urethr (o): urethra
urethritis = inflammation of urethra

5 Recognize, pronounce, define, and spell some common suffixes.

Super Suffixes

suffix: meaning
medical term = definition

-cyte: cell
leukocyte = white blood cell

-ectomy: excision, removal of
splenectomy = removal of spleen

-emia: blood condition
anemia = lack of red blood cells

-emesis: vomiting
hyperemesis = excessive vomiting

-ism: a condition
hyperthyroidism = condition caused by an excessive production of thyroid hormones

-itis: inflammation
stomatitis = inflammation of the mouth

-logy: study of
hematology = study of the blood

-megaly: enlargement
splenomegaly = enlarged spleen

-oma: tumor
melanoma = mole or tumor, may be cancerous

-osis: condition
halitosis = bad breath

-ostomy: creation of an opening
ileostomy = creation of an opening into the ileum

-otomy: cut into
laparotomy = cutting into the abdomen

-pathy: disease
myopathy = disease of the muscle

-penia: lack
leukopenia = a lack of white blood cells

-phagia: to eat
dysphagia = difficulty swallowing

-phasia: speaking
aphasia = absence of speaking

-phobia: exaggerated fear
acrophobia = fear of high places

-plasty: surgical repair
angioplasty = surgical repair of a vessel using a balloon

-plegia: paralysis
paraplegia = paralysis of lower portion of the body

-rrhage: excessive flow
hemorrhage = excessive flow of blood

-scopy: examination using a scope
colonoscopy = examination of the large intestine or colon with a scope

-stomy: creation of an opening
colostomy = opening into the colon

-tomy: incision, cutting into
thoracotomy = incision into chest wall

-uria: condition of the urine
dysuria = painful urination

Do CMS on your AKA ASAP!

When you take care of your residents, do not use medical terms or medical abbreviations. It is a form of abuse to use terms that a resident does not understand. Residents may be harmed physically if they do not understand a word, and they may also feel foolish or stupid.

6 Recognize, pronounce, define, and spell some common abbreviations.

When communicating with your residents and their families, you should use simple, non-medical terms. When you communicate with your supervisor or other members of the healthcare team, using medical terminology will help you give more precise and complete information.

Abbreviations are another way to communicate more efficiently with other caregivers. Learn the standard medical abbreviations your facility uses, and use them to report information briefly and accurately.

Following is a list of abbreviations of terms you may need to be familiar with. It is not a complete list. Check with your facility to see if there are others you will need to know.

abd.	abdomen
ABR	absolute bedrest
a.c.	before meals (L. ante cibum)
ad lib	as desired (L. ad libitum)
adm.	admission
ADLs	activities of daily living
AFB	acid-fast bacillus (Tb)
AIDS	acquired immune deficiency syndrome
AKA	above-knee amputation
AL	assisted living
ALF	assisted living facility
Alz. dis.	Alzheimer's disease
am, AM	morning (L. ante meridiem)
AMA	against medical advice, American Medical Association
amb	ambulate
AODM	adult onset diabetes mellitus
AP	apical pulse
approx.	approximately
AROM	active range of motion
ASAP	as soon as possible
ASHD	arteriosclerotic heart disease
as tol	as tolerated
ax	axillary
BID, b.i.d.	two times a day (L. bis in die)
bilat	bilateral
BKA	below-knee amputation
bld	blood
BM	bowel movement
BP, B/P	blood pressure
BR	bedrest
BRP	bathroom privileges
BS	blood sugar
BSC	bedside commode
BSE	breast self exam
c̄	(L. cum) with
Ca	calcium, cancer
cath	catheter
CBR	complete bedrest
cc	cubic centimeter
CCU	coronary care unit
CDC	Centers for Disease Control
CHF	congestive heart failure
cl liq	clear liquid
CMS	circulation, motion, sensation
c/o	complains of, in care of
CNA	certified nursing assistant
CNS	central nervous system
CPR	cardiopulmonary resuscitation
CVA	cerebrovascular accident, stroke
CVP	central venous pressure
CVS	cardiovascular system
DAT	diet as tolerated
dc	discontinue
dischg	discharge
DJD	degenerative joint disease
DM	diabetes mellitus
DNR	do not resuscitate
DOA	dead on arrival
DOB	date of birth
DON	director of nursing
Dr.	doctor
DRG	diagnostic related group
drsg	dressing
DVT	deep vein thrombosis
ECG, EKG	electrocardiogram
EEG	electroencephalogram
ER	emergency room
ETOH	alcohol
FBAO	foreign body airway obstruction
FBS	fasting blood sugar
FF	force fluids
fld	fluid
FSBS	fingerstick blood sugar
ft	foot
FUO	fever of unknown origin
FWB	full weight-bearing
FYI	for your information
F/U, f/u	follow-up
fx	fracture
geri chair	geriatric chair
GI	gastrointestinal
h, hr	hour (L. hora)
H_2O	water

H/A	headache
HBV	hepatitis B virus
HIV	human immunodeficiency virus
HOB	head of bed
HOH	hard of hearing
hs	hour of sleep
ht	height
HTN	hypertension
hyper	above normal, too fast, rapid
hypo	low, less than normal
hs	hour of sleep
ht	height
HTN	hypertension
hyper	above normal, too fast, rapid
hypo	low, less than normal
I & O	intake and output
ICU	intensive care unit
IDDM	insulin-dependent diabetes mellitus
inc	incontinent
irr., irrig	irrigation
I.V.	intravenously
isol	isolation
JCAHO	Joint Commission on Accreditation of Health Care Organizations
K+	potassium
kg	kilogram
l (*Fr. litre*)	liter
L	left
lab	laboratory
lb	pound (L. libra)
LLE	left lower extremity
lg	large
liq	liquid (L. liquor)
LLQ	left lower quadrant
LOC	level of consciousness
LPN	Licensed Practical Nurse
lt.	left
LTC	long-term care
LUQ	left upper quadrant
LVN	Licensed Vocational Nurse
M.D.	medical doctor
meds	medications
MI	myocardial infarction
min	minute
ml	milliliter
mm Hg	millimeters of mercury
MMR	measles-mumps-rubella vaccine
mod	moderate
MRSA	methicillin-resistant staph aureus
MS	multiple sclerosis
N/A	not applicable
N.A.	nursing assistant
N/C	no call
neg	negative
NF	nursing facility
NIDDM	non-insulin dependent diabetes mellitus
NKA	no known allergies
NPO	nothing by mouth (L. nils per os)
N, V, and D	nausea, vomiting, and diarrhea
NWB	non-weight-bearing
O_2	oxygen
OBRA	Omnibus Budget Reconciliation Act
OOB	out of bed
occ	occasionally
OJ	orange juice
OPD	outpatient department
O.R.	operating room
os	mouth
OSHA	Occupational Safety and Health Administration
oz	ounce
p̄	after
PACU	post-anesthesia care unit
P.A.S.S.	pull, aim, squeeze, sweep (acronym)
pc, p.c.	after meals (L. post cibum)
PCA	patient-controlled anesthesia
PEG	percutaneous enteral gastrostomy
per os	by mouth
peri care	perineal care
pm, PM	afternoon
PNS	peripheral nervous system
p.o.	by mouth (L. per os)
post op	after surgery
PPE	personal protective equipment
pos.	positive

pre op	before surgery
prep	preparation
p.r.n., prn	when necessary (L. pro re nata)
PROM	passive range of motion
PSA	prostatic specific antigen (blood test for cancer)
Pt.	patient
pt.	pint
PVD	peripheral vascular disease
PWB	partial weight-bearing
q̄	every (L. quaque)
qd	every day (L. quaque die)
qh, qhr	every hour (L. quaque hora)
qhs	every night at bedtime
q2h, q3h, q4h	every two hours, every three hours, every four hours
q.i.d., qid	four times a day (L. quarter in die)
q.o.d.	every other day
Q.S.	every shift or once a shift
quad	four, quadriplegic
R	respirations, right
R/A	rheumatoid arthritis
R.A.C.E.	Remove people closest to fire; Alarm pulled; Close doors and windows; Extinguish fire (acronym)
RBC	red blood cell/count
reg.	regular
rehab	rehabilitation
req.	requisition
res.	resident
resp.	respiration
R.I.C.E.	Rest, Ice, Compression, Elevation (acronym)
RLE	right lower extremity
RLQ	right lower quadrant
RN	Registered Nurse
R/O	rule out
ROM	range of motion
RR	respiratory rate
rt.	right
RUE	right upper extremity
RUQ	right upper quadrant
s̄	without (L. sine)
ss	one-half (L. semi, semisse)
sm.	small
SNAFU	situation normal, all fouled up (slang)
SNF	skilled nursing facility
spec.	specimen
SOB	shortness of breath
S & S, S/S	signs and symptoms
SSE	soapsuds enema
staph	staphylococcus
stat	immediately (L. statim)
STD	sexually transmitted diseases
strep	streptococcus
std. prec.	standard precautions
T.	temperature
TB	tuberculosis
T, C, DB	turn, cough and deep breathe
temp	temperature
TIA	transient ischemic attack
t.i.d., tid	three times a day (L. ter in die)
TLC	tender loving care
TPN	total parenteral nutrition
T.P.R.	temperature, pulse, and respiration
TURP	transurethral resection of the prostate
TWE	tap water enema
Tx	traction, treatment
U/A, u/a	urinalysis
UGI	upper gastrointestinal
unk	unknown
URI	upper respiratory infection
UTI	urinary tract infection
vag.	vaginal
VRE	vancomycin-resistant enterococcus
vs, v.s.	vital signs
WBC	white blood cell/count
w/c	wheelchair
WNL	within normal limits
wt.	weight

7 Recognize some common symbols used in the medical field.

Symbols

We see many **symbols** in our daily lives. Here are some of the more common symbols you may see in your new field.

&	and	↓	decreased
@	at	<	less than
☣	biohazard	>	greater than
Δ	change, heat	X	multiply
✓	check	No. #	number
C/O	complains of	±	plus/minus
©	copyright	%	percent
°	degree	☢	radiation
$	dollars	lt	left
♀	female	rt	right
♂	male	ss	one-half
↑	increased		

Summary

Medical terms are interesting and can be fun to learn. As you learn the language of medicine, your job as a nursing assistant becomes much easier. Unfamiliar terms start making sense and enable you to care for residents in a safer and more efficient fashion. Once you have learned the language of medicine, you will never have to learn it again!

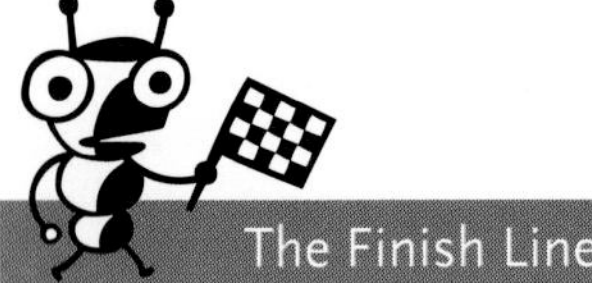

The Finish Line

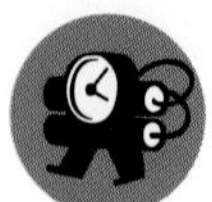

What's Wrong With This Picture?

Find all of the medical terms' spelling errors in this short story.

At the time of her admission to Linwood Home, Maidy had cordiac problems along with a phlebitus in her left leg. By the time Maidy was 90 years old, she needed a nefrectomy. After that experience, she developed noctoria. Also at that age, her hart problems caused tachcardia. When she was 95, Maidy had a proctoscupy. The doctors discovered colon cancar. She was treated with surgery and her condition improved.

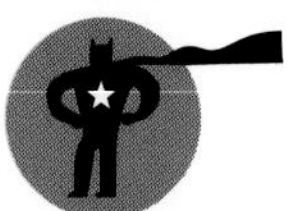

Star Student Central

Complete the following exercises.

1. Using many of the new terms you have learned, write your own short story for your class. It should not be longer than two paragraphs. Make the story interesting and full of funny mistakes. Your classmates can correct it.
2. Form a study group of not more than four people. Divide the medical terminology into four groups: Prefixes, Roots, Suffixes, and Abbreviations. Each person develops a fun game of "Who am I?" For example: "I am one of the Prefixes. I have something to do with the color red. Who am I?" Another example would be: "In Latin, my phrase would be nils per os. When I am written as an order, the poor resident can't eat or drink."

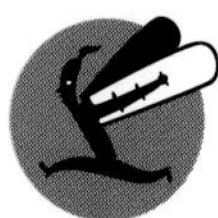

You Can Do It Corner!

Complete the following sentences by filling in the blanks with the missing prefixes. (LO 3)

1. The resident in room 343 developed low blood pressure, known as ____________ tension.
2. Mrs. Molly Ivy started to breathe rapidly in the night, developing ____________ pnea.
3. The ____________ operative resident, Ashley Stephan, came back to our facility once the surgery was completed.
4. Deena Sampson was admitted with ____________ tension, or high blood pressure.
5. Miss Martinez developed a slow heart rate

known as ____________ cardia last night.

6. Both of Katrina's parents had to wear glasses with two lenses, or ____________ focals.

7. Mrs. Hernandez was NPO ____________ operatively, for eight hours before her surgery.

8. Red blood cells called ____________ rocytes, carry the oxygen in our blood.

9. Resident Max Singer developed ____________ uria, increased amounts of urine.

By choosing True or False, decide whether each sentence uses the correct root. (LO 4)

1. Cardiology is the study of the blood. T F
2. Neuritis means inflammation of the kidney. T F
3. A bronchoscope is a scope for viewing the bronchi. T F
4. The word cephalgia means "headache." T F
5. Hepatomegaly means "enlargement of the hip." T F
6. The word stomatitis is a word meaning "inflammation of the stomach." T F
7. A craniotomy is an incision into the skull. T F
8. A gastrectomy means "removal of the adrenal glands." T F
9. An angioplasty is surgery on the arteries. T F
10. Toxicology is the study of poisons. T F

Circle the word that shows the correct spelling of this medical term.

1.	psoriasis	psoriesis
2.	splenectomy	splenectome
3.	nephritis	nephrittis
4.	rhinoplaisty	rhinoplasty
5.	ileostramy	ileostomy
6.	endoscopy	endoscoppy
7.	thermometer	thermomeater
8.	cardiolagy	cardiology
9.	myopathy	myopathey
10.	neuralygia	neuralgia

Fill in the missing letters.

1. ____.c. after meals
2. ___.i.d twice a day
3. q.___.d. every other day
4. R.I.___.E. Rest, Ice, _ompression, Elevation
5. W.___.L. within normal limits
6. T.L.___ tender loving care
7. L.O.___. level of consciousness
8. R.___.Q. right upper quadrant
9. N.___.A. no known allergies
10. ___.i.d. three times a day
11. ___.O.M range of motion
12. a.___. before meals
13. T.W.___. tap water enema
14. q___s every night at bedtime
15. ___KO to keep open
16. A.__.A.P. as soon as possible
17. __.i.d. four times a day
18. p.__.n. when necessary
19. S.__.E. soapsuds enema
20. N__O nothing by mouth

Star Student's Chapter Checklist

1. I have read my textbook chapter.
2. I have reviewed my own "Pocketful of Terms."
3. I have listened to my tutor tape.
4. I have reviewed and highlighted my class notes.
5. I have read and completed any handouts from this chapter.
6. I have completed "The Finish Line."
7. Star Time! Choose your reward!

Your Goal: Sharpening Your Communication Skills

Look Like a Star!

Look at the Learning Objectives and The Finish Line before you begin reading this chapter.

Look at your pocket calendar.
With your pencil, put a bracket (   ) around a study period every single day.

Look at your homework for this chapter.
Plug each piece of homework into a certain time slot.

Look at the Star Student's Chapter Checklist at the end of this chapter. Check off each item as it is completed.

"A wise old owl sat on an oak
The more he saw the less he spoke:
The less he spoke the more he heard;
Why aren't we like that wise old bird?"

Edward Hersey Richards, 1874-1957
from *Wise Old Owl*

"The important thing is to not stop questioning."

Albert Einstein, 1879-1955

Learning Objectives

1. **Spell and define all STAR words.**
2. **Identify the most common causes of errors in healthcare facilities and discuss six sample errors in workplace communication.**
3. **Describe the "Five Star Communication Chain."**
4. **Describe the Minimum Data Set (MDS) manual, including its purpose and how it is used.**
5. **Name the five steps in the nursing process and give examples of objective data and subjective data.**
6. **Describe the "Five Rights of Delegation."**
7. **List the four "Basic Observations at a Glance" and two examples of each.**
8. **Define the terms "critical thinking" and "conflict resolution" in resident care.**
9. **List four guidelines for critical thinking in observing and reporting.**
10. **Describe the importance of strict confidentiality with all resident information.**
11. **Identify the people you will communicate with in a facility and how you will communicate with them.**
12. **Describe verbal and nonverbal communication.**
13. **Describe a standard resident chart.**
14. **Describe the SOAP charting style and discuss rules for effective charting.**
15. **Identify the components of a standard Kardex.**
16. **Discuss the nursing assistant's role in care planning and at care conferences.**
17. **List the seven steps to expert telephone etiquette.**
18. **Describe the correct use of the resident call system.**
19. **Describe the nursing assistant's role in change-of-shift reports and "rounds."**
20. **List the information found on an assignment sheet.**

The Morse Code

The Morse Code was invented by Samuel Finley Breese Morse (1791-1872), U.S. artist and inventor. He created this code, an alphabet composed of dots (shorts) and dashes (longs), in the 1800s. He also built the first telegraph line in the U.S.A., from Baltimore, Maryland, to Washington D.C. The first message sent between Washington and Baltimore was: "What hath God wrought!" In 1861, the telegraph line connected the two coasts of the United States.

1 Spell and define all **STAR** words.

Advance Directive: in health care, identifies the resident's wishes during an emergency regarding life-saving efforts.

arbitration: the act of bringing in an outside person or group to help solve a dispute.

assessment: the collection and organization of objective and subjective data from a variety of sources to identify resident problems.

body language: all of the conscious or unconscious messages your body might send as you communicate with others.

care conference: a method of meeting, sharing, and gathering information about residents in order to develop a plan of care.

care plans: written plans developed by the nurse that outline the steps taken by the staff to reach the goals or outcomes set.

chart: written record of all care received within a facility or form used to highlight certain information.

charting: the act of making notes of care and observation; documenting.

code: when a group of specially-trained staff is called to provide advanced life support to a resident.

code status: whether a resident has a signed advance directive or not.

delegation: the transferring of authority to a specific individual to perform a task.

diaphoretic: sweating or perspiring heavily.

domestic violence: type of violence relating to the family and family situations in which harm may be done to an individual.

evaluation: a careful examination and judgement.

implementation: putting into action.

intervention: the act of coming in to change an action or condition.

Kardex: a brand name of a card file that is used to keep resident information organized and easy to locate.

LIFELINE: a call system that connects a person to help when needed.

mediation: the act of bringing about a settlement between parties.

medical record: resident chart or record of all care received in the facility.

nonverbal communication: communication without words.

nursing diagnosis: the identification of a resident's health problems; done with the intent to determine a plan of care.

nursing process: five organized steps that nurses use to try to solve the health problems of residents (assessment, nursing diagnosis, planning, intervention, and evaluation).

plan of care: plan that identifies the interventions that will be taken in order to meet the needs of the residents.

objective data: also known as signs; data we collect using our senses of sight, hearing, smell, and touch.

oriented x 3: the ability to understand and adjust to the environment regarding person, place, and time; person knows who he is, what year it is, where he is located.

oxygen therapy: the giving of oxygen for the treatment of a condition due to a lack of oxygen.

Range of motion (ROM): the normal range of movement of a joint.

record: (noun) a written account of information; (verb) to set down information in permanent form, especially to write down permanently.

report: (noun) an account, usually verbal, of departing staff to incoming staff at the change of shift; (verb) to relate or tell about.

rounds: movement of staff members from room to room to discuss each resident and the plans of care.

SOAP: a method of charting; includes subjective, objective assessment, and plan of care.

subjective data: also called symptoms; information we collect from the residents, their family members and friends.

verbal communication: communication involving the use of words or sounds, spoken or written.

vital signs: the temperature, pulse, respiration, blood pressure, and pain level of a person.

2 Identify the most common causes of errors in healthcare facilities and discuss six sample errors in workplace communication.

"I MADE A MISTAKE!"

What sentence could be more bloodcurdling in health care? Almost instantly, a set of reactions occurs. People immediately mobilize and try to correct the problem with a minimum amount of harm to the resident. What probably causes more mistakes than anything else? Errors in communication and/or carelessness.

Some mistakes are life-threatening and can cause serious injury or even death. Others are smaller and simply inconvenience people. Whatever the scope of the mistake, if people were more careful and communicated better, fewer mistakes would happen in facilities and everywhere else.

Consider the following examples:

Problem 1: Leah Nottingham, an 89-year-old resident, receives her treatment on the wrong leg.

Mistake: The nurse gave an incomplete instruction to the nursing assistant: "You have to do the treatment on Mrs. Nottingham's leg." The nursing assistant did not ask the nurse which leg.

Problem 2: Tommy Morgan, a 79-year-old resident, receives the wrong diet tray. Because he just had the "stomach flu," the diet made him feel ill and he vomited his lunch.

Mistake: The dietary department prepared the wrong diet for Tommy Morgan. A diet order sent from the unit was not written correctly. "Full liquid diet" was written instead of "clear liquid diet." There is a big difference between the two diets. (See Chapter 22 for information about special diets.)

Problem 3: Tristine Hyland, a 100-year-old resident, slips and falls in the hallway, breaking a hip.

Mistake: The nurse asked the front desk to call housekeeping to mop up a major spill in the hallway. The housekeeping department never gave the message to the housekeeper, and the people on the floor did not follow up to make sure it was cleaned up promptly.

Problem 4: The new resident, Emma Turner, has an order for **oxygen therapy** (giving oxygen for the treatment of a condition due to a lack of oxygen). The oxygen is put on Ms. Turner by the nurse and the gauge is set by the nurse at two liters per minute. A half-hour later, the nursing assistant notes that Ms. Jones is still having some trouble breathing. She reports this to the nurse immediately.

Mistake: Mark Rogers, the doctor, carefully wrote oxygen to be give at "5 liters per minute." The ward clerk wrote it as a "2," and the nurse checked it off as correct.

Problem 5: Nurse Ray Atkins asks nursing assistant Kathy Smith to have Frank Harper, a 60-year-old resident, sit up after a feeding given through a tube for "a while."

Mistake: Mr. Harper begins choking after the nursing assistant lays him back down after only 10 minutes have passed. Mr. Harper was supposed to sit up for at least 30 minutes, but the instructions given by the nurse were not specific and the nursing assistant did not clarify them. Due to this error, Mr. Harper develops a type of pneumonia that can be caused by fluid getting into the lungs.

Problem 6: Two staff members, David Carrizo and Tonya Stafford, take two residents on a local outing. While on the outing, they become separated. One of the residents starts walking toward the entrance and is stopped by a security guard and returned to the staff members.

Mistake: David and Tonya both "assumed" the resident was being watched over by the other person. They did not clarify who would have the responsibility for watching the resident. A real tragedy could have occurred because of this miscommunication.

Each of these situations could have been prevented with proper communication. Nursing assistants provide the majority of resident care and must be extremely careful every day to try to prevent mistakes from occurring. The healthcare team must communicate clearly with all persons within the facility in order to reduce errors in communication.

3 Describe the "Five Star Communication Chain."

When we communicate, we wear many "hats." We can be the "sender" or the "receiver." The person who communicates first is the "sender," sending a message. The person who receives the message is called the "receiver." Receiver and sender are constantly switching roles as they communicate. The image below shows an example of the many hats we wear as we communicate with others in the health-care facility. The following steps are crucial to effective communication:

1. Sender: I have the CORRECT MESSAGE!
2. Sender: I have the CORRECT RECEIVER!
3. Sender: I have the CORRECT CHOICE OF METHOD!
4. Receiver: CONFIRMATION: MESSAGE RECEIVED AND UNDERSTOOD!
5. Sender: Makes sure of CORRECT RESPONSE/ACTION.

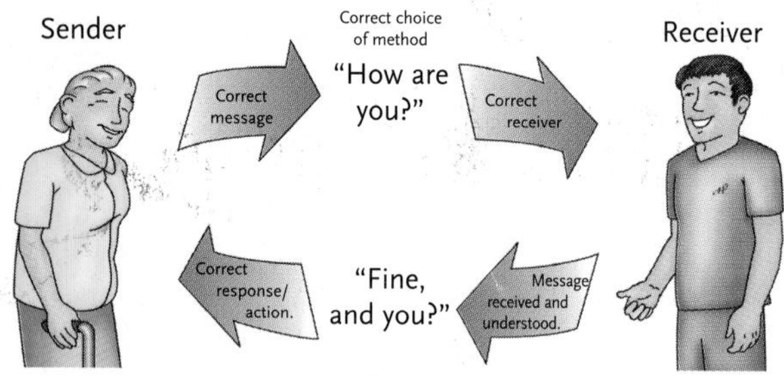

Figure 6-1. **Important steps in effective communication.**

In each of the earlier examples listed, a breakdown in the "chain" of communication occurred somewhere in the sequence of events. Figure 6-2 puts the above five steps into the chain. These must all be successfully completed for effective communication to take place.

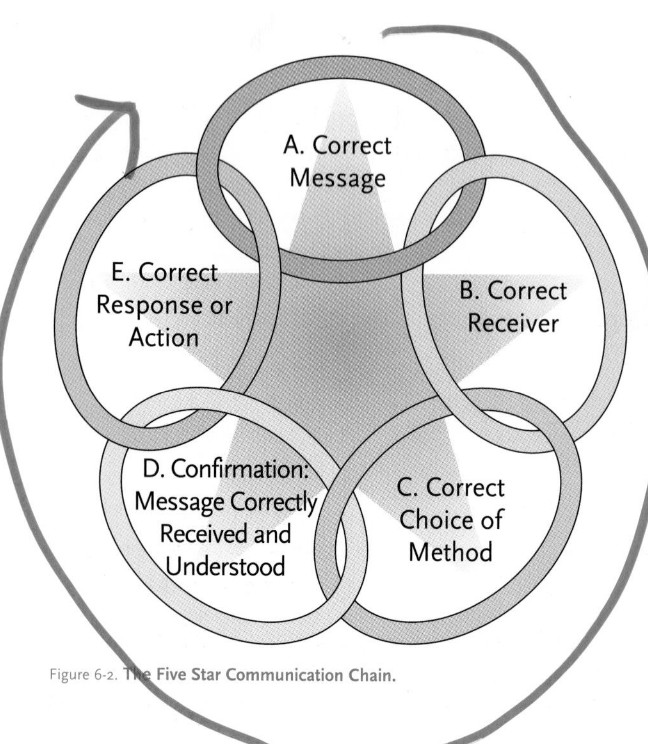

Figure 6-2. **The Five Star Communication Chain.**

Let's now apply the "Five Star Communication Chain" to Problem 5 within Learning Objective 2.

1. Nurse Ray Atkins decides he wishes to give the nursing assistant instructions on what to do after the tube feeding is finished. The nurse reviews the instructions in his mind to keep Mr. Jones sitting up for 30 minutes after the tube feeding is completed.
2. Nurse Atkins determines Kathy Smith is the nursing assistant assigned to Mr. Jones.
3. Nurse Atkins decides that verbal communication would be the best method for instructing Kathy Smith. The nurse tells Kathy to keep Mr. Jones sitting up for not less than 30 minutes after the tube feeding has stopped and is removed.
4. Nurse Atkins determines that the message has been properly received. Kathy repeats the message back to him.
5. Nurse Atkins checks on the resident twice within 30 minutes after the tube feeding has ended; Frank Jones is fine after the tube-feeding.

The end result of good communication, then, is for the right or best action or response to take place. The action could be as simple as a hug from a family member or a smile from a resident. You might be trying to switch a day with a fellow staff member so that you can attend a wedding. Whatever you wish to accomplish, understand that the precise way you communicate the information to others is crucial to your success as a "**STAR** communicator."

4 Describe the Minimum Data Set (MDS) manual, including its purpose and how it is used.

The MDS manual is an assessment tool developed by the federal government to provide long-term care (LTC) facilities with a structured, standardized approach to caring for their residents. The original edition was produced in 1990. The manual is revised periodically.

The assessment tools consist of:

1. RAPs (Resident Assessment Protocols)
2. MDS (Minimum Data Set) - A very detailed assessment which is completed upon admission to a LTC facility, then yearly, and whenever a resident exhibits a significant change.

3. Quarterly Assessment - A shortened version of the MDS, completed every three months on all LTC residents.

SECTION V. RESIDENT ASSESSMENT PROTOCOL SUMMARY Numeric Identifier__________

Resident's Name: | Medical Record No:

1. Check if RAP is triggered.
2. For each triggered RAP, use the RAP guidelines to identify areas needing further assessment. Document relevant assessment information regarding the resident's status.
   - Describe:
     - –Nature of the condition (may include presence or lack of objective data and subjective complaints).
     - –Complications and risk factors that affect your decision to proceed to care planning.
     - –Factors that must be considered in developing individualized care plan interventions.
     - –Need for referrals/further evaluation by appropriate health professionals.
     - –Need for referrals/further evaluation by appropriate health professionals.
   - Documentation should support your decision-making regarding whether to proceed with a care plan for a triggered RAP and the type(s) of care plan interventions that re appropriate for a particular resident.
   - Documentation may appear anywhere in the clinical record (e.g., progress notes, consults, flowsheets, etc.).
3. Indicate under the Location of RAP Assessment Documentation column where information related to the RAP assessment can be found.
4. For each triggered RAP, indicate whether a new care plan, care plan revision, or continuation of current care plan is necessary to address the problem(s) identified in your assessment. The Care Planning Decision column must be completed within 7 days of completing the RAI (MDS and RAPs).

A. RAP Problem Area	(a) Check if Triggered	Location and Date of RAP Assessment Documentation	(b) Care Planning Decision–check if addressed in care plan
1. DELIRIUM	☐		☐
2. COGNITIVE LOSS	☐		☐
3. VISUAL FUNCTION	☐		☐
4. COMMUNICATION	☐		☐
5. ADL FUNCTIONAL/ REHABILITATION POTENTIAL	☐		☐
6. URINARY INCONTINENCE AND INDWELLING CATHETER	☐		☐
7. PSYCHOSOCIAL WELL-BEING	☐		☐
8. MOOD STATE	☐		☐
9. BEHAVIORAL SYMPTOMS	☐		☐
10. ACTIVITIES	☐		☐
11. FALLS	☐		☐
12. NUTRITIONAL STATUS	☐		☐
13. FEEDING TUBES	☐		☐
14. DEHYDRATION/FLUID MAINTENANCE	☐		☐
15. ORAL/DENTAL CARE	☐		☐
16. PRESSURE ULCERS	☐		☐
17. PSYCHOTROPIC DRUG USE	☐		☐
18. PHYSICAL RESTRAINTS	☐		☐

B.__________ 2. Month Day Year
1. Signature of RN Coordinator for RAP Assessment Process

__________ 4. Month Day Year
3. Signature of Person Completing Care Planning Decision

Figure 6-3. **Resident Assessment Protocol Summary.**

The MDS manual helps the nurse complete the assessment accurately. The manual offers a very detailed guide on how to assess each resident and record that assessment as accurately as possible. The manual also offers examples and definitions for the nurse who fills out the MDS assessment.

Nursing assistants will have different degrees of familiarity with the MDS tool according to each facility's policy. However, the reporting you will do regarding changes in your residents may "trigger" a needed assessment. Always **report** changes you notice in your residents.

5 Name the five steps in the nursing process and give examples of objective data and subjective data.

The nurse must look at all of the data gathered by the staff each day and develop a plan of care for each resident based upon this information. Many people on the healthcare team contribute to this plan of care. As the nursing assistant on the "front lines," you will contribute to the plan of care for each of your residents. You will do this by gathering and reporting important information or data about each of your residents to the care team.

The **nursing process** is an organized method of ensuring the best nursing care possible. The following terms are used in the nursing process:

- **assessment**
- **nursing diagnosis**
- **implementation**
- **intervention**
- **plan of care**
- **evaluation**

In order to develop a plan of care, the nurses must collect data, or information, from all of the staff. This information will be in the form of signs and symptoms. Important data can be described as either objective or subjective. The way to distinguish between these two methods is described below.

Objective Information	*Subjective Information*
What you observe	What residents, family members, and/or friends tell you

Objective information has to do with our senses. **Objective data**, also known as signs, are data we collect using our senses. We use four of our five senses to gather objective information:

Sight **Hearing** **Smell** **Touch** (or feeling)

We do not use the fifth sense, taste. (That's a relief!)

Subjective data, also called symptoms, are pieces of information we collect from residents, and also their family members and friends. This is information the "subject" is telling you, so it is an opinion. The objective data we collect may confirm this information.

OBJECTIVE	SUBJECTIVE
1. Connan Davis has an emesis (vomits).	1. Connan Davis states: "I feel nauseous."
2. Sandy Sotello yells so loudly she can be heard 50 feet away.	2. Sandy Sotello states: "I have pain in my chest."
3. Anastasia Romano has a bumpy, red rash all along the backs of his arms and legs.	3. Anastasia Romano states: "I itch all over."
4. Samuel Cohen's toe is blue and swollen.	4. Samuel Cohen states: "My toe hurts a lot."
5. Shellie Martin trips and falls.	5. Shellie Martin states: "I am really dizzy."

The goal of gathering this information is to successfully help a resident. This is done by developing a plan of care, which might be developed in this way:

1. The nurse determines that Rosie Cerrullo keeps falling asleep at bingo games. The nurse reports this to the doctor who looks at possible medical causes for this problem. Nothing is found medically that could be causing the problem.

2. The nurse identifies "sleep pattern disturbance" as the nursing diagnosis.

3. The staff all meet and share observations regarding this resident. It is determined that there is a brand new neighbor in the next room who snores quite loudly.

4. Two possible methods can be used to try to help Rosie sleep better. One is to identify a nursing diagnosis for the resident who snores and try to decrease his snoring, if possible. Another is to offer Rosie a glass of milk each night (milk can sometimes help people go to sleep), or keep Rosie's door shut tightly at night. In an extreme case, the staff may look into moving Rosie to a new room.

5. Rosie has been drinking the milk for one week now. The staff has made sure they keep the door shut tightly each night. Rosie no longer falls asleep at her bingo games. We have a successful nursing plan of care.

6 Describe the "Five Rights of Delegation."

Not only will the nurse be developing the plan of care, but nurses also have to decide which tasks to delegate to others, including you. **Delegation** means transferring authority to a specific individual to perform a task. Everything you do in your job is delegated to you by a licensed healthcare professional. Licensed nurses are accountable for all aspects of nursing care, including all delegation decisions. The National Council of State Boards of Nursing identified "The Five Rights of Delegation," which can be used as a mental checklist to assist nurses in the decision-making process.

The Five Rights of Delegation include the Right Task, Right Circumstance, Right Person, Right Direction/Communication, and Right Supervision/Evaluation. Before delegating certain tasks, nurses may consider these questions.

- Is there a match between the resident's needs and the nursing assistant's skills, abilities, and level of experience?
- What is the level of resident stability?
- Is the nursing assistant the right person to do the activity?
- Can the nurse provide the nursing assistant with appropriate direction and communication?
- Is the nurse available to provide the supervision, support and assistance that the nursing assistant needs?

There are questions you may want to ask yourself before accepting a delegation. Consider the following questions.

- Do I have all the information I need to do this job? Are there questions I should ask?
- Do I believe that I can perform this activity? Do I have the necessary skills?
- Do I have access to the necessary supplies, equipment and other needed support?
- Do I know who my supervisor is, and how to reach him/her?
- Have I informed my supervisor of my special needs for assistance and support?
- Do we both understand who is doing what?

Never be afraid to ask for help! Always ask if you need any more information or if you are unsure about something. If you feel that you do not have the skills necessary to perform a task, explain this to your supervisor.

7 List the four "Basic Observations at a Glance" and two examples of each.

The observations of a nursing assistant are vital to the health and well-being of the residents within each facility. Gathering objective and subjective information will assist the nurse in assessing changes. When nursing assistants constantly watch over their residents, residents are safer and more secure. The four "Basic Observations at a Glance" follow with an example of each. This is a method to quickly assess your residents each time you check on them by asking if any of the following have changed:

1. **Orientation:** Is the resident "**oriented x 3**" (to person, place and time)? In other words, does he know who he is, who you are, where he is, and what year it is?

Examples:

Cyrus Golden walks to the desk in a locked dementia unit and calls you by your correct name. He has not done this for at least a year. You understand he has been taking a new medication.

Resident Marilyn McCoy starts talking about the upcoming election, stating, "I am voting for Roosevelt." Yesterday she had discussed current politics and mentioned current leaders by name.

2. Vital Signs: Are the resident's **vital signs**, or the temperature, pulse, respiration, blood pressure, and level of pain normal or abnormal? (Vital signs will be covered in depth in chapter 16.)

Examples:

Resident Roberta Enriquez has a temperature of 101.6 degrees right now. Her last temperature was normal—98.6 degrees.

Resident Matt Williams has a pulse this evening of 92 beats per minute. You know his regular pulse has been 86 to 88 beats per minute.

3. Evaluation of the Resident from the Outside: Is there any change in the way the resident looks today versus yesterday? (For example, changes in the outside appearance of the skin, the eyes, or the ears?) Has there been a change in the resident's ability to move any part of her body? Can the resident still perform all of her regular daily activities that she could yesterday?

Examples:

Resident Danielle Singer has bright-red bleeding on her dressing.

Resident Peter Velasquez is extremely **diaphoretic** (displays heavy sweating or perspiration).

4. Evaluation of the Resident from the Inside: Has the resident had a change in weight or overall appetite, or the ability to go to the bathroom (urinating, bowel movement)? Can the resident see, hear, smell, touch, and taste the same today as he did yesterday? Has his mood changed?

Examples:

Resident Daniel Levine, usually a good eater, does not eat any of his dinner tonight.

Resident Biff Randall has not had a bowel movement for three days and says he is feeling discomfort in his abdomen.

8 Define the terms "critical thinking" and "conflict resolution" in resident care.

If you have ever heard the phrase, "She can't think on her feet," you may know that it means the person cannot look at a problem and quickly come up with the best response. Nursing assistants do not deal in problem-solving or decision-making regarding the health and well-being of residents; this is the nurse's role. However, a nursing assistant often must look at a situation with a resident and decide if the nurse needs to be notified. You sometimes hold the "magic key" to a prompt staff response to a resident's health emergency. Critical thinking, then, in the world of the nursing assistant, is the ability to make good observations in order to report them and get help for a potential problem before harm comes to the resident.

When you work with a team of people, conflict occurs. The key to handling a conflict is for you to understand that most people do not like to disagree. Sometimes it just cannot be helped. If a person seems difficult to get along with, he may not have slept well last night or may have had a fight with a member of his family. If a resident does not want to cooperate, she may be in pain or may be lonely.

When you disagree with a policy made by your facility, remember that the people who are in charge of the facility have information you do not have. They make the best decisions they can even though these decisions may not always be popular with staff. If you have a conflict with your boss or supervisor, try to understand that this person really wants to help you; however, a boss cannot change a policy for you at the expense of other staff. In short, it works best if you try to be reasonable with your requests.

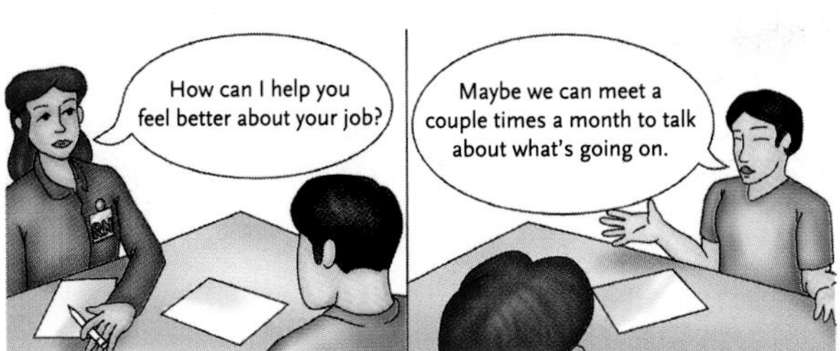

Figure 6-4. **Always try to be reasonable with your requests.**

Sometimes resolving a conflict means you have to compromise. One method of handling a conflict is shown in the three steps below.

1. Ask yourself how important this problem is "in the scheme of things." What is the worst that could happen if it is not solved your way?

2. Identify what may happen if you decide to work together to solve this issue. Could the outcome be better if you work together?

3. Is there anyone who can be brought in to assist you in this situation? This type of person is known as an "arbitrator" or a "mediator." **Arbitration** or **mediation** can sometimes be of great help in a difficult situation. So remember: conflicts will sometimes occur in the workplace. The key is to know when to stand firm, when to walk away, and when it's time to compromise.

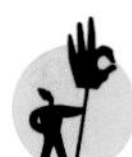

Don't delay! Report right away!

When you are caring for your residents, there are certain observations and situations that should be reported to the nurse immediately. In this textbook the following phrase will be used to help you identify one of these situations:

★ *"Don't Delay. Report Right Away!"*

9 List four guidelines for critical thinking in observing and reporting.

Careful gathering of observations is important to the health and well-being of all of your residents. How do you determine what observations to report immediately to the nurse and which ones can wait until later? This involves critical thinking, the ability to make good observations in order to get help for a potential problem before harm comes to the resident. Nursing assistants have to decide frequently when to notify the nurse about a change.

Critical Thinking and the Nursing Assistant: Is the Change Serious?

1. Look at the CHANGE in the resident.

2. Decide if the CHANGE could mean something SERIOUS. This text will teach you many of these potentially serious changes.

3. Notify the nurse IMMEDIATELY with any CHANGE that could be serious.

4. For any CHANGE that may not seem serious, write down the information in your pocket notebook and report it to the nurse later in your shift.

Sometimes a nurse will ask you to report every change, no matter what the change is. A resident's condition will need to be monitored closely. If this is the case, you will simply report each change in a resident's condition to the nurse as it happens.

10 Describe the importance of strict confidentiality with all resident information.

Have you ever heard the phrase, "The walls have ears?" It means secrets are easily discovered, and gossip has a way of getting around when people do not guard what they say.

It can be easy to make a mistake regarding resident privacy and confidentiality. However, it is important that you do not make this mistake. Each resident deserves our respect and the privacy and confidentiality outlined in the "rights" section of Chapter 3. A "STAR nursing assistant" does not repeat resident information to anyone. The observations you gather about your residents are private pieces of information that must not be repeated to anyone except the nurse in charge of that resident. During the end-of-shift report, the nurses may discuss important changes in resident care. *This information is also private and must not be repeated to anyone not directly involved with the care of the resident.* So, every time you are tempted to repeat information you may see or hear, ask yourself the following question: "Is this confidential information?" If the answer is yes, "zip your lips," and stop right there!

Consider these situations:

1. Nursing assistant Roberto Chavez gets on an elevator and is greeted by another staff member, Nicole Maples. Nicole asks Roberto if resident Moira Sinclair's tests for cancer have come back yet. Roberto says "Oh yes, she has cancer." They did not know that Moira's cousin was also on the elevator with them. Her cousin did not know about the cancer.

2. Nursing assistants Patrick and Cindy are eating lunch in the cafeteria. They begin discussing the fact that the new 73-year-old resident, Mr. Thompson, has been diagnosed with a serious sexually-transmitted disease (STD). They do not

realize that Mr. Thompson's wife is seated behind them in the next table and overhears their conversation. She was not aware that her husband has an STD.

3. Resident Aaron Little asks you what is wrong with the new resident, Mrs. Lane. You answer, "They found that she's got hepatitis." Mr. Little tells everyone this information, and the other residents are all now fearful that they may get hepatitis.

In each of these situations, had the nursing assistants asked themselves the question above regarding confidential information, it would have prevented them from repeating it.

You would not want anything repeated about yourself or any of your family members or friends to other people. Always remember: the resident is someone's mother, father, sister, brother, or friend, and his family members and friends feel the same way. However, confidentiality is not only about promoting respect and dignity. Keeping residents' information confidential is the law, and you must follow it.

11 Identify the people you will communicate with in a facility and how you will communicate with them.

There are many people you will communicate with in different ways on a daily basis while working in a healthcare facility. Some of these people are identified below.

Doctors, Nurses, Supervisors, Managers, and Other Staff Members

Nursing assistants will communicate with the nursing team in a variety of ways. You will communicate verbally and nonverbally. You will chart information and may use a computer. You will use the telephone, a call system, and possibly a Kardex or a cassette recorder. You may be involved in care planning. You need to become familiar with each of these methods in order to effectively communicate with the team on a regular basis.

Other Departments

Nursing assistants will communicate with other departments. This may occur over the telephone or in person. The inter-relationship between departments in a facility is very important. It makes the difference between excellent, organized care and problems. You must deal with other departments in a positive manner in order to keep communication lines open and friendly. If a staff member from another department treats you badly, you can inform your nurse in charge. He may need to follow up on the problem.

Residents

The most important communication you will have with your residents occurs each time you greet them. At that time, you will introduce yourself and identify (ID) the resident. You will explain the procedure you are going to be doing and encourage the resident's participation. You will do this for every resident each time you provide care. Residents may or may not wear name bands on their arms in facilities. If your facility does not require name bands, you will use another method for identifying your residents. Many facilities use up-to-date photos outside or inside the resident's room to help identify residents. Explaining each procedure is vital in the communication process. It is a part of the "rights" section in Chapter 3.

Families and Visitors

The nursing team should always try to have a good, open relationship with families and friends of residents. One way to keep a good relationship is to always respond immediately whenever a resident calls for assistance. This will let the family or friends know that you are taking excellent care of their loved one. It could comfort them knowing that their loved one is safe and secure. Families are also a rich source of information regarding your residents' likes, dislikes, and histories. By asking about these things, you learn more and are able to provide better care.

The Community

When you deal with the people in the community, it is usually over the telephone or in person. Team members may receive calls from doctors' offices or clinics, or one of their staff may visit the facility. Members of the media may inquire about a resident. The way you present yourself to the community is vital to your reputation and the reputation of your facility. You are considered "representatives" of the facility and must present yourself in a positive and professional manner. Using foul language or slang, or speaking rudely or harshly will have a negative affect on the way you and your facility are viewed by the community.

12 Describe verbal and nonverbal communication.

When we verbally communicate, we use words. Speaking and writing are two ways of communicating verbally. **Verbal communication** also includes the WAY in which we speak or write. How your voice sounds when you speak says as much as what you say. The words you choose to use, whether in speaking or writing, convey a message as well. For instance, if you sound harsh or blunt when speaking to a resident or another staff member, that person may think you are mad at him. If you use foul language, the person may be insulted. If someone speaks too loudly or sounds like she is "talking down" to you, you may feel foolish, disrespected, and upset. So, always consider the way you sound, and carefully consider your choice of words.

Five techniques for effective communication are:

1. Are your words appropriate? Are the words at the right level so your resident can understand them?
2. Is your body language appropriate? (good eye contact?)
3. Are you using an acceptable tone of voice? (concerned and caring?)
4. Do you wait for a response? (avoiding interrupting the person?)
5. Do you only deal in facts? (avoiding giving your opinion?)

Showing off is rude!

Using medical terminology when speaking to residents or residents' families or friends may be considered abusive behavior if they do not understand the terms you use. This prevents residents or family members from understanding a procedure or important information regarding the health and well-being of their loved one. These individuals may not tell you that they do not understand. They may simply not want to appear as if they do not know something. It is best to never use medical terms when speaking or writing to residents, family members, or friends. Also, do not hold a personal conversation with a coworker in front of a resident, or talk over a resident's head while performing care.

When writing information, a person must consider each and every word that he writes. It is truly amazing how a simple word can be misunderstood by another person. When you write anything in the healthcare industry, whether it be a note to your supervisor, a request to another department, or a note asking another staff member to switch a day with you, take great care in the way you write the note. Be clear and direct in your communication.

Check to see if you are using the appropriate:
- words, so that you will be understood
- clear handwriting, so it can be read correctly

Nonverbal communication is also called **body language**. Body language has to do with all of the conscious or unconscious messages your body might send as you communicate with others. It consists of things like your posture, body movements, facial expressions, and gestures. Your body language can add positive or negative messages to your attempts to communicate with people. Residents, staff, families, and friends may be very sensitive to changes in body language and can have their feelings easily hurt.

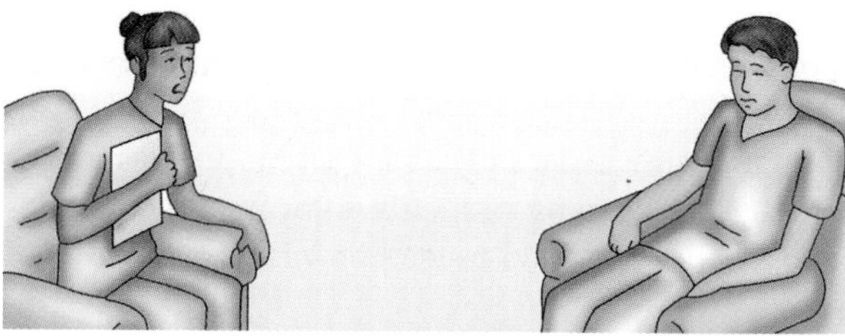

Figure 6-5. **Body language often speaks as plainly as words. Which of these people seems more interested in the conversation they are having?**

Touch is another important method of nonverbal communication. Nursing assistants need to touch residents frequently during daily care. When deciding whether or not to touch a resident, asking permission is always acceptable if the person understands you. If the person pulls away, this can be a sign he does not want to be touched. With the resident's permission, holding a hand or touching a shoulder may help comfort the resident.

Touch practices differ greatly from one culture to another. Some cultures accept the touch of strangers, while others have strict rules regarding touch.

Below are some examples of positive and negative nonverbal communication.

Positive Nonverbal Communication
- smiling in a friendly manner
- leaning forward to listen
- with permission, putting your hand over a resident's hand while listening to her

Negative Nonverbal Communication
- rolling your eyes or crossing your arms
- tapping your foot while talking
- pointing your finger in someone's face while speaking

As you read these examples of body language, imagine someone doing this to you and think about how it would make you feel. If the resident is behaving as if he is offended by your behavior, think about what you might be doing with your body. People can successfully change their body language. It will greatly improve the way you relate to other people.

13 Describe a standard resident chart.

The **chart**, or resident **medical record**, is the legal **record** of the resident's care while in the facility. This record is saved for a specified number of years. After a specific amount of time has passed, the chart may be converted into a different format, like microfilm, in order to save valuable space. The record is saved so that it can be obtained by a future healthcare provider, who might need the chart someday to gather important information about a resident's past medical history. Information might be needed regarding an **Advance Directive**, the wishes or directions given by a resident for an emergency regarding life-saving efforts. It may also be obtained by a court should a legal situation arise in the future. The chart includes information such as:

- admission forms
- resident history and physical forms
- Advance Directives
- physician's orders
- care plans
- physician's progress notes
- nursing assessment or history
- nurse's notes
- flow sheets
- graphic record
- intake and output record
- consent forms
- lab and test results
- surgery reports

Your responsibility regarding the resident chart is primarily to gather information and report it to the nurse. The nurse may then write this data in the chart in the nurse's notes.

A few facilities allow nursing assistants to chart in a medical record. Most facilities limit nursing assistants' writing in the chart, or charting, to certain forms. The "intake and output" form is commonly used by the nursing assistant. Remember, all of the information you see or add to a resident's medical record, or chart, is covered under confidentiality and the privacy rights of residents.

Intake & Output Record

Client Name: ____________ HCA Name: ____________
Address: ____________ Record Date: ____________

Intake			Output		
Time	Type	Amount	Time	Urine Amount	Incontinent Episode

Output	Time	Approximate Amount
Vomiting		
Heavy Perspiration		
Diarrhea		

Figure 6-6. You may be asked to document intake and output.

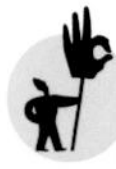

The Medical Record — A possible lifeline.

Some facilities allow nursing assistants to carry charts from one place to another within a facility. If you are ever asked to bring a chart to another unit or to a different department, you must never let the chart out of your sight. Remember, the information within that chart could be vital information used in emergencies. You must never put that information at risk in any way. While you are transferring the chart, it is not appropriate for you to read any part of the chart or to let anyone else read it. It is also important that you give the chart to the designated individual and not just place it on a counter.

14 Describe the SOAP charting style and discuss rules for effective charting.

Charting usually revolves around the nursing process. There are different methods of charting used in various facilities. One method we will review here is the SOAP method of charting.

SOAP

S= Subjective data, symptoms (The subject tells you.)

O= Objective data, signs (Observe, see, hear, smell, feel)

A= Assessment (Organize conclusions from S & O)

P= Plan care

The following is an example of SOAP charting: problem identified, problem viewed and assessed, problem cared for.

Case Study

William L. Pickard, Male
54 years old, D.O.B . 11/22/23
1400 #1 Unusual Spots

S- "All of a sudden my skin has spots!"
O- Skin appears to have dime-sized black spots
on many areas.
A- No previous history of spots.
P- Lotion applied to spots.

- Referred to physician for assessment.

Figure 6-7.

All facilities will have policies and procedures for charting. Everyone must follow them.

Elements of Effective Charting

Confidentiality: Remember to treat all information within the chart as confidential information.

Permanence: When you chart in any way, use black ink. People must be able to read your writing, so be careful to write neatly. In addition, draw a line through areas where no writing exists. Remember, a resident's chart is a legal record. When documenting care given, always wait to document until after you have completed your care. Never record any care before it is performed.

Signature: You must always sign each recording you make within the chart. This is done in the following manner: Max Johnson, NA (or CNA). Other agencies might allow a first initial, such as: M. Johnson, NA.

Accuracy: You must use only facts, never opinions, when charting. Chart exactly what the person has said (subjective), or what you see, hear, smell, or touch (objective). The words "seems," "appears to be," or "looks like" are not used in charting. An example of an opinion is: "The resident seemed angry at her relatives." That is your opinion of the resident's behavior. If you said: "The resident was speaking loudly and angrily to her relatives," this would be more factual.

Never use correction fluid to fix errors. The way to correct an error is to draw one line through it and write the correct word or words. Follow your facility's policy. (Figure 6-8)

Standard Terminology: Use only accepted abbreviations and other medical symbols and terminology. You must never make up your own abbreviation. A comprehensive list of medical abbreviations can be found in Chapter 5.

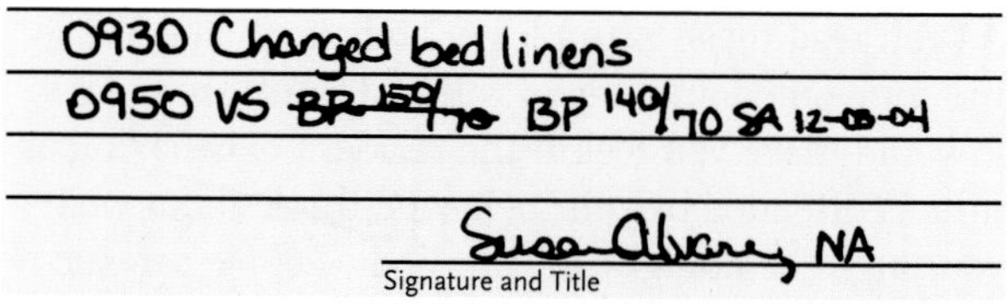

0930 Changed bed linens
0950 VS ~~BP 150/70~~ BP 140/70 SA 12-08-04

Susan Alvarez, NA
Signature and Title

Figure 6-8.

Use size to describe data instead of words like "large," "moderate or medium," or "small." For example, you may consider using a coin size to describe the approximate size of a spot or an amount of bleeding on a bandage.

15 Identify the components of a standard Kardex.

A **Kardex** is a brand of card file that keeps resident information organized and easy to locate. This card file is usually kept at the nurse's station so that staff can access it. There may be two separate Kardex files for a unit, depending upon the size of the unit.

The Kardex includes the resident's plan of care as written and ordered by the healthcare provider (doctor or nurse practitioner). Figure 6-9 outlines a sample Kardex.

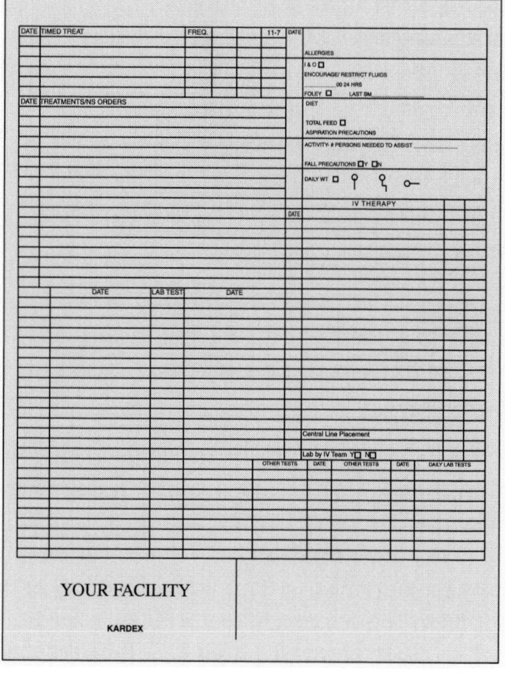
DATE | TIMED TREAT | FREQ. | 11-7 | DATE
ALLERGIES
I & O ☐
ENCOURAGE/ RESTRICT FLUIDS
______ 00 24 HRS
FOLEY ☐ LAST BM______
DATE | TREATMENTS/NS ORDERS
DIET
TOTAL FEED ☐
ASPIRATION PRECAUTIONS
ACTIVITY- # PERSONS NEEDED TO ASSIST ______
FALL PRECAUTIONS ☐Y ☐N
DAILY WT ☐
IV THERAPY
DATE
DATE | LAB TEST | DATE
Central Line Placement
Lab by IV Team Y☐ N☐
OTHER TESTS | DATE | OTHER TESTS | DATE | DAILY LAB TESTS
YOUR FACILITY
KARDEX

Figure 6-9.

16 Discuss the nursing assistant's role in care planning and at care conferences.

The nursing assistant has an important role in the development of resident care plans. **Care plans** are prepared using all of the observations from all of the staff caring for the resident. They may be written at a special **care conference**, and you may be asked to attend this conference. During the conference, you will add important observations to assist the nurses in preparing the care plans. Many residents have several different problems that are put into care plan form. An example of a care plan that could be developed to improve a resident's care is listed below.

Sample Care Plan for Rosie Cerrullo (see Learning Objective 5)

Problem: Sleep disturbance pattern
Goal/Outcome: Resident will sleep at least seven hours per night and report that she feels more rested within two weeks.
Goal/Outcome to be reviewed: Date listed here
Nursing Actions:
1. Close door to room.
2. Provide milk before bedtime.
3. Close door to neighbor's room.
Evaluation: Within one week, resident is sleeping at least seven hours per night and reports feeling more rested.

The care conference is a method of meeting to share, and gather information about residents in order to develop plans of care. Team members include nurses, nursing assistants, social workers, dietitians, physical therapists, and other important staff members. Each of these team members may share important information to be used to create or add to the plan of care. Residents, family members, and friends may also attend all or a part of the care conference. Members of the community, such as ombudsmen, who participate in a care conference share helpful information too. Care plans developed at the care conference are kept at the nurse's station or next to the resident's room in an individual station.

17 List the seven steps to expert telephone etiquette.

Earlier in this chapter, we discussed the importance of good relationships with your facility's community. When you use the telephone in any way during your shift, you are representing your facility to the surrounding community. It is vital that you follow strict rules for telephone etiquette. Seven steps to expert telephone etiquette in a healthcare facility follow:

1. Cheerfully say, "Good morning", "good afternoon", or "good evening."
2. Identify your facility: "Lincolnwood Facility."
3. Identify yourself and your position: "Nancy Jones, Nursing Assistant."
4. Listen closely to the caller's request. In emergencies, take action immediately.
5. Have a pad and pen handy to write down messages. Ask for correct spelling of names.
6. Get a telephone number, if needed.
7. Say "Thank you," and "Goodbye."

A few general rules for the use of telephones at healthcare facilities are listed below:

1. Never give out any information regarding staff members or residents over the telephone. This means if someone calls and says, "Does Susie Hawkins work there?" you respond in this way: "Please hold and I will get my supervisor to assist you." Most facilities have this policy due to the increase in **domestic violence** (violence related to the family or family matters) and other problems, like stalking, in recent years. Creditors may also call facilities looking for people who owe them money. All resident and staff information is confidential and must never be given out over the telephone. Refer this type of phone call to a supervisor.
2. You may place a caller on hold if you need to get someone to take the call. Make sure you ask the caller if she can hold first. Ask for help and additional training if you need it.
3. You may have to transfer a call at times. If you do not know how to transfer, ask for training on transferring calls.
4. Know your facility's policy on personal phone calls. If they are not allowed, you may use a pay phone, when available. Do not put your job at risk by making personal calls during work.
5. Know your facility's policy on personal cellular phones and pagers. These may be prohibited in the workplace.

18 Describe the correct use of the resident call system.

You can communicate with residents, family, and other staff using the facility call system. Other terms for this system are "signal light," or "call light." This system enables residents to call you whenever they are in need. You must think of this system as your resident's **LIFELINE**. A lifeline is something that connects another person to help when needed. A lifeline can literally save someone's life. Nursing assistants should always take calls promptly and must never disregard any call for help from any resident. There are many kinds of call systems available.

Types of Call Systems — Box 6-1

1. The first, and simplest, type of call system is the "bell" style, which you may have seen at a store. The main drawback to this style is that you cannot speak to the resident and the bell is not always loud enough to hear.
2. The intercom call system is the most common type of system. In this system, the resident (or visitor or other staff member) presses a button of some kind and a sound is heard at the nurse's station. When the button is pressed, a light goes on at the station identifying the room number of the resident calling. The staff member can speak to the person from the station and then follow up in any way needed.
3. A newer call system involves the use of staff pagers. The signal for help goes directly to the person assigned to care for that resident.

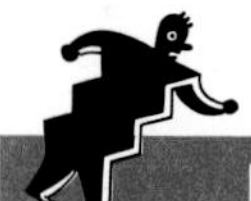

Principal Steps

The Correct Use of the Call System

1. *A resident, visitor, or healthcare team member presses the call button.*
2. *Light goes on outside of door.*
3. *Person at nurse's station desk turns on intercom and asks "What can I do for you?" or "How may I help you?" OR team member goes to room to ask, "What can I do for you?"*
4. *Person in the room turns off call light if problem or request is taken care of at the nurse's station over the intercom OR team member turns off call button if he or she comes to the room.*
5. *Always leave a call button within reach of resident before leaving room. Timely response to call lights is important for both resident safety and satisfaction.*
6. *Staff provides the services requested or gets appropriate help.*

19 Describe the nursing assistant's role in change-of-shift reports and "rounds."

There are two types of shift reports: start-of-shift report and end-of-shift report. Nursing assistants usually are asked to be present for the start-of-shift reports; the nurses are present for both types of reports. The nursing team gathers to discuss and plan resident care for a particular shift, approximately 8 to 12 hours in length.

Start-of-Shift Report

1. Arrive on time for this report.
2. Each staff member is given his or her assignment for the shift. This assignment identifies the residents each staff member will be primarily responsible for during that shift. However, remember, each resident is "your" resident, and you must listen for important information about all of the residents in your area.
3. The staff listens to a nurse (or a cassette recording of a nurse) from the prior shift who reports on the care of each resident. Examples of information passed to the next shift are appetite problems, difficulties with urination, complaints of pain, or a change in the ability to move about.
4. The nurses give special instructions to the other staff members, nurses, and nursing assistants who will be providing resident care. This is the time to ask important questions about your residents. Special information shared during a report may include new admissions to the facility and transfers or discharges from the facility.

End-of-Shift Report

1. Nursing assistants report to the nurses before the end-of-shift report. They will give the nurses any important information about their residents gathered during their shift. Examples of this information are change in pulse or temperature, change in the amount of fluids the resident has taken in or output, rashes or skin changes signaling the start of a pressure sore.

2. The nurses bring all of the information they have gathered from the nursing assistants and other staff to the end-of-shift report. This information is shared with the staff for the next shift.

Some facilities use a method of reporting called "**rounds**," where staff members move from room-to-room and discuss each resident and the plan of care. As a nursing assistant, you may be involved in rounds at your facility. If you participate in rounds, the key is to listen closely. Take notes on your assignment sheet using a clipboard under it to make writing easier. Offer valuable information to the other staff when you have it. Sometimes, this method of walking from room to room makes residents feel better cared for because they are reassured that many people are available to help them when needed.

20 List the information found on an assignment sheet.

An assignment sheet identifies residents and contains all of the tasks that you must perform for them. Certain things are done for each of your residents on a daily basis. These daily tasks are called the activities of daily living (ADLs), which include activities such as dressing and eating. Another section you may find on an assignment sheet is **ROM (Range of Motion)**, which are the exercises done to bring joints through a full range of movement. **Code status** is a section that tells the staff whether the resident has an Advance Directive or not. Advance Directives are documents that allow people to choose what kind of medical care they wish to have in the event they are unable to make those decisions themselves. A "**code**" is when a group of specially-trained staff provide advanced life support during an emergency with a resident.

NURSING ASSIGNMENT SHEET

TEAM MEMBER: | BREAK: CONFERENCE: LUNCH: DATE:

TEAM LEADER: | ASSIGNMENT:

ROOM	PATIENT	BATH	ACTIVITY	DIET	FLUIDS	TO BE CHECKED	TREATMENTS	SPECIMEN	COMMENTS
		BED SELF * SHOWER TUB SITZ	BED DANGLE BRP BRP HELP AMB AMB HELP WALKER CRUTCHES WC	REGULAR SOFT SURG LIQ FULL LIQ SPECIAL FASTING TUBE FEEDING	FORCE NPO LIMIT SIPS WATER ICE CHIPS IV DIST WATER	BLOOD PRESSURE TPR TEST URINE AC & HS SLIDING SCALE I&O LEVIN TUBE CHEST TUBE FOLEY OXYGEN	ENEMA DOUCHE PERI CARE LIGHT WEIGH ORAL HYGIENE SPECIAL BACK CARE PREPARE FOR SURG PREPARE FOR X-RAY OT PT ECT	STOOL URINE SPUTUM BLOOD CULTURE TISSUE	
		BED SELF * SHOWER TUB SITZ	BED DANGLE BRP BRP HELP AMB AMB HELP WALKER CRUTCHES WC	REGULAR SOFT SURG LIQ FULL LIQ SPECIAL FASTING TUBE FEEDING	FORCE NPO LIMIT SIPS WATER ICE CHIPS IV DIST WATER	BLOOD PRESSURE TPR TEST URINE AC & HS SLIDING SCALE I&O LEVIN TUBE CHEST TUBE FOLEY OXYGEN	ENEMA DOUCHE PERI CARE LIGHT WEIGH ORAL HYGIENE SPECIAL BACK CARE PREPARE FOR SURG PREPARE FOR X-RAY OT PT ECT	STOOL URINE SPUTUM BLOOD CULTURE TISSUE	
		BED SELF * SHOWER TUB SITZ	BED DANGLE BRP BRP HELP AMB AMB HELP WALKER CRUTCHES WC	REGULAR SOFT SURG LIQ FULL LIQ SPECIAL FASTING TUBE FEEDING	FORCE NPO LIMIT SIPS WATER ICE CHIPS IV DIST WATER	BLOOD PRESSURE TPR TEST URINE AC & HS SLIDING SCALE I&O LEVIN TUBE CHEST TUBE FOLEY OXYGEN	ENEMA DOUCHE PERI CARE LIGHT WEIGH ORAL HYGIENE SPECIAL BACK CARE PREPARE FOR SURG PREPARE FOR X-RAY OT PT ECT	STOOL URINE SPUTUM BLOOD CULTURE TISSUE	
		BED SELF * SHOWER TUB SITZ	BED DANGLE BRP BRP HELP AMB AMB HELP WALKER CRUTCHES WC	REGULAR SOFT SURG LIQ FULL LIQ SPECIAL FASTING TUBE FEEDING	FORCE NPO LIMIT SIPS WATER ICE CHIPS IV DIST WATER	BLOOD PRESSURE TPR TEST URINE AC & HS SLIDING SCALE I&O LEVIN TUBE CHEST TUBE FOLEY OXYGEN	ENEMA DOUCHE PERI CARE LIGHT WEIGH ORAL HYGIENE SPECIAL BACK CARE PREPARE FOR SURG PREPARE FOR X-RAY OT PT ECT	STOOL URINE SPUTUM BLOOD CULTURE TISSUE	
		BED SELF * SHOWER TUB SITZ	BED DANGLE BRP BRP HELP AMB AMB HELP WALKER CRUTCHES WC	REGULAR SOFT SURG LIQ FULL LIQ SPECIAL FASTING TUBE FEEDING	FORCE NPO LIMIT SIPS WATER ICE CHIPS IV DIST WATER	BLOOD PRESSURE TPR TEST URINE AC & HS SLIDING SCALE I&O LEVIN TUBE CHEST TUBE FOLEY OXYGEN	ENEMA DOUCHE PERI CARE LIGHT WEIGH ORAL HYGIENE SPECIAL BACK CARE PREPARE FOR SURG PREPARE FOR X-RAY OT PT ECT	STOOL URINE SPUTUM BLOOD CULTURE TISSUE	

CODE					
*	YOU WASH BACK AND LEGS	WC	WHEELCHAIR	ECT	ELECTRICAL CONVULSIVE THERAPY
BRP	BATHROOM PRIVILEGES	BP	BLOOD PRESSURE	OT	OCCUPATIONAL THERAPY
AMB	AMBULATORY	NPO	NOTHING BY MOUTH	PT	PHYSICAL THERAPY
I & O	INPUT AND OUTPUT	DIST	DISTILLED WATER		

Figure 6-10. **A sample assignment sheet.**

Some facilities fill out assignment sheets for the nursing assistants. Others allow each nursing assistant to complete his or her own assignment sheet. A sample assignment is shown in Figure 6-10. Either way, during the change-of-shift report you must listen closely to all of the information given about the residents on your assignment sheet. Assignment sheets contain the following information:

- names and room numbers of residents
- the medical diagnosis of each resident
- code status
- activity level
- range of motion (ROM) exercises
- bathing
- diet
- fluid order
- bowel and bladder information
- vital signs: frequency of measurement
- treatments to be performed
- special tests/miscellaneous (other things) to be performed

Carrying out your own special assignments each day is done by gathering all of your organizational skills. There is no "magic wand" that gives you the ability to organize your work; this comes through experience. Do not expect to be perfect the first week, or even the first month, on the job.

Remember earlier in the textbook when we discussed the way you organize your life at home? Things like paying the bills, buying the food, doing the laundry, picking up children, and remembering cards and gifts on special days may be part of your daily life. Feeling organized at home is the same as feeling organized on the job. Look to others for guidelines on how to plan your daily care and create the perfect mix for you. Before you know it, you will be a supremely skilled, organized nursing assistant, a vital part of the healthcare team.

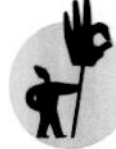

Show up!

Assignments primarily depend upon the number of residents and the number of staff members available to care for them during that shift. It is very important for you to work every day you are scheduled. Missing a day without good reason can put your residents in danger and can also put the staff at risk due to having too many residents to care for. This happens because there simply is not enough staff to provide good quality care that day. If you must be absent, call your facility as early as possible to inform them of your absence. This allows your supervisor to start trying to replace you as soon as possible.

Summary

The use of effective communication is one of the most important ways to provide quality care to residents. Good communication can prevent serious errors in the facility. Learning how to use different communication methods correctly can help a nursing assistant become more professional.

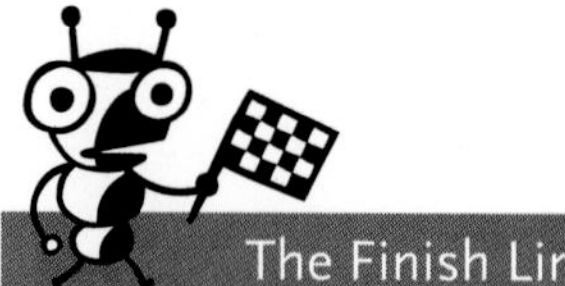

The Finish Line

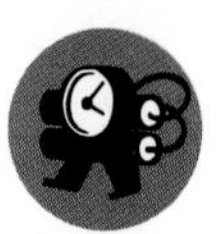

What's Wrong With This Picture?

Identify the errors in charting in the following notes found in sample charts (medical records):

Miss Joyce McGinley 141-2. Appears to be feeling some pain. J. Wilder N.A.

Mr. Scott Cota 132-2. States: "I have a sore area on my leg.", Davis N.A.

Mrs. Eileen Carreras 147-2. States: "I have a pain in my big toe." C. Tran N.A.

Ms. Aubrey Holbrook 154-1. Looks like her leg is weaker today. D. Rodriguez N.A.

Mr. R.J. Harrison 143-1. Moderate amount of bleeding on dressing. K. Elliot N.A.

Mr. Sean Menager 125-2. Seemed angry this morning. M. Proctor N.A.

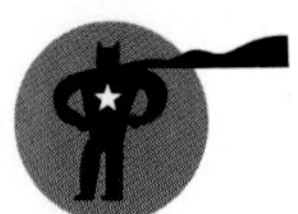

Star Student Central

1. Try to make arrangements to spend one half-hour volunteering at a facility answering the telephone. Answer the phone using all of the appropriate facility information and identify yourself as a student, if required. This exercise will help you practice proper telephone etiquette.

2. While at home or in the classroom, write a sample end-of-shift report for a nurse-in-charge. Each of your sample residents should be reported on in some way. You can role-play by reporting the information to your classmates or to the instructor.

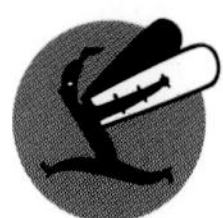

You Can Do It Corner!

The following sentences describe either objective or subjective data. Write an "S" for subjective or an "O" for objective in the space to the right of each sentence (LO 5).

1. You note Erin Gallardo is having trouble swallowing. O__________
2. Resident Laura Watson says she has a sore throat. S__________
3. Gary Meyers states, "I have a hard time catching my breath." S__________
4. You see Mrs. Heather Magnuson holding her abdomen. O__________
5. When Mr. Holmes urinates, you notice it's a dark red color. __________

Answer the following questions.

6. What is the MDS manual? Why would you be involved with it? (LO 4)
7. What are the four basic observations at a glance? (LO 7)
8. Why is it important that you keep all of your residents' information confidential? (LO 10)
9. What is body language? What is an example of good body language? (LO 12)
10. What would you do to contribute at a care conference? (LO 16)
11. Why is a call light a resident's lifeline? (LO 18)
12. What items are found on an assignment sheet? (LO 20)
13. What does the acronym "SOAP" mean? (LO 14)
14. What is a resident's chart? (LO 13)
15. Who are five groups with whom you may com-

municate in a long-term care facility? (LO 11)

16. What does critical thinking mean in terms of being a nursing assistant? (LO 8)

17. What are questions you may ask yourself before accepting a delegation? (LO 6)

18. What are five steps to effective communication? (LO 3)

19. What are the five steps in the nursing process? (LO 5)

20. What are four steps that can help you decide if a change needs to be reported immediately or later? (LO 9)

21. What are examples of problems that are reported on a start-of-shift report? (LO 19)

22. What is the most common cause of errors in healthcare facilities? (LO 2)

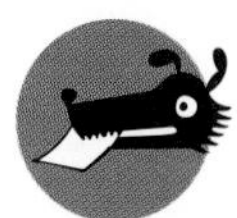

Star Student's Chapter Checklist

1. I have read my textbook chapter.
2. I have reviewed my own "Pocketful of Terms."
3. I have listened to my tutor tape.
4. I have reviewed and highlighted my class notes.
5. I have read and completed any handouts from this chapter.
6. I have completed "The Finish Line."
7. Star Time! Choose your reward!

Your Guide: Communication Challenges

Look Like a Star!

Look at the Learning Objectives **and** The Finish Line
before you begin reading this chapter.

Look at your pocket calendar.
With your pencil, put a bracket (   ) around a study period every single day.

Look at your homework for this chapter.
Plug each piece of homework into a certain time slot.

Look at the Star Student's Chapter Checklist
at the end of this chapter. Check off each item as it is completed.

"Think before thou speakest."

Miguel De Cervantes, 1547-1616, from Don Quixote

"I have often regretted my speech, never my silence."

Syrus, Maxim 633

Learning Objectives

1. Spell and define all STAR words.
2. Identify nine barriers to communication.
3. Describe communication challenges related to other cultures.
4. Identify four communication guidelines for the resident with a visual deficit.
5. Identify seven communication guidelines for the resident with a hearing deficit.
6. Identify ten communication guidelines for the resident with the inability to smell or feel.
7. Identify six communication guidelines for the resident with a cognitive barrier.
8. Identify five communication guidelines for the comatose resident.
9. Identify seven communication guidelines for the disoriented and/or confused resident.
10. Identify eight communication guidelines for residents with dementia and define behaviors related to Alzheimer's disease.
11. Explain reality orientation and identify nine guidelines for using it.
12. Explain validation therapy and give two examples of it.
13. Identify twelve communication guidelines for the resident with functional barriers.
14. Identify seven communication guidelines used with a paralyzed resident.
15. List seven defense mechanisms used as methods of coping with stress.
16. List four levels of anxiety and identify eight communication guidelines used with the anxious or fearful resident.
17. Identify five communication guidelines used with the depressed resident.
18. Identify seven communication guidelines used with the angry resident.
19. Identify seven communication guidelines used with the combative resident.
20. Explain why residents may show sexually-aggressive behavior and identify six communication guidelines for handling it.

The Navajo Code Talkers

In 1942, a young Navajo named Philip Johnson approached top-ranking U. S. military staff with an idea of how to use the Navajo language as a code during World War II. Many Navajos, including some teenagers, became Marines and went to work as Navajo Code Talkers. They used a form of the Navajo language to send top-secret messages during the war. Carl Gorman, Sr., the oldest of the Code Talkers, is the father of R.C. Gorman, a famous Navajo artist from New Mexico. In 1943, there were about 200 Navajo Code Talkers, and ultimately, around 400 Code Talkers went to the Pacific to serve in World War II. The Navajo Code Talk remained Top Secret until 1968. The code was never broken. The Navajo Code Talkers played a vital role in the victory of the United States in World War II.

The 29 original Navajo Code Talkers were awarded Congressional gold medals in 2001.

1 Spell and define all **STAR** words.

airway: the natural passageway for air to enter into the lungs.

Alzheimer's disease: progressive and irreversible deterioration of the brain causing loss of memory, disorientation, and other difficulties.

aphasia: the inability to communicate through speech, writing, or signs.

artificial airway: an airway formed artificially to bring air into the lungs.

cerebrovascular accident, CVA: a stroke; sudden loss of consciousness and possible paralysis caused by a hemorrhage, clot within the brain, or rupture of a blood vessel to the brain.

cognitive impairment: when the ability to communicate is affected by a disorder of the brain and may change a resident's ability to speak and understand language.

coma: abnormal state that occurs, usually in illness or injury, in which a person is unable to respond to any change in the environment, including pain.

communication barrier: something preventing or blocking good communication.

confusion: temporary or permanent inability to think in an organized or logical manner.

deficit: a lack of something.

dementia: a mental disorder due to a structural change in the brain; not a normal result of the aging process.

defense mechanisms: coping mechanisms used to deal with some kind of stress.

disoriented: not aware of person, place, or time.

gait: manner of walking.

hearing-impaired: unable to hear adequately; loss of some or all ability to hear sounds.

hemiplegia: paralysis on one side of the body.

integrated: included or incorporated.

intimidating: frightening.

multi-infarct dementia: numerous strokes causing reduced blood flow and damage to the brain.

paralysis: temporary or permanent loss of sensation or voluntary movement.

paraplegic: a person having paralysis of the lower portion of the body and both legs.

Parkinson's disease: a chronic nervous system disease with tremors, muscle weakness and rigidity, and an unusual walk or gait.

perseveration: frequent repetition of words, phrases, questions, or actions by residents with dementia.

quadriplegic: a person having paralysis of the arms, legs, and trunk of the body.

reality orientation: a group of techniques incorporated into daily routines in long-term care facilities used to try to re-orient certain residents with dementia to person, place, and time.

scent-impaired: unable to smell.

stroke (cerebrovascular accident, CVA): a sudden loss of consciousness and possible paralysis caused by a hemorrhage, clot within the brain, or rupture of a blood vessel.

tracheostomy: opening into the trachea to keep an open airway.

validation therapy: type of therapy that focuses on validating the experiences of residents with dementia rather than trying to orient them to reality.

visually-impaired: unable to see adequately.

2 Identify nine barriers to communication.

Sometimes residents will have difficulty understanding or using verbal (spoken or written) communication. This occurs due to a barrier or block preventing adequate communication. For example, a person who has a hearing **deficit** has lost some or all ability to hear sounds and may not be able to understand you when you are explaining a care procedure. This is called a sensory deficit because the person has lost the ability to use one of his five senses.

Following are nine **communication barriers** and ways to avoid them:

Resident does not hear you, does not hear correctly, or does not understand. Stand directly facing the resident. Speak slowly, making sure each word is spoken clearly, especially if your resident is hard of hearing or has a different native language. You do not need to shout. Speak in a low, pleasant voice. Do not whisper or mumble. If your resident says he or she cannot hear you, speak more loudly, but maintain a pleasant, professional tone of voice. If your resident wears a hearing aid, check to make sure it is on and working properly.

Resident is difficult to understand. Be patient and take the time to listen. Ask the resident to repeat or explain. Try to repeat or rephrase the message in your own words to make sure you understood.

Message uses words receiver does not understand. Do not use medical terminology with your resident or your resident's family. Speak in simple, everyday words so that you are easily understood. Do not pretend to understand the meaning of a word; ask what a word means if you are not sure.

Using slang confuses the message. Avoid using slang words and expressions that may not be understood or are unprofessional.

Using clichés makes your message meaningless. Clichés are phrases that are used over and over again and do not really mean anything, for example: "You'll be fine," or "It'll all work out." Instead of using a cliché, listen to what your resident is really saying. Respond with a meaningful and thoughtful message. For example, if a resident is afraid of having a bath, say "I understand that it seems scary to you. What can I do to make you feel more at ease?" instead of saying "Oh, it'll be over before you know it."

Asking "why" makes the resident defensive. Try not to ask "why" when a resident makes a statement. "Why" questions make people feel defensive. For example, a resident may say she does not want to attend a scheduled activity. If you ask "why not?" you may receive an annoyed or limited response. Instead, ask, "Are you too tired to do this, or is there something else you want to do?" Your resident may then be willing to discuss the issue.

Giving advice is inappropriate. Do not offer your personal opinion or give advice. Residents and family members should make important decisions on their own or with help from their doctors and nurses. Giving medical advice is not within the scope of your practice and could be dangerous.

Yes/no answers end a conversation. Unless you are seeking direct information, ask open-ended questions that need more than a yes or no answer. Yes and no answers bring any conversation to an end. For example, if you want to know what your resident likes to eat, do not ask "Do you like meatloaf?" Instead, try "What are some of your favorite foods?"

Nonverbal communication changes the message. Be aware of your body language and gestures when you are speaking. Be alert to nonverbal messages from your residents and clarify them. For example "Ms. Gold, you say you're doing well but you seem to be in pain. Can I help in any way?"

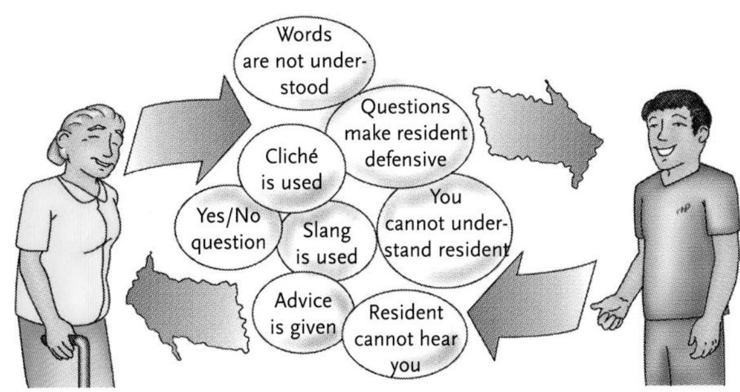

Figure 7-1. **Barriers to communication.**

3 Describe communication challenges related to other cultures.

There are certain cultural differences you need to be aware of in order to communicate effectively. The first difference is in the words or language spoken or written. Verbal communication is vital to understanding your residents. You must be sure that they understand everything you say to and do for them. In Chapter 4, the use of an interpreter was introduced. An interpreter can make resident care run more smoothly. Never hesitate to request an interpreter when you believe your resident does not understand something.

The second consideration concerns nonverbal communication. Touch, you will remember from chapter 6, is a part of nonverbal communication or body language . Each culture has its own distinct habits and practices regarding touch.

The distance people stand or sit apart from each other varies widely between cultures. Some cultures encourage both men and women to hug and kiss when meeting others. Some cultures prefer shaking hands upon meeting, while other cultures bow or smile.

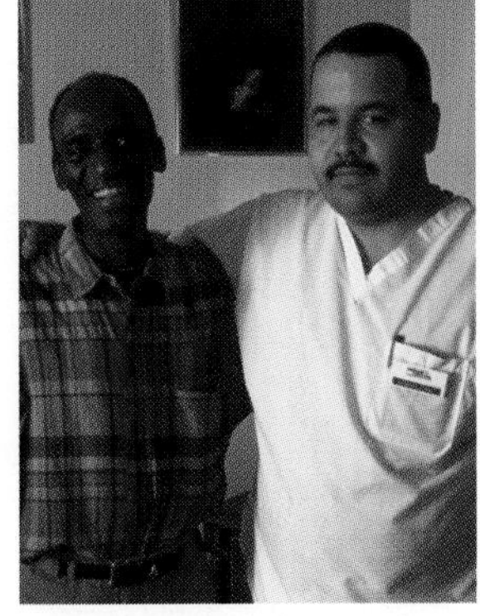

Figure 7-2. **How a resident perceives your touch may depend on his cultural background.**

Some people establish eye contact quickly and maintain it for an entire conversation, while other people in other cultures consider this rude.

Touching members of the opposite sex may also be dealt with differently. Some groups have no problem with unmarried members of the opposite sex touching or sitting next to each other. Other cultures have rules that unmarried people must stay a certain distance apart from members of the opposite sex.

4 Identify four communication guidelines for the resident with a visual deficit.

When you are assigned to care for a resident who has a visual deficit, there are specific things you can do to help communication. Try to imagine what it feels like to be **visually-impaired**. It can be very **intimidating** to have lost the ability to see.

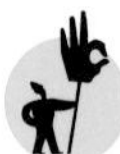

Put yourself in their shoes.

To try and understand what it feels like to have a visual deficit of some kind, try this activity. With your instructor present, find a student partner and a wheelchair. One of you will sit in the wheelchair and be the "resident" and the other will be the "nursing assistant." The "resident" must close his eyes while the "nursing assistant" wheels him around the room or through the hallway. You may find that you have quite a bit more empathy with people who can't see very well after this exercise.

Communication Guidelines - Visual Deficit

1. Speak to the resident when greeting him. (Never touch first.)
2. Look at the resident the entire time you are speaking with him. Make sure there is adequate lighting in the room.

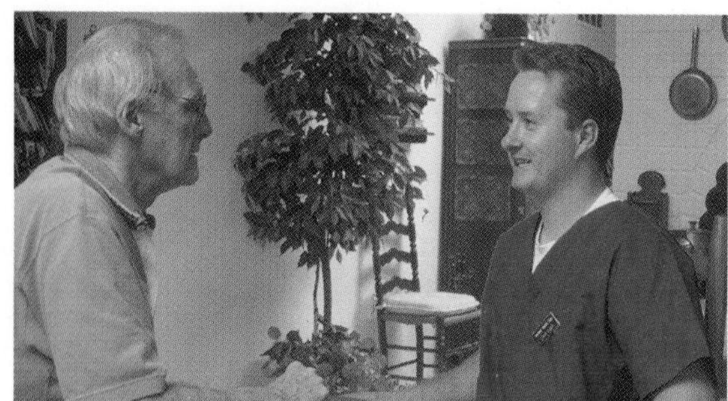

Figure 7-3. **Speak face-to-face, in good light.**

3. Do not shout.
4. Announce when you are going to leave the area where the resident is.

5 Identify seven communication guidelines for the resident with a hearing deficit.

Communicating with a resident who cannot hear can be a challenge. Residents have different kinds of hearing losses. Hearing may also be temporarily impaired due to noises in the room. Become familiar with any hand gestures a **hearing-impaired** resident might use. When you are assigned a resident who has trouble hearing, use the following guidelines to provide better care:

Communication Guidelines - Hearing Deficit

1. Stand or sit so that the resident can see you.
2. Look at the resident the entire time you are with her. A hearing-impaired resident may read lips. Make sure there is adequate lighting in the room.
3. If the resident uses a hearing aid, make sure it is turned on.
4. If the TV or radio is on, turn it off.
5. Speak clearly in a low tone of voice. Do not shout. If the person favors one ear, speak to that side.
6. Do not chew gum or cover your mouth with your hand while speaking.
7. Do not exaggerate pronunciation of words.

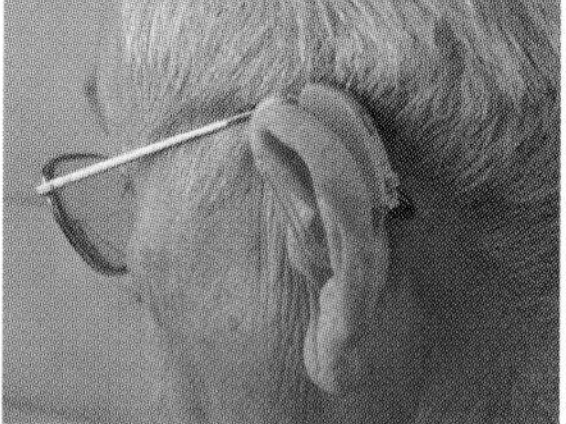

Figure 7-4. **Make sure hearing aids are turned on.**

6 Identify ten communication guidelines for the resident with the inability to smell or feel.

A resident who is **scent-impaired** may not be able to smell and recognize unsafe substances in the air. To aid in the care of a resident who cannot smell, review the following guidelines:

Communication Guidelines - Inability to Smell

1. Notify the resident of any strong cleaning fluids being used nearby. Some heavy cleaning fluids, waxes, or other products can upset the stomach or affect the lungs. If the resident cannot smell these substances, he will be unable to ask you to

move him to another area.

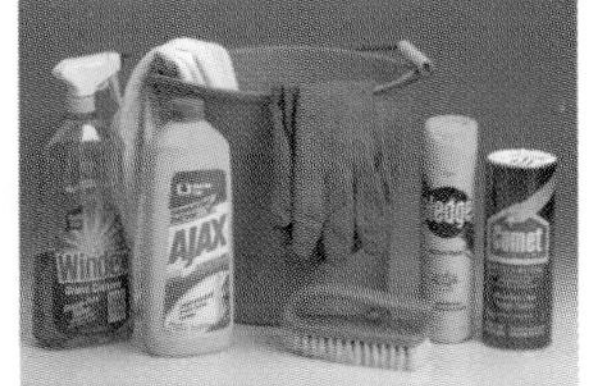

Figure 7-5. **A resident who cannot smell may not be aware of cleaning fluids.**

2. In case of a gas leak or a fire, this resident may not smell the smoke or gas. She should be one of the first to be told of the problem and removed from the area.
3. When food is served, it is polite to go first to this resident's room to bring him to the dayroom.

Communication Guidelines - Inability to Feel

The resident who has a problem feeling sensations can be at risk of injury from heat, cold, and sharp objects. One reason a resident has this problem is poor circulation to certain body parts. Another reason is **paralysis**. When dealing with a resident who has an inability to feel, the guidelines below should be followed:

1. Alert the resident whenever the temperature becomes colder or warmer than usual. Provide an extra blanket or extra clothing, or remove heavier or extra clothing.

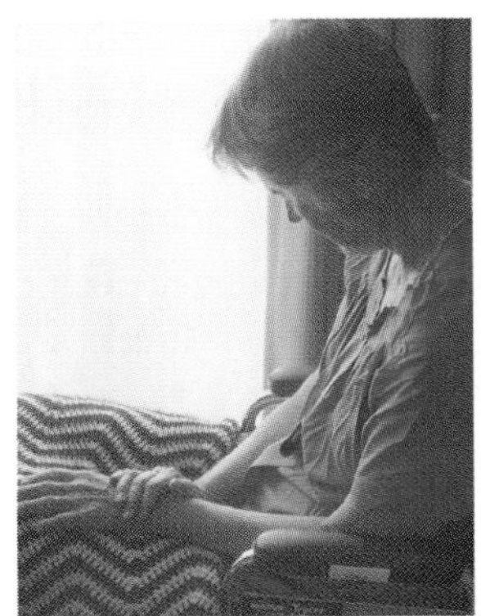
Figure 7-6. **An extra blanket can provide much-needed warmth.**

2. Notify the resident if any hot or cold treatments are to be used on a body part. Communicate with and check the resident every five minutes while the pack is on the skin. In some cases, the nurse will ask that you stay with the resident the entire time the pack is on the body.

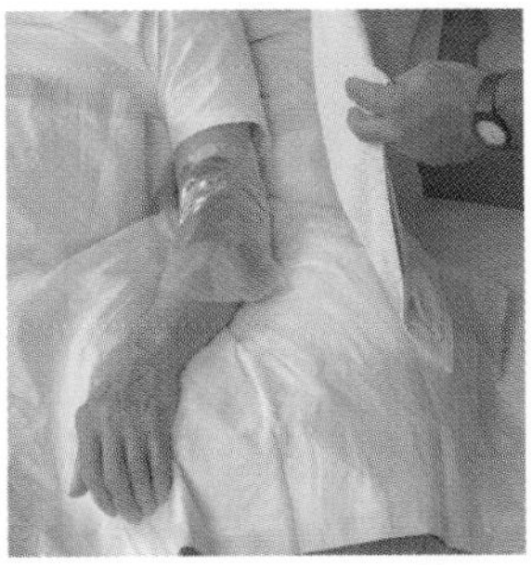

Figure 7-7. **When a hot or cold pack is on the skin, check with the resident often.**

3. Remind the resident to never sit too close to a space heater or radiator.
4. Tell the resident you will stay with her at all times should she choose to use the stove or microwave.
5. Check resident and reposition as ordered to reduce pressure on bony skin areas.
6. Check on and communicate with the resident often during your shift. A resident unable to feel pain can be at extreme risk for injury.
7. Limit access to sharp objects.

7 Identify six communication guidelines for the resident with a cognitive barrier.

The resident with a **cognitive impairment** may have damage to an area of the brain. This damage can be due to a blood clot, trauma, or the closure of blood vessels. The resident's ability to speak and/or understand spoken or written words may be affected. The medical term for this deficit is **aphasia**. There are two types of aphasia. Receptive aphasia is the inability to *understand* what others are communicating through speech or written words. Expressive aphasia is the inability to *express* needs to others through speech or written words. A person with aphasia may be referred to a speech therapist or pathologist for therapy to help him improve his ability to communicate. If the therapist leaves directions for the nursing team on dealing with the person with aphasia, you need to follow your nurse's guidelines regarding those directions.

Communication Guidelines - Aphasia

1. Stand or sit so that the resident can see you.
2. Look at the resident the entire time.
3. Do not shout.
4. Speak clearly.
5. Do not rush the resident.
6. Use special methods as directed by the nurse, such as special communication boards.

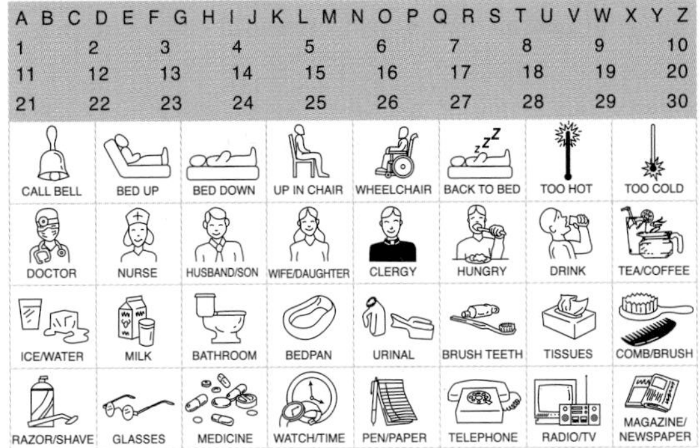

Figure 7-8. **A sample communication board.**

8 Identify five communication guidelines for the comatose resident.

You may be assigned to care for a resident who is comatose. **Coma** is a condition that usually occurs with an illness or injury, in which a person is unable to respond to any change in the environment, including pain. Comatose residents deserve your respect in the same way that an alert resident deserves your respect. Many comatose people come out of their coma and identify that they could hear everything being said while in the coma. So, when caring for a comatose person, remember to follow the guidelines below:

Communication Guidelines - Comatose Resident

1. Introduce yourself when entering the resident's room.
2. Explain each procedure before beginning it.
3. Use touch when explaining a procedure.
4. Do not hold personal discussions during the care of a comatose resident.
5. Announce when you are going to leave the comatose resident's room.

Their ears may still hear!

When caring for a comatose or unconscious resident, appropriate language and topics of conversation should be chosen. Inappropriate personal conversations can be seen as a form of abuse. Leave personal situations and problems at home when caring for all residents.

9 Identify seven communication guidelines for the disoriented and/or confused resident.

A cognitive impairment may also cause a resident to become **disoriented**. This condition may be permanent, due to an injury or disorder in the brain. It can also be a temporary state, due to dehydration or medication. We first discussed orientation in Chapter 6. When a resident is "oriented x 3", it means he can identify who he is and who you are (person), the city, state, and facility he is in (place), and the correct year (time). A resident who is disoriented may not be able to express one or more of these things. A resident may be oriented x 1 to person, or oriented x 2 to place and time. Reality orientation methods (Learning Objective 11) are helpful in reducing a resident's disorientation.

Confusion is a situation where a resident is temporarily or permanently unable to think in an organized or logical manner. Confused residents may not remember to finish eating a meal or may be unable to locate their room. Confusion is often due to a physical problem, such as a lack of proper blood flow to the brain due to not taking medication correctly. It can also be a result of the inability to see or hear well. Other causes include being placed in a strange facility or having a language barrier.

As providers of care, communicate with disoriented or confused residents in the best manner possible.

Communication Guidelines - Disoriented and/or Confused Resident

1. Speak to the resident when greeting him. (Never touch first; this may upset the person.)
2. Look at the resident the entire time you are speaking with him.
3. Do not speak loudly.
4. Use touch if it does not upset the resident.
5. Repeat directions if needed. Use short, simple sentences. Break tasks into steps.
6. Listen to and be patient with the resident. Look at the resident's method of communication and the entire message rather than focusing on the words alone.
7. Announce that you are leaving the area the resident is in. Repeat it twice.

10 Identify eight communication guidelines for residents with dementia and define behaviors related to Alzheimer's disease.

Dementia is defined as a mental disorder resulting from a structural change in the brain. It is *not* a normal result of the aging process. There are different causes of dementia. One cause is a **stroke** or **cerebrovascular accident (CVA)**, a sudden loss of consciousness and possible paralysis caused by a hemorrhage or clot within the brain or a rupture of a blood vessel.

Another cause is **Alzheimer's disease**, a disease which usually strikes people anywhere from middle age to old age. Alzheimer's residents will require more and more care as the illness progresses. They may spend a some time at home being cared for by home caregivers. When this is no longer possible, they are usually placed in a living environment that offers more supervision and care. Eventually the resident will require complete care and will be admitted to a secure unit. Alzheimer's disease is covered in detail in Chapter 27 on nervous system disorders.

Dementia may also be caused by other disorders, including the following:

- **Multi-Infarct Dementia**: numerous strokes causing reduced blood flow and damage to the brain
- Acquired immunodeficiency syndrome (AIDS)
- **Parkinson's Disease**: a chronic nervous system disease with tremors, muscle weakness and rigidity or stiffness and an unusual walk or **gait**

Figure 7-9 identifies the causes of dementia and shows what percentage is due to each of the causes.

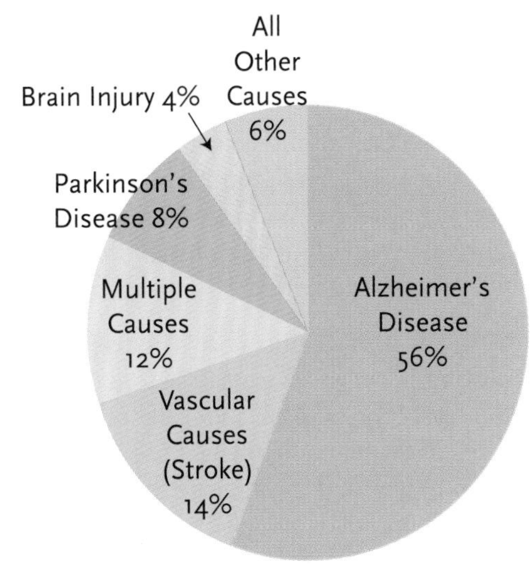

Figure 7-9. **Causes of dementia.**

Dementia can cause a resident to lose his ability to perform activities of daily living (ADLs). Dementia can also put the resident at risk of serious harm because he is no longer able to make good decisions.

Communication Guidelines - Dementia

1. Speak to the resident when greeting him. (Never touch first; this may upset the person.)
2. Look at the resident the entire time you are speaking with him.
3. Do not speak loudly. Be calm.
4. Use touch and gestures if appropriate.
5. Only do one task or talk about one subject at a time. Be patient. Use simple, short sentences.
6. Repeat directions and answers as many times as needed.
7. Use pictures.
8. Praise often.

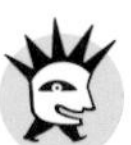

By Carolyn Barge, CNA

Working with Alzheimer's and dementia residents is a very challenging experience. It is important to address individual behaviors. Each resident is different, and you will learn which method works with each one.

I experience something new every day in my unit. You can never walk into the unit and expect the shift to start the same way every day. There are some routines, but I find that no matter how well you plan your time, there is going to be an unexpected event of some sort. You can't allow yourself to get frustrated.

When dealing with residents with Alzheimer's and dementia, you have to be very flexible. They may wake up thinking that their children need to get ready for school. You should simply reassure them that their children have been taken care of and are at school.

Most of all I believe that you have to really listen to what your residents are saying. They may say something like "I hurt," and telling them that you will ask the nurse to give them something may not be an adequate response. Be specific. Ask where it hurts and see how the person responds.

There are many ways to work effectively with these residents. Be flexible, calm, friendly, and know when to leave and re-approach if a resident is agitated or upset.

I have become very attached to my residents. The love they give back is tenfold to anything that I can provide for them. They are like another family to me. I've had some wonderful conversations with them, and each has meant so much.

Understand your residents, and you will have one of the best and most fulfilling experiences of your life. I do!

Behaviors associated with Alzheimer's disease include the following:

- **agitation**: restless or excited behavior.
- **anxiety**: apprehension, worry, uneasiness.
- **catastrophic reactions**: an overreaction to a stimulus or trigger.
- **clinging**: holding onto others.
- **combativeness**: attacking others in some way.
- **delusions/hallucinations**: believing things that are not true; seeing things that are not there.
- **inappropriate sexual behaviors**: disrobing, touching others or themselves inappropriately.
- **perseveration**: frequent repetition of words, phrases, questions, or actions.
- **rummaging/hoarding**: hiding trivial things like medicine cups, straws; going through drawers and closets.
- **sleep disturbance**: inability to sleep or waking up suddenly.

- **sundowning**: increased agitation and restlessness in the evening hours.
- **suspiciousness**: accusing others of stealing.
- **wandering/pacing**: walking around constantly; walking back and forth over and over again.

11 Explain reality orientation and identify nine guidelines for using it.

Reality orientation is a method of reducing confusion or disorientation in some residents. These methods are usually **integrated** into the everyday care of the residents. It is used with residents who are confused, disoriented or in the early stages of Alzheimer's disease. Reality orientation uses calendars, clocks, signs, and lists to reorient the resident to person, place, and time.

Guidelines - Reality Orientation

Awareness of person

1. Call the resident by name.
2. Always identify yourself.
3. Ask about family, pictures, or personal items.

Awareness of place

4. Ask about activities.
5. Inquire about recent meals.
6. Use newspapers, magazines, TV, and radio to reorient the resident to current events.

Awareness of time

7. Use clocks and calendars to reorient the resident to time. Maintain the day-night cycle.
8. Use the date and time when providing care.
9. Mention seasons or months when selecting clothes or when looking out the window.

Remember that reality orientation happens all day during all kinds of care activities.

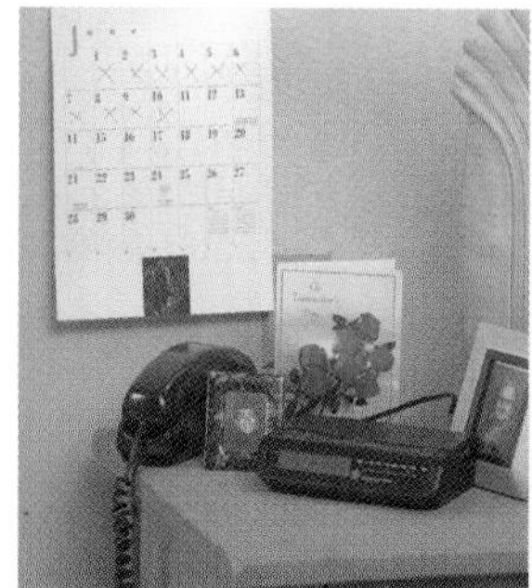

Figure 7-10. A calendar and clock can help a resident remain oriented.

12 Explain validation therapy and give two examples of it.

Validation therapy is an approach used for residents with advanced dementia. "Validating" means giving value to or approving, and making no attempt to reorient the resident to actual circumstances. Validation therapy attempts to "play along" with your resident's fantasies. Some examples of validation therapy are listed below.

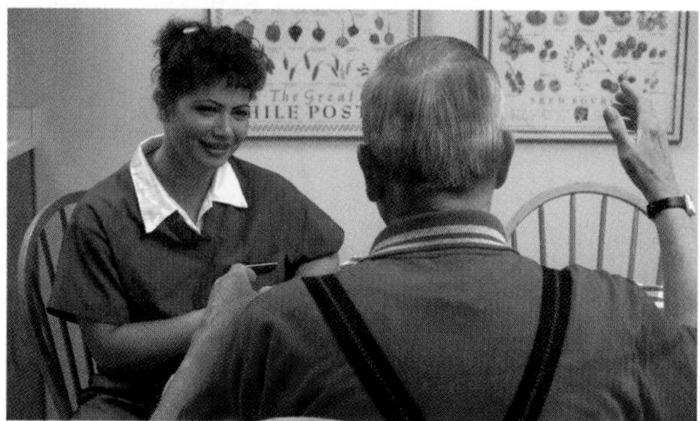

Figure 7-11. Validation therapy is accepting a resident's fantasies without attempting to reorient him to reality.

1. Resident Amy Montego comes to you and says she is late for "prom." You quietly ask her about the color of her dress and to describe it. This allows her to work through the memory without forcing her back to reality.
2. Resident Josiah Hinson says he has to finish picking his crop of broccoli before the upcoming frost hits. You ask about the number of acres of farmland he owns. He expresses his accomplishments as a farmer and speaks with pride about his land.

Handling these situations in this fashion combines validation therapy with reminiscence therapy, a technique used to discuss memories from long ago in a positive manner. The resident may emerge from the episode feeling good about herself and her past. This can improve the resident's self-image.

Reality may be too much to handle!

Using reality orientation for residents in advanced stages of dementia can be frustrating for these residents. It can result in catastrophic reactions. Creating a stressful environment must be avoided. Validation therapy may be a better approach for these residents.

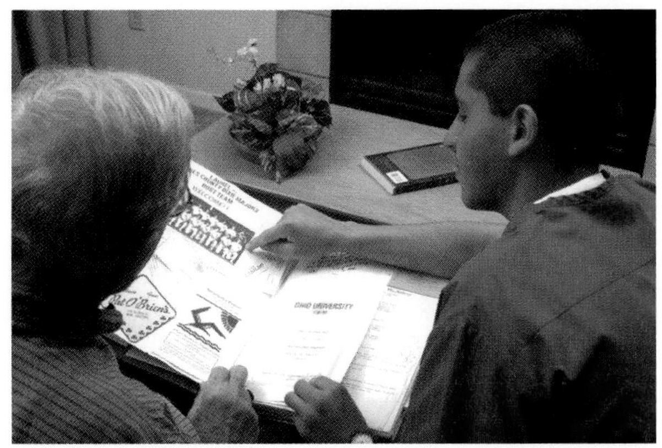

Figure 7-12. **Reminiscence therapy is encouraging a client to remember and talk about an important time in his past.**

13 Identify twelve communication guidelines for the resident with functional barriers.

Residents may have a functional problem that interferes with their ability to speak. Some of the main causes of problems are difficulty in breathing, physical problems with the mouth or lips, or an **artificial airway**.

Difficulty Breathing

When dealing with a resident who has difficulty breathing, never push the resident to speak. It can make breathing even more difficult. Allow plenty of time between words and sentences. Help a resident with breathing problems using the following:

1. Allow the resident enough time to speak. Be patient.
2. Ask the resident to write down anything you do not understand.
3. Do not tire the resident. Use a writing board if the resident becomes tired.
4. Never remove a resident's oxygen for any reason. Only nurses do this.
5. If needed, ask the nurse to apply oxygen if ordered p.r.n. (when necessary.)

Physical Problems with the Lips, Mouth and Tongue

Some of the problems with the mouth area that make speech difficult include the following:

- lip, mouth or tongue sores of any kind
- dental problems of any kind, including missing teeth and dental work, poorly-fitting dentures
- birth defects like cleft palate
- paralysis of one side of the mouth

Communication guidelines for a resident with physical problems related to the mouth are:

1. If able to speak, allow enough time to speak. Be patient.
2. Ask the resident to write down anything you do not understand.
3. Never tire the resident. Use a writing board if resident becomes tired.
4. Report mouth sores, poorly-fitting dentures, or complaints of mouth pain to the nurse.

Artificial Airway

An **airway** is the natural passageway for air to move into and out of the lungs. A resident with an artificial airway will have a tube placed into the airway to allow him to breathe through an opening in the neck. Residents will sometimes have an artificial airway due to a blockage somewhere in their natural airway. This blockage prevents them from breathing normally.

One type of artificial airway is called a **tracheostomy**. An opening is made surgically directly into the trachea (windpipe) for the air to reach his lungs. This may be done because a resident cannot breathe normally through the nose.

Communication guidelines for a resident with a tracheostomy include the following.

1. If able to speak, allow time to speak. Listen closely and be patient.
2. If able to write, use a writing board, pad, or a communication board.
3. If unable to speak or write, use other methods such as nodding or eye-blinking for "Yes" and "No." (One blink for "yes," and two blinks for "no.")

14 Identify seven communication guidelines used with a paralyzed resident.

A person who is paralyzed may not be able to communicate effectively. The area of the body that is paralyzed will determine the extent of the communication problem. A person with **hemiplegia** has paralysis on one side of the body. A **paraplegic**, a person who has paralysis of the lower portion of the body and both legs, may have the full use of his hands and his speech.

A **quadriplegic**, a person who has paralysis of the arms, legs, and trunk of the body, may require special methods of communication. Methods for communicating with paralyzed residents are outlined below.

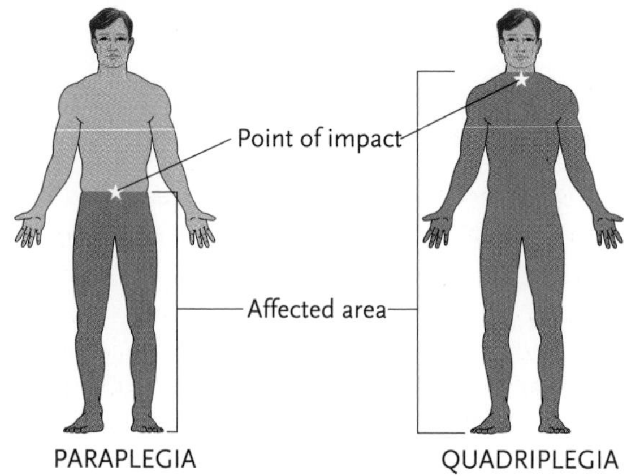

Figure 7-13.

Communication Guidelines - Paralyzed Resident

1. Determine whether the resident can speak and/or write.
2. If able to speak, allow time to speak. Listen closely and be patient.
3. If able to write, allow enough time.
4. Politely ask to repeat or rewrite anything you do not understand.
5. If unable to speak or write, use other methods such as nodding or blinking for "Yes" and "No."
6. Use a communication board for more complex questions.
7. Use praise often.

15 List seven defense mechanisms used as methods of coping with stress.

Communicating with residents under stress must be done with a great deal of empathy and sensitivity. Words must be carefully chosen so that you do not increase the person's stress level. Residents who are under a great deal of stress may use **defense mechanisms**, unconscious behaviors used to help a person cope with conflict or stress. Defense mechanisms allow a resident to release tension that has built up due to stress. To help you communicate with residents under stress, it is helpful to understand defense mechanisms.

Defense mechanisms prevent the person from facing the real reason some situation has occurred. For example, when a resident complains of a stomachache for three days, the focus tends to be on that ache. The real reason she may be complaining is that she is afraid to go to the dayroom due to the unwanted attentions of another resident.

Here are some definitions and examples of defense mechanisms:

Conversion: changing a conflict within to a physical symptom. A male resident develops a stomachache each day before dinner to avoid a new resident he finds obnoxious.

Denial: blocking reality. A resident tells the staff that the lab made a mistake with her diagnosis of cancer.

Displacement: transferring a strong feeling to a less threatening object. A female resident who had a fight with her son might yell at the nursing staff.

Projection: identifying feelings in others that are actually feelings within oneself. A resident calls a friend "gossipy" while she is telling secrets about that friend.

Rationalization: making excuses. An elderly man fails a driving test and says the tester was "unfair."

Repression: excluding painful events from conscious thought. A woman develops amnesia about abuse she suffered as a child.

Regression: going back to behavior from the past for comfort. A male resident who is stressed starts to rhythmically rock, a childhood coping mechanism.

16 List four levels of anxiety and identify eight communication guidelines used with the anxious or fearful resident.

When one becomes anxious, one develops an uneasy or apprehensive feeling. Feeling anxious is not the same as feeling afraid. With fear, one is dealing with the present time. Anxiety comes in dealing with the future, which is unknown. The resident who is fearful is dealing with a threat of some kind. The resident's fear may or may not be real.

There are four levels of anxiety:

1. Mild anxiety

2. Moderate anxiety
3. Severe anxiety
4. Panic

The signs and symptoms increase from one level to another, and a person who is panicking (Level 4) may not be able to focus on reality. There are physical symptoms of intense anxiety which include shakiness, sweating, and a racing heart. The goal of communicating with the anxious person is to reduce the overall level of anxiety and stress.

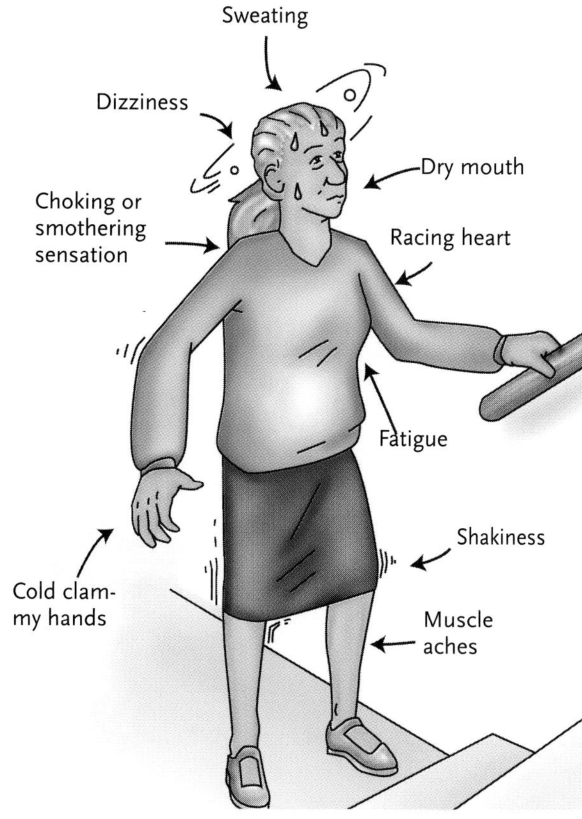

Figure 7-14. **Common symptoms of anxiety.**

Communication Guidelines - Anxiety or Fear

1. Speak to the resident when greeting him. (Never touch first; this may upset the person.)
2. Do not speak loudly, as it may upset the person. Reduce noise.
3. Speak slowly and calmly.
4. Use touch if it does not upset the person.
5. Listen to and be patient with the resident. Ask gentle questions to try to identify the fear.
6. Be empathetic. Be calm and reassuring.
7. Avoid demanding behavior.
8. Reassure resident he is safe.

17 Identify five communication guidelines used with the depressed resident.

You will care for many residents who show some signs of depression. Depression is an illness that can be controlled or even cured. Residents who have recently relocated to a facility may begin to show some signs of depression. Consider for a moment the changes and personal losses the resident has experienced. Personal losses include loss of spouse, family, and friends. Other losses include the loss of health, independence, mobility, and the ability to care for oneself. People may have to move out of a lifetime home and into a facility full of strangers.

Residents may not have any family members nearby, or close family may not choose to visit them. They will probably have to share a room with someone for the first time in their lives. One of these factors can be enough to make a person depressed. However, residents may have to deal with all of these problems. It is not surprising if they become depressed. Your role is to be there for your residents to help them through depressed periods. Try to make each day as pleasant an experience as possible.

Communication Guidelines - Depression

1. Greet the resident with a smile if appropriate. Be pleasant and supportive.
2. Use touch cautiously to help comfort the resident. Consider cultural differences before using touch.
3. Sit down and listen to the resident. Lean forward and keep good eye contact. This body language helps show you are interested.

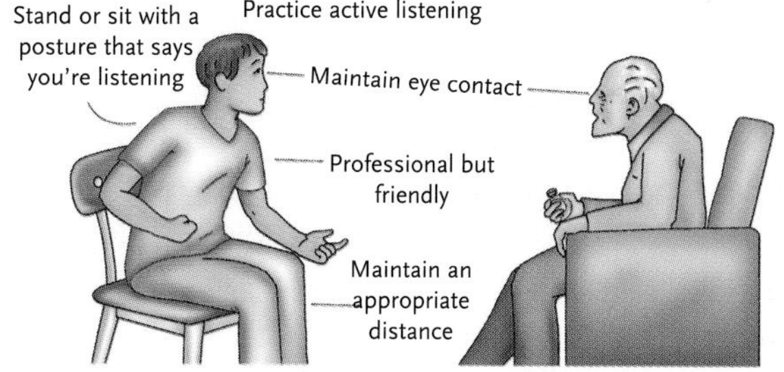

Figure 7-15. **Practice good communication skills with depressed residents.**

4. Think before you speak. Try to empathize with the resident's feelings and situation.

5. Report a depressed resident to the nurse immediately. The staff may contact a physician, a family member or friend, or a clergy member. Watch for any signs of depression in your residents. Use the acronym "SOMBER," identified below to remember these signs. The word "somber" means dark or shadowy, or having feelings of gloom or melancholy.

SOMBER

Sleep: unusual fatigue or tiredness, insomnia

Other physical changes: headaches or constipation

Mood: a feeling of sadness that may seem overwhelming, irritability, crying, suicidal feelings or thoughts

Behavior: lack of an ability to make simple decisions, lack of concentration, socially withdrawing from others, lack of desire to join in activities, repetitious behavior, feelings of low self-esteem or worthlessness

Eating: anorexia, weight loss

Relationships: lack of sexual desire, lack of interest in socializing

Depression may also cause low blood oxygen levels, malnutrition, fever, and infections.

18 Identify seven communication guidelines used with the angry resident.

Anger can be difficult to defuse. It has to be handled very carefully in order to not increase the person's anger. At the first sign of anger in a resident, it may be best to inform the nurse so that he can be aware and assist you with the situation. Sometimes it will be necessary to call for security, if that is an option within your facility.

At times, a resident's anger makes the person seem overly demanding, requiring more time than the average person. When this occurs, the nursing staff may schedule a care conference to discuss the demanding behavior. Care plans can be developed to reduce the behavior. Your input at a care conference is valuable. Offer any helpful ideas and suggestions to identify the cause of the anger and to relieve it.

Communication Guidelines - Anger

1. Greet the resident. Be pleasant and supportive.
2. Say to the resident, "I am here for you. What can I do to help you?"
3. Listen closely to the exact words the resident chooses. Determine what triggered the anger.
4. Watch the resident's body language.
5. Think before you speak. Try to empathize with the resident's feelings and situation. Remain calm and speak in a normal tone. Consider your responses carefully.
6. If the resident's anger increases, get the nurse and/or security immediately.
7. Try to involve the resident in activities if she is willing, such as taking a walk, drawing pictures, or listening to music.

19 Identify seven communication guidelines used with the combative resident.

When anger increases, a resident may become combative. A combative resident is a threat to you, other staff, residents, and visitors. Your responsibility is to keep everyone safe. If you sense a resident's anger is worsening, call for the nurse immediately to assist you with the situation. Combative behavior requires special techniques.

Communication Guidelines - Combative Residents

1. Call the nurse when you sense anger increasing.
2. A decision may need to be made to call security (if available to you).
3. Keep yourself and other people at a safe distance from the resident.
4. Stay calm. Do not appear threatening to the resident. NEVER HIT BACK!
5. Offer reassurance to the resident.
6. Follow direction of the nurses.
7. When anger passes, sit with the resident for a while to provide comfort if instructed to do so.

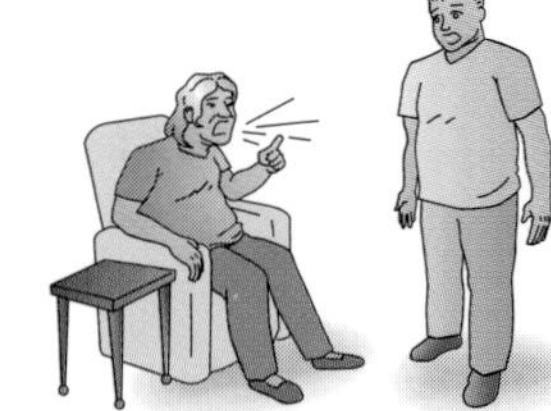

Figure 7-16. **Stay calm and keep yourself at a safe distance when dealing with a combative resident.**

Never hit a resident!

Unfortunately, it is not uncommon to read or hear about physical abuse of the elderly by paid or unpaid caregivers. These caregivers may be family, friends, or healthcare team members. Many times, physical abuse is due to stressful situations causing the caregiver to lash out quickly. It is important that you know you can never hit a resident, NO MATTER WHAT. Even if a resident strikes you first, you may not strike back. Hitting residents can cause serious physical harm. Residents are usually quite frail. Bones may be broken and other serious internal injuries may occur.

In addition, if you strike a resident, you will most likely be terminated. Serious charges may be filed by the authorities. Hitting a resident is inappropriate and against the law.

If you feel that your impulses are out of control, get help, or ask for advice. Put some distance between you and the situation.

20 Explain why residents may show sexually-aggressive behavior and identify six communication guidelines for handling it.

Older adults, like all humans, are sexual. They have the right to express their sexuality, and their choices about sexuality are as varied as those of any other age group. However, sometimes residents' behavior does not seem normal or makes you or others uncomfortable. This behavior may be identified as sexually aggressive. Sexually-aggressive behavior in front of the staff or other residents is due to many reasons.

1. Illness or disability may cause residents to be unable to perform sexually. They may wish to try to attract the attention of others to show that they are still able to function sexually.
2. Illness may make the person behave much differently than he would have in the past. Dementia may be a factor, because a person with dementia loses certain abilities of reasoning and judgment. When a person has difficulty distinguishing between appropriate and inappropriate behavior, errors in judgement may occur. Prior to the changes in the brain caused by dementia, certain behaviors would never have occurred. Some of these behaviors are sexual in nature.

Communication Guidelines - Sexually-Aggressive Residents

1. Ask a co-worker to go into the room with you, if advised.
2. Report all sexually-aggressive behavior to your supervisor.
3. Inform the resident that this behavior is inappropriate and ask that he or she stop.
4. Reinforce positive behavior of the resident.
5. Listen to the resident if he or she shows a sign of wishing to talk.
6. Do not judge the resident's behavior.

All human beings need love and affection. Aging can affect a person's ability to express sexual needs and limit his access to partners. Residents have the right to engage in mutually-agreed-upon sexual relationships. Residents also have the right to masturbate, which means sexual self-stimulation. If you witness either of these situations, be sensitive. Provide privacy. Do not make fun of the situation.

Summary

Communicating effectively can be a challenge with some residents. Residents must all be treated in such a fashion that they understand everything that will be done to them each and every day. In order to make sure that your residents understand all that you will do, you must become familiar with the different communication challenges you will encounter in a facility. Once you are familiar with these special communication needs and methods, you will feel more prepared when dealing with the various types of residents in a facility.

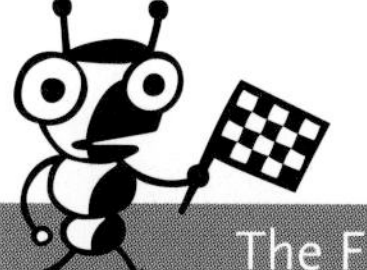

The Finish Line

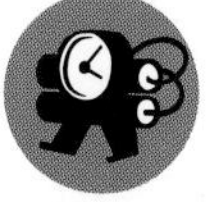

What's Wrong With This Picture?

The following are all examples of defense mechanisms. The wrong defense mechanism has been identified. Correct the errors.

1. A resident has been diagnosed with lung cancer. The resident chooses not to believe this. The nurse recognizes that the resident is using the defense mechanism called displacement.
2. A resident avoids going to her favorite activity,

shuffleboard, by saying she has shoulder pain because she does not like the new activity director. The nurse recognizes that the resident is using the defense mechanism called denial.

3. A nursing staff member comes to work in a very angry mood after coming her divorce hearing. The other staff members recognize that this team member is using the defense mechanism called repression.

4. A new resident was just weighed. She informed the staff that the scale must be broken because she has never been that weight. You note the weight prior to admission to be within two pounds of this new weight. The nurse recognizes that the resident is using the defense mechanism called conversion.

5. A resident comes back from church, throws her sweater on the bed, and promptly yells at her roommate to turn her music down. You find out her close male friend did not sit next to her in church; he in fact sat next to another female resident. You recognize that this resident is using the defense mechanism called projection.

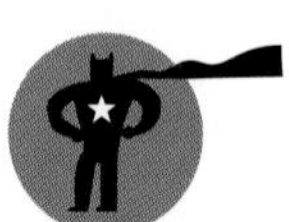

Star Student Central

1. Spend some time with a person you know who has a visual deficit. Take notes on the difficulties and risks associated with having a visual deficit and share them with your class.

2. Spend some time with a person who has a hearing deficit. Take notes on the difficulties and risks associated with having a hearing loss and share them with your class.

3. Role-play using some of the types of residents covered in this chapter. Each student should choose one type of resident and "be the resident." Make up different scenarios, and decide how the person being the caregiver should respond. Choose from:
   - resident with a visual deficit
   - resident with a hearing deficit
   - fearful resident
   - depressed resident
   - angry or demanding resident
   - combative resident

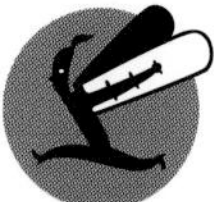

You Can Do It Corner!

1. What should you do first when dealing with a resident with a visual deficit? (LO 4)

2. What is reality orientation? Should it be used in the early or late state of Alzheimer's? (LO 11)

3. What are nine barriers to communication? (LO 2)

4. What types of dangers would a resident with the inability to feel have? (LO 6)

5. What steps should you take upon arriving at the bedside of a comatose resident? (LO 8)

6. If a resident is unable to speak or write, what are two other methods of communication you can use? (LO 13)

7. What are the two types of aphasia? What do they mean? (LO 7)

8. If a resident becomes combative, what steps can you take? (LO 19)

9. What is the leading cause of dementia? (LO 10)

10. What is the difference between paraplegia and quadriplegia? (LO 14)

11. What does the acronym "SOMBER" mean as it relates to signs of depression? (LO 17)

12. What is the defense mechanism "projection"? (LO 15)

13. What does validation therapy attempt to do? (LO 12)

14. What are two considerations you must make concerning other cultures? (LO 3)

15. What kind of input would be valuable for you to have at care conference concerning a resident's anger? (LO 18)

16. What are six steps to take with a sexually aggressive resident? (LO 20)

17. What are four levels of anxiety? (LO 16)

18. What does "disoriented" mean? (LO 9)

19. What is the first step in communicating with a resident who has a hearing deficit? (LO 5)

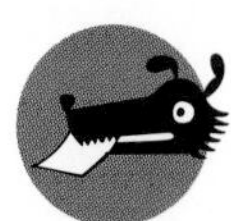

Star Student's Chapter Checklist

1. I have read my textbook chapter.
2. I have reviewed my own "Pocketful of Terms."
3. I have listened to my tutor tape.
4. I have reviewed and highlighted my class notes.
5. I have read and completed any handouts from this chapter.
6. I have completed "The Finish Line."
7. Star Time! Choose your reward!

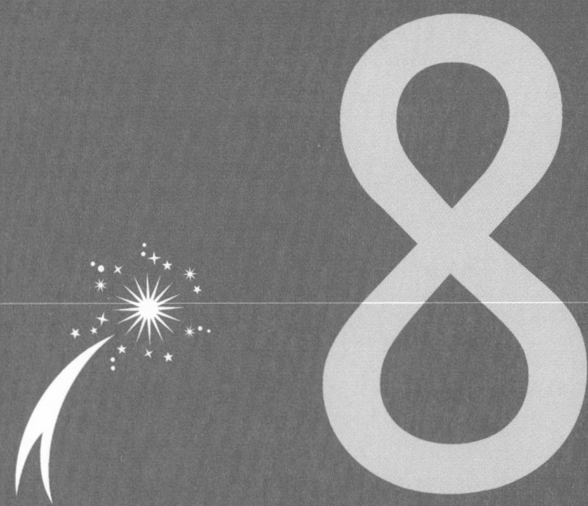

A View from the Top: The Healthy Mind

Look Like a Star!

Look at the Learning Objectives and The Finish Line before you begin reading this chapter.

Look at your pocket calendar.
With your pencil, put a bracket ( ) around a study period every single day.

Look at your homework for this chapter.
Plug each piece of homework into a certain time slot.

Look at the Star Student's Chapter Checklist at the end of this chapter. Check off each item as it is completed.

"Old age, especially an honored old age, has so great authority, that this is of more value than all the pleasures of youth."

Marcus Tullius Cicero, 106-43 B.C.

"The harvest of old age is the recollection and abundance of blessings previously secured."

Marcus Tullius Cicero, 106-43 B.C.

Learning Objectives

1. **Spell and define all STAR words.**
2. **Explain the concepts of health and wellness.**
3. **Define "holistic care" and explain its importance in health care.**
4. **Discuss Maslow's Hierarchy of Needs.**
5. **Identify Maslow's 15 traits of a self-actualizing person.**
6. **Define and discuss psychology and personality.**
7. **Identify two attitudes or personality types shown by most people.**
8. **List the eight basic types of human emotions.**
9. **Discuss Erikson's eight stages of psychosocial development.**
10. **Describe the stages of growth and development and the developmental tasks that relate to each stage.**

The Roots of Psychology

The science of psychology started in the mid-1800s. Psychology is the science that deals with mental processes. An early philosopher named Wilhelm Wundt founded the first psychological laboratory in 1879 and wrote that the mind needed to be studied. Another early professor of psychology, Edward Titchener, who earned a position at Cornell University, said that psychology is "the science of consciousness." The work of Sigmund Freud did not become well-known until the 1920s. Freud developed "psychoanalysis," the idea that behavior is controlled by hidden motives and unconscious desires, and that it may be treated with psychotherapy.

1 Spell and define all STAR words.

adulthood: the period when a person is fully developed and mature.

developmental psychology: the study of the developmental changes that occur in people as they age.

developmental task: a task a person must accomplish in one of the developmental stages.

emotions: strong feelings.

extrovert: an outgoing person.

health: sound physical and mental condition.

holistic: care involving the entire person, including her physical, emotional, spiritual, and social needs.

inferiority complex: when one feels inferior to (less important than) others.

introvert: a reserved or shy person.

need: something necessary or required.

persona: outer attitude or appearance, the one shown to others.

personality: emotional and behavioral traits that characterize a person.

psychology: science dealing with mental processes.

psychosocial: relating to the mental and social aspects of a human.

puberty: the period when a male or female becomes capable of reproduction.

trait: characteristic of an individual.

wellness: state of well-being.

2 Explain the concepts of health and wellness.

The World Health Organization has defined the word **health** as "a state of complete physical, mental, and social well-being, and not merely the absence of disease or infirmity." This view of health looks at the functioning of the whole person. It also takes the focus off disease and redirects it to healthy attitudes and lifestyle. In recent years, we have seen an explosion of information on health, wellness, and healthy living.

Wellness has to do with successfully balancing everything that happens in our everyday lives. Five dimensions of wellness have been defined: physical, social, emotional, intellectual, and spiritual. The physical dimension of wellness includes things like being able to complete everyday tasks. The social dimension has to do with relating to other people. The emotional dimension covers managing stress and expressing feelings. The intellectual dimension deals with growing and learning throughout life. The spiritual dimension includes a person's religious beliefs, ethics, values, and moral development.

3 Define "holistic care" and explain its importance in health care.

The nursing profession looks at a resident from a **holistic** standpoint. The term "holistic" comes from the Greek term that means "whole." Health care today is formed around the thought that harmony in one's life promotes good health. If a disturbance of some kind occurs, the disharmony that results can cause illness. So when we care for a resident, we look at the entire person, including her physical, **psychosocial**, and spiritual needs. This can improve a resident's chances of living to the fullest extent possible.

4 Discuss Maslow's Hierarchy of Needs.

Abraham Maslow, a psychologist, developed a model to describe what he believed to be the five basic human needs. A **need** is something necessary for a person in order to survive and grow. The lower-level needs on the pyramid are the ones that must be met in order to survive. These needs must be met before higher needs can be attempted. Figure 8-1 shows Maslow's Hierarchy of Needs.

The first needs you must help your residents meet are physical needs, like air, food and water, rest, and sleep. If a resident cannot breathe, this becomes the focus of every waking moment. He cannot reach the next level until he is able to meet that basic need and take a simple breath. We cannot understand how terrifying it is to be unable to take a breath until we see someone in that position.

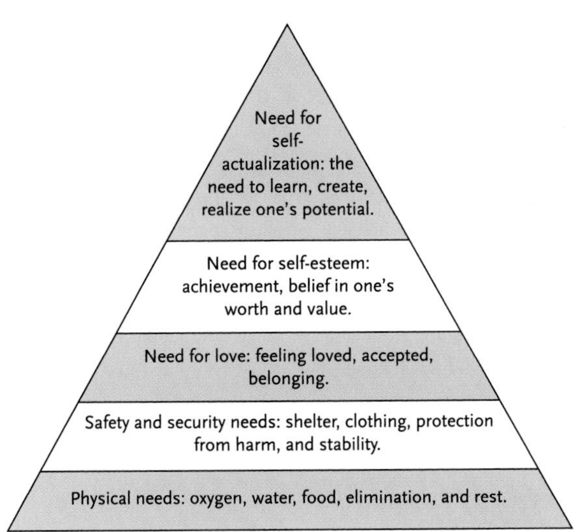

Figure 8-1. Maslow's Hierarchy of Needs.

Ensuring Easy Access to Food and Drink

Refusing to help residents meet some of their basic needs—eating and drinking—is abuse. When food is delivered to residents' rooms, the trays must be set up in a timely manner. Residents must have their trays prepared so they can eat as easily as possible. Not bothering to open a milk carton or to cut the meat on a plate can prevent a resident from eating all of the food needed. This can be considered abuse.

The second level is safety and security, which has to do with a resident's feelings of being secure throughout each day. When a resident no longer has the security of being in her own home, she may feel very uneasy. It can be upsetting to suddenly move to a care facility filled with strangers. New residents may find it difficult to adapt to this new environment, and they may need a lot of time to get used to it.

If residents are unable to feel comfortable, safe, and secure throughout the day, this prevents them from reaching the next step on the needs chart. Nursing assistants can assist residents in their adjustment to their new home by providing excellent care and encouraging them to interact with other residents and staff.

The third level is love and belonging. In your life, you may hug and kiss family members, friends, and even pets often. When people move into a care facility, they may be separated from their loved ones. If they were used to hugs, kisses, and other physical expressions of love and caring, then living in a new place full of strangers could be very lonely.

Residents need to feel as if they belong in their new home. This is why it is so important for you to welcome them and try to help them develop relationships with as many other residents and staff members as possible. The relationships between residents and staff are different from the resident-to-resident relationships, but they are just as important.

The fourth level is the need for self-esteem. Residents may feel less of a sense of self-worth due to the fact they are more dependent on others. They will need help with tasks they have performed alone all their lives. This is one of the reasons that they must be allowed to continue to be as independent as possible. The more your residents can care for themselves, the better they will feel about themselves. Praising achievements, no matter how small, maintains dignity and self-esteem.

Self-actualization is the highest need a person can achieve. In order to get to this level, the person must reach maximum potential. Human beings rarely reach this level in every single part of their lives. Residents will each be at different stages in this process. Some residents may seem content with the level they have reached in life, spending their days quietly watching television or reading. Other residents might still be striving to do more, whether by helping other residents read mail or write letters, or helping out at the facility gift shop.

Spiritual Needs

Residents will have different spiritual needs. Spirituality or spiritual belief has been defined as believing in a higher power, creative force, divine being, or infinite source of energy. Spirituality has also been defined as all behaviors that give meaning to life and provide strength for individuals.

Residents may have strong beliefs in God or very little or no belief in a higher power. Residents may consider themselves spiritual, but may not believe in God or a higher power. The important thing for nursing assistants to remember is to respect all residents' beliefs, **whatever they are.** Making judgments regarding residents' spiritual beliefs or trying to push your beliefs upon any resident is not appropriate.

Older residents may begin to consider the life they have led as a whole and may start coming to terms with the end of life. There are many things a nursing assistant can do to assist residents with their spiritual needs. Some of these things follow.

1. When a resident asks for a clergyperson, you must handle this request immediately.

★ *"Don't Delay. Report Right Away!"*
A nursing assistant who receives such a request must follow the proper channels to obtain the services of the religious person as soon as possible. Any delay may mean the clergyperson could arrive after it is too late.

2. Sometimes residents may ask to pay a visit to a chapel. Many facilities have chapels available for use by residents and staff. A request such as this must also be handled promptly. Residents may wish to say prayers, and these prayers might be very important to the residents. Residents may also wish to bring religious items such as books, beads, or jewelry with them. Make sure you handle these items carefully.
3. Residents may simply want to talk to someone about their fears or concerns. Sometimes you are the single best person to meet this need. It may be important for you to spend time **listening** to the resident's concerns. You may want to respond only when it seems important, such as when comfort is needed by the resident.

Spiritual needs are different for each person. When you respect and provide support for each resident's individual spiritual concerns, you are helping to meet their needs.

Sexual Needs

Humans are sexual beings, and will have sexual needs until they die. Sexuality is a very important part of every human being. Sexuality is not just about having sex. Sex and sexuality have been defined in the following way: sex is defined as something we do, while sexuality is something we are. Sexual identity or orientation, defined as a person's desire for one sex or the other, plays a big part in each individual's sexuality.

Sexual Orientation: Terms Defining Sexual Identity

Heterosexual: A person who has a desire for a person of the opposite sex.

Homosexual: A person who has a desire for a person of the same sex.

Bisexual: A person who has a desire for persons of both sexes.

Transsexual: A person who believes he or she was not born in the "correct" physical body. This person may seek a sex-change operation.

A common myth is that elderly people no longer have sexual needs or desires. On the contrary, residents living at home or in a facility continue to have sexual needs. They do not leave their sexuality at the door of the facility. Many things can affect residents' sexuality and sexual needs. Culture and religion may play a big part in determining a resident's sexual identity. The way a person is raised also plays a part in his or her sexuality, along with experiences in school and in the surrounding community.

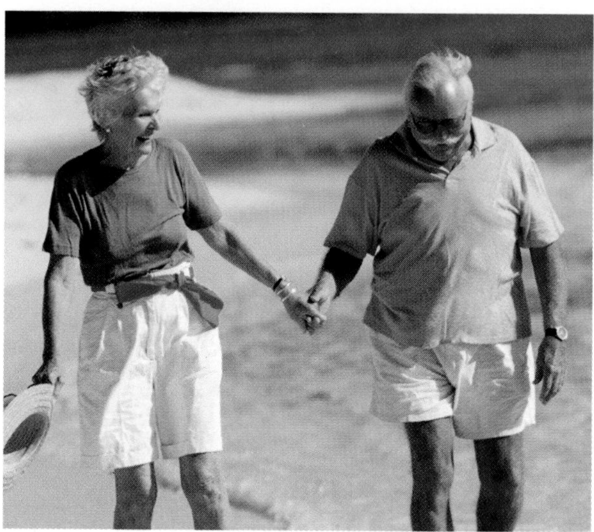

Figure 8-2. **Human beings continue to have sexual needs throughout their lives.**

Because residents continue to have sexual needs, healthcare team members may frequently have to deal with situations that can cause embarrassment for staff and other residents. *The best way to handle sexual needs is to remember that the facility in which your residents live is their home.* People in a facility may behave in a somewhat free and open manner sexually, as if it were the home they had lived in for a long time. It is best not to judge any resident's sexual behavior and to allow for privacy whenever a sexual situation occurs. If a situation is disturbing or inappropriate, ask your supervisor for assistance. Tips on dealing with the sexually-aggressive resident are discussed in Chapter 7.

Illness may affect residents' sexual expressions. A resident's ability to express him- or herself sexually may have changed due to illness or disease. If you encounter this situation, it is best to report it to the nurse. The nurse may arrange for the resident to receive special help from an expert on sexuality, who may be able to assist the resident in adapting to the illness or disease in the best way possible. This may decrease residents' chances of becoming depressed or upset due to the physical and sexual changes.

5 Identify Maslow's 15 traits of a self-actualizing person.

Abraham Maslow also developed a chart describing "the self-actualizing person" as someone who is well-adjusted. People differ on the definition of "well-adjusted." Maslow believed that people who appear well-adjusted try to maximize their own growth and potential. Some view the well-adjusted person as someone who can fit into society as a whole. For example, when a person disregards his neighbors and has loud parties, some might feel he has not adjusted well to **adulthood** and its responsibilities.

In Box 8-1, you will see that Maslow identified 15 traits of a self-actualizing person. He put this list together by looking closely at certain famous people and a set of students in college. It would be difficult for someone to show all of these traits all of the time. In addition, a person who shows all of these traits is not necessarily the "perfect" being. This simply means that the person is interested in self-actualizing and striving every day to accomplish it.

Traits of a Self-Actualizing Person — Box 8-1

EFFICIENT PERCEPTIONS OF REALITY: The self-actualizing person is realistically oriented and comfortable with his perceptions of reality.

ACCEPTANCE OF SELF AND OTHERS: The self-actualizing person accepts herself, other people, and the world the way they are.

SPONTANEITY: The self-actualizing person is spontaneous.

PROBLEM CENTERING: The self-actualizing person focuses on problems outside of himself. He is problem-centered rather than self-centered.

PRIVACY: The self-actualizing person is comfortable being alone and needs her privacy.

AUTONOMY: The self-actualizing person is not controlled by others or by outside forces. He is independent.

FRESHNESS OF APPRECIATION: The self-actualizing person is continually appreciating people and things. This appreciation is fresh, rather than stereotypical.

PEAK EXPERIENCES: The self-actualizing person has profound and transforming spiritual and mystical experiences. These experiences are not necessarily religious.

IDENTIFICATION WITH HUMANITY: The self-actualizing person identifies with others.

INTERPERSONAL RELATIONSHIPS: The self-actualizing person has deeply meaningful, intimate relationships with a few beloved people.

DEMOCRATIC VALUES AND ATTITUDES: The self-actualizing person has democratic values and attitudes and is able to learn from everyone.

DISCRIMINATION BETWEEN MEANS AND ENDS, GOOD AND EVIL: The self-actualizing person knows the difference between good and evil. She does not confuse means with ends. She is able to appreciate doing good as end unto itself and does not require appreciation or acknowledgment.

UNHOSTILE SENSE OF HUMOR: The self-actualizing person has a philosophical, rather than hostile, sense of humor. He does not make jokes that hurt other people.

CREATIVITY: The self-actualizing person is driven to create. She is original and less conventional.

RESISTANCE TO ENCULTURATION: The self-actualizing person resists conforming to the culture. He is able to look past his environment.

6 Define and discuss psychology and personality.

Psychology is defined as the scientific study of behavior and mental processes. The goal of psychology is to use scientific methods to obtain answers to psychological questions. Psychologists collect information through observation. There are many divisions in the field of psychology. For example, physiological psychology deals with the way the physical body affects a person's behavior. The study of abnormal behavior is identified as clinical psychology.

Developmental psychology is the study of how people change throughout their lives. This study looks at the stages in a person's life and the way a person develops in each stage. Personality psychology looks at the different **traits** people exhibit.

Personality is described as a person's unique pattern of behavior over a period of time. Each person has his or her own unique personality. This is what makes us so different from one another.

Sigmund Freud, founder of psychoanalysis, who lived from the late 1800s until the early 1900s, developed well-known theories about personality. Psychoanalysis is based on the belief that the meanings of personal experiences often remain unacknowledged. Freud believed that these meanings contribute greatly to the factors that determine emotions and behavior. He believed that the behavior of humans comes from drives, or unconscious instincts. Some of the terms first used by Freud are ego, id, superego, and the unconscious. The id deals with urges and desires. The ego is concerned with thinking and reasoning skills. The superego refers to the conscience of an individual. The unconscious has to do with hidden thoughts—thoughts of which we are not aware.

Freud thought that sexual instinct has a great deal to do with personality development. He believed there is a relationship between the energy a child produces from the sexual instinct, also known as the "libido," and the child's overall development. He divided personality development into the following stages: oral, anal, phallic, latent, and genital. Each stage is concerned with a child's focus on a particular area of the body. He placed great importance on these stages in the development of the personality.

7 Identify two attitudes or personality types shown by most people.

Attitude is important in today's workplace. Carl Jung, born in 1875, was a Swiss psychologist who studied attitudes. He divided people into different groups and studied them. He believed people show both male and female types of behavior depending upon the situation.

Jung also identified two main attitudes in individuals—the introvert and the extrovert. **Introverts** tend to be shy and reserved. They are mostly concerned with their own inner thoughts and feelings and may appear somewhat aloof or antisocial at times. It may be difficult for an introvert to go to a social function like a dance or a family reunion. **Extroverts**, on the other hand, are quite outgoing and very interested in the outside world. They tend to enjoy being members of various groups and love participating in outside events. Extroverts may be involved in many organizations. People are usually a combination of both of these attitude types. One type, however, is usually dominant.

Jung developed the idea that our persona is something we show to others. The word **persona** comes from the Latin word for mask. Our persona is our "public face." Jung believed that our persona helps shape our personality.

8 List the eight basic types of human emotions.

Think for a minute about all of the emotions you and your friends and family show in one day.

Emotionally, we are constantly changing from one extreme to another. In 1980, Robert Plutchik identified eight primary categories of human **emotions**: disgust, anger, anticipation, joy, acceptance, fear, surprise, and sadness. Figure 8-3 shows some of the emotions we exhibit each day.

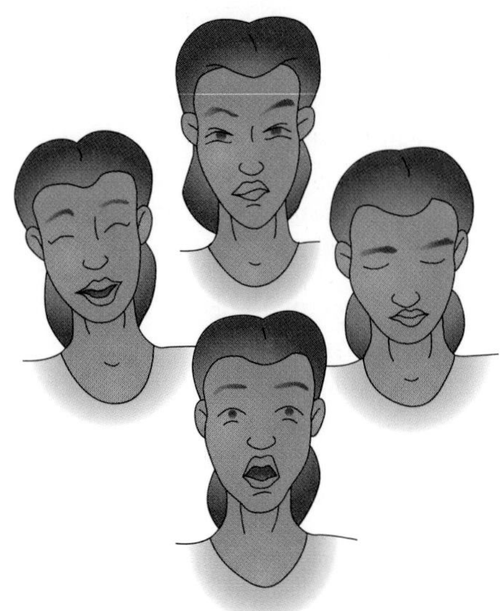

Figure 8-3. Anger, sadness, fear, and joy are some of the emotions we show every day.

Physiological changes, the physical changes in our body, may be the cause of sweeping changes in emotions. Chapter 7 outlines methods of dealing with residents showing certain types of emotions, such as anger, fear, apprehension, or anxiety. You will see these emotions occur in your residents. The best way to help residents deal with all of the different emotions they feel is to be there to provide any support they need. You should get help from a nurse if any situation becomes too much for you to handle.

This too shall pass.

Always remember: "This, too, shall pass." When you become stressed in a given day or week, life can seem overwhelming. If you have moments when your responsibilities seem to be getting the best of you, sit for a moment and LOOK at your pocket calendar. SEE the goals you have set for the week. Then promise to do ONE thing at a time, check it off, and go on to the next task. If you divide up, or compartmentalize, your day into small pieces, you will accomplish much more with less stress!

How is your sense of humor?

During the time of Hippocrates around 400 B.C., the idea of four "humors" became popular in the practice of medicine. The four humors were identified as follows: blood, having to do with the liver; phlegm, having to do with the lungs; yellow bile, referring to the gallbladder; and black bile, referring to the spleen. When a person was in a state of good health, the humors were thought to be balanced. Unfortunately, this method of trying to balance the four humors was not successful in solving the various health problems of Hippocrates' time.

9 Discuss Erikson's eight stages of psychosocial development.

Erik Erikson developed the eight stages of psychosocial development in 1963. "Psychosocial" means the mental and social aspects of a human being. Erikson believed very strongly that humans continue to develop and change as they grow older. He thought that life occurs in stages and that people attempt to move through these stages as they age. In his theory, each stage consists of a conflict that must be resolved before a person is able to move to the next stage. Each conflict is a turning point. Erikson believed that successful resolution of the conflicts leads to a healthier psychosocial development and personality.

One of the ways nursing personnel help residents move through these stages is by assisting them in times of stress. If a nursing assistant becomes aware of a resident's fear of death, the nurse can be alerted. Staff may then secure people to help the resident cope with that particular fear.

The first stage, "**trust vs. mistrust**," is when babies learn to depend on their families and the ability of the family unit to meet their needs. The inability to trust a parent to bring a bottle of milk when hunger occurs causes frustration, and the child may eventually fear the start of each day. Trust in infancy sets the stage for an expectation that the world will generally be a good place to live.

"**Autonomy vs. shame and doubt**" is the second stage, which usually occurs in late infancy and toddlerhood. When children learn to move about on their own, they develop a sense of autonomy, or independence. When children are restrained too much, they are likely to develop shame and to doubt their ability to do tasks well. This situation can lead to the beginning of an **inferiority complex**, a feeling of being inferior, that may exist throughout their lives.

The third stage, "**initiative vs. guilt**," outlines childrens', usually preschoolers', ability to accept challenges in their lives. If children are not encouraged to take on new projects and develop responsibilities, they may not seek challenges later in life. Developing a sense of responsibility increases initiative.

"**Industry vs. inferiority**" involves childrens' ability to live and interact in the world of adults. Children must learn to dress themselves, learn the value of work, and start making friends in order to understand the importance of social skills. When parents always tie their children's shoes, they encourage dependence. By not promoting independence, parents stifle their children. Children may then simply lose hope in the ability to "do" for themselves.

The fifth stage, "**identity vs. role confusion**," has to do with a person's ability to create a "self." We all have many roles in life. Each person has roles, such as daughter or son, employer or employee. People must learn to flow freely back and forth from role to role. Unique abilities and professions must be identified and chosen based on these strengths. We are all good at one thing or another; however, we cannot do everything well. When people are unable to move from role to role or cannot find an occupation that suits them, they may become frustrated or confused.

"**Intimacy vs. isolation**" is the sixth stage. This stage outlines a person's quest for intimacy with another person. When a person forms a healthy and intimate relationship with another person, intimacy will be achieved. If people are unable to form close relationships in life, they may become lonely and isolated.

The seventh stage "**generativity vs. stagnation**" deals with people, usually in middle adulthood, assisting younger generations to develop useful lives. The feeling of having not done anything to help the next generation, according to Erikson, is called stagnation.

The final stage, "**integrity vs. despair**," is generally experienced in late adulthood. When people reflect on what they have done with their lives and identify their lives as successful, they have a feeling of worth and a sense of satisfaction. If people have not developed a positive outlook in most of the previous stages of development, they may have little confidence and experience doubts and unhappiness.

10 Describe the stages of growth and development and the developmental tasks that relate to each stage.

Human development progresses through stages from infancy to late adulthood. Growth and development move along together at slightly different speeds for different people, but ultimately they continue up to the end of life. There are many stages of development. Cognitive development focuses on how children learn and process information. Language development focuses on the development of language skills for the purpose of communicating with others. Moral development has to do with forming a sense of right and wrong. Motor development is the process of gaining the ability to do such things as grasp, walk, cut with scissors, and draw with crayons. Physical development deals with the many changes that happen to the body during growth. Sexual development has to do with the reproductive changes that occur when young people reach **puberty**. Social development is the process of learning to relate to other people.

As people move through the cycles of life, they must master certain **developmental tasks** from stage to stage. These tasks are important because individuals must accomplish each before moving on to the next stage. Figure 8-4 outlines the developmental tasks that are required throughout all of the stages of life.

Developmentally Disabled Residents

A small number of people you will care for will be developmentally disabled. This is a chronic condition that limits normal function. Causes vary from injury and disease to mental retardation. People who are developmentally disabled require the same respect, preservation of dignity, and great care as your other residents. Treat them as adults, regardless of the behavior they exhibit. Praise and encourage them often. Repeat words to make sure they understand, and always be patient when this situation arises. People who are developmentally disabled have the same needs as the rest of the people in your care.

Summary

In this chapter, we have learned how the mind works and how the growth of our personality may relate to our overall behavior. While caring for your residents, you will recognize some of the things we have discussed in this chapter. The key to helping your residents stay mentally alert and healthy is to try to help each resident cope with the various problems that may occur. You can help them focus on living life to the fullest extent possible.

Infancy					Toddler	Preschool	School Age
Birth–4 Weeks	**4 Weeks–3 Months**	**3–6 Months**	**6–9 Months**	**9–12 Months**	**1–3 Years**	**3–6 Years**	**6–12 Years**
Physical •may lift/turn head •behavior based on reflexes •rapid physical growth	Physical •rapid physical growth •grasps, may squeeze finger/thumb	Physical •rapid physical growth •may sit with or without support •usually rolls over	Physical •rapid physical growth continues •moves about •usually sits by self	Physical •rapid physical growth continues •may begin to crawl, climb	Physical •learns to walk •may be toilet-trained by 3 years	Physical •physical growth slows •may run, climb stairs •learns to dress self •may start tying shoes	Physical •may begin losing baby teeth
Relating to Others •may smile	Relating to Others •smiles, coos, cries •turns toward you may startle	Relating to Others •may try to mimic your sounds •laughs	Relating to Others •babbles •understands word "no"	Relating to Others •words may make more sense	Relating to Others •learning more words •may put a few words together	Relating to Others •may be bossy or shy •begins to speak in sentences	Relating to Others •learns to write and starts to tell time •may be bossy or shy •starts to develop study skills
Care •help parents meet needs •keep control of infant's surroundings	Care •keep control of infant's surroundings	Care •keep control of infant's surroundings	Care •keep control of infant's surroundings	Care •keep control of infant's surroundings	Care •encourage practice walking •encourage verbal communication with others	Care •encourage play •encourage independence in some daily activities, such as dressing •encourage increasing vocabulary	Care •encourage hobbies and activities •praise accomplishments •continue increasing vocabulary

Adolescence	Adult	Middle Age	Older Adults	Old Age	Very Old Age
12–18 Years	**18–40 Years**	**40–65 Years**	**65–75 Years**	**75–85 Years**	**85 years and older**
Physical •may have growth spurts •growth may end for girls=18 •growth may end for boys=21-25	Physical •females may have children	Physical •some physical signs of aging may appear	Physical •more physical signs of aging	Physical •physical changes may intensify •may become more dependent upon others and require care	Physical •physical problems multiply •physical changes may cause need for increased level of care
Relating to Others •develops morals and values •may have mood swings •very interested in appearance •may become infatuated •independence expands	Relating to Others •life relationship formed with another person •chooses career •adjusts to life independent from parents •may have children	Relating to Others •"empty nest" feelings may occur •may care for children and aging parents—"sandwich generation" •may volunteer in addition to career •one or both parents may die •may provide some care for grandchildren •may travel	Relating to Others •adapts to being retired •may increase volunteering •may form social groups w/ other older adults •may travel	Relating to Others •may begin to settle life and prepare for death	Relating to Others •may lose friends and family members as they die •begin the process of coping with death
Care •help cope with challenges they will face in life	Care •promote good health habits	Care •promote good health habits	Care •encourage participation in groups and activities •promote good health habits	Care •keep safe	Care •maintain independence •assist with care as necessary

Figure 8-4. The stages of growth and development.

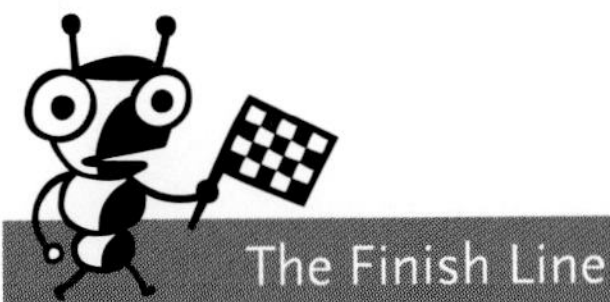

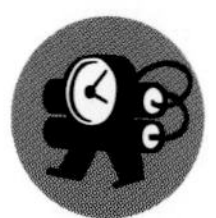

What's Wrong With This Picture?

Look at Maslow's triangle below. Some of the basic needs have mixed-up words, and some are in the wrong spots in the triangle. Write the basic needs as they should appear.

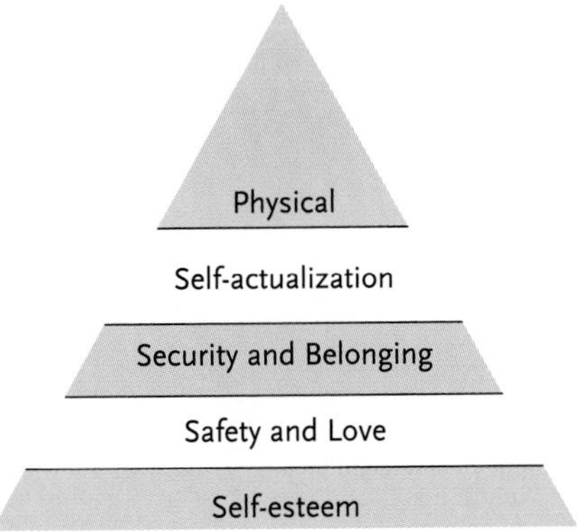

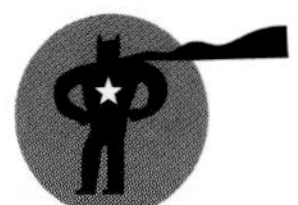

Star Student Central

1. Write some ideas for helping your residents cope with the emotions they show each day. For example, consider your response to a resident's anger at receiving a cold dinner tray.
2. Make a list of two introverts and two extroverts you know. Think about whether you are an extrovert or an introvert, and identify one way your particular attitude may help your residents.

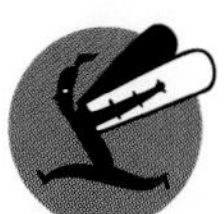

You Can Do It Corner!

Fill in the blanks in the sentences at right.

1. An individual who is a shy, quiet person, has an ____________ personality. (LO 7)
2. Erikson's stage describing a baby's dependence on the parents to meet the basic needs is called " ____________ vs. ____________." (LO 9)
3. The type of development dealing with a child's ability to form a sense of right and wrong is known as ____________ development. (LO 10)
4. The self-actualizing person has been described as someone who is ____________. (LO 5)
5. According to Maslow, the first needs that must be met are ____________ needs, such as air, food and water, rest, and sleep. (LO 4)
6. Looking at the functioning of the whole person takes the focus off ____________ and redirects it to healthy attitudes and lifestyles. (LO 2)
7. Eight primary human emotions include fear, surprise, anger, disgust, anticipation, joy, sadness, and ____________. (LO 8)
8. Caring for a resident by meeting physical, emotional, spiritual, and social needs is called ____________ care. (LO 3)
9. A person's unique pattern of behavior that continues over a period of time is called a ____________. (LO 6)

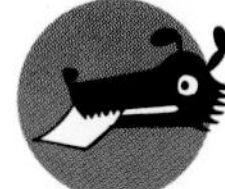

Star Student's Chapter Checklist

1. I have read my textbook chapter.
2. I have reviewed my own "Pocketful of Terms."
3. I have listened to my tutor tape.
4. I have reviewed and highlighted my class notes.
5. I have read and completed any handouts from this chapter.
6. I have completed "The Finish Line."
7. Star Time! Choose your reward!

9

A View From The Inside: **The Healthy Human Body**

Look Like a Star!

Look at the **Learning Objectives** and **The Finish Line** before you begin reading this chapter.

Look at your pocket calendar.
With your pencil, put a bracket (   ) around a study period every single day.

Look at your homework for this chapter.
Plug each piece of homework into a certain time slot.

Look at the **Star Student's Chapter Checklist** at the end of this chapter. Check off each item as it is completed.

Learning Objectives

1. Spell and define all STAR words.
2. Define six sciences that study the human body.
3. Classify the human being in the scientific world.
4. Compare the human organism to other animals.
5. Identify six structural levels of organization in humans.
6. Define the term "homeostasis" and discuss how it relates to normal body function.
7. Briefly review principles of basic chemistry and the chemical elements found in the human body.
8. Discuss the pH scale and how it relates to homeostasis.
9. Discuss the importance of body fluids and electrolytes in homeostasis.
10. Describe cell theory and cell division.
11. Identify the four types of tissues in the human body.
12. Name the major organs, explain their structure and functions, and discuss some of the aging changes for each body system.
13. Define and locate anatomical terms relating to position and location.
14. Define and locate body regions and cavities inside the body.

"What a piece of work is man! How noble in reason! How infinite in faculty! In form and moving, how express and admirable! In action, how like an angel! In apprehension how like a God! The beauty of the world! The paragon of animals."

William Shakespeare, 1564-1616
from *Hamlet*

"An unlearned carpenter of my acquaintance once said in my hearing: 'There is very little difference between one man and another; but what little there is, is very important.' This distinction seems to go to the heart of the matter."

William James, 1842-1910

Aristotle put the "love" in our hearts.

The warm blood and arrangement of blood vessels are obviously a governing system within the body, and this influenced the search for the soul. When excessive blood is lost, the body dies. Therefore, some concluded, blood must contain a vital, life-giving force. The scholars of Mesopotamia were influenced by this idea, as was Aristotle, the Greek scientist and philosopher, who lived centuries later. Aristotle believed that the seat of the soul was the heart and that the brain functioned in cooling the blood that flowed from the heart. The association of the heart, in song and poetry, with the emotions of love and caring has its basis in Aristotle.

1 Spell and define all STAR words.

alimentary canal: digestive tract in its entirety; spans from the mouth to the anus.

alveoli: tiny, grape-like sacs in the lungs where the exchange of oxygen and carbon dioxide occurs.

anatomy: the study of the human body structure.

antibody: a protein that defends the body against certain microscopic, foreign substances in the blood.

artery: a vessel that carries oxygen-rich, carbon dioxide-poor blood from the heart; the aorta is the largest artery.

atria: the upper two chambers of the heart.

biochemistry: the study of the chemical reactions of living things.

biology: the study of all life forms.

bladder: a sac that serves as storage for urine until it is released from the body during urination.

blood: the fluid circulating through the body within the heart and all blood vessels; the main means of transport within the body.

blood vessels: the tubes that transport the blood; arteries, veins, and capillaries.

bone marrow: soft material in the cavities of the bones where blood cells are made.

brain: the part of the nervous system primarily responsible for memory, thought, and intelligence, along with regulation of vital functions, such as heart rate, blood pressure, and breathing.

bronchi: branches of the passages of the respiratory system that lead from the trachea into the lungs.

capillaries: tiny, extremely thin blood vessels where the exchange of gases, nutrients, and waste products occurs between blood and tissue fluid.

cartilage: a fibrous connective tissue of the skeletal system.

chemistry: the study of the structure of matter.

chyme: semi-liquid substance made as a result of the chemical breakdown of food in the stomach.

colon: large intestine; has four sections—ascending, transverse, descending, and sigmoid colon.

cytology: the study of the cell.

dehydration: excessive loss of body fluids.

dermis: the inner, or second, layer of the skin; positioned beneath the epidermis.

diffusion: the exchange of nutrients and wastes.

digestion: the internal mechanical and chemical breakdown process that converts food into nutrients which can be utilized at the cellular level.

digestive tract: tract that spans from the mouth to the anus; alimentary canal.

disorders: conditions or diseases that impact and change homeostasis.

duodenum: the first part of the small intestine where the common bile duct enters the small intestine; location where the chyme (partly digested mixture of food) enters the intestine from the stomach.

electrolytes: chemical substances that are essential to maintaining fluid balance and homeostasis within the body.

epidermis: the outer layer of the skin.

extension: the stretching and lengthening of a muscle, e.g. when a muscle straightens a limb.

fight or flight response: the sympathetic nervous system's response to a stressor.

flexion: the contraction and shortening of a muscle, e.g. when a muscle flexes.

gland: an organ that produces and secretes a substance of some kind, e.g. endocrine glands secrete hormones.

heart: four-chambered pump that is responsible for the flow of blood in the body.

homeostasis: the ability of the human body to maintain internal conditions that are necessary for life; dynamic response to an internal or external change affecting the body.

homo sapiens: a Latin term meaning "wise human being."

hormone: a chemical secreted by the endocrine glands.

joint: the point where two bones meet; provides movement and flexibility; types include immovable, sliding, hinged, and saddle.

kidneys: two organs that lie in the back of the abdominal cavity just above the waist; responsible for filtering the blood, forming and excreting the urine, and regulating the electrolytes of body fluids.

ligament: a band of fibrous tissue that connects bones and supports the joints.

lungs: main organs of respiration responsible for the exchange of oxygen and carbon dioxide gases.

mammal: any of various warm-blooded animals of the class Mammalia, including human beings; characterized by a covering of hair on the skin and, in the female, milk-producing mammary glands for feeding the young.

mass: amount of matter a body or object contains.

meiosis: cell division of the reproductive system; ova and sperm are formed; reproduction occurs via fertilization.

melanin: dark pigment found in hair and skin.

membrane: something that covers, protects, lines, or separates internal parts of the body.

mitosis: body cell division; enables the body to grow.

muscles: a group of tissues that contract and produce motion, support the body, protect organs, and create heat.

nerve impulses: electrical impulses sent to and from the brain to communicate with all parts of the body.

ova: female sex cells; eggs.

pathophysiology: the study of various disorders that occur in the functioning of the body.

peristalsis: muscular contractions that push food through the alimentary canal (digestive tract).

pharynx: the throat.

physiology: the study of how body parts function.

pituitary gland: the master gland of the endocrine system; called the "master" because it has the ability to control hormone production of other glands.

primate: a mammal of the order Primates; characterized by refined development of the hands and feet, a shortened snout, and a large brain.

puberty: transitional time when body development transforms boys and girls (non-reproductive beings) into men and women (capable of reproducing) by maturing the reproductive systems.

sperm: male sex cells.

spinal cord: the part of the nervous system inside the spinal canal from which 31 pairs of nerves grow; nerve impulses are transmitted through this cord to and from the brain; also triggers special reflexes to respond quickly to changes in the environment.

stimulus: (pl. stimuli): an agent that causes an activity of some kind in an organism or an organ.

stressor: something that causes stress.

tendons: tough bands of connective tissue that anchor or connect a muscle to a bone.

tissues: groups of cells that perform certain functions together.

trachea: the windpipe; an air passage that goes from the throat (pharynx) to the bronchi.

vein: vessel that carries carbon dioxide-rich blood towards the heart (venous return).

ventricles: the two lower chambers of the heart.

2 Define six sciences that study the human body.

Biology is the study of all life forms. Humans, animals, plants, and cellular organisms are all part of the science of biology. Anatomy and physiology are a part of the science of biology. **Anatomy** is the study of body structure, while **physiology** looks at how body parts function.

Pathophysiology is the study of the disorders (conditions or diseases) that occur in the functioning of the body. **Chemistry** studies the structure of matter. **Biochemistry** looks at the chemical reactions of living things.

3 Classify the human being in the scientific world.

Humans have a special place in the animal kingdom and the scientific world. The human being is known as "**homo sapiens**." This is a Latin term which means "wise human being." The first people who were identified as "modern human beings" or "modern man" and looked like we do now have been named "homo sapiens sapiens." This means "wise, wise human being."

A human being is a part of the animal kingdom in the class known as **mammals**. Some of the characteristics of mammals include hair, teeth that differ in size, and mammary glands that provide milk for feeding their young. Within the class of mammals, there are orders. Humans belong to the order of **primates**. Monkeys and apes also belong to this order. Primates have large brains and the ability to grasp objects. The family that humans belong to is called Hominidae. Homo sapiens are a part of this family. Homo sapiens have a large cerebrum, the part of the brain responsible for thought and intelligence.

4 Compare the human organism to other animals.

Human beings have many characteristics similar to other animals. For example, many animals develop in a similar way to humans. See Figure 9-1.

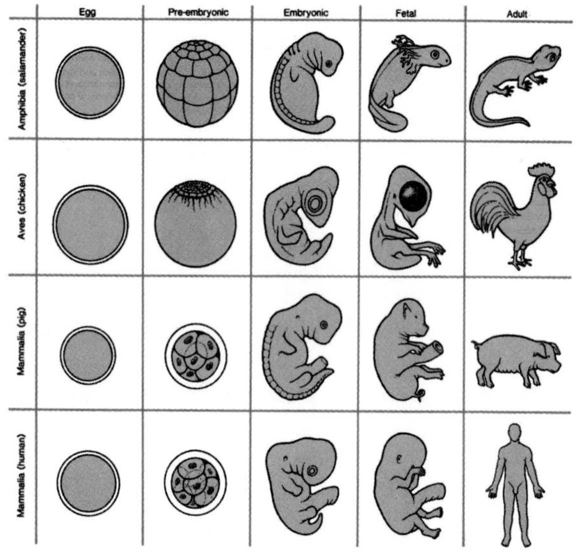

Figure 9-1. Stages of development of the human and other animals. (From *Human Anatomy* by Kent Van De Graaf. Reprinted with permission of The McGraw-Hill Companies. Copyright © 1988.)

The human organism also has many features that separate it from other animals. For example, a human has a large and well-developed brain. This brain has developed to the point that humans are able to reason and remember things in remarkable ways. The human organism has developed the ability to speak due to the vocal cords. Humans can walk upright, which is quite different from other animals. Walking upright allows humans to use their hands to do just about anything. The thumb, only seen in the order of primates, can be used to grasp and use various objects. Think for a moment about your thumbs. Could you hold a fork or a knife without them? Try this and see what happens.

5 Identify six structural levels of organization in humans.

The human organism is made up of many different levels. This is essentially how the human body is organized. An overview of the many levels within the human body is shown in Figure 9-2.

- Level 1 Chemical
- Level 2 Cellular
- Level 3 Tissues
- Level 4 Organs
- Level 5 Body Systems
- Level 6 Organism

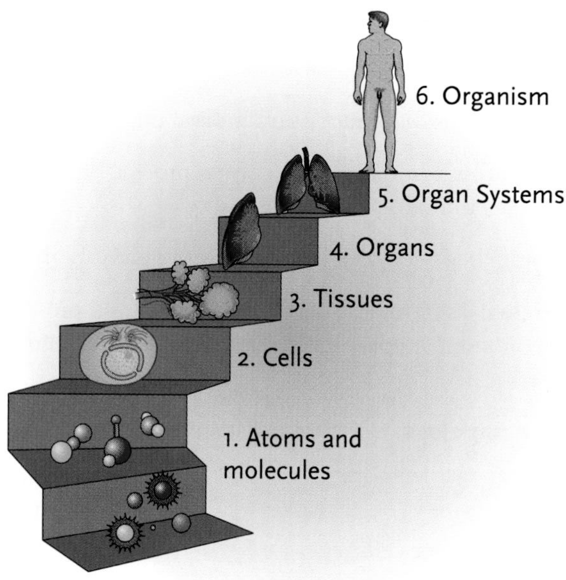

Figure 9-2. The different levels of the human organism.

Everything begins with atoms and molecules. **Level one**, called the chemical level, is composed of atoms and molecules. In the proper balance and amounts, chemicals are required to keep the human organism alive and functioning normally.

Level two is the cellular level. The human body is made up of many different kinds of cells. Some examples of cells are blood, nerve, and muscle cells. Each cell looks quite different and has very specific functions.

Level three is the tissue layer of the body. Tissues are made up of layers of cells. Once these layers of cells come together, they are able to perform specific body functions. Examples of tissues are epithelial, connective, muscle, and nervous.

System	Organ Example	Functions	Related Word
integumentary	skin	protection	dermatology
skeletal	bones / joints	body shape	osteology / arthrology
muscular	muscles	movement	myology
nervous	brain	controls body activity	neurology
endocrine	glands	regulation of organs	endocrinology
circulatory	heart	oxygen and nutrition delivery to cells	cardiology
lymphatic	lymph nodes	protection from disease	immunology
respiratory	lungs	oxygen/carbon dioxide exchange	pulmonology
digestive	stomach	food absorption	gastroenterology
urinary	kidneys	waste removal	urology
reproductive	ovaries / testes	creates new human beings	gynecology

Level four is the organ level of the body. Groups of tissues come together to form organs. Organs are very important to well-being. The heart is an example of an organ. The heart beats approximately 42 million times in a single year.

Level five is the system level in the body. Systems are made up of different kinds of organs so that each system can accomplish complex body functions. Two examples are the circulatory system, consisting of the heart and blood vessels, and the urinary system, consisting of the kidneys, ureters, bladder, and urethra. The table above shows the body systems, sample organs, basic functions, and the word(s) describing one type of study of that particular system. Chapters 24 through 34 discuss the systems and related care.

Level six is the organism level: a complete, unique, individual being. We are living organisms called human beings. We are made up of many complex systems that function in exact ways, creating an organism that is able to survive for many decades.

The temperature of the body must remain close to the normal level of 98.6°F or 37°C. If the body's temperature rises, there is usually a reason for this change. An illness of some kind may be developing within the body, or perhaps the person has been out in the sun too long. When the temperature rises, the body will try to regulate the temperature and bring it back down to a normal level by using processes, such as increasing blood vessel size, to help cool the body.

The term "homeostasis" will be used frequently throughout this textbook. It will be used to help explain how changes that occur inside us, such as an illness, and around us, such as temperature changes, can affect the normal functioning of the body. Each system in the body plays a unique part in maintaining homeostasis. However, some systems are more involved than others. Understanding how the body restores homeostasis will help you become a better nursing assistant. **Ultimately, this understanding improves your ability to observe residents and recognize any changes that need to be reported.**

6 Define the term "homeostasis" and discuss how it relates to normal body function.

Staying well and functioning normally during a lifespan is important. In order to do this, bodies must keep certain internal conditions stable. This is called **homeostasis**. Temperature, oxygen, the amount of fluid in the body and what the fluids are made of, along with the amount of salt in the body, are examples of things that can change from moment to moment. For each, there is an ideal range for optimal functioning. The body tries very hard to keep these ranges at fairly stable levels in order to remain healthy and well.

7 Briefly review principles of basic chemistry and the chemical elements found in the human body.

To maintain homeostasis, a body must maintain stable levels of all of the chemicals inside. Body fluids are made up of chemicals. Being familiar with the chemicals in bodies will help you better understand how the human body works.

All matter takes up space and has mass. **Mass** is defined as how much matter each substance holds. The atom is the basic unit of matter, and every substance is made up of atoms. Atoms are made of protons, neutrons, and electrons. Molecules are formed when two or more atoms unite.

In chemistry, there are 109 different substances that are made of a single atom. These are called "elements." These elements are the building blocks of all living and non-living things. Ninety-two elements are typically found in nature. Each element is identified by a chemical symbol.

Chemistry: It's Symbolic!

1. *Usually symbols are made up of the first few letters (usually the first one or two) in the name of the chemical. The second letter is always lower case.*
   oxygen = O
   carbon = C
   calcium = Ca
   iodine = I
2. *Sometimes Latin terms are used:*
   sodium = natrium = Na
   potassium = kalium = K
   gold = aurum = Au
   silver = argentum = Ag

When elements combine, compounds are formed. A compound like sodium chloride (NaCl) has one part sodium and one part chlorine. This is more commonly known as simple table salt. Water (H_2O) has two parts hydrogen and one part oxygen.

There are 26 elements found in the human body. Box 9-1 shows 99.9% of the chemicals and the percentage of them in the human body. Most of the body's mass, about 96%, is made up of just four elements: oxygen, carbon, hydrogen, and nitrogen. There are nine elements that make up another 3.9% of the body's mass, and the balance, or 0.1% of the body is made up of 13 elements. These elements combine to make up organic and inorganic compounds. Both types of compounds are found in the human body.

Chemical Elements Found in the Body Box 9-1

Element/Symbol	% of Body Mass	Function in Body
These four elements make up about 96% of body mass:		
Oxygen (O)	65.0%	Part of water, needed for cell respiration
Carbon (C)	18.5%	Found in every organic molecule; a part of carbohydrates and lipids
Hydrogen (H)	9.5%	Part of water, all foods, and most organic molecules; a part of carbohydrates and lipids
Nitrogen (N)	3.2%	Part of all proteins
These elements make up about 3.9% of body mass:		
Calcium (Ca)	1.5%	Bone and tooth hardness
Phosphorous (P)	0.4%	Bone and tooth structure
Potassium (K)	0.4%	Nerve and muscle function
Sulfur (S)	0.3%	Part of many proteins
Chlorine (Cl)	0.2%	Water balance
Sodium (Na)	0.2%	Water balance
Iodine (I)	0.1%	Hormone production
Iron (Fe)	0.1%	Part of hemoglobin (the oxygen-carrying element of the blood)
Magnesium (Mg)	0.1%	Enzyme function

These "trace elements," with their chemical symbols in parentheses, make up about 0.1% of body mass:

Aluminum (Al)	Boron (B)	Chromium (Cr)
Cobalt (Co)	Copper (Cu)	Fluorine (F)
Manganese (Mn)	Molybdenum (Mo)	Selenium (Se)
Silicon (Si)	Tin (Sn)	Vanadium (V)
Zinc (Zn)		

8 Discuss the pH scale and how it relates to homeostasis.

The term "pH" means "parts Hydrogen." The pH scale ranges from 0 to 14. The lower the number, the more acidic the fluid; the higher the number, the more alkaline, or basic, the fluid. Thus, 0 would be acid and 14 would be basic or alkaline. A pH of 7 is considered neutral; pure water has a pH of 7, so it is considered neutral.

Body cells and fluids generally have a pH close to neutral, or 7.0. For the human body to maintain homeostasis, the pH level must be kept at a fairly stable level. Bodies have buffers like sodium bicarbonate ($NaHCO_3$) that maintain pH levels. These are found in certain body fluids. Buffers adjust acids and bases in body fluids as needed. This very important process helps a body maintain homeostasis.

Box 9-2 shows some examples of body fluids and other substances on a pH scale.

pH values of common substances and human body fluids Box 9-2

Substance/body fluid	pH Value
Gastric juice (stomach acid)	1.2–3.0
Lemon juice	2.2–2.4
Carbonated soft drink	3.0–3.5
Vaginal fluid	3.5–4.5
Tomato juice	4.2
Coffee	5.0
Urine	4.6–8.0
Saliva	6.35–6.85
Milk	6.6–6.9
Distilled (pure) water	7.0
Blood	7.35–7.45
Semen	7.20–7.60
Pancreatic juice	7.1–8.2
Eggs	7.6–8.0

9 Discuss the importance of body fluids and electrolytes in homeostasis.

Body fluids, such as cellular fluids and plasma, make up about 55% to 60% of body weight. Water is the primary component of body fluids. In a normal adult male, water makes up about 60% of body weight. Because the female body contains more fat, total body water is lower in the adult female than it is in adult males.

Body fluids contain chemicals. Organic compounds like glucose are found in body fluids. Electrolytes are found in body fluids as well. **Electrolytes** are vital to survival. They are so named because they conduct an electric current. Molecules that form ions (electrically-charged atoms) when dissolved in water are called electrolytes. Acids, bases, and salts are electrolytes. Some electrolytes are minerals that the body needs for homeostasis.

The major electrolytes in the body are sodium, potassium, calcium, magnesium, and chloride. Sodium, potassium, and magnesium assist in nerve and muscle function. Calcium helps bones and teeth, blood clotting, and nerve and muscle function. Chloride, along with hydrogen, makes up the gastric (stomach) juice, hydrocloric acid (HCL).

When body fluids decrease due to **dehydration**, they must be restored. Figure 9-3 shows a method of restoring body water and returning to homeostasis.

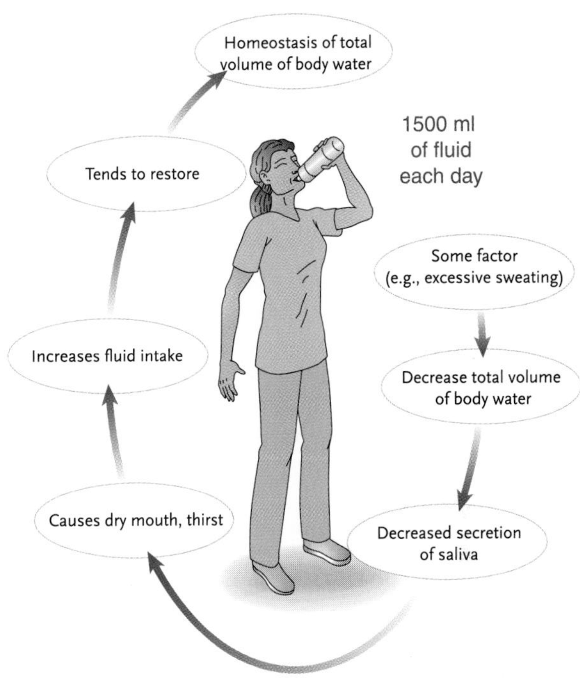

Figure 9-3. Homeostasis of body water.

10 Describe cell theory and cell division.

The cell theory proposes that all living organisms are made up of cells. In 1838-1839, two scientists named Matthias Schleiden and Theodor Schwann laid the foundation for this theory, which eventually became the study of the cell, or **cytology**.

The primary parts of the cell are the cell membrane, the cytoplasm and the nucleus. The cell membrane controls the movement of chemicals in and out of cells. The cytoplasm consists of the material between the nucleus and the cell membrane. The nucleus is the control center of the cell. Within the cell nucleus are the 46 chromosomes, which carry genetic material, or genes.

Cells divide in two different ways: mitosis and meiosis. As a cell ages or becomes damaged, it must be replaced. This process, known as cell division, is called **mitosis**. When mitosis occurs, two daughter cells are formed having the identical genetic formula as the mother cell. Figure 9-4 shows mitosis.

Meiosis is the process by which the specialized sex cells divide; reproduction can then follow. This type of cell division occurs with two cells, sperm and ovum (egg, ova is plural), each having 23 chromosomes. When an egg, or ovum, becomes fertilized, they come together to form a full cell, or zygote, with 46 chromosomes.

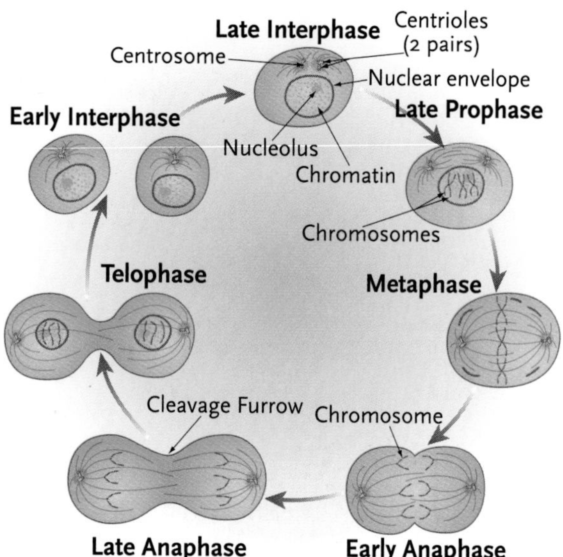

Figure 9-4. **Mitosis.**

Slides and Cells

Three centuries ago, Robert Hooke observed part of a plant under a microscope. He could see many tiny sections. Hooke chose the name "cell" because the tiny parts reminded him of the cubicles of ancient monasteries that the monks lived in .

11 Identify the four types of tissues in the human body.

Tissues are groups of cells. Each type of tissue has a specific function. There are four types of tissues: epithelial, connective, muscle and nerve.

Epithelial tissue is tissue that lines and covers many body parts. There are no **blood vessels** located in epithelial tissue. However, it is still living tissue and must receive nutrients and eliminate wastes in order to survive. Epithelial tissue protects the body and serves as the lining of many organs. The exchange of nutrients and waste products occurs with the neighboring connective tissue. This movement is accomplished through a process called **diffusion**.

Connective tissue makes up the majority of the tissues in the body. This type of tissue connects, binds, and supports. Examples of connective tissue are adipose (fat) tissue, which provides a cushion and an insulation for the body, and bone tissue, which supports and protects the body.

Muscle tissue works by contracting. **Muscles** function by providing support for the body, creating heat, and giving protection to internal organs. There are two types of muscle: voluntary and involuntary. Skeletal muscles are called voluntary muscles because they move by receiving nerve impulses from our brain. The four chambers of the heart are made up of cardiac muscle. Cardiac muscle is an involuntary muscle because you do not tell your heart to beat. It does so automatically. Smooth muscle is another involuntary muscle. It makes up the walls of arteries, **veins**, the stomach, and the intestines. It also constricts (closes or narrows) and dilates (widens or expands) the pupils in the eyes depending upon the amount of light around us.

The neuron and neuroglia are the two types of nerve tissue. This type of tissue reacts to **stimuli**, or agents from the environment that can cause reactions. Nerve tissue provides the communication between all parts of the body through nerve impulses. **Nerve impulses** are similar to little electric currents sent to and from all of the body's organs. Nerve tissue controls many body functions in this manner. The neuron is the nerve cell. These cells conduct the nerve impulses. The neuroglia are the supporting cells that protect neurons and bind them together.

12 Name the major organs, explain their structure and functions, and discuss some of the aging changes for each body system.

Note that this section discusses the structure and function, as well as age-related changes, of each body system. Diseases and disorders of each system, along with the appropriate care, will be discussed in Chapters 24 through 34.

System 1 The Integumentary System

Points of Interest

The integumentary system consists of the skin, the hair, the nails and the glands of the skin. It is considered an organ because it is a group of tissues that has defined functions. The skin is the largest organ in the body. In adults, the skin is the heaviest organ, weighing about 10–11 pounds or more and covering an area of about 22 square feet. The skin makes up about 16% of a person's body weight. We find an amazing number of structures within one square inch of the skin: 500 sweat glands, more than 1000 nerve endings, many yards of tiny blood vessels, almost 100 oil glands, and millions of cells!

Structure of the Skin

The skin is a membrane. A **membrane** is a tissue that covers, protects, lines, or separates parts of the body. There are three types of epithelial membranes in the body: cutaneous membranes (the skin); serous membranes (pleura), and the mucous membranes (reproductive tract lining). The skin covers and protects the body, provides sensation, and also has other functions.

The two basic layers of the skin are the epidermis and the dermis. The **epidermis**, or outer layer of the skin, is where mitosis occurs. New cells are made and the aging cells are forced upward to the surface of the skin. When they lose their blood supply, these skin cells become dry, flaky, and eventually die and fall off the skin. Keratin is a substance found in the dead skin cells of the epidermis. Keratin has waterproof qualities that protect the inside of the body when we get wet. Beneath the very top of the epidermis lie other types of cells. One is the melanocyte, which contains **melanin**, the substance that gives skin its color. The more melanin your skin produces, the darker your skin color is.

Receptors are found in the skin that give us the ability to feel and touch. One type of receptor is found near the surface of the skin and the other is found within the dermis.

The **dermis** is the deeper layer of the skin. Within the dermis lie the structures responsible for unique fingerprints. These are called the dermal-papillae. These ridges form before a baby is born. Fingerprints and footprints, which grow as a child becomes an adult, will always have the same pattern and can identify people throughout their lives. Also included in the dermis are hair and nail follicles, sweat and oil glands, blood vessels, and receptors for touch, temperature, pressure, and pain.

Collagen fibers, which make skin tough, are found within the dermis. Elastic fibers are also found in the dermis. They give the skin its elasticity, or ability to stretch.

The subcutaneous layer is positioned immediately underneath the dermis. This is the area of the body where fat, or adipose, tissue lies. This adipose tissue also serves as a cushion over bone and provides some protection as it insulates us from cold weather. Humans' fat layer is thinner than the fat layer in some other animals.

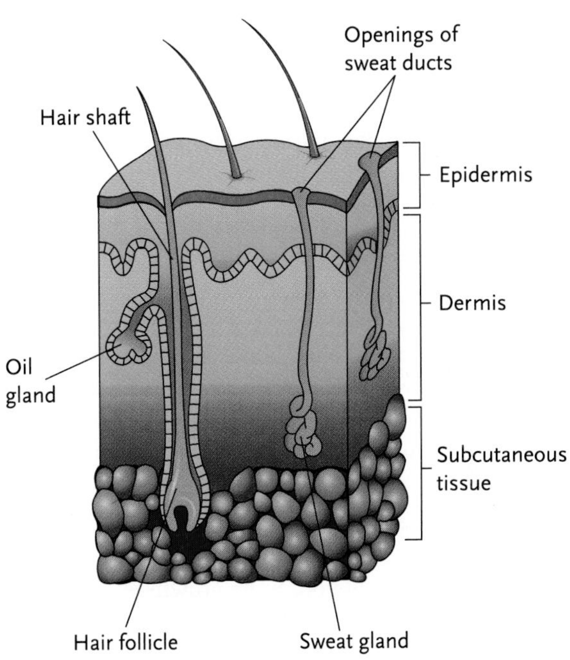

Figure 9-5. Cross-section showing details of the integumentary system.

Functions of the Skin

- protects the body from things like cuts and ultraviolet radiation from the sun
- regulates body temperature
- responds to heat, cold, pain, pressure, and touch
- excretes waste products in sweat
- helps formation of vitamin D

Destination: Homeostasis

When cells die or become damaged, the homeostasis so vital to health and wellness is disturbed. The body responds by attempting to regain homeostasis. When the surface of the skin is cut, clotting factors sent out into the blood plasma begin their work. The platelets also do their important job by temporarily closing the blood vessel. This repair process causes a substance, fibrin, to be released to seal the cut by forming a scab, a hard protective structure. The healing process completes itself when new connective tissue develops over the injury. Epithelial tissue cells begin to divide and multiply, ultimately growing over the scabbed area until it is completely healed. When tissue repair is complete, the injured area returns to homeostasis.

Aging and the Integumentary System

Normal age-related changes include the following:

- decrease of collagen and loss of elasticity in elastic fibers, causing wrinkles
- slower growth of hair and nails
- decrease in size of oil glands, causing fragile skin
- decrease in the number of certain melanocytes, causing gray hair
- occurrence of age or "liver" spots due to the increase in the size of other melanocytes
- loss of protective fatty tissue

System 2 The Skeletal System

Points of Interest

Contrary to popular belief, bones are living structures. Living bone cells called osteocytes lie within the bones. Before birth, the skeleton consists primarily of **cartilage**, a fibrous connective tissue. Newborn babies generally have about 270 bones. As bone development or formation occurs, the bones harden and fuse together to form the 206 bones of the human adult skeleton. Bone growth is usually complete by the age of 25. In a male, bone growth can continue into the twenties, while in the female bone growth may end before 20 years of age.

The male skeleton has bones that are usually bigger and heavier than the female skeleton. However, the female pelvis must be larger in order to accommodate the birth of a baby. The word "pelvis" comes from a Latin word meaning "basin." In comparison, the male pelvic opening is narrower. Figure 9-6 shows a comparison of the male and female pelvis. Note the size of the openings, or pelvic inlet and pelvic outlet, in the male versus the female.

Structure of the Skeletal System

The skeletal system is composed of cartilage, bone, bone marrow, periosteum, and the joints, also known as articulations. These are all types of connective tissue. Osteocytes are the mature bone cells that make up bone tissue. Cartilage cushions the bones at the joints. The outer layer of a bone is referred to as hard or compact, while the inner layer at the end of a long bone is referred to as soft and spongy. **Bone marrow** lies within the spongy area, or bed, of the long bones. Bone marrow is responsible for the production of red and white blood cells and the platelets. The periosteum is a membrane that covers part of the surface of bones. **Joints** are found at the places where two bones meet.

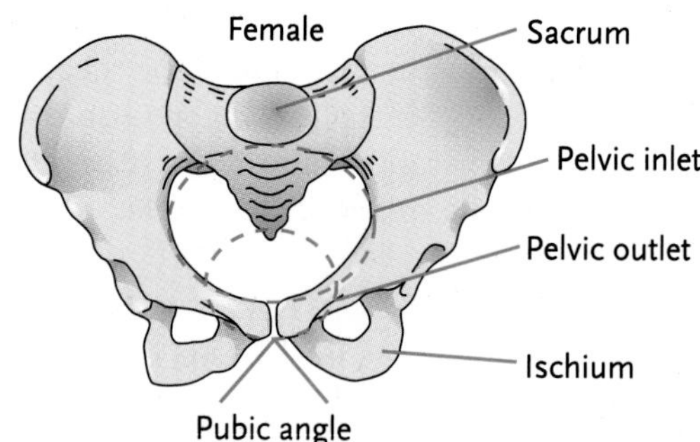

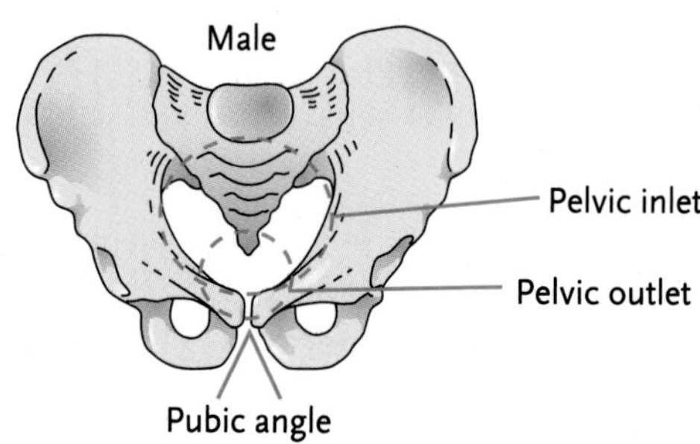

Figure 9-6. **Comparison of the male and female pelvis.**

The skeletal system is made up of four types of bones:

1. Long bones–the humerus (upper arm bone), the femur (thigh bone)
2. Short bones–the carpals (wrist bones), the tarsals (ankle bones)
3. Flat bones–the sternum (chest)
4. Irregular bones–bones of the vertebrae

The skeleton, or framework, of the human body has 206 bones. Bones are hard and rigid, but are made up of living cells. Bones allow the body to move and protect the organs.

The joints, or articulations, are important structures that hold

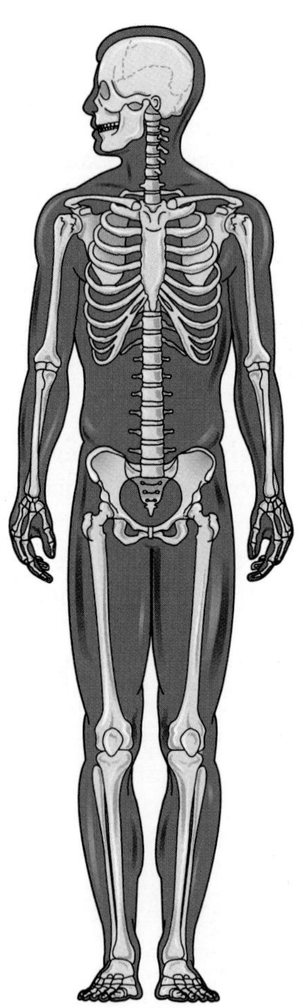

Figure 9-7. **The skeleton is composed of 206 bones that facilitate movement and protect organs.**

bones together. There are three types of joints: movable, slightly movable, and immovable. Examples of immovable joints are the bones of the cranium (skull). They are also called sutures because they sit between the bones and hold them together. An example of a slightly movable joint is the symphysis, or joint between the pubic bones. The joint between the scapula and the humerus is an example of a freely movable joint. Within the joint itself is the synovial membrane. The synovial membrane makes synovial fluid, which prevents friction when the bones move. Figure 9-8 shows examples of movable joints.

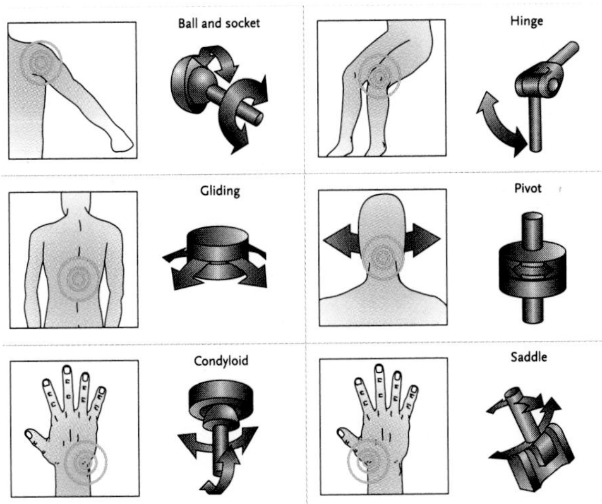

Figure 9-8. **Types of movable joints.**

A **ligament** is a band of fibrous tissue that connects bones together and supports the joints. Ligaments can become injured during sports or other strenuous activities. Torn ligaments can take a long time to heal following an injury.

Functions of the Skeletal System

- provides a framework for the body
- aids in mobility; helps move the body
- protects internal organs
- creates new blood cells in bone marrow
- stores minerals—calcium and phosphorous

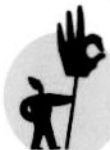

My joint hurts!

Why does swelling occur when we have an injury to a joint? After an injury, synovial fluid is produced to act as a cushion and keep the injured joint still. Within a joint, there is a limited area. The added fluid causes pressure inside the enclosed space, which leads to swelling and pain. It is always important to see a doctor after an injury to determine the severity of the injury.

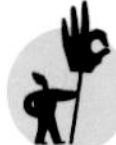

No swinging by the arms!

Pulling too hard on a person's arm can easily dislocate shoulder joints. Because of this, never jerk a resident's arm or attempt to lift or reposition a resident by pulling on the arm. Dislocations can cause extreme pain and may cause permanent damage.

Destination: Homeostasis

The skeletal system helps to regulate the calcium levels in blood. Bones serve as a storage area. When blood calcium decreases to abnormally low levels, bones are alerted to release some of the stored calcium back into the blood, and the calcium level then returns to normal range. Homeostasis is restored.

Aging and the Skeletal System

Normal age-related changes include the following:

- porous and brittle (easily broken) bones
- loss of space between vertebrae; potential loss of height
- less flexible joints, causing slower body movements and increased chance of pain

System 3 The Muscular System

Points of Interest

Without muscles, bodies would be unable to move, people could not breathe, and hearts would not beat. There are over 600 muscles in the human body. Muscles help bodies move by contracting and relaxing.

Structure of the Muscular System

Three types of muscle tissue are found within the body: skeletal, smooth, and cardiac.

A skeletal muscle is a voluntary muscle. It works by contracting and shortening, causing the bones to move closer together. As skeletal muscles pull the bones together, the bones move. **Flexion** of a muscle causes it to bend. **Extension** of a muscle will make it straighten. The normal range of motion for the joints that allow the bones to move is fully covered in Chapter 18.

Muscle cells, or myofibers, are the basic cells of the muscular system. These cells cause contraction and relaxation of muscles. The number of skeletal muscle fibers that move when we do a task depends on the type of task we choose. When a small task is chosen, just a few skeletal muscle fibers may move. A bigger task will require more skeletal muscle fibers to contract to complete the task. Some skeletal muscle fibers are contracting and others are relaxing at any point in time. Once a person turns 30, he or she begins losing skeletal muscle mass. This is slowly replaced by fat. The person may also lose certain types of muscle fibers.

Tendons are tough bands of connective tissue that anchor or connect a muscle to the bones. It is like a link that transfers the contraction from the muscle to the joint to the bone so that the bone ultimately moves. Fascia binds muscles together.

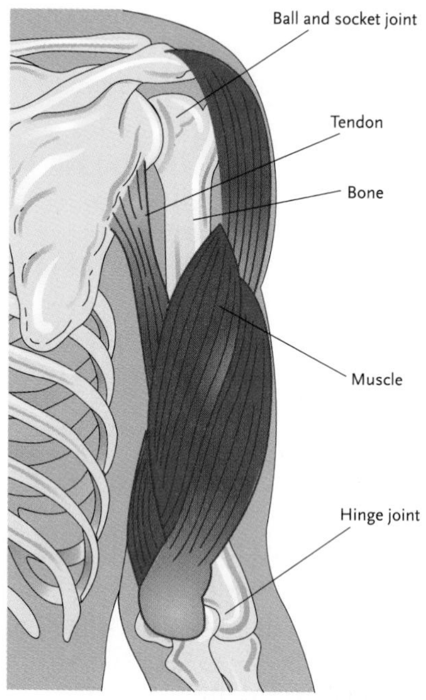

Figure 9-9. Muscles are connected to bone by tendons. Bones meet at different types of joints, including the ball and socket joint and the hinge joint shown here.

A smooth muscle is an involuntary muscle. These muscle fibers are not as big as skeletal muscle fibers. This type of muscle has the ability to stretch without putting a lot of stress on the muscle. Examples of smooth muscles are the walls of the uterus and the stomach. The uterus has to stretch tremendously in order to accommodate a growing baby, and the stomach has to stretch to adjust to a changing intake of food and drink.

Cardiac muscles make up the heart. This type of muscle is also involuntary and contracts and relaxes anywhere from 60 to 100 times each minute. The average heartbeat is 75 times per minute in the normal adult. Cardiac muscle requires a great deal of oxygen to accomplish this task.

Functions of the Muscular System

- moves body
- moves certain substances inside the body, such as **chyme** in the **digestive tract** or blood in the heart
- produces heat
- maintains posture
- protects organs

Why are rusty nails dangerous?

Tetanus is a bacterial disease caused when bacteria enters the body, usually through a puncture wound in the skin, such as when you step on a rusty nail. The bacteria is carried to the spinal cord, which then sends impulses back to the muscles, causing them to contract or spasm. The muscles in the jaw are affected first, which is why tetanus is sometimes called "lockjaw." Tetanus is often fatal. If the victim does survive, his quality of life may be greatly reduced due to paralysis and other complications. It is very important to keep your family's tetanus immunizations up-to-date.

Destination: Homeostasis

The muscular system contributes to homeostasis in different ways. One way is by restoring homeostasis when muscle fatigue occurs. Consider the stiffness you may feel when you run or jog. When muscles are stimulated and moved for a long period of time, the muscles may suffer from overuse. This is commonly called "oxygen debt" because there is not enough oxygen to supply the muscles, preventing normal contracting ability. A substance called lactic acid collects in the muscles. This lactic acid has to be eliminated in order for the muscles to return to normal, eliminating soreness and stiffness. The removal of lactic acid occurs when metabolism increases. When the excess lactic acid has been removed, oxygen is supplied to the muscles. Homeostasis is restored, and muscle soreness is relieved.

Aging and the Muscular System

Normal age-related changes include the following:
- loss of muscle tone and strength
- decreased ability to do strenuous tasks

System 4 The Nervous System

Points of Interest

What an amazing organ the human brain is! It is made up of about 100 billion neurons and 1000 billion neuroglia. The brain, weighing about three pounds, is only about two percent of a person's body weight. However, it needs about twenty percent of the body's blood supply. The brain has long been considered the "final frontier" when it comes to understanding the human body. Because there is so much about the brain that we still do not understand, it is realistic to predict that we will be studying the brain and its functions for years to come.

Imagine a control center that sends out orders to millions of cells within the human body. That is essentially what the nervous system is responsible for: controlling the health and well-being of the body. It's an enormous task. The nervous system is separated into two major kinds of cells, which carry out this task every day. They are neurons and the neuroglia.

Neurons are the basic working units of the nervous system, the nerve cells. They are responsible for sending and receiving the nerve impulses from the receptors, located in different parts of the body, through the spinal cord to the brain. Neurons are also involved in thought processes, directing the functioning of glands, and the movement of muscles. The role of the neuroglia is to hold together, support and protect the neurons. This appears to be an appropriate name for this cell since "glia" comes from the Greek word for "glue."

Structure of the Nervous System

The nervous system is divided into two main divisions, the central nervous system (CNS) and the peripheral nervous system (PNS). The **brain** and the **spinal cord** are in the central nervous system. The nerves to and from all other body parts are a part of the peripheral nervous system.

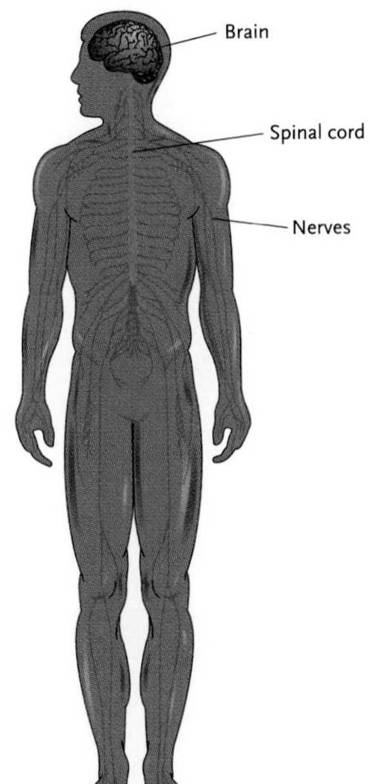

Figure 9-10. The nervous system includes the brain, spinal cord, and nerves throughout the body.

The Central Nervous System (CNS)

The brain, as indicated before, weighs approximately three pounds, making it one of the largest organs in the human body. The brain is divided into four parts: the brainstem, the diencephalon (hypothalamus and thalamus), the cerebellum, and the cerebrum.

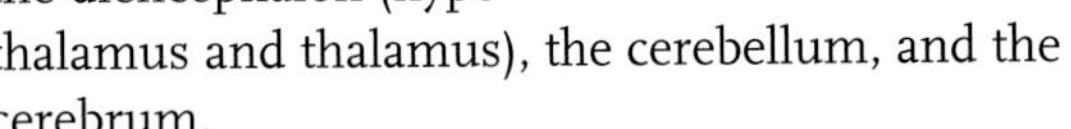

There are two sides, or cerebral hemispheres, in the brain. The right side of the brain, or right hemisphere, controls the motor activity on the left side of the body. The left side, or left cerebral hemisphere, controls the motor activity on the right side of the body.

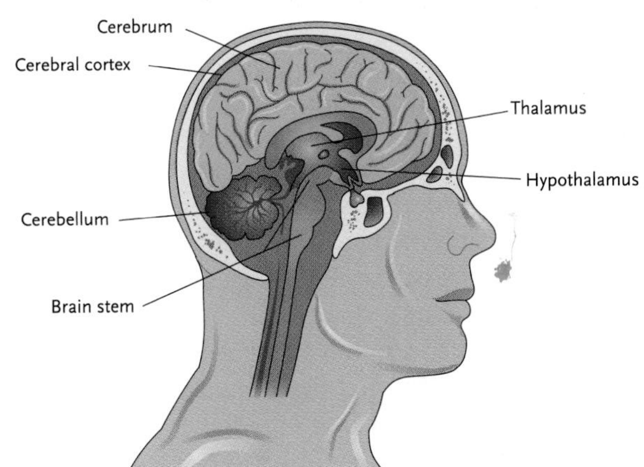

Figure 9-11. The four main sections of the brain are the brainstem, the diencephelon, the cerebellum, and the cerebrum.

Men and woman really are different!

Males seem to have the ability to express emotions only in the right side of the brain, or the right cerebral hemisphere. Females appear to have emotional capability in both the right and the left cerebral hemisphere. This may be the reason why some people believe that males have a more limited ability to express their emotions than females.

The spinal cord is located inside the vertebral canal in the spinal cavity of the body. It is about eighteen inches long. The spinal cord has two types of tissue: white matter and gray matter. The areas of white matter are the pathways for the conduction of nerve impulses. The gray matter receives and coordinates messages.

The spinal cord is also the center that controls the body's reflexes. Examples of reflexes include blinking an eye when a particle of dust touches it and removing a finger from a hot object.

The brain and the spinal cord are protected by the cerebrospinal fluid (CSF). The CSF cushions the brain and the spinal cord from shocks, serves as a delivery system for certain types of nutrition, and eliminates waste products and toxins. A membrane called the meninges also protects the brain and the spinal cord. The meninges is protected by the bone that surrounds it.

The Peripheral Nervous System (PNS)

The peripheral nervous system (PNS) consists of the spinal and the cranial nerves. The twelve cranial nerves mainly serve the head and neck region, with one nerve also having branches to the heart. The peripheral nerves are also classified as the autonomic nervous system (ANS) because the nerves respond automatically. They are either sympathetic or parasympathetic, depending upon their response to stimuli and **stressors**—anything that causes stress—on the body.

The sympathetic division activates the **fight or flight response**. This occurs when a person must act quickly during some kind of an emergency. Some of the changes that occur are increases in blood pressure and heart rate, a surge in adrenalin (epinephrine), and an increase in blood glucose (sugar) to be used for energy. You may have heard incredible stories of a person lifting a car off another person in an emergency. This amazing feat may be caused by the fight or flight response.

The parasympathetic nervous system is primarily responsible for the control of normal body processes such as heart rate and blood pressure. This division also relaxes the body after the sympathetic fight or flight response is no longer needed.

The 3 Rs vs. Art

The left hemisphere of the brain is usually involved in a person's ability to do the "3 Rs," in this case, reading, writing and 'rithmetic, or mathematics. The right hemisphere of the brain is more generally involved in a person's artistic and creative abilities.

The Senses

The five senses are considered a part of the nervous system. They are touch, taste, smell, sight, and hearing. The sense of touch exists in the dermis of the skin. The touch receptors mentioned earlier are responsible for the ability to feel and touch.

The taste buds are found on papillae located on the tongue. These papillae make the tongue bumpy.

The nasal cavity is the receptacle of smell. Within the upper part of the nasal cavity, there is an area called the olfactory area. That area begins the process of sensing odors. It then sends messages to the centers for smell in the brain, where the odors are identified.

Within the eye are the receptors that give us the ability to see. The thickest layer of the eyeball is called the sclera, or the white of the eye. The front part of the sclera is called the cornea, which is transparent. The cornea is positioned over the iris, the part of the eye that is genetically colored and gives eyes their unique color. The pupil is a dark structure found in the center of the iris, which dilates (opens) and constricts (closes) to adjust to the amount of light coming into the eye. Inside the back of the eye is the retina. It contains cells that respond to light and send a message to the brain, where the picture is interpreted so you can "see."

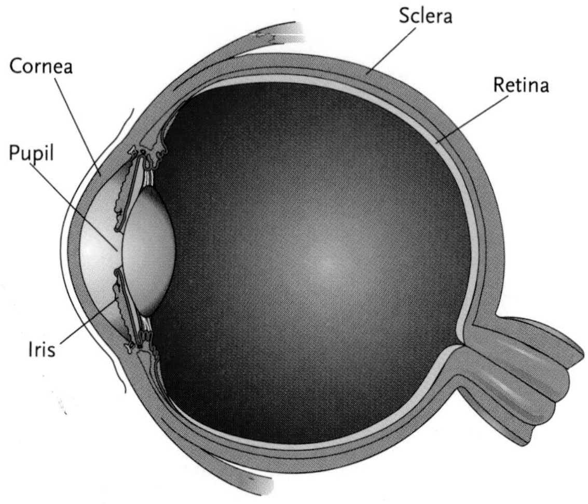

Figure 9-12. **The parts of the eye.**

The ear is the sense organ that provides balance and hearing. It is divided into three sections: the outer, middle and the inner ear. Hearing occurs when the sounds enter the ear canal and vibrations are transferred by the structures of the middle ear into the inner ear. This occurs when the eardrum or tympanic membrane vibrates. The three tiny bones within the middle ear, known as the ossicles, pick up these vibrations and cause fluid to move within the inner ear. When this fluid moves, hair cells bend on the spiral organ, or organ of Corti, the hearing organ; these hair cells send nerve impulses to the brain.

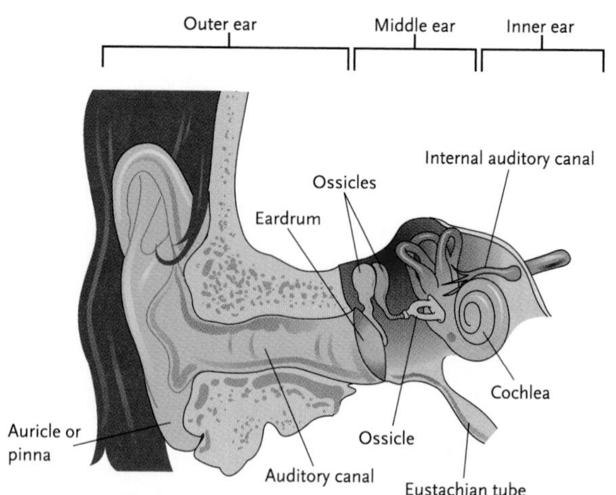

Figure 9-13. **The outer ear, middle ear, and inner ear are the three main divisions of the ear.**

The greater number of hair cells that are moved or bent, the more nerve impulses are sent to the brain.

Functions of the Nervous System

- senses changes occurring both inside and outside of the body
- decides on the best response to the change
- calls the body to action to initiate the best response
- controls mental processes of all types, including sensations, memory, and voluntary control of movements
- provides reflex centers; for example, for heartbeat and respirations

Destination: Homeostasis

Those incredible stories of a person lifting a car off another person in an emergency happened due to the sympathetic nervous system's fight or flight response, outlined earlier. A person confronted with a great fear or emergency will immediately have an increase in the secretion of epinephrine (adrenalin), increased heart rate and blood pressure, a surge of energy due to the increase in blood glucose, dilated pupils, and dilated tiny tubes in the lungs called bronchioles, allowing more air, and thus oxygen, to enter the body. After the car has been lifted off the person trapped beneath it, the parasympathetic nervous system returns all of the above systems to normal levels, restoring homeostasis.

Aging and the Nervous System

Normal age-related changes include the following:

- reduced ability to send impulses to and from the brain, decreasing sensitivity of nerve endings
- slower voluntary and involuntary movements
- structural changes to inner ear, causing reduction in the ability to hear certain frequencies
- reduction in nerve cells which can affect hearing, vision, and smell

System 5 The Endocrine System

Points of Interest

The endocrine system regulates many vital body functions. The endocrine glands play a significant role in determining both size and male and female sex characteristics in humans. The ability to trigger the uterus to begin the contractions necessary for childbirth is due to a hormone called oxytocin.

The growth of children is controlled by growth hormones. Without hormones, we would not be able to switch into the fight or flight response outlined in the section on the nervous system.

Structure of the Endocrine System

The endocrine system is composed of many glands in different areas of the body. A **gland** is an organ that produces and secretes chemicals called **hormones**. The endocrine glands secrete these hormones into the blood circulation for delivery to target tissues or organs.

The **pituitary gland** is often called the "master gland" due to its ability to control the hormone production of other glands. It is located at the base of the brain and attached to the hypothalamus. There are two parts of the pituitary gland, the anterior (front) and the posterior (behind) section. The anterior releases the hormones while the posterior section stores hormones for release when needed.

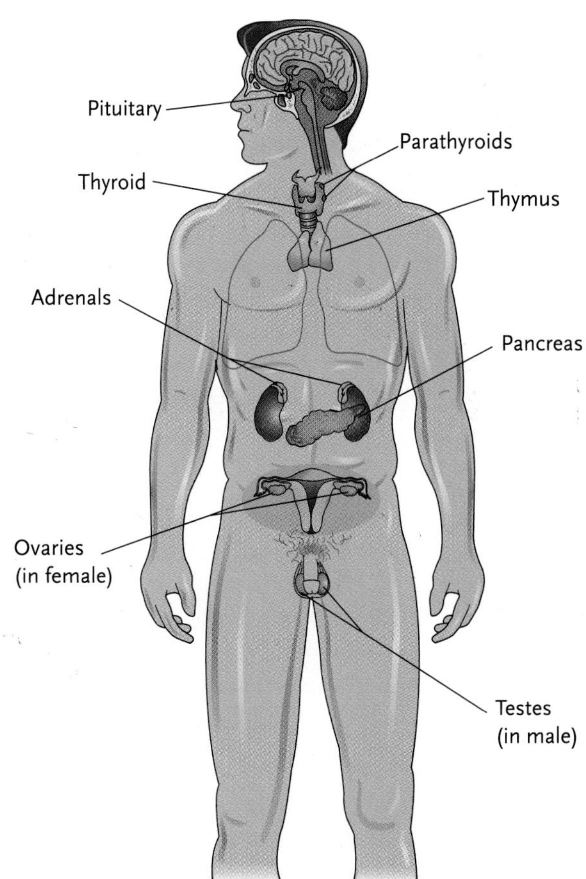

Figure 9-14. The endocrine system includes organs that produce hormones that regulate body processes.

The thyroid gland is found below the larynx, or voice box. Thyroid hormones primarily regulate growth and metabolism. If a child has a deficiency of thyroid hormones, he may be short for his age. Thyroid hormones also stimulate the growth of nervous tissue. The overall growth of a baby's brain and nervous system may be affected if there is a lack of thyroid hormones during fetal development.

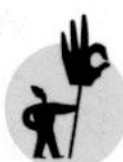

Iodine Allergy and Dye: A Life-Threatening Combination

Iodine is important to the normal functioning of the thyroid gland. Common table salt is where people usually get their daily intake of iodine. If you are allergic to iodine, you must tell your doctor to list iodine as an allergy in your medical record or chart. People who are allergic to iodine should tell their doctor about the allergy if they are ever scheduled to have any test that requires dye to be injected into the body. Serious life-threatening allergic reactions can occur when people who are allergic to iodine have dye injected during tests.

Four tiny parathyroid glands are attached to the thyroid gland. They are responsible for the production of parathyroid hormone. This hormone is vital for regulating the levels of calcium and phosphate in the bloodstream.

The adrenal glands are located on top of the kidneys. They secrete epinephrine (adrenaline) and norepinephrine (noradrenalin), aldosterone, and cortisol.

Aldosterone is involved in electrolyte balancing of sodium, potassium, and water in the body. Essentially, aldosterone acts when a stressor, like hemorrhage or dehydration, occurs by increasing the sodium and decreasing potassium in the blood. These changes cause the body to increase its overall volume of blood. It also causes the blood pressure, which may have dropped during the stressor, to return to normal levels.

Cortisol (hydrocortisone) is a hormone that works to maintain metabolism. It is also produced by the cortex, or "outer layer" of the adrenal gland. It does this by regulating the amount of glucose in blood. Cortisol also has a role in increasing blood pressure during a stressor like hemorrhage.

The pancreas is found in the upper left area of the abdomen. The islets of Langerhans are the cells within the pancreas that produce insulin. Insulin works like a key to "unlock" the blood and allow for the release of glucose to be used by the cells for energy.

The sex glands of the male and female are endocrine glands. The female sex glands are the ovaries, located on either side of the uterus. The ovaries produce estrogen and progesterone.

Testosterone, the male hormone, is responsible for the development of male sex characteristics, such as the deepening of the voice and growth of a beard.

Functions of the Endocrine System

- assists in the regulation of metabolism and energy levels
- acts to preserve homeostasis
- plays a major part in human growth and development
- is essential for human reproduction

Destination: Homeostasis

When a stressor causes the level of thyroid hormone to decrease in the blood, the control centers in the brain turn on to increase the amount of thyroid hormone released into the blood. Homeostasis is restored when the level of thyroid hormone returns to normal.

Aging and the Endocrine System

Normal age-related changes include the following:

- decrease in male and female sex hormones
- less efficient production of insulin

System 6 The Circulatory System

Points of Interest

Blood is the life-giving substance that keeps us healthy, vibrant, and alive. An adult male will have about five to six liters (five to six quarts) of blood, while an adult female will have about four to five liters (four to five quarts). Blood makes up seven to eight percent of the body's total weight. The color of blood within your arteries is bright red because it carries the oxygen that your cells need to stay alive. Blood within your system of veins is darker red in color when it is low in oxygen and high in carbon dioxide as it carries the wastes and carbon dioxide from the cells. Blood in the veins is not really the color blue; this is a common way to differentiate it from blood in the arteries.

The heart has to accomplish the enormous task of delivering blood to every inch of blood vessels each day to keep cells alive. There are over 60,000 miles of blood vessels in the body.

A healthy heart will beat about 100,000 times per day for a person's lifetime. (75 times per minute x 60 minutes in an hour x 24 hours in a day = 108,000 times a day).

Structure of the Circulatory System

The heart is positioned between the lungs, slightly to the left of the middle of the chest. The **heart** is composed of four main chambers: the **atria** (the upper left and right chambers) and the **ventricles** (the lower left and right chambers). The right atrium receives carbon-dioxide-rich blood from the body. It is delivered via the superior vena cava from the head and upper extremities and the inferior vena cava, which delivers blood from the rest of the body.

Blood is pumped from the right atria to the right ventricle. The right ventricle pumps the carbon-dioxide-rich blood into the lungs via the pulmonary arteries. These are the only arteries in the body that carry carbon-dioxide-rich blood; the other arteries carry oxygen-rich blood. The exchange of carbon dioxide for oxygen is made during this process. The blood then travels back into the heart through the pulmonary vein. These are the only veins in the body that carry oxygen-rich blood.

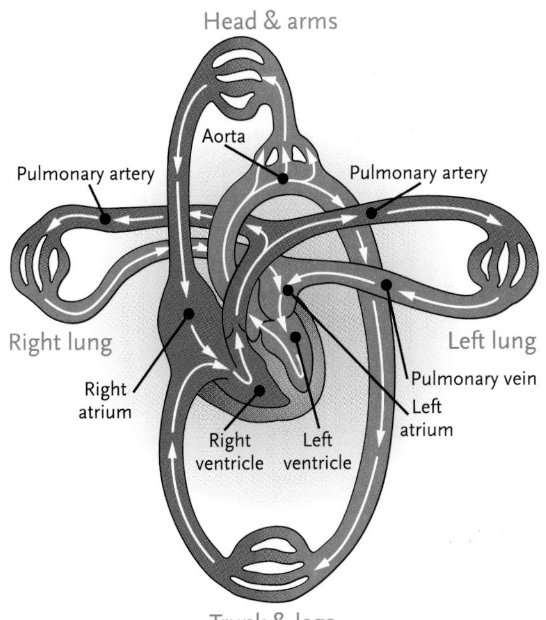

Figure 9-15. **The flow of blood through the heart.**

While in the lungs, carbon dioxide is removed when we exhale, or breathe out, and oxygen is added when we inhale, or take a breath. This exchange of gases returns oxygen-rich blood to the left ventricle. The left ventricle then ships the oxygen-rich blood out of the heart via the largest **artery** in the body, the aorta. The blood is delivered to all of the arteries in the body through the arterial system.

With the exception of the pulmonary arteries, the arteries carry oxygen-rich blood away from the heart to deliver the oxygen to the cells. When the blood arrives at the cell level, the blood moves into arterioles, the tiniest of the arterial vessels. Gas, nutrient, and waste exchanges happen within the capillaries. **Capillaries** connect to the venules, small veins. The vessels get smaller as they move into the limbs. The venules collect the carbon-dioxide-rich blood from the capillaries and then drain this blood into the veins. The veins carry the carbon-dioxide-rich blood back to the heart and the whole process begins again.

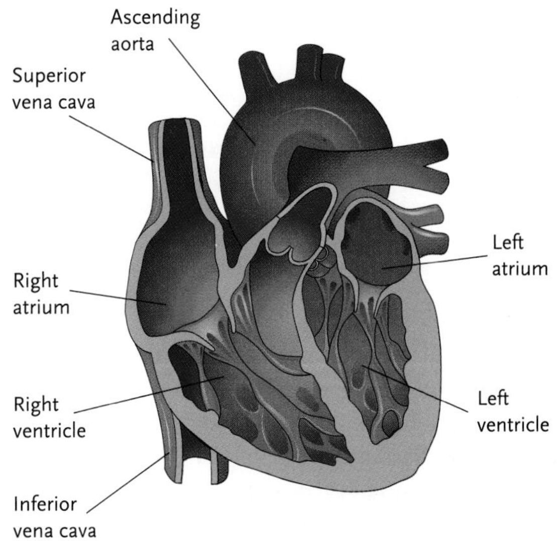

Figure 9-16. **The four chambers of the heart connect to the body's largest blood vessels.**

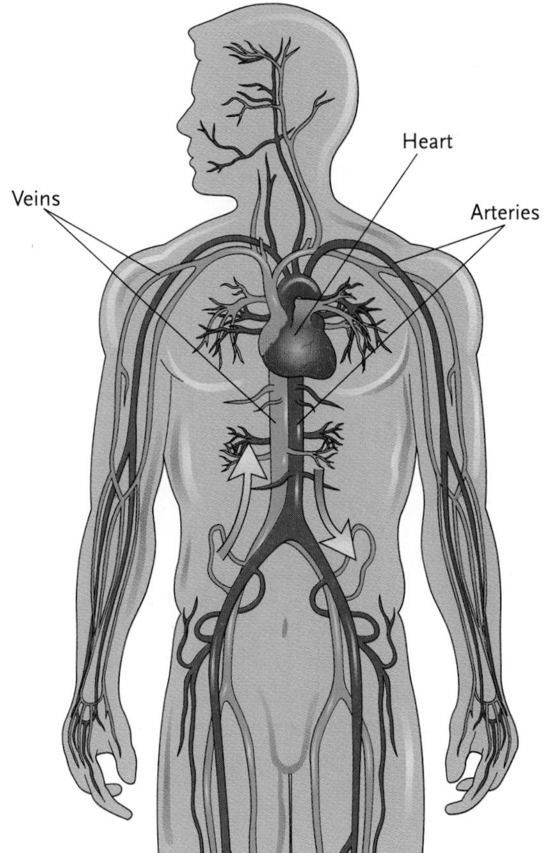

Figure 9-17. **The heart, blood vessels, and blood are the main components of the circulatory system.**

Blood is made up of solids and liquids: the cells and the plasma. The plasma makes up about 55% of the blood and the blood cells make up the remaining 45%. Blood is composed of three different types of blood cells: the red blood cells, or erythrocytes; the white blood cells, or leukocytes; and the platelets, or thrombocytes. Hemoglobin is contained within red blood cells. Hemoglobin carries the oxygen through the blood vessels.

Red blood cells also transport carbon dioxide from the cells through the heart to the lungs where it is eliminated from the body through exhaling.

White blood cells (leukocytes) protect bodies from the invasion of dangerous microorganisms. Some white blood cells "eat" bacteria.

Platelets, or thrombocytes, are vital in the clotting of our blood. The red bone marrow found in the long and flat bones forms the red blood cells, certain white blood cells, and our platelets. Lymphatic tissue produces our lymphocytes and monocytes, certain types of white blood cells. The lymphatic system will be covered later in this chapter.

The Most Famous Carrier

One of the most famous "carriers" of any disease is Queen Victoria of England. She reigned from 1837 to 1901. She carried the disease "hemophilia." Hemophilia is also known as the "bleeding disorder" because the blood fails to clot and abnormal bleeding occurs. Descendants of Queen Victoria brought hemophilia to the royal families all over Europe into which they married.

Plasma, the liquid portion of the blood, is made up mostly of water. The plasma carries nutrients, waste products, hormones, salts, antibodies, and the substance necessary for the blood to clot.

Functions of the Circulatory System

The heart:

- pumps blood through the blood vessels to every cell in the human body

The blood:

- transports oxygen, food, and hormones
- removes carbon dioxide and other waste products
- controls pH level and body temperature
- clots our blood and fights pathogens (bad microorganisms) and poisons

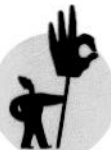

Rh Negative Moms: Rh Positive Baby #2 May Be at Risk!

The blood type you have is determined by your genes. Blood types were first identified by Karl Landsteiner early in the 20th century. Around 1940, he helped in the discovery of the Rh factor in blood. Some people are Rh positive; others are Rh negative.

When a mother is Rh negative and her first baby is Rh positive, the baby will usually be born without incident regarding the Rh factor. However, the mother's blood may form antibodies. A second Rh positive baby may then be at risk. The antibodies formed during the first pregnancy will try to destroy the red blood cells of the second baby.

To avoid destruction of the second baby's red blood cells, a treatment called RhoGam may be given to the mother within 72 hours after delivery of the first baby to prevent the production of the antibodies.

Destination: Homeostasis

When we have a sudden decrease in our blood pressure, perhaps due to shock (decrease in amount of blood to organs and tissues) or a severe hemorrhage (loss of blood), our body's homeostasis is upset. One of the body's responses to this change is to trigger the sympathetic nervous system to increase the heart rate along with the force of the contraction of the heart. This increases the overall cardiac output of blood. The blood vessels then become smaller, increasing the blood pressure. The heart tries to restore an adequate volume of blood to all of the body tissues. When blood volume is back to normal levels, the body has returned to homeostasis.

Aging and the Circulatory System

Normal age-related changes include the following:

- heart pumps less efficiently
- blood vessels narrow and become less efficient

System 7 The Lymphatic System and Immunity

Points of Interest

Picture a S.W.A.T. (Special Weapons and Tactics) team rushing to the rescue when a company is being invaded by a band of armed robbers. Now imagine a S.W.A.T. team living within our bodies, made up of cells responsible for rushing to the rescue when your body is invaded by dangerous microorganisms. This is one of the functions of the immune system.

Immunity is the body's defense against harmful substances. There are two types of immunity. One, nonspecific immunity, produces a response which allows additional red and white blood cells to begin fighting the disease-causing organisms. Other aids in nonspecific immunity are intact (unbroken) skin, saliva, mucous membrane secretions, and tears.

The second type of immunity is specific immunity. Specific immunity consists of both natural and artificial immunity. An example of natural immunity is the formation of antibodies following the recovery from a certain disease, such as the mumps. An example of artificial immunity is a vaccination.

Structure of the Lymphatic System

The lymphatic system is composed of the lymph, lymph vessels, lymph nodes, spleen and the thymus gland. Lymph is a clear yellowish fluid that moves into the lymph system from the tiny capillaries in our circulatory system. Lymph carries disease-fighting cells called lymphocytes.

The lymph nodes are clumps of lymphatic tissue found in groups along the lymph vessels. These nodes work to cleanse the lymph fluid of microorganisms, such as bacteria, along with other foreign substances. Lymph nodes are strategically located in places where pathogens can be trapped and prevented from harming the body.

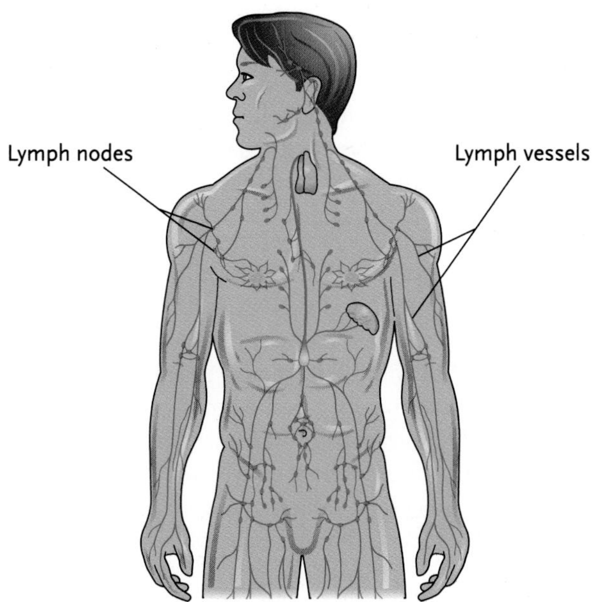

Figure 9-18. **Lymph nodes are located throughout the body.**

Tonsils are large clumps of lymphatic tissue at the back of the oral cavity at the entrance to the throat (**pharynx**). Tonsils work to protect us against bacteria that tries to enter the body, especially through the mouth or nose.

Do you still have your tonsils?

The tonsils combat infection in the ear, nose and throat areas. When children have repeated infections of the tonsils, sometimes the tonsils themselves become a source of infection. Today, doctors do not routinely remove the tonsils. Doctors will sometimes try antibiotics or ear tubes first in an attempt to keep the tonsils. This is quite different from years ago when the first step was frequently to remove the tonsils.

The spleen, an organ, is the biggest cluster of lymph tissue in the human body. One of its main functions is as a storage unit for blood. When the blood is in the spleen, the spleen cleanses the blood of old red blood cells and bacteria.

The thymus is found between the lungs. Its duty is to make the very important T-cells, or T-lymphocytes. Chapter 35 has more information on T-cells. These cells attack and destroy specific types of pathogens. The thymus reaches its greatest size at puberty and shrinks as we become adults. Once its work is completed, the gland turns into fat and other tissue. Normally, most of its work has been completed early in childhood.

Antibodies are proteins manufactured by the liver and found in the plasma. Antibodies are manufactured in response to an antigen, or foreign substance, in the body. Antigens come into the body in many forms. Examples include bacteria, allergens, dust, and pollen. Antibodies then work to prevent the foreign invader from doing our body harm. How the antibody works depends upon the invader. Sometimes an antibody will make a poison or toxin harmless. Other times, antibodies will cause foreign cells to stick together, which makes it easier for special white blood cells, phagocytes, to gobble them up.

Vaccines cause our bodies to produce antibodies against a particular disease. Vaccines can be made with live organisms or with organisms killed by heat or chemicals. Vaccines can also be made with a living, very mild form of the disease, which is altered with heat or chemicals. When the person is given the vaccine, it will cause the individual to create antibodies. These antibodies will usually protect the person from getting the disease in the future. For example, the live mumps vaccine usually prevents a child from coming down with the very painful and dangerous disease known as mumps. Since the consequences of having mumps can be severe—deafness and possibly sterility in males—the immunization is not only encouraged but required in many states for admission to school.

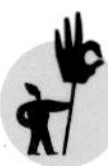

Hepatitis B: Avoiding a Hidden Danger

The three-step hepatitis B vaccine is normally given free of charge to nursing assistants and other healthcare workers. When you begin your job, your employer must offer you the opportunity to take the vaccine. You must return for the second and third dose for the maximum immunity to occur.

Functions of the Lymphatic and the Immune Systems

- protect against the invasion of foreign substances and pathogens
- return extra fluid to the circulatory system

Destination: Homeostasis

A hemorrhage is when the body loses a great deal of its blood. When a hemorrhage occurs, the spleen gears up for action. The blood that the spleen has held for the body in its "storage shed" (as much as a full pint), is released into the bloodstream. This release of blood helps our body's volume of blood return to normal and helps restore the blood pressure to normal levels. When the body's blood supply and blood pressure have returned to normal, homeostasis is restored.

Aging and the Immune and Lymphatic System

Normal age-related changes include the following:

- slower antibody response
- decrease in T-lymphocytes
- less effective response to vaccines

System 8 The Respiratory System

Points of Interest

The human body must have oxygen delivered constantly to each of its billions of cells or death will occur within a few minutes. Many people have experienced choking when eating or drinking. When the airway is blocked, oxygen cannot reach the lungs. A choking person may have only seconds before becoming unconscious due to the lack of oxygen.

Oxygen is our first and foremost basic need; it comes before water, food, elimination, or rest. For example, consider whether you would be able to use your hand to lift a glass of water to your lips if you could not take a breath. It would be impossible.

A healthy person will breathe about 12 to 20 times per minute. A person who has difficulty breathing on his own might breathe 24 times per minute or up to 40, 50, or even more times per minute in order to take in sufficient oxygen to nourish the cells.

Structure of the Respiratory System

The respiratory system is composed of the nose, pharynx, larynx, trachea, bronchi, lungs, and alveoli. The nose serves as the front line of the body's air filtration. It will remove particles like dust and bacteria from the air as it moves through the nasal cavity. The nose also warms and humidifies the inhaled air before it continues along toward the pharynx, or throat. The air winds through this passageway down to the larynx, or voice box. The larynx is made up of nine pieces of cartilage, including the thyroid cartilage (sometimes known as the Adam's apple) and the epiglottis. The epiglottis acts like a lid, shutting off the larynx during the swallowing process. This blocks food from entering the **trachea** or windpipe and causing us to choke.

The larynx enables us to speak. Exhaled air passes over the vocal cords and causes them to vibrate. Males have lower voices because they have thicker and longer vocal cords than females. This causes their vocal cords to vibrate more slowly, which lowers the overall pitch of their voice.

The trachea or windpipe transfers air from the outside of the body to the lungs. From the trachea, the air travels into the **bronchi**, the branches that will enter into the lungs. It is often said that the trachea and its branches resemble an upside-down tree. The bronchi turn into the tiniest branches, called the bronchioles. These tiny branches end in the grape-like clusters called **alveoli**. These are known as the air sacs of the lungs.

The **lungs** are large organs within the chest cavity. They are covered by a membrane called the pleura, which covers and protect the lungs. The pleura is made up of two layers that have fluid in between them. This fluid allows the pleura to move easily without rubbing together as the lungs expand and contract. The lungs expand when we breathe in (inhalation) and contract when we breathe out (exhalation). The process of inhaling uses more energy than the process of exhaling. Exhaling, then, is considered a passive process using very few muscles.

The oxygen and carbon dioxide gas exchanges occur in the lungs and in the cells of the body. The exchange inside the lungs is called external respiration. During external respiration, oxygen moves into the blood, and carbon dioxide moves into the alveoli. The carbon dioxide is transported from the alveoli when we exhale out through the nose and the mouth.

The exchange of gases inside the cells in the rest of the body is called internal respiration. During internal respiration, oxygen moves into the cells and carbon dioxide moves into the blood. The second exchange is now complete. The cells have their oxygen and the carbon dioxide is headed to the lungs to be exhaled. This process of breathing air in and out is continuous; it never stops. Our cells must constantly be filled with a fresh supply of oxygen.

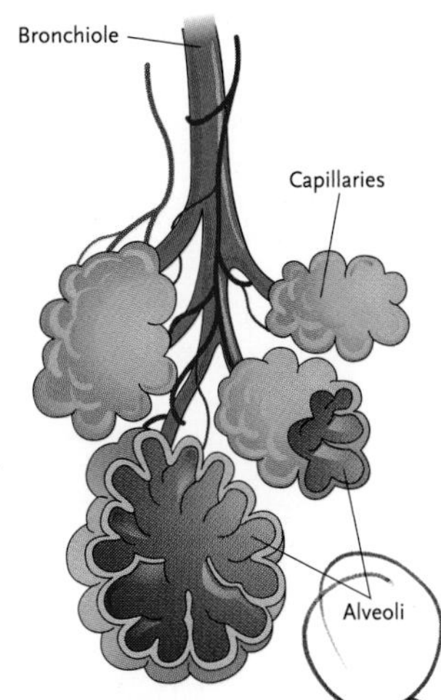

Figure 9-19. **Oxygen and carbon dioxide are exchanged between the alveoli and the capillaries that supply them with blood.**

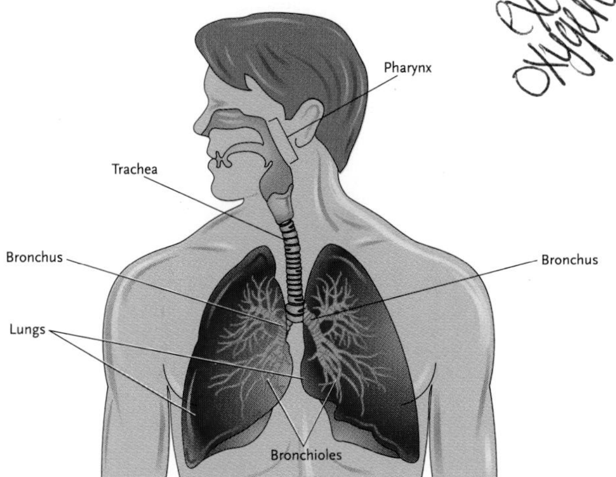

Figure 9-20. **The respiratory process begins with inspiration through the nose or mouth. The air travels through the trachea and into the lungs via the bronchi, which then branch into bronchioles.**

Functions of the Respiratory System

- serves as an air filter, cleansing the inhaled air
- supplies oxygen to body cells
- removes carbon dioxide from the cells
- produces the sounds associated with speech

Destination: Homeostasis

When the blood oxygen level falls due to a stressor, the area in the brain responsible for respiratory control, the medulla, sends out nerve impulses. These impulses cause our diaphragm and the other respiratory muscles to contract more forcefully and more often. This is known as hyperventilation, or rapid and deep breathing. This increase in breathing causes the blood oxygen level to increase. When the blood oxygen level returns to normal, homeostasis is restored. If the blood oxygen level does not return to normal, body cells may suffer permanent damage due to a lack of oxygen.

Aging and the Respiratory System

Normal age-related changes include the following:

- air sacs (the alveoli) become less elastic
- airways become less elastic and stiff
- lung capacity decreases
- blood level of oxygen decreases
- decreased lung capacity can cause voice to weaken

System 9 The Gastrointestinal System

Points of Interest

Lobster, lasagna, barbecued ribs. Are you hungry yet? Food is a source of joy and signals togetherness for some people. Others may think of food as the enemy. Some people feel they need to count every calorie. Others can eat anything without gaining a pound. Whether a person loves or hates food, or perhaps is somewhere in between, food is a basic need and vital to survival.

The consistency of food changes as we chew, swallow, and digest it. The gastrointestinal or digestive system must work efficiently to change food into a substance that can be absorbed by our cells. There are many organs involved in the absorption of our food. The gastrointestinal tract (GI tract), also called the **alimentary canal**, is a tube consisting of many of the organs of **digestion**. The GI tract is probably much longer than you thought. It is almost 30 feet in length. This tube is coiled up inside of each person. The many organs of digestion work together to provide the energy body cells need each day.

Structure of the Gastrointestinal System

The gastrointestinal system is made up of two sections: the GI tract and the accessory organs. The GI tract is a continuous tube from the opening of the mouth all the way to the anus, where solid wastes are eliminated from the body. The mouth, or oral cavity, is where the food enters the body when we eat. The tongue begins by moving food around in the mouth.

The salivary glands secrete a fluid called saliva which begins lubricating and dissolving the food. The teeth break up food during a process called mastication (chewing). Food forms a bolus, a mass of food that is easier to swallow. The bolus moves into the pharynx or throat, where it travels down to the esophagus, a tube about ten inches in length. This occurs as part of the swallowing reflex. We pause in our breathing when we swallow because we cannot breathe and swallow at the same time. As we learned in the respiratory system section, the epiglottis acts like a lid shutting off the larynx during the swallowing process. This blocks food from entering the trachea or windpipe and causing us to choke. Food moves into the stomach from the esophagus because of muscular contractions that push it toward the stomach. This is called **peristalsis**.

When the food reaches the stomach, it mixes with gastric juice, a fluid that has a pH of between one and two. This pH makes gastric juice a strong acid capable of killing most of the microorganisms that come into the stomach. The stomach changes the food into a substance called chyme (from the Greek word chymos, meaning juice). Food usually stays in the stomach for about two to six hours after eating. From there, the chyme passes into the first part of the small intestine, called the **duodenum**. The small intestine is about 20 feet long and is approximately an inch in diameter.

The small intestine receives secretions from the liver and the pancreas. The small intestine also secretes intestinal digestive juice from its walls. The liver produces bile, a substance that breaks down fats, and releases bile into the gallbladder. When needed, the gallbladder sends the bile to the small intestine through the common bile duct. The pancreas produces juices that digest carbohydrates, proteins, and fats. These juices are sent to the small intestine through the pancreatic duct, which joins the common bile duct.

The small intestine is lined with villi, tiny fingerlike projections that absorb our food and fluids. Absorption takes place because the food is broken down into tiny molecules that are able to travel through the cells into the blood and lymph. Approximately 90% of our food and fluids is absorbed in the small intestine.

The rest of absorption occurs in the large intestine. It is about two and one-half inches in diameter and about five feet long. The large intestine helps regulate water balance by absorbing water and electrolytes and eliminates solid wastes as feces. The first part of the large intestine, the cecum, has a valve that prevents the feces from moving backward into the small intestine. The appendix is attached to the cecum. The exact function of the appendix is not known. The rest of the large intestine consists of the ascending, transverse, and descending **colon** along with the rectum and anus. The chyme takes three to ten hours to become feces within the colon. Feces can be about 40% bacteria. Feces are eliminated from the body through the waves of muscle contractions called peristalsis.

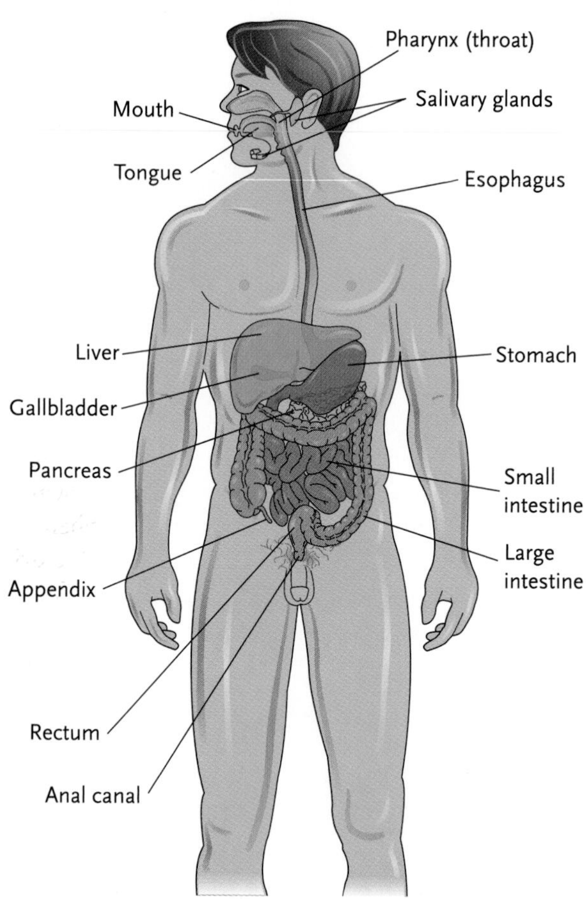

Figure 9-21. The gastrointestinal tract consists of all the organs needed to digest food and process waste.

Bacteria Beware!

The body protects itself against things that could cause harm if absorbed into the bloodstream. The stomach and the lymph system kill many harmful bacteria. Vomiting and diarrhea are other types of responses that rid the body of irritating or harmful substances.

Functions of the Gastrointestinal System

- ingests food
- digests food
- absorbs food
- eliminates waste products from food/fluids

Destination: Homeostasis

When a person becomes dehydrated, he may experience a dry mouth, along with other symptoms. Having a drink will wet the mouth and, hopefully prevent the body from suffering any ill effects due to the temporary lack of fluids. The body must regain its fluid balance in order to return to homeostasis.

Aging and the Gastrointestinal System

Normal age-related changes include the following:
- decrease in ability to taste
- difficulty with digestion of certain foods
- constipation
- difficulty chewing
- decreased absorption of vitamins
- decrease in saliva and digestive fluids

System 10 The Urinary System

Points of Interest

Most of us know what it's like to have to go to the bathroom and be nowhere near a restroom. Perhaps you have had to wait for the bathroom in your own home! Ideally, people should always urinate when they first feel the need to do so. This protects the urinary system, which is vital to our survival and plays a key role in homeostasis.

Our kidneys cleanse wastes from our body cells that build up in our bloodstream by using a self-cleaning filtration system. In fact, all of our blood is cleansed and filtered about 60 times in a day. Approximately 99% of the fluid that comes out of the blood each day returns to the blood. About 180,000 cubic centimeters (180 liters or almost 48 gallons) of fluid is filtered each day! We make only 1000 cc (one liter) to 2000 cc (two liters) of urine in a 24-hour period, despite the incredible amount of blood the kidneys filter every day.

Structure of the Urinary System

The urinary system consists of two kidneys, two ureters, the urinary bladder, and the urethra. The **kidneys** are kidney-bean-shaped organs. They lie slightly above the waist against the rear wall of the abdominal cavity and on either side of the spine. Each kidney is about four to five inches in length, one inch thick, and weighs between four and six ounces. The kidneys are partially protected by the back muscles and the lower ribs. The kidneys cleanse and filter the waste products and toxic materials from our blood. They also regulate the amount of electrolytes within the body and help to regulate blood pressure and water balance.

Substances needed by the body are reabsorbed and the substances not needed—toxins and waste products—stay in the kidney and form urine. The urine is then transferred to the bladder through tubes called the ureters. The ureters are narrow tubes about one foot in length. When we urinate, the ureters also prevent the backflow of urine into the kidneys.

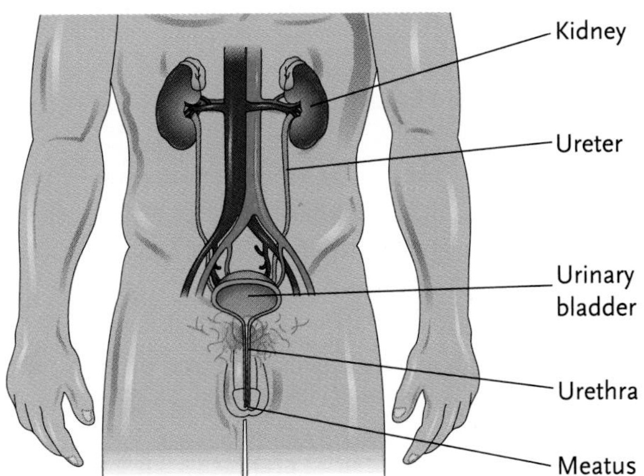

Figure 9-22. The urinary system consists of two kidneys and their ureters, the bladder, the urethra, and the meatus.

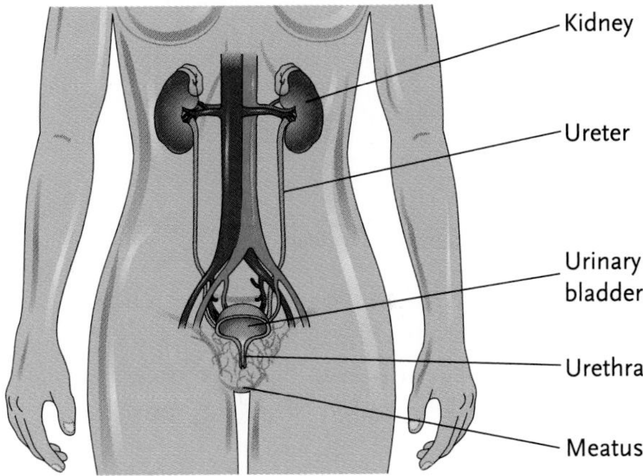

Figure 9-23. The female urethra is shorter than the male urethra. Because of this, the female bladder is more likely to become infected by bacteria traveling up the urethra.

The urinary **bladder** serves as a type of "storage shed" for our urine. When the bladder has collected about 200 to 400 cc of urine, nerve impulses are transferred to the lower portion of our spinal cord. The spinal cord sends nerve impulses back that cause the muscles of the bladder to contract and relax our internal sphincter. The urine moves into the urethra, the tube that carries the urine out of the body. In the male, the urethra is approximately seven to eight inches long. In the female it is approximately one and one-half inches long. We also have an external sphincter. We need to voluntarily relax this external sphincter in order to pass urine from our body. This is the process of urinating. When this sphincter is damaged, weakened, or loses contact with the nervous system, it can cause incontinence. Incontinence is the inability to control urination.

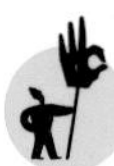

Tiny stones can be a big pain!

Kidney stones, also called renal calculi, may block a ureter and can cause extreme pain. Urine production may also be decreased during a blockage because of a reflex that causes tiny vessels in the kidney to get smaller or constrict.

Functions of the Urinary System

- removes waste products from the blood
- regulates the levels of electrolytes in the body
- assists in the regulation of blood pressure
- helps maintain water balance in the body

Destination: Homeostasis

When we have a low intake of water and other fluids, homeostasis is threatened. The kidneys will try to continue filtering the blood. They have to keep the water balanced in the body while continuing to remove all of the wastes from the blood. They do this by increasing the amount of water that is returned to the bloodstream. This causes less water to be transferred into the urine and more concentrated urine to be produced. Thus, when water intake decreases, the body adjusts so that the water balance in our body remains stable, and we return to homeostasis.

Aging and the Urinary System

Normal age-related changes include the following:

- kidneys do not filter the blood as efficiently
- more bladder infections due to incomplete emptying of the bladder caused by weaker muscle tone

System 11 The Reproductive System

Points of Interest

Consider for a moment how safe, warm, and comforting the womb is for a growing baby. Now, consider what a shock it is to suddenly be brought into the world with all of its loud noises and strange people! It's hard to believe that we have all been through this experience. The body is truly an incredible machine to be able to accomplish such a feat: the reproduction of itself.

Puberty is the time when the reproductive system becomes fully developed and able to reproduce. It comes from the Latin word meaning "grown up." In the male, it usually begins at about the age of 13 to 15 years and causes the secondary sex characteristics to develop. These are the deepening of the voice, the growth of body hair, rapid weight gain and increases in height and size of the shoulders, increase in penis and testicle size, and sometimes the occurrence of nocturnal emissions, known as "wet dreams."

In females, puberty usually occurs sometime between the ages of 9 and 16 but can be delayed up to the age of 18. The height and weight increase in a growth spurt and breast enlargement occurs. The growth of body hair under the arms and in the pubic area is seen, along with a slight clear to whitish discharge from the vagina. During this time period, the female will have her first menstrual period, called menarche.

Structure of the Reproductive System

The male reproductive system consists of the penis, testes, and glands, such as the prostate gland. The testes are found within the sac of skin known as the scrotum. The scrotum is usually slightly cooler in temperature than the rest of the male's body. This cooler temperature is necessary for the production of **sperm**. The male hormone testosterone is produced within the testes. Sperm travel from the testes to the epididymis, a coiled tube that can be as long as 20 feet! Sperm become fully mature within this tube and then move into the ductus (or vas) deferens, a tube that sperm travel through in order to reach the ejaculatory duct.

From the ejaculatory duct, sperm empty into the urethra, where they are released from the body through the penis. During this trip through the male reproductive organs, the sperm mix with fluid produced in three glands, the seminal vesicles, the prostate gland, and Cowper's glands. Each of these glands produces a portion of the semen that mixes with the sperm to assist the sperm in meeting its final destination. Semen is released during ejaculation in small amounts, anywhere from about two to five cubic centimeters at a time. Every cubic centimeter of semen has about 50 to 100 million sperm.

The female reproductive system is made up of the ovaries, fallopian tubes, uterus, vagina, the external genitals—the vulva—and the mammary glands or breasts. The female egg cells or **ova** are produced within the ovaries. At birth, there are originally hundreds of thousands of follicles within an ovary that may someday turn into mature ova or eggs. By the time a young girl reaches the age of puberty, the number of follicles that may turn into mature ova ranges from 300 to 500. Ova are released from ovaries (usually alternating ovaries) each month during the process called ovulation. The ovum or egg cell then travels into the respective fallopian tube, one of two tubes that open into the uterus.

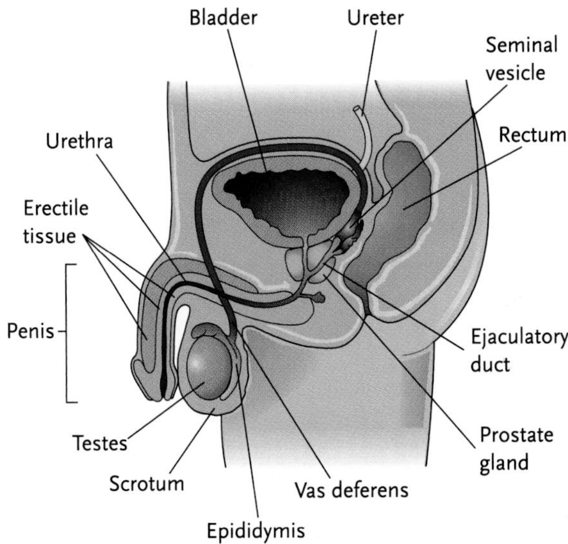

Figure 9-24. **The male reproductive system.**

As the ovum reaches the fallopian tube, it may be fertilized by a sperm that will swim its way up into the tube. If it is not fertilized, the ovum will die within about 24 to 48 hours. Sperm usually die within two days. If an ovum is fertilized, it moves into the uterus, or womb, where it implants into the lining of the uterus and grows into a baby. If an ovum is not fertilized, the secretion of female hormones decreases and menstruation occurs. The vagina acts as the receiver of sperm during intercourse and as the canal for the birth of a baby. It also serves as the outlet for the menstrual blood during a woman's period.

The breasts or mammary glands are the glands that nourish a new baby. They are responsible for the production of milk within the alveolar glands inside the breast. These glands send the milk into milk ducts that come together at the nipple in the area called the areola. This process is called lactation.

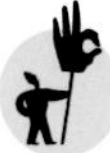

Saunas and Hot Tubs: Not Baby's Best Friend!

Male infertility may occur when the testes are exposed to higher than normal temperatures. Things that may destroy sperm and cause a low sperm count include tight clothing, hot baths, and saunas.

When pregnant, the female vulva, especially the part of the external genitals called the labia minora, usually becomes swollen and bluish due to the increase in blood flow to this area. This physical change appears around the eighth to the twelfth week. It can help diagnose pregnancy.

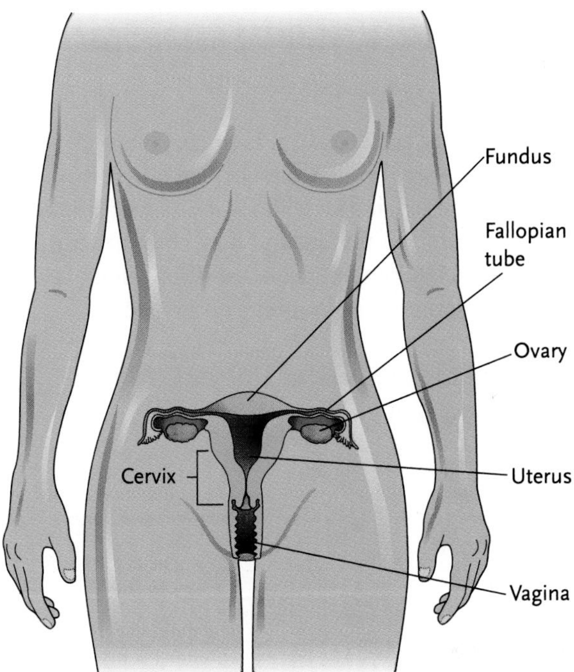

Figure 9-25. **The female reproductive system.**

Functions of the Reproductive System

Male
- manufactures sperm and the male hormone testosterone

Female
- manufactures ova (eggs) and female hormones, estrogen and progesterone
- develops babies
- produces milk (lactation) for the nourishment of a baby after birth

Destination: Homeostasis

Homeostasis can be affected by changes in the male and female reproductive systems. The levels of male and females hormones can increase due to a stressor. This causes the brain to send a message to the reproductive glands to decrease production of testosterone. Blood level of the male hormone will then return to normal; the body returns to homeostasis.

Aging and the Reproductive System

Normal age-related changes in men include:
- prostate gland enlarges
- number and capability of sperm decreases

Normal age-related changes in women include:
- occurrence of menopause when the menstrual period ends, usually between the ages of 35 and 55
- decrease in production of estrogen and progesterone leading to osteoporosis
- drying and thinning of vaginal walls

13 Define and locate anatomical terms relating to position and location.

When looking at the body, it is important to be able to identify where an area or specific body part is located. Terms that deal with location and position that may help you understand how body structures relate to each other are identified below. Box 9-3 describes some of the locations of the body.

Terms of Location and Position Box 9-3

Term	*Definition*	*Example*
Superior	*above, or higher*	The lungs are superior (above) to the knees.
Inferior	*below, or lower*	The knees are inferior (below) to the lungs.
Anterior	*toward the front*	The navel is on the anterior (front) surface of body.
Posterior	*toward the back*	The buttocks are on the posterior (back) surface of body.
Ventral	*toward the front*	The navel is on the ventral (toward the front) surface side of the body.
Dorsal	*toward the back*	The buttocks are on the dorsal (toward the back) surface side of the body.
Medial	*toward the midline*	The lungs are medial to (at the midline of) the arms.
Lateral	*away from the midline*	The arms are lateral to (away from midline of) the lungs.
Internal	*within, or interior to*	The tonsils are internal (within, interior) to the lips.
External	*outside, or exterior to*	The lips are external (outside, exterior) to the tonsils.
Superficial	*toward the surface*	The skin is superficial (surface) to the ribs.
Deep	*within, or interior to*	The ribs are deep (away from surface of) to the skin.
Central	*the main part*	The brain is part of the central (main part of) nervous system.
Peripheral	*extending from the main part*	Nerves in the arm are part of the peripheral (extending from main part of) nervous system.
Proximal	*closer to the origin*	The shoulder is proximal (nearer to point of attachment) to the elbow.
Distal	*further from the origin*	The elbow is distal (further to point of attachment) to the shoulder.
Parietal	*pertaining to the wall*	The parietal pleura lines the chest cavity.
Visceral	*pertaining to the organs*	The visceral pleura covers the lungs.

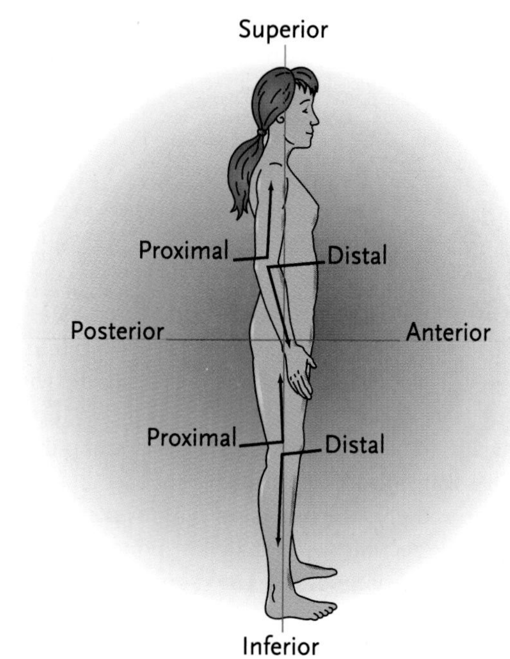

Figure 9-26. **Directions of the body.**

14 Define and locate body regions and cavities inside the body.

Body cavities are the areas that hold the organs of the body. The two primary body cavities are the dorsal and the ventral cavities. Figure 9-27 shows the two body cavities. Some of the organs within the two body cavities are identified in Box 9-4.

Body Cavities Box 9-4

Body Cavity	Organ(s)
Ventral Body Cavity	
Thoracic cavity	Trachea, heart, blood vessels, lungs

Abdominal cavity	Liver, gallbladder, stomach, spleen, pancreas, small intestine, parts of large intestine
Pelvic cavity	Lower (sigmoid) colon, rectum, urinary bladder, reproductive organs
Dorsal Body Cavity	
Cranial cavity	Brain
Spinal cavity	Spinal cord

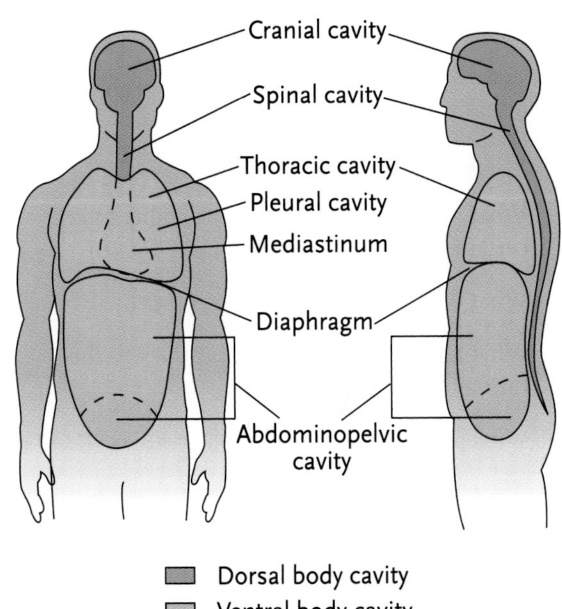

Figure 9-27. **Body cavities.**

Summary

The human body is full of fascinating structures, performing amazing functions. When nursing assistants are familiar with the normal structure and function of the bodies of their residents, they will understand and recognize important changes in their residents more rapidly. Your ability to promptly recognize changes in residents enables nurses and doctors to quickly restore the resident's body to homeostasis or provide a measure of comfort. Nursing assistants on the front lines of care have a tremendous role in the health and well-being of all of their residents.

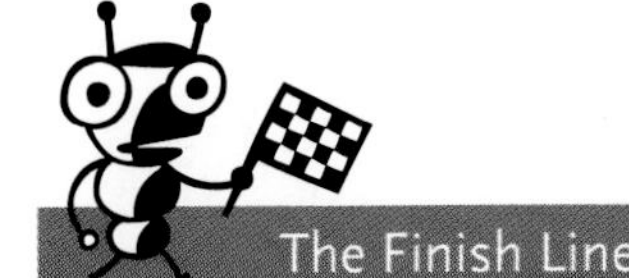

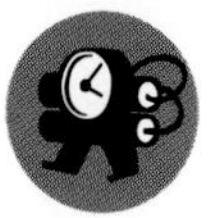

What's Wrong With This Picture?

Each paragraph below has various errors. Correct the errors and list the normal changes of aging for each system.

System 1: Integumentary System

The integumentary system consists of the muscles, the joints, and the tendons. The skin is the smallest organ in the body. In adults, the skin is the heaviest organ weighing about 50–60 pounds or more. The skin makes up about 76% of a person's body weight.

System 2 Skeletal System

The skeletal system is made up of two types of bones: long bones and short bones. The skeleton, or framework, of the human body has 506 bones. Bones are soft and flexible.

System 3 Muscular System

Two types of muscle tissue are found within the body: smooth and cardiac. A smooth muscle is a voluntary muscle. Cardiac muscles make up the liver. Flexion of a muscle causes it to straighten. Extension of a muscle makes it bend.

System 4 Nervous System

The brain consists of two sides or hemispheres. The left hemisphere controls the left side of the body. The right hemisphere controls the right side of the body. The four senses are considered a part of the nervous system. They are taste, smell, sight, and touch.

System 5 Endocrine System

The parathyroid gland regulates growth hormone. The adrenal glands control calcium levels in the body. Insulin is a vital hormone that regulates the salt level in the body; it is produced in the pituitary gland.

System 6 Circulatory System

The heart is positioned a little to the right of the center of the chest or sternum in most people. The heart has six chambers. The ventricles are the upper chambers and the atria are the lower chambers.

System 7 Lymphatic System

Lymph nodes are sometimes able to catch dangerous bacteria before they enter the bloodstream. The thymus stores and cleanses blood. The hepatitis B vaccine is a one-dose vaccine that is given free to many healthcare workers.

System 8 Respiratory System

The lungs remove oxygen from the blood and release it when we exhale. When people inhale, they breathe in carbon dioxide and it is passed into our blood by the trachea. The larynx opens and closes when we eat and breathe.

System 9 Gastrointestinal System

The stomach collects food from the pharynx, the hollow tube that goes from the throat to the stomach entrance. The small intestine is primarily responsible for the absorption of water. The gallbladder is responsible for the excretion of solid waste products.

System 10 Urinary System

The urinary system removes solid wastes from the body. The ureters are organs that form urine. The bladder filters waste products out of urine. The kidneys are the storage shed for urine.

System 11 Reproductive System

The ovaries are the structures where the ova or egg cells of the female develop. The ova or egg cell and the sperm unite within the uterus and the fertilized cell digs its way into the cervix where it develops into a baby.

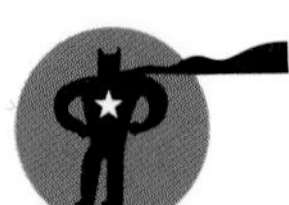

Star Student Central

1. Create a crossword puzzle with not more than five to ten words from this chapter. Share this crossword with your classmates.
2. Find a fascinating fact on the human body in a newspaper, magazine, book, or on the Internet. Bring it in and share it with your class.

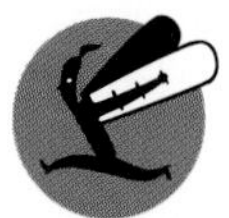

You Can Do it Corner!

Answer the questions below.

1. What is the Latin term for wise human being? (LO 3)
2. What are the six human structural levels of organization? (LO 5)
3. What is formed when elements combine? (LO 7)
4. What is the term for the body's ability to keep certain internal conditions stable? (LO 6)
5. What does the pH scale tell us? (LO 8)
6. What are four major types of tissues in the human body? (LO 11)
7. What are the two primary body cavities? (LO 14)
8. What are the six sciences related to the human body? What are their definitions? (LO 2)
9. What are some characteristics of the class known as mammals? (LO 3)
10. What are some differences between the human organism and other animals? (LO 4)
11. In terms of the pH scale, what number is most alkaline or base? Most acidic? (LO 8)
12. What are three primary parts of the cell? (LO 10)
13. What do the following terms mean: ventral, superior, inferior, medial, lateral, and dorsal? (LO 13)
14. As it relates to chemistry, what does mass mean? (LO 7)
15. What is the primary component of body fluids? (LO 9)
16. What are the two ways cells divide? (LO 10)
17. What two cavities make up the dorsal body cavity? (LO 14)
18. How many chromosomes form a full cell or zygote? (LO 10)

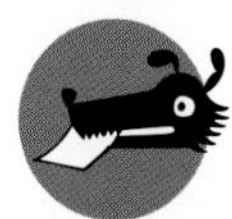

Star Student's Chapter Checklist

1. I have read my textbook chapter.
2. I have reviewed my own "Pocketful of Terms."
3. I have listened to my tutor tape.
4. I have reviewed and highlighted my class notes.
5. I have read and completed any handouts from this chapter.
6. I have completed "The Finish Line."
7. Star Time! Choose your reward!

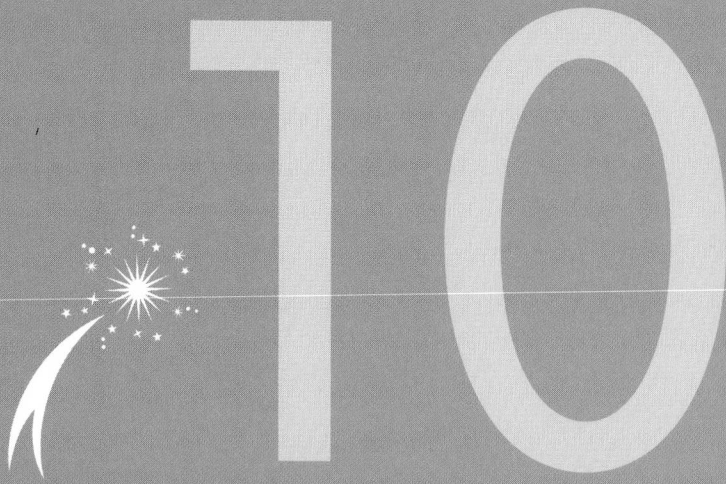

Your Facility:
The Place Your Residents Call Home

Look Like a Star!

Look at the Learning Objectives and The Finish Line before you begin reading this chapter.

Look at your pocket calendar.
With your pencil, put a bracket (   ) around a study period every single day.

Look at your homework for this chapter.
Plug each piece of homework into a certain time slot.

Look at the Star Student's Chapter Checklist at the end of this chapter. Check off each item as it is completed.

"There is no place more delightful than home."

Marcus Tullius Cicero, 106-43 BC

"I grow old learning something new every day."

Solon, Valerius Maximus, 640-560 BC

Learning Objectives

1. **Spell and define all STAR words.**
2. **Compare long-term care, assisted living, home care, and adult daycare centers.**
3. **Explain the Centers for Medicare & Medicaid Services (CMS) and identify how long-term care facilities are paid for services.**
4. **Describe the long-term care survey process.**
5. **Define the roles of eight members of the healthcare team.**
6. **Identify the six qualities of a nursing assistant who is a team player.**
7. **Describe four methods of nursing care.**
8. **Discuss the facility chain of command.**
9. **Explain the importance of the policy and procedure manuals.**
10. **Discuss a standard resident unit and list the equipment usually found in a unit.**
11. **Identify the special department used to obtain new equipment for a resident.**
12. **Compare the operation of manual and electric beds.**
13. **Describe wheelchair, geri-chair, and basic stretcher use.**

The Good Old Days?

In the past, job descriptions for nursing staff included many rules and regulations that will seem strange and even laughable to the nursing staff of the 21st century. Nurses had to act as "warden" to prevent patients from playing cards, stealing from one another, drinking, or fighting. All cleaning of the wards was done by the nursing staff, which meant long, tiring hours washing and waxing floors along with other tedious chores. The heating and lighting of the hospital were usually the nurses' responsibility. They had to carry coal and fill lamps with oil. In some places, they had to be the chimney sweeps as well!
Nurses were not allowed to openly smoke, drink, or go out socially. In some institutions, nursing staff were forbidden to meet or see anyone of the opposite sex. So, whenever you think about the challenges of today, consider the difficulties of the past!

1 Spell and define all **STAR** words.

acute care: care of people having an acute or short-term illness.

adult daycare: care given to adults during daytime hours only.

assisted living: a setting for people who require a certain amount of supervised assistance in meeting basic needs, but less assistance than a long-term care facility.

Central Supply: department for storing supplies and obtaining new equipment for residents.

chain of command: the order of authority within a facility.

charge nurse (nurse-in-charge): a nurse responsible for a team of healthcare workers.

chart: a resident's medical record.

continuity of care: beneficial method of caring for a resident. All staff who provide any care for residents work towards a similar goal of maintaining or restoring good health to the fullest extent possible. This type of care does not end on the weekends or during holidays. Hard-working staff are scheduled 365 days a year in order to provide the best and most comprehensive care possible for every person.

functional nursing: method of care assigning specific tasks to each team member.

geriatric (or geri-) chair: a special chair with an attached lap table.

healthcare team: the group of individuals providing resident care.

inter-generational care: mixing children and the elderly in the same care setting.

Licensed Practical Nurse (L.P.N.): licensed nurse educated to assist the registered nurse in the giving of care.

Licensed Vocational Nurse (L.V.N.): licensed nurse educated to assist the registered nurse in the giving of care. Some states identify L.P.N.s in this way.

long-term care: care provided to individuals primarily in nursing homes; usually provided for an extended period of time.

Nurse Practitioner (R.N.N.P.): a nurse with advanced education able to see patients and write prescriptions.

pet therapy: the practice of bringing pets into a facility or home to provide stimulation.

policy manual: the book of rules related to the care of residents.

primary nursing: method of care in which the registered nurse coordinates individual resident's care.

procedure manual: the book of resident procedures at a facility.

private room: a room with only one resident.

registered nurse (R.N.): licensed, professional nurse trained to plan and oversee care.

record: a written accounting of care; chart.

resident-focused care: method of care in which resident is primary focus; team members are cross-trained in skills, allowing residents to see many of the same faces performing care.

sandwich generation: people responsible for the care of both their children and aging relatives.

semi-private room: a room that houses more than one resident.

state-of-the-art: current.

subacute care: continued acute care required after discharge from a hospital.

team leader: a nurse in charge of a group of residents for one shift of duty.

team nursing: method of care in which a nurse acts as a leader of a group of individuals giving care.

2 Compare long-term care, assisted living, home care, and adult daycare centers.

The nursing assistants of today have endless job opportunities. The facility in which you will work depends on you, your schedule, and the type of resident you prefer. A job applicant can literally pick and choose among positions because there are so many available. You will see local job fairs held frequently at various facilities along with numerous advertisements listed in the Sunday newspaper. More information on finding and securing jobs can be found in Chapter 37.

In this textbook, we will focus on facilities that provide **long-term care** primarily for elderly residents. Since we are concentrating on long-term care settings, **acute care** facilities, like hospitals and ambulatory surgery clinics, will not be covered in depth. **Subacute care**—continued care required by people after discharge from a hospital—will be covered in depth later in the textbook.

The long-term care facilities of today provide health care for people who are no longer eligible for hospital care and are unable to stay in their homes. This type of facility may be large or small. Other terms for this type of facility are:

- nursing home
- nursing facility
- skilled nursing facility
- extended care facility

A long-term care facility is the resident's HOME. This is why we call people in these facilities "residents." This will continue to be the resident's home until the person is able to return home, is moved to another facility, or dies. You must always remember that when you knock on the door and walk into a resident's room, it is the very same thing as knocking on the door of your neighbor's home. Always treat residents' rooms must with respect.

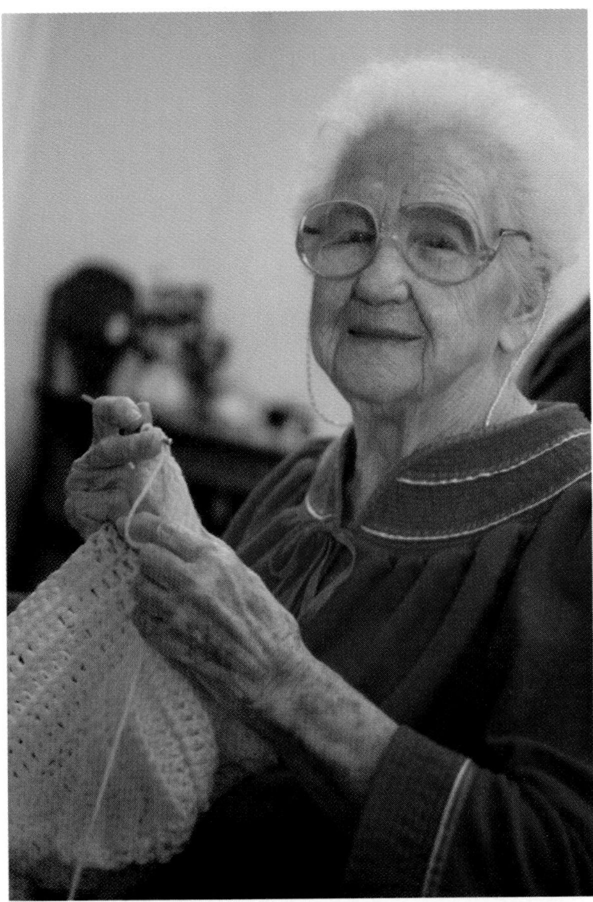

Figure 10-1. A person who is admitted to an assisted living facility is still relatively independent. Some assisted living centers will be able to place her in a higher care unit within the same facility when she requires it.

An **assisted living** facility may be attached to a long-term care facility or it may stand alone. This type of home usually offers residents an apartment-style or condominium-style set of rooms. An assisted living facility may also be set up in a free-standing home.

Staff members are available to provide whatever daily care the resident needs. Residents who are admitted to assisted living facilities are generally more independent and do not require as much care, at least initially, as they would in other types of facilities. Many assisted living centers have a stair-step method of handling their residents' needs. The stair-step method means that a person is admitted to a facility when he is still fairly independent. As he requires more care, the level of placement within the facility changes. The advantage of being able to place a loved one in an assisted living facility which has the stair-step method is that the resident is not shuffled around from place to place.

Home health care is care that takes place within a person's home. In some ways, working as a home health aide is similar to working as a nursing assistant in a long-term care facility. Almost all care learned in this textbook applies to home health aides. Most of the personal care procedures and basic medical procedures are the same. However, home health aides may also clean the home, shop for groceries, do laundry, and cook meals. They will generally have more contact with the family and will work more independently with clients, although a supervisor monitors their work. The advantage of receiving home health care is that clients do not have to leave their homes. They may have lived in those homes for many years, and everything is familiar. Staying at home may be more comforting.

An **adult daycare** center may be a part of another facility, or it may be housed in a free-standing location. This type of facility is gaining popularity as more and more families require two incomes to make ends meet. In the past, aging family members were cared for primarily in the home. Today, the **sandwich generation**—the generation caring for children and aging parents at the same time—is frequently unable to spend the necessary time at home. If no one is available to care for an elderly relative at home, or if a spouse or family member needs a break from caregiving, another option must be chosen. Adult daycare is quickly becoming this option for many busy families.

The daily fee for an adult daycare center is usually significantly less than the cost of a long-term care facility. These fees may be easier for families to handle. At the same time, families like being able to bring their loved ones home each evening. Some centers have merged their adult and child daycare facilities, offering **inter-generational care**. This is considered the "best of both worlds" as the young and old spend their days together. It is not hard to imagine the joy an elderly person would have being close to young children. Many elderly people live far away from close family and may never get to see their grandchildren. This works to provide "grandparents" or "grandchildren" for those who have none or who live too far away from their own families.

The Importance of Activities — Box 10-1

Residents, like many people, are happier when they are busy. Many facilities have an activity department. Daily schedules are normally posted with activities for that particular day. Some available activities include arts and crafts, board games, newspapers, magazines, books, TV and radio, exercise, inter-generational therapy, pet therapy, gardening, and group religious events.

Your responsibility regarding activities and residents is to have residents ready to go when an activity is scheduled. They may need a reminder, along with a trip to the bathroom, change of incontinent brief, or additional grooming. Make sure residents feel comfortable before they leave their room.

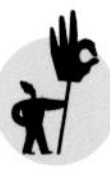

Pet Therapy

Another addition to adult daycare, inter-generational care, or nursing home care is pet therapy. ***Pet therapy*** *provides different kinds of animals to brighten the days of older adults. The Delta Society, founded in 1977 by a physician and a veterinarian, is a national organization dedicated to the therapeutic bond between animals and humans. The group welcomes inquiries from owners interested in volunteering good-natured dogs for participation in a therapy program. You can contact the society by visiting their web site, www.deltasociety.org. Most people love having the animals nearby and become quickly attached to them. Remember to take into account any pet allergies or fear of pets residents may have when using pet therapy.*

Early Nursing Homes

Some of the early nursing homes in the United States were built because many homes for the elderly had to close down due to the Social Security Act of 1935. The number of private nursing homes grew so much that states were forced to develop standards of care for these facilities because of the 1950 amendments to the Social Security Act. In 1987, the OBRA Act further expanded these standards of care.

3 Explain the Centers for Medicare & Medicaid Services (CMS) and identify how long-term care facilities are paid for services.

The Centers for Medicare & Medicaid Services (CMS), formerly the Health Care Finance Administration (HCFA), is a federal agency within the U.S. Department of Health and Human Services. CMS runs two national healthcare programs, Medicare and Medicaid, which help pay for healthcare and health insurance for millions of Americans. CMS has many other responsibilities as well.

Medicare is a program that covers a percentage of the costs of health care for people who are 65 years of age or older. Once a person reaches the age of 65, he is automatically eligible. However, there is a time frame, or a "window," for each person to sign up for this coverage. Thus, each person has to return all necessary forms promptly. Medicare also provides insurance assistance for certain people below the age of 65 who are permanently disabled or handicapped or have certain covered disorders.

Medicaid is a program funded by both the federal government and each state. It covers specific healthcare costs for people who have no means to pay for their care. Medicaid eligibility is determined by income and special circumstances. Participants have to qualify for this assistance.

Long-term care facilities are paid a fixed amount by Medicare and Medicaid for services performed for residents, based on the resident's need upon admission. This makes facilities cost-conscious. If care takes longer than the estimated time for a particular service, facilities lose money. This is why you will not be able to spend as much time as you want with one resident or may even feel rushed at times. If facilities lose money on too many residents, they may be forced to close.

4 Describe the long-term care survey process.

To ensure that long-term care facilities (and home health agencies) are following state and federal regulations, inspections are conducted every 9 to 15 months by the state agency that licenses facilities. These inspections are called surveys. Inspections may be done more often if a facility has been cited for problems, or less often if the facility has a good record. Inspection teams include a variety of trained healthcare professionals.

Surveys evaluate how well the facility provides care to its residents, focusing on how their nutritional, physical, psychosocial, and spiritual needs are being met. The surveyors do this by interviewing residents and family, observing the staff's interactions with residents and care provided, reviewing resident charts, and observing meals. Surveys are one reason the "paperwork" part of your job is so important.

If a facility needs to be cited for being out of compliance with a federal regulation, surveyors use federal tags (F-tags) to note these problems.

When surveyors are in your facility, try not to be intimidated. Provide the same great care you do every day. Answer any questions they may have to the best of your ability. If you do not know the answer to a question, be honest. Never guess! Tell the surveyor that you do not know the answer but will find out as quickly as possible and do just that. Do not offer any information unless asked.

5 Define the roles of eight members of the healthcare team.

The **healthcare team** you will work with consists of many different members. Box 10-2 outlines the many team members at a facility. Healthcare teams provide care for the whole resident. The resident is the most important part—the center—of the healthcare team. Members of the healthcare team may include the following:

Team Members Box 10-2

Activities Director: The activities director plans activities such as bingo or special performances for the residents. The activities are designed to help residents socialize and keep them physically and mentally active.

Medical Social Worker (MSW): A medical social worker determines residents' needs and helps them get support services, such as counseling and financial assistance.

Nursing Assistant or Certified Nursing Assistant (NA/CNA): The nursing assistant performs specific tasks, such as taking vital signs, bathing residents, and performing skin care. As a nursing assistant, you are truly on the front lines of the healthcare team. You are one of the most important team members because you have the most direct contact with residents. Thus, if a resident's health changes from day to day, you will most likely be the first one to notice this change. Some of the differences that occur may not easily be seen by a person who is not close to the resident throughout the day. A nursing assistant must communicate frequently with the nurse-in-charge in order to report any changes in residents' conditions promptly.

Nurse: Your immediate supervisor may be a registered nurse (R.N.), a licensed practical nurse (L.P.N.), or a vocational nurse (L.V.N.). An explanation of the different types of nurses and their training follows. A nurse assesses resident status, monitors progress, and administers treatments, particularly drug therapies, as prescribed by a physician.

> **Registered Nurse** (R.N.): A person with a license by examination who has completed two, three, or four years of education to become a nurse.
>
> **Registered Nurse, Nurse Practitioner** (R.N.N.P.): A person with advanced training in nursing who may see patients at offices and is able to write prescriptions. Usually the nurse must complete at least five years of education to become a nurse practitioner.
>
> **Licensed Practical** or **Vocational Nurse** (L.P.N./L.V.N.): A person with a license by examination who has completed one to two years of education to become a practical nurse.

Physician (MD): A physician diagnoses disease or disability and prescribes treatment. MDs have graduated from four-year medical schools, which they attended after receiving a bachelor's degree. Many physicians also attend specialized training programs after medical school.

Physical Therapist (PT): A physical therapist administers therapy in the form of heat, cold, massage, ultrasound, electricity, and exercise to muscles, bones, and joints in an effort to improve circulation of blood to the body part, promote healing, and help the resident regain or maintain mobility.

Registered Dietitian (RDT): A registered dietitian or nutritionist assesses the resident's nutritional status and plans a program of nutritional care. A dietitian also teaches residents and their families about special diets that will improve their health and help manage their illness.

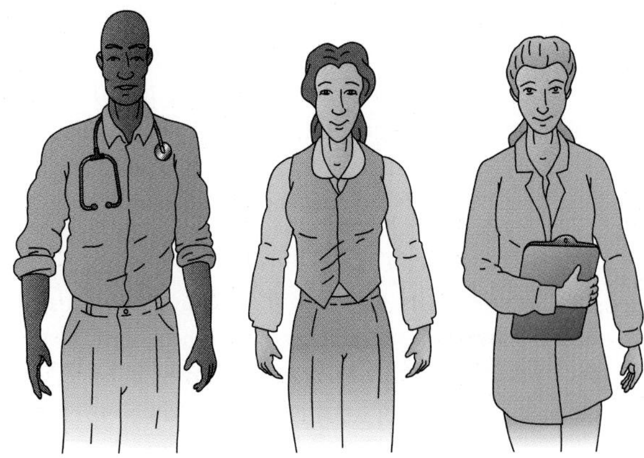

Figure 10-2. A physician, dietician, and a physical therapist are some of the team members with whom you will work.

Speech Language Pathologist (SLP): A speech language pathologist teaches exercises that will help the resident improve or overcome speech problems.

6 Identify the six qualities of a nursing assistant who is a team player.

The concept of the "team player" has been discussed for years in the employment world. To understand this concept, consider your impression of a good employee. For example, one of the employees in a local store is talking about a personal problem rather than assisting customers. This is poor customer service. In the healthcare field, managers want team members who offer excellent service to their residents. To join the ranks of the team players, remember the following rules:

1. Stay focused on work. Leave personal problems at home.
2. Never gossip about anyone–residents, staff members, or visitors.
3. Speak positively about your facility at all times. Never say anything bad about your facility, fellow employees, or supervisors.
4. Accept constructive criticism gracefully. Learn from it.
5. Offer constructive criticism when it will benefit the team. Your opinion counts.
6. Be willing to help others p.r.n. (when necessary).

7 Describe four methods of nursing care.

Over the years, the nursing field has seen many changes. Many different types of nursing care have been used at various facilities. There are four basic types of nursing care outlined below. Each facility chooses the type of nursing care that would provide the best and most efficient care for their residents.

1. **Team Nursing**: This method is used in many facilities. A registered nurse has the role of the **team leader**. Assignments are made, care is given and the team members report back to the team leader throughout the day to keep communication open. In this organized method of nursing care, the resident's care is managed in an efficient way. This is the true "team" approach to care.
2. **Primary Nursing**: In this method, the registered nurse is responsible for giving more of the overall care to residents. This type of care allows for a closer relationship between the nurse and the resident. The nurses are able to manage residents' care in a more organized fashion. Consistency and **continuity of care** are positive results of this method.
3. **Functional Nursing**: In this method, staff members provide care to large numbers of residents throughout the day. Each staff member is given one or more specific tasks to complete on a large number of residents living in a unit. For example, one nursing assistant makes all of the beds on the entire floor, while another completes all of the daily weights. Some people believe this method of care is disorganized because there is less continuity of care. Staff members may not have the time or the opportunity to truly observe and spend quality time with each resident. Changes that occur in the resident's condition may be overlooked due to this fragmented style of nursing care.
4. **Resident-Focused Care**: This style of nursing care focuses on the resident, not the staff members. Each resident's care is carefully planned with the resident's comfort in mind. Some members of this team may be trained in many skills. This is called cross-training. For example, one caregiver may be a skilled nursing assistant along with having the ability to draw blood (phlebotomy). When a resident on a particular unit needs blood drawn, a familiar face can perform the procedure. This can reduce some of the fear of having a stranger perform this type of procedure. Cross-training provides continuity of care and allows residents to see many of the same team members regularly. Residents tend to like seeing the same staff members, as it makes the facility feel more like a home.

8 Discuss the facility chain of command.

Facilities have a **chain of command** that outlines the line of authority in the facility. The nursing assistant will usually have a nurse as an immediate supervisor. If a nursing assistant has a problem with the x-ray department, the nursing assistant will report this situation to the appropriate person—usually an immediate supervisor or the **charge nurse**. The nursing assistant would never go directly to the x-ray department to notify them of the problem. That would not be following the chain of command. A nursing assistant may get into trouble by not following the chain of command. When handling any problem, it is best to check with your immediate supervisor first. When you carefully follow the chain of command, you are following the team player guidelines discussed earlier. Figure 10-3 shows a chain of command.

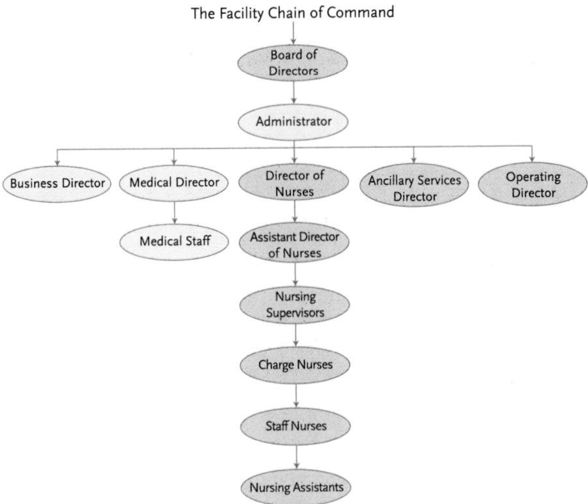

Figure 10-3. **The facility chain of command.**

Quitting without Notice: A Losing Combination!

You must never quit a job without proper notice! Always check to see what notice is required and give your employer at least that much time to hire and begin training a replacement. When you quit a job without notice, this poor decision can stay with you for a long time and cause problems for you in a future job search.

9 Explain the importance of the policy and procedure manuals.

All facilities are required to have manuals outlining policies and procedures. A policy is a course of action that should be taken every time a certain situation occurs. A procedure is a particular method, or way, of doing something.

The **policy manual** will keep a complete list of each and every policy for a particular facility. For example, a very basic policy is that the chain of command must always be followed.

The **procedure manual** will provide you with information on the correct way to complete every procedure for your residents. For example, your facility will have procedures on how to give a bed bath to a resident.

Everyone needs a reminder on how to perform a task from time to time. This manual can serve as a guide if you want to review the steps in a given procedure. You must never feel embarrassed or hesitant to sit down and pull out a procedure manual. Nursing assistants who accept their limitations and ask questions when they are unsure provide safer resident care. Acting too confident when you are unsure of a procedure is dangerous to your residents and possibly even to you. Always ask if you have questions.

These manuals are usually separate from each other and are kept in an easy-to-reach spot in the facility. It is important that you know where these manuals are kept so that you may refer to them when necessary.

10 Discuss a standard resident unit and list the equipment usually found in a unit.

A resident room, or unit, will include everything a person needs to get through the day. A unit is either a **private room** or a **semi-private room**. Private rooms are usually the more popular and sought-after rooms. They have a single bed and provide the resident with valued privacy. Semi-private rooms usually have two beds set up parallel to each other. Beds are usually numbered "Bed A" and "Bed B" or "Bed 1" and "Bed 2." The bed closest to the door is always "Bed 1" or "Bed A," while the bed by the window or on the opposite wall is called "Bed B" or "Bed 2." Serious mistakes have been made due to team members performing procedures on the wrong residents because they mixed up the bed numbers. Residents do not always wear identification bands, so these mistakes can and do occur. You must always identify residents before providing care and check identification bands when available. If you are not sure which bed number and resident requires your assigned care, double-check with the charge nurse. Never guess and perform a procedure without being absolutely sure!

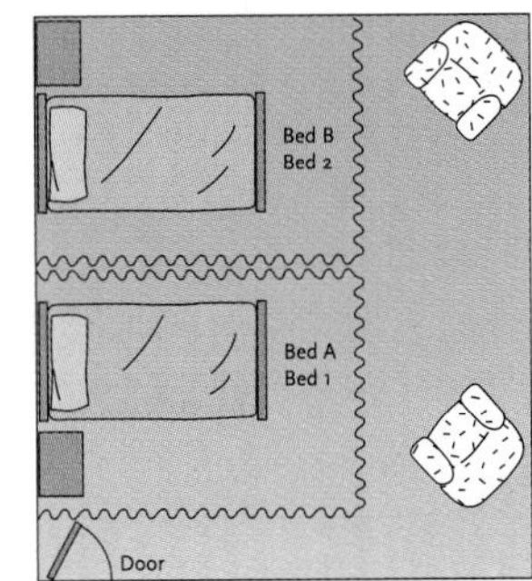

Figure 10-4. **Bed numbers are important.**

Some extroverted residents actually prefer a semi-private room and would prefer having company to being alone. Residents who are more introverted may need to feel more like they are in their own homes and may like being alone. Box 10-3 shows an example of the standard equipment in a resident unit.

Standard Unit Equipment — Box 10-3

1. Bed
2. Bedside stand and possibly a dresser
3. Overbed table
4. One or two chairs
5. Washbasin for bathing
6. Emesis or kidney basin
7. Bedpan for both men and women and a urinal for men
8. Water pitcher and cup
9. Privacy screen or privacy curtain
10. Call system or call light

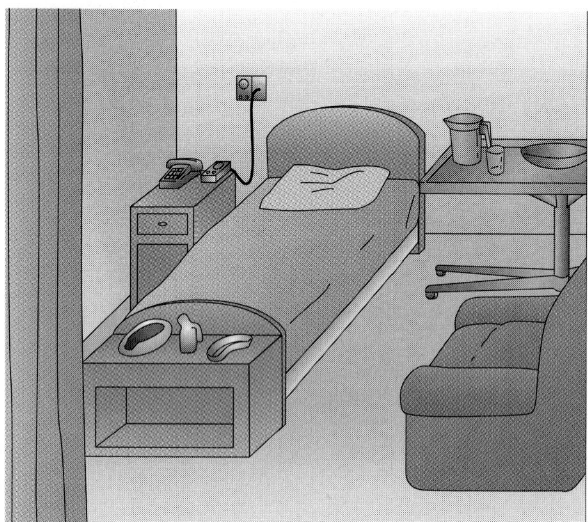

Figure 10-5. **Resident unit, showing typical supplies and equipment.**

11 Identify the special department used to obtain new equipment for a resident.

When a resident enters a facility, he or she usually brings personal items from home. Any equipment the resident needs can be obtained by ordering it from a special department called **Central Supply**, or Supply, Processing, and Distribution (SPD). New **state-of-the-art** methods for obtaining supplies are now being used in some facilities.

12 Compare the operation of manual and electric beds.

Residents' rooms should have comfortable, inviting beds. There are different types of facility beds, from simple and relatively inexpensive beds to state-of-the-art electric models. Box 10-4 describes the two most common styles of beds used in facilities. The more features a bed has, the more expensive it becomes.

Facility Beds: A Comparison — Box 10-4

Safety Note: All four facility bed wheels must always be locked before a resident is moved to or from the bed!

The Manual Bed

1. May have full or partial-length side rails.
2. May not have controls attached, such as TV control or bed control.
3. May not have openings for intravenous (IV) poles
4. Operation may be difficult for residents and staff alike.

The Electric Bed

1. Often has partial-length side rails.
2. Bed and TV controls attached to bed.
3. Openings for equipment like IVs.
4. Operation tends to be a simple process.

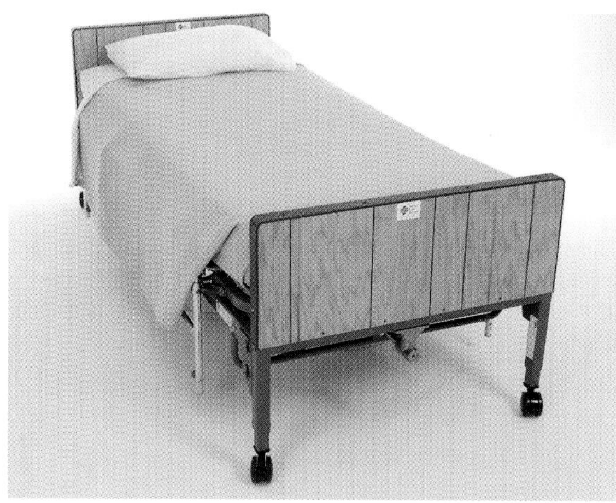

Figure 10-6. **An electric bed.**

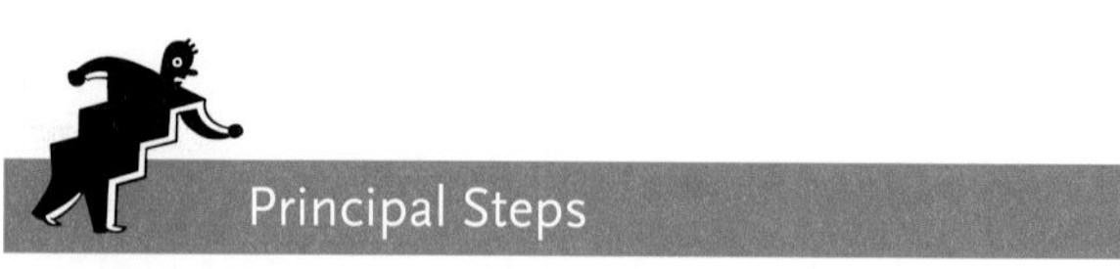

Using Manual Bed Cranks

1. *"Left Head": The left crank moves the head of the bed up and down.*
2. *"Center Body": The center crank moves the entire bed or "body" up and down.*

3. *"Right Knee" or "Right Foot": The right crank moves the foot of the bed up and down.*

13 Describe wheelchair, geri-chair, and basic stretcher use.

Many residents eventually reach the point where they are no longer able to stand and support their weight safely. At this time, the safety options available for the resident will be examined. Residents who require more support may choose a wheelchair to move about more safely. Wheelchairs come in many colors, styles, and sizes. There are basic, less expensive wheelchairs and top-of-the-line wheelchairs that may be extremely expensive. The healthcare team will look at the overall needs of the resident and choose the best wheelchair to meet these needs.

The **geri-chair** is a specialty chair that provides a comfortable, easy-to-clean seat and back, and has the added feature of an attachable tray table. However, when the tray table is in place, the chair becomes a restraint and must be documented as such.

Principal Steps

Basic Wheelchair Use

SAFETY NOTE: Wheelchair wheels must always be locked on both sides before a resident is moved to or from the wheelchair.

1. *Opening and closing (collapsing) a standard wheelchair: To open a wheelchair, pull on both sides to make the arm rests separate and the seat flatten. To close the wheelchair, lift the center of the seat and pull upward until the chair collapses.*
2. *To remove an armrest on a standard wheelchair, usually one or two buttons must be pressed in order to lift the armrest. To attach an armrest, line up the button, and slip into place until the buttons "click."*
3. *To remove the footrest, locate the lever, pull back, and pull the footrest off the knobs. To re-attach the footrest, line up the knobs, and slide footrest into place until it clicks.*
4. *To lift or lower footrest on a standard wheelchair, support the leg or foot, squeeze lever and pull up or push down.*
5. *If there is a pocket in the back of the wheelchair, this can be used during the transport of a resident to temporarily store a resident* ***record****, or* ***chart****.*
6. *When moving down a ramp, you should go down backwards, with the resident facing the top of the ramp, also going down backwards. It is possible that the resident and the wheelchair could "get away from you" if you allow the wheelchair to face forward and go down first.*

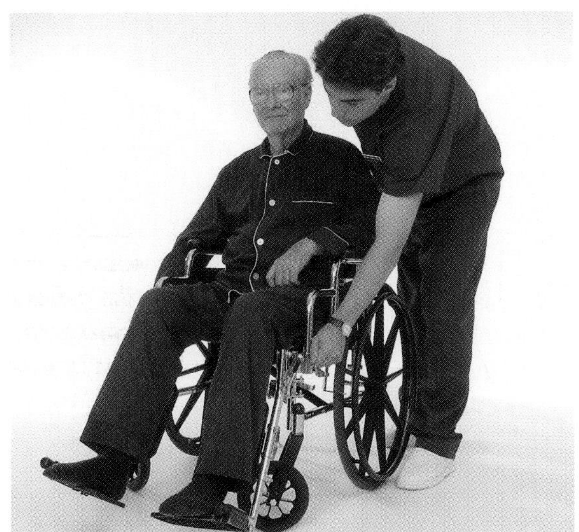

Figure 10-7.

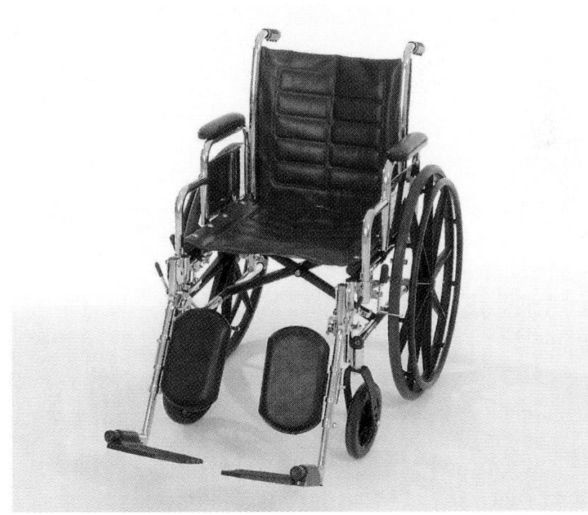

Figure 10-8.

Principal Steps

Safe Use of the Geri-Chair

SAFETY NOTE: Geri-chair wheels must always be locked on both sides before a resident is moved to or from the geri-chair.

1. *When using a geri-chair, remember a resident may slide through the chair and fall to the floor. Team members must evaluate whether this chair is best for each resident.*
2. *The tray table on certain geri-chairs can be extremely heavy. Use caution when raising and lowering this tray table. Do not catch your fingers OR your resident's fingers in the tray when attaching or releasing the tray table. Always receive directions on using the tray table, as these trays are viewed as restraints, and residents who need them require special care. Geri-chairs can be considered restraints. Restraints are discussed further in Chapter 12.*

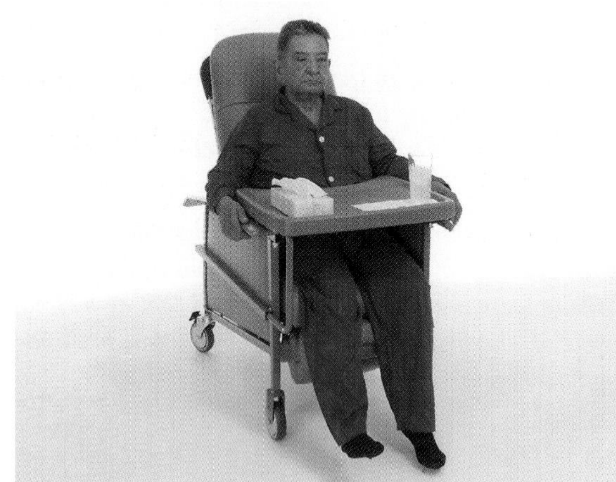

Figure 10-9.

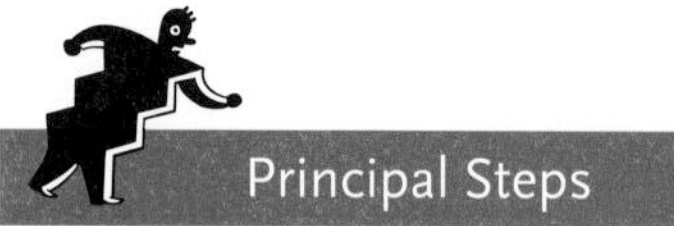

Principal Steps

Basic Stretcher Use

SAFETY NOTE: Stretcher wheels must always be locked on both sides before a resident is moved to or from the stretcher.

1. *Belongings may be moved using the bottom section of the stretcher, if available. Do not forget to double-check this area after transferring a person from the stretcher to any other area. Valuable belongings can easily be left behind.*
2. *The stretcher may have safety straps connected to it or you may have to add facility straps of some kind to the stretcher for safety. Side rails may also be a part of the stretcher. BOTH side rails and safety straps should be used for each resident to prevent accidents and falls.*
3. *Never leave any person alone on a stretcher for any reason, even if someone tells you to do so. Stretchers are high off the ground and can be very dangerous.*
4. *Move residents with the head of the resident closest to you. Then you can observe the person's breathing and overall condition during the move.*
5. *When moving down a ramp, you should go down backwards, with the resident facing the top of the ramp, also going down backwards. It is possible that the resident and the stretcher could "get away from you" if you allow the stretcher to go down first.*

Summary

The place your residents live is very important to them and their families. Your goal is to make this place as safe and home-like as possible for each resident. The policy and procedure manuals can be of great assistance to you when you are asked to perform an unfamiliar procedure. By understanding how to use the special equipment in some facilities, you will help ensure the safety of all residents. The nursing assistant has a very important role in making each resident's stay in a long-term care facility safe, comfortable, and pleasant.

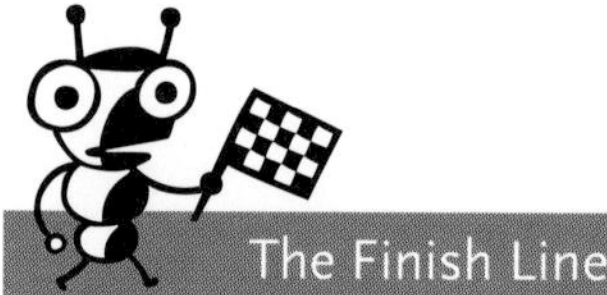

The Finish Line

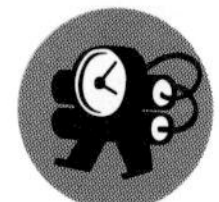

What's Wrong With This Picture?

Look at the following sentences. Correct the errors in each.

1. Marissa Sandler is a registered dietician (RDT). She is an important member of the healthcare team. Most of her duties include diagnosing residents' diseases and disorders and prescribing treatment for them.
2. Christina Simpson is a speech language pathologist (SLP). The bulk of her duties include administering therapy in the form of heat, cold, massage, ultrasound, electricity, and exercise. She is mostly responsibly for helping the resident regain or maintain mobility.
3. Cicely McDermott is an activities director. She

teaches exercises that will help residents improve or overcome speech problems.

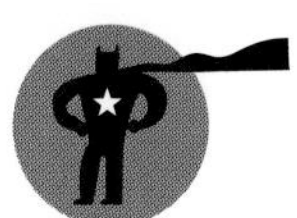

Star Student Central

1. Do you have a relative working in a healthcare facility? Look into obtaining permission from his or her employer to go with him or her as a sort of "Volunteer for a Day." You may have to have a current negative TB test in order to visit the facility. This is a great opportunity to become familiar with a healthcare facility.
2. Look in your telephone book and find listings for adult daycare facilities and assisted living facilities. Pick up the telephone and call one facility and ask whether you may visit for an hour one day soon. Explain that you are currently training to be a nursing assistant. This will give you some exposure to a new type of facility.

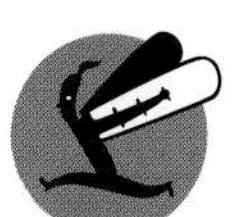

You Can Do It Corner!

1. Identify five qualities of a team player. (LO 6)
2. Describe the four methods of nursing care. List how the duties are divided between staff members. (LO 7)
3. Name four different terms used to identify a long-term care facility. (LO 2)
4. Describe what the chain of command in a facility does. (LO 8)
5. Define policies and procedures. (LO 9)
6. Identify one safety precaution when using a wheelchair. (LO 13)
7. Identify two safety precautions when using a geri-chair. (LO 13)
8. Describe how beds are usually identified in a facility. (LO 10)
9. List four ways electric and manual beds generally differ. (LO 12)
10. List the two major programs regulated by the CMS. (LO 3)
11. Identify a department used to obtain new equipment for residents. (LO 11)
12. List some of the ways surveyors evaluate care provided in a LTC facility. (LO 4)

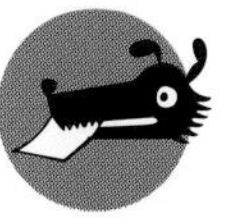

Star Student's Chapter Checklist

1. I have read my textbook chapter.
2. I have reviewed my own "Pocketful of Terms."
3. I have listened to my tutor tape.
4. I have reviewed and highlighted my class notes.
5. I have read and completed any handouts from this chapter.
6. I have completed "The Finish Line."
7. Star Time! Choose your reward!

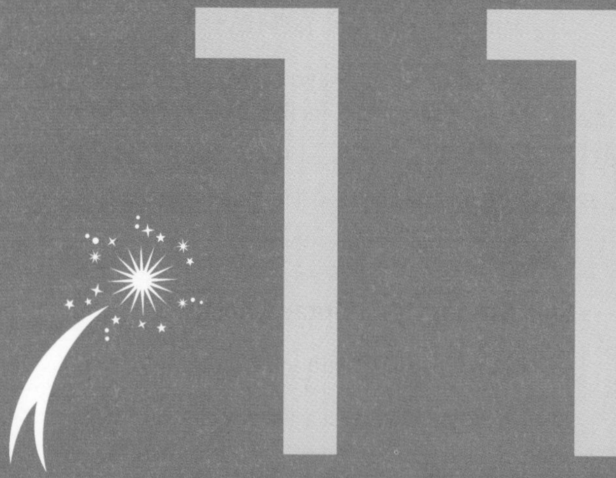

11

Quality Infection Control: Breaking the Chain of Infection

Look Like a Star!

Look at the Learning Objectives and The Finish Line before you begin reading this chapter.

Look at your pocket calendar.
With your pencil, put a bracket (   ) around a study period every single day.

Look at your homework for this chapter.
Plug each piece of homework into a certain time slot.

Look at the Star Student's Chapter Checklist at the end of this chapter. Check off each item as it is completed.

Learning Objectives

1. Spell and define all STAR words.
2. Define the three types of infections and identify symptoms of an infection.
3. Define "infection control" and related terms and list methods of infection control in facilities.
4. Define the "chain of infection" and describe infection control practices for each link.
5. Identify when to wash hands.
6. Discuss the basic principles of using personal protective equipment (PPE) in the healthcare facility.
7. Explain OSHA and describe five guidelines OSHA requires that employers follow for the Bloodborne Pathogen Standard.
8. Define the Centers for Disease Control and Prevention (CDC) and explain standard precautions.
9. Summarize the current CDC transmission-based precautions.
10. Describe overall care of the resident in an isolation unit.
11. Define the terms "MRSA" and "VRE."

Successfully perform these Practical Procedures

Handwashing

Applying and Removing Non-Sterile Gloves

Applying and Removing a Gown

Applying and Removing a Face Mask

Applying an N95 Respirator Mask

Applying and Removing Goggles/Face Shield/Combo Face Shield

Applying and Removing the Full Set of PPE in the Correct Order

"The sick are the greatest danger to the healthy; it is not from the strongest that harm comes to the strong, but from the weakest."

Friedrich Wilhelm Nietzsche, 1844-1900

"Always be on the look-out for the unusual."

Alexander Fleming, 1881-1955, on the discovery of penicillin

Semmelweis and Childbed Fever: It was handwashing, plain and simple!

Imagine having the "cure" to a deadly disease that killed thousands of women after childbirth and being unable to convince the medical community and the world of your discovery! Ignaz Semmelweis, 1818-1865, was a Hungarian doctor who practiced and taught medicine in Vienna, Austria during the mid-1800s. He noted that the death rate on a certain maternity ward was higher than on a similar ward at the same facility. The only difference he could find was that doctors and medical students came to the ward where the death rate was higher right after dissecting corpses in the autopsy rooms. The second ward, where the midwives worked, had a much lower death rate. The midwives did not go into the autopsy rooms.

Semmelweis asked the doctors and the medical students to first wash their hands and then soak them in a special solution before and after examining the maternity patients. After this process was initiated, the death rate from childbed fever dropped dramatically. Semmelweis eventually wrote a book on his discovery.

1 Spell and define all **STAR** words.

autoclave: machine creating steam or a type of gas that kills all microorganisms.

barrier: block or obstacle of some kind; object worn by healthcare provider to prevent the transmission of infectious diseases.

biohazard container: container used for disposal of objects potentially harmful to people.

bloodborne pathogen: microorganism found in the blood of humans that may cause disease in humans when they have contact with blood or body fluids like tears, saliva, respiratory secretions, perspiration (sweat), vomit, urine, feces, vaginal fluid, or semen.

Bloodborne Pathogen Standard: federal law requiring that healthcare facilities protect employees and all other people who enter or live in a facility from disease-producing microorganisms.

body fluids: tears, saliva, respiratory secretions, perspiration, vomit, urine, feces, vaginal fluid, or semen.

carrier: person who carries a pathogen without signs or symptoms and who can spread the disease.

catheter: a tube passed through the body for removal of or injection of fluids into body cavities.

CDC (Centers for Disease Control and Prevention): federal government agency responsible for improving the overall health and safety of the people of the United States.

clean: not contaminated by the microorganisms called pathogens.

clean technique: medical asepsis; the methods used to reduce pathogens or to prevent their spread in a facility.

communicable disease: disease transmitted directly or indirectly from one person to another.

contagious disease: communicable disease; disease easily spread from one person to another.

contaminated: soiled, unclean; having disease-causing organisms or infectious material on it.

direct spread: transmitted from one person to another.

dirty: contaminated by the microorganisms called pathogens.

disinfection: introducing a substance that kills bacteria; using an agent that frees an object from infection.

drainage: flow of fluids from a wound or cavity.

enterococci: naturally occurring flora (living microorganisms) that inhabit the digestive tract and female genital tracts; these organisms can cause infections when they are accidentally transferred to other parts of the body.

exposure control plan: a written plan kept in a particular spot on the unit that explains how to prevent exposure to blood or body fluids and procedures to follow if exposed.

exposure incident: situation when a person is exposed to a bloodborne pathogen.

fomites: something that connects or attaches to and transmits infectious material.

immunity: resistance to infection by a specific pathogen.

immunizations: the process of causing a patient to become immune.

incubation period: the period of time between exposure to infection and the appearance of the first symptom.

indirect spread: the spread of infectious disease through a vehicle or a vector (carrier).

infection: state of being invaded by a pathogen, a microorganism causing disease.

infection control: methods and practices used to prevent the spread of infection.

infectious disease: any disease caused by growth of pathogens in the body.

isolation: limitation of the movement and social contact of a resident suffering from a communicable disease.

localized: restricted to a limited area.

medical asepsis: clean technique; methods used to reduce pathogens or prevent their spread in a facility.

microbe: microorganism.

microorganism (MO): a tiny living thing not visible to the naked eye without a microscope.

mouth-to-mouth resuscitation: rescue breathing.

MRSA: Methicillin-Resistant Staphylococcus Aureus; an infectious disease caused by a pathogen that is resistant to many antibiotics.

mucous membranes: the membranes that line body cavities, such as the mouth or nose.

non-communicable disease: disease that is not contagious, or easily passed from one person to another.

non-intact skin: any skin that is broken, such as open sores (including acne) and dry, cracked skin.

non-pathogen: microbe that ordinarily will not cause a person to get an infection.

normal flora: the microorganisms within the body that normally live and grow in certain locations; when they enter a different part of the body, they may cause an infection.

nosocomial infection: infection caught or acquired while in a healthcare facility.

Occupational Safety and Health Administration (OSHA): A federal government agency that sets rules and policies to protect workers on the job.

PPE: personal protective equipment; includes gowns, gloves, masks, and eye shields.

pathogen: the microorganisms that cause disease.

portals of entry: spots that allow entry into a host.

portals of exit: spots that allow exit from a host.

reservoir: place where an infectious agent normally lives and multiplies.

resistance: total of the body's barriers to the invasion of an infectious agent.

sterilization: the process of completely removing or destroying all microorganisms by heat or steam.

sterile technique or surgical asepsis: methods that completely remove all microorganisms, both pathogenic and non-pathogenic, from supplies and equipment.

susceptible host: a person having little resistance to an infectious disease.

systemic: pertaining to the whole body.

transmission: transfer of a disease.

vaccines: agents given for the purpose of establishing resistance to an infectious disease.

vector: a carrier, usually an insect, that transmits disease-causing microorganisms.

VRE: Vancomycin-resistant Enterococcus; enterococci that are resistant to Vancomycin, a powerful antibiotic designed to prevent or kill bacterial infections.

2 Define the three types of infections and identify symptoms of an infection.

An **infection** is caused by a **microorganism,** a small organism also called a **microbe.** A **pathogen** is a microorganism which causes infection. For an infection to develop, this pathogen must invade and start growing within the human body. There are two main types of infections, localized and systemic. A **localized** infection might be an infection in, for example, the eye, while a **systemic** infection happens when the pathogen invades the bloodstream and moves throughout the body.

A special type of infection that can be localized or systemic is called a **nosocomial infection.** A nosocomial infection, an infection spread inside a facility from one resident, staff member, or visitor to another resident, can be mild or life-threatening. Residents can become severely ill due to an infection obtained in a facility. There are many ways you can prevent nosocomial infections, but the best way to prevent infection is proper handwashing. Since these infections may be particularly dangerous to the elderly, your residents are at risk. Follow all guidelines for reducing infection. It may save the life of one or more of your residents someday.

The three types of infections and examples of each are identified in Box 11-1.

Types of Infections — Box 11-1

Type	*Place Found*	*Example*
Localized Infection	Limited to one area of body	• Cystitis (bladder infection) • Conjunctivitis (eye infection)
Systemic Infection	Spreads throughout body by the blood or lymph fluid	• Advanced syphilis • AIDS
Nosocomial Infection	Localized or systemic Resident gets it after entering the facility.	• urinary tract infection (UTI) due to catheterization

An **infectious disease** is a disease caused by a pathogen. The pathogen "brings its suitcases" and "sets up housekeeping" within the host. The pathogen will cause an infection as long as the host has low **resistance**, the ability of the human body to resist the pathogens. There are two types of infectious diseases: communicable and non-communicable. A **communicable disease** is a disease that occurs when a pathogen is spread from one person to another. A **contagious disease** is a communicable disease that is spread easily from person to person. A **non-communicable disease** is a disease not easily spread from one person to another. This type of a disease may be caused when certain things happen. For example, the E. coli microbe can be accidentally moved from the colon to the urinary tract where it may cause a bladder infection. When it stays in the colon, it usually is not harmful.

There are certain signs and symptoms of an infection that you need to be able to observe and report. Some of these symptoms are outlined in Box 11-2. Should you ever observe a fever, **drainage** such as pus, or bleeding, immediately inform the nurse. Minutes count when dealing with localized versus systemic infections. For example, imagine you forgot to report your resident's symptoms and left the facility. By the time you return the next day, certain types of infections could have traveled into the bloodstream and become systemic. This would put your resident at a much greater risk. Reporting symptoms of infection promptly is vital to the health and well-being of all of your residents. So with possible infections, remember these important words:

★ *"Don't Delay. Report Right Away!"*

Symptoms of Infection — Box 11-2

★ *"Don't Delay. Report Right Away!"*

Type	*Symptoms*
Localized Infection	Redness, swelling, pain, heat, and drainage (the flow of fluid from a wound or a cavity)
Systemic Infection	Fever, chills, headache, change in other vital signs, nausea, vomiting, or diarrhea (N, V, and D)

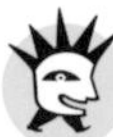

By Debra Medders, CNA

One of the most important things nursing assistants can do for themselves, their families, and their residents is to wash their hands! We can never be too cautious in our efforts to control and prevent the spread of infection. For bacteria to spread, certain things have to be in place. These things include a place where it starts, a place for it to grow, a way for it to move from one place to another (a cut, for example), and someone who is susceptible to catching it. A favorite place for microorganisms to hide is under the fingernails. Those extra few seconds it takes to clean under the nails may someday save someone's life. We all need to be more careful about our handwashing practices. When we are, we can reduce the spread of infection and make everyone around us healthier because of it!

3 Define "infection control" and related terms and list methods of infection control in facilities.

Infection control consists of methods used to control and prevent the spread of disease. Infection control is the responsibility of all members of the healthcare team.

Infection control is about breaking the chain of infection, which is discussed in Learning Objective 4. The links in the chain of infection can be blocked by quality infection control. This is done by using a method called the **clean technique**, also called **medical asepsis.** Medical asepsis is used in all healthcare facilities. Before we outline medical asepsis, some terms must be understood.

When any object can be called **clean**, it means it is not **contaminated** by the microorganisms which cause infection called pathogens. Contamination is when an object has come into contact with pathogens. An object that is considered **dirty** has been contaminated by pathogens.

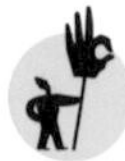

Clean and Contaminated Utility Rooms

Each facility usually has two separate areas for handling clean and contaminated items. These areas are normally called the "clean" and the "dirty" or "contaminated" utility rooms. The clean utility room may have large carts that hold all of the supplies you may need for your residents. Before you enter the clean utility room, you must wash your hands. This helps keep the equipment clean inside this room.

The contaminated or dirty utility room is usually separate from the clean utility room. This room is used to place equipment that may not be needed for a resident anymore. Supplies may be kept in this room that are not considered "clean," such as trash bags. It is extremely important that you wash your hands before leaving the contaminated utility room so that you do not transfer bacteria from that area to another area of your unit. A sink is usually inside this room. After you have washed your hands, you must not touch ANYTHING inside this room. If you do, you must wash your hands a second time.

Measures like disinfection and sterilization are used to decrease the spread of pathogens. **Disinfection** means pathogens are destroyed. **Sterilization** means all microorganisms are destroyed, not just pathogens. Special hard-shelled, microorganisms, called spores, that may not be killed by disinfection are killed by sterilization. An **autoclave** is usually used to sterilize equipment. This machine creates steam or a type of gas that kills all microorganisms.

The goal of medical asepsis is to prevent the spread of pathogens by keeping a facility as clean as possible. This does not mean that the facility is free from microorganisms. The only way to make an area or object completely free of microorganisms is to use **surgical asepsis.** Another way to describe surgical asepsis is **sterile technique.** This is a technique that completely removes all microbes, both pathogenic and **non-pathogenic**, from supplies and equipment. Surgical asepsis makes an object or area sterile, completely free of all microorganisms. There may be times when you will be asked to assist a nurse or other staff member in a procedure that requires sterile technique. You must have special in-service training in order to help with this type of procedure. Chapter 24 has more information on the sterile field, sterile gloves, and sterile dressings. These are all measures used in surgical asepsis.

At the end of each shift, the following will usually be cleaned and disinfected. They are then placed in a facility-approved site.

- wheelchairs
- geri-chairs
- stretchers
- shower chairs and other items
- portable tubs

Nursing assistants who clean the equipment usually wear heavy-duty cleaning gloves and work in a well-ventilated area.

Methods of Infection Control for a Facility

- Handwashing is the single most important method to reduce the spread of infection.
- Use gloves whenever necessary.
- Clean a cut or break in your skin immediately with a facility-approved disinfecting product.
- Cover your mouth and nose when coughing or sneezing. Immediately wash your hands afterward.
- Keep yourself as healthy as possible.
- Never use one resident's personal items for another resident. Keep all personal items separate.
- Never transfer personal items or any kind of equipment from one room to another. An exception is something like your stethoscope. You must disinfect the part of your stethoscope that touches a resident in between residents.
- Hold all equipment or personal care items you carry away from your uniform while walking.
- Completely clean objects before using them if they have dropped to the floor.
- Clean all equipment used by a resident after use. Follow the facility's guidelines for disinfection.
- Clean all common areas (areas used by more than one resident) after use.
- Remove food or soiled eating utensils in residents' rooms after food trays have been picked up.
- Change water cups often.
- Clean resident toothbrushes and shaving equipment often.
- Never place contaminated items like bedpans or any other dirty items on the overbed table. Remember that residents' FOOD is placed on this table.
- Do not shake linen of any kind. This could move dangerous dust into the air.
- Fold linen so that the most soiled (dirtiest) area is toward the inside.
- Never place dirty linen on the floor for any reason.
- Never touch your uniform with linen you may be carrying.
- When cleaning anything, move from the cleanest to the dirtiest area.

Residents are at greater risk for acquiring an infection while living in a facility than when they are in their own homes. One method of reducing the overall rate of infection is to keep the residents as healthy as possible by promoting good health habits. This requires organization and caution on the part of all staff members. Ways to keep residents healthy and reduce or prevent nosocomial infections are identified in Box 11-3.

Keeping Residents Infection-Free — Box 11-3

Integumentary: Keep the skin clean and dry at all times. Wet or dirty skin can increase the risk of infection. When cleaning any part of the body, move from the cleanest to the dirtiest part.

Muscular/Skeletal: Stimulate muscles with activities and regular exercise. Muscles, bones, and joints stay strong with regular exercise and activity.

Circulatory: Blood circulation is stimulated with exercise and activity. The risk of blood clots is reduced. Cells that work to fight infection move more quickly to the site of dangerous pathogens with improved circulation.

Digestive (GI): Encourage residents to drink adequate fluids and eat food on their diet tray. Keep track of food and fluid intake and output. Fluids help cleanse the body of microorganisms.

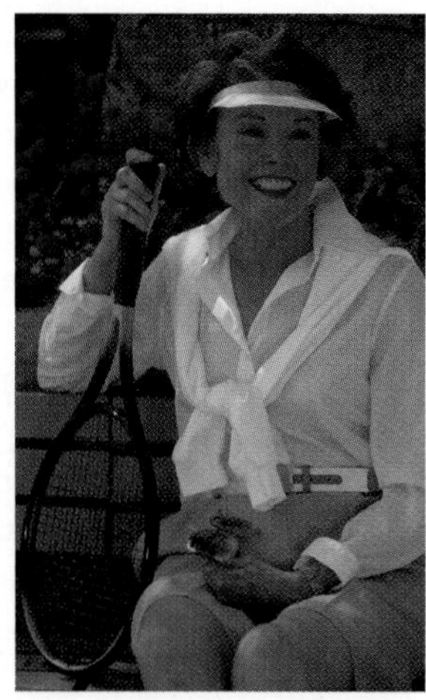

Figure 11-1. **Everyone benefits from regular exercise.**

Exercise helps keep residents' bowels regular. Encourage regular schedule for moving bowels. Wipe from front to back when cleaning feces.

Endocrine: The level of hormones can affect our urine output and our energy levels. Report signs or symptoms such as increase or decrease in urine output, increase or decrease in overall energy, increase or decrease in appetite. Lack of nutrition or adequate urine output can increase risk of infection.

Urinary: Take residents to the bathroom regularly. This keeps the urinary system running smoothly. Clean residents thoroughly after urinating. Wipe from front to back (cleanest to dirtiest).

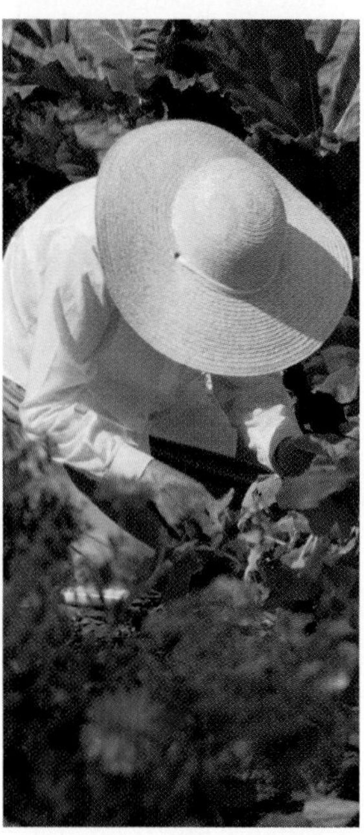

Figure 11-2. **Activities help residents remain mentally alert.**

Do catheter care as ordered by the doctor. A **catheter** is a tube used to drain urine from the bladder. Never disconnect the tubing used in a catheter system.

Nervous : Keep residents mentally alert by involving them in activities and promoting independence. When people become depressed or lonely, their resistance to infection can decrease.

Respiratory: Encourage deep breathing and coughing when needed to stimulate the person's respiratory system and inflate the lungs. This prevents fluid from gathering in the lungs, which can cause an infection.

Reproductive: Encourage relationships among residents. Love and affection have been shown to improve emotional state and decrease depression. Depression increases the risk of infection.

Lymphatic: Decrease stress and fatigue in residents' daily routines. Stress and fatigue may increase the risk of infection by lowering resistance.

4 Define the "chain of infection" and describe infection control practices for each link.

There are six links in the chain of infection:

Link 1: Common agents/sources of infection
Link 2: Reservoir
Link 3: Portal of exit
Link 4: Mode of transmission
Link 5: Portal of entry
Link 6: Susceptible host

If there is a break in any one of the links, the infection can be prevented.

Chain Link 1: Common agents/sources of infection

Microorganisms are small living bodies that cannot be seen without a microscope. They can cause infection and disease by entering the body and changing cells. They are everywhere around us—on our skin, in food, air, and water. The microorganisms that cause infection are called pathogens.

Types of Microorganisms — Box 11-4

1. Bacteria: organisms that are made of a single cell; may cause disease. Example: Salmonella enteritidis: causes food poisoning from eating contaminated chicken or eggs.
2. Fungi: organisms that sometimes cause disease. Example: Candida: causes yeast infections, oral or vaginal.
3. Protozoa: organisms made up of a single cell; may cause disease. Example: Giardia lamblia: causes Giardiasis (diarrhea); spread by contaminated water or food.
4. Viruses: the tiniest organisms; may cause disease. Example: Mumps: causes fever, swelling of the salivary glands; vaccine available for mumps.
5. Worms: made of more than one cell; may cause disease. Example: Pinworms: cause itching of anal skin; most common worm problem in the United States.
6. Arthropods: made of more than one cell; may cause disease. Arthropods can transmit Rickettsia, a microorganism that causes many diseases. Example: Ticks: can cause Lyme disease

Normal flora are the microorganisms within the body that normally live and grow in certain locations. When they enter a different part of the body, they may cause an infection.

There is a waiting period between the time the pathogen moves in and the time it causes a "full-blown" infection. This time period is called an **incu-**

bation period. Here are some examples of incubation periods.

- Chicken pox: 2-3 weeks, usually about 14 days
- Influenza: 1-3 days
- Measles: 10-21 days

Infection Control Example for Link 1: Vaccines.

Vaccines can give a person **immunity** to a disease without causing the symptoms of the particular disease. The immunity may not last forever. Box 11-5 identifies the required **immunizations** (shots or injections) for different ages.

Required Immunizations — Box 11-5

United States, January - December 2001

Vaccines are listed under the routinely recommended ages. Bars indicate range of acceptable ages for immunization. Catch-up immunization should be done during any visit when feasible. Shaded ovals indicate vaccines to be assessed and given if necessary during the early adolescent visit.

Age ▸ / Vaccine ▾	Birth	1 mo	2 mos	4 mos	6 mos	12 mos	15 mos	18 mos	24 mos	4-6 yrs	11-12 yrs	14-18 yrs
Hepatitis B[2]	Hep B #1											
		Hep B #2			Hep B #3						Hep B[2]	
Diphtheria, Tetanus, Pertussis[3]			DTaP	DTaP	DTaP		DTaP[3]			DTaP	Td	
H. influenzae type b[4]			Hib	Hib	Hib	Hib						
Inactivated Polio[5]			IPV	IPV	IPV[5]					IPV[5]		
Pneumococcal Conjugate[6]			PCV	PCV	PCV	PCV						
Measles, Mumps, Rubella[7]						MMR				MMR[7]	MMR[7]	
Varicella[8]						Var					Var[8]	
Hepatitis A[9]									Hep A-in selected areas[9]			

Chain Link 2: Reservoir

The **reservoir** is the place microorganisms grow. Microorganisms grow best in these conditions:

1. A warm place
2. A dark place
3. A place that is moist
4. A place where food is available
5. A place that has oxygen (some microorganisms do not require oxygen to survive)

The reservoir may be a human or an animal reservoir, or it may be an object of some kind. There are two primary ways of spreading an infection from a reservoir: direct and indirect.

Direct spread occurs when a person gets a disease directly from another person (reservoir). The human reservoir may be one of the following:

- A person with active disease
- A person carrying the disease (a **carrier**). A human carrier "carries" the disease and does not show symptoms at the time he or she spreads the disease. This "carrier" may or may not get the disease at a later time.

Indirect spread occurs when a person gets a disease from an object or insect, rodent or other animal (reservoir). Objects are also called "fomites." A **fomite** is an object that has picked up a pathogen and can now spread the pathogen to another person. Fomites may be things like infected food, water, utensils we eat with, or bed linens. **Vectors** (insect or animal) are actually special kinds of reservoirs that spread a disease from one human to another. Think of them as special "carriers of bad news." The vector picks up the bad news (pathogen), carries it, and then infects another human.

Infection Control Example for Link 2: Keeping surfaces clean and dry.

Chain Link 3: Portal of exit

There can be different exit routes, or **portals of exit**, from a reservoir. These are places the microorganism can leave the body of the human or animal and spread to a person. Figure 11-3 outlines the portals of exit from a human reservoir.

Infection Control Example for Link 3: Covering the mouth when sneezing.

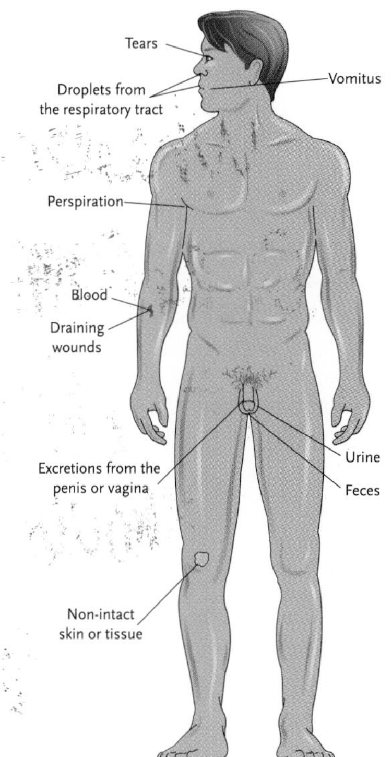

Figure 11-3. **Portals of exit.**

Chain Link 4: Mode of transmission

The actual **transmission,** or transfer, of an infectious disease occurs in different ways. It is important to become familiar with the various methods of transmission in order to protect yourself and your residents from infections.

Contact Transmission

- Contact with person's blood
- Contact with person's **body fluids** (tears, saliva, respiratory secretions, perspiration, vomit, urine, feces, vaginal fluid, or semen)
- Direct Contact Transmission: One person's body has direct contact with a contaminated person's body.
- Indirect Contact Transmission: When a **susceptible host** has contact with a contaminated object, such as a needle, instrument, or dressing.

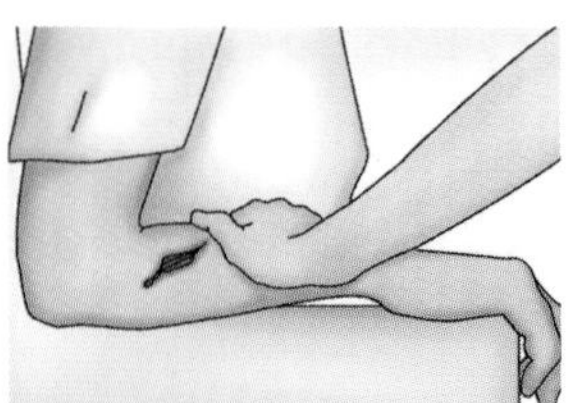

Figure 11-4. **Infections can be transferred from an open area on the skin.**

Droplet Transmission

- Infected person coughs, sneezes, or talks while very close to another person (within three feet). It is also possible that singing, laughing, or spitting may transmit droplets.
- A susceptible host inhales droplets and gets an infection.

Airborne Transmission

- Pathogen is carried a distance (more than three feet) by moisture in the air; some pathogens can stay alive in these moisture particles for quite some time.
- Pathogen is carried a distance (more than three feet) by dust; some pathogens can stay alive in dust particles for quite some time.
- Host inhales moisture or dust and gets an infection.

Common Vehicle Transmission

- Pathogen from human contaminates substance or object, like food, water, medications, devices, or equipment.
- Pathogen is transferred by eating, drinking, or touching substance or object and transferring the infection.

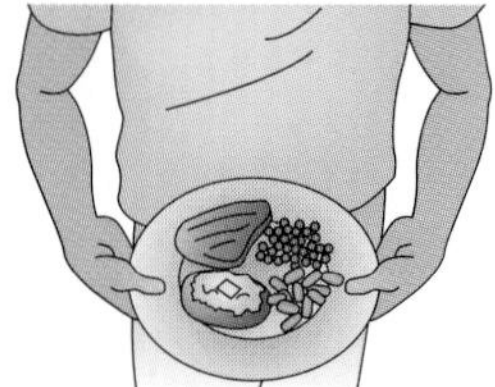

Figure 11-5. **Pathogens can be transferred from humans to food.**

Vector Transmission

- Pathogen is transferred from infected human to a vector (animal, such as a rat; or flying or crawling insect such as a mosquito or fly).
- Vector transfers infection to another person through a bite or into an open area on the skin.

Infection Control Example for Link 4: Handwashing.

Chain Link 5: Portal of entry

Pathogens enter the human host through different **portals of entry.** Figure 11-6 outlines the portals of entry into a human host.

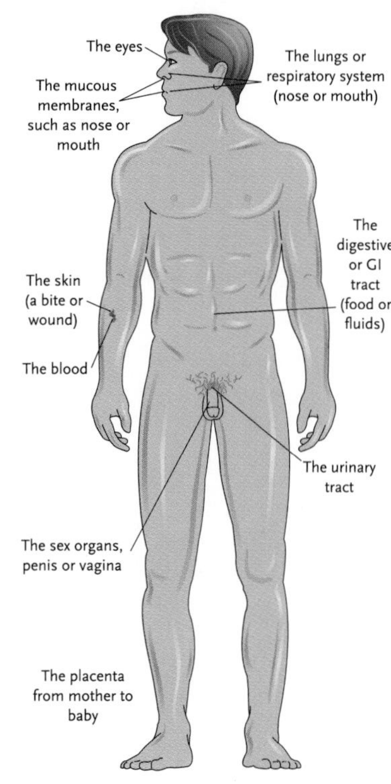

Figure 11-6. **Portals of entry.**

When a pathogen invades the body, it causes an infection. Many areas of the body are protected by a sort of "armor" that prevents pathogens from invading and causing infection. This armor works along with the immune system as a whole to help protect the body from harmful bacteria. Box 11-6 identifies the various types of "armor" on the body that helps keep it healthy.

Infection Control Example for Link 5: Wearing gloves.

The Human Body's Defensive Armor (Box 11-6)

Nasal Passages: **Mucous membrane** has cilia, tiny hairs in the nose that trap microorganisms.

Epidermis: As long as skin stays unbroken and undamaged, microorganisms cannot get inside.

Lungs: Lungs have phagocytes, cells that gobble up microorganisms.

Mouth: Saliva has a protein called Lactoferrin that blocks the growth of bad microorganisms.

Eye: The eyes have tears that protect them by cleaning out microorganisms.

GI tract: The GI tract has good microorganisms that prevent the growth of bad microorganisms.

Vagina: The vagina has a low pH of about 3.5 to 4.5, which blocks the growth of pathogens.

Urethra: Urine rinses out pathogens from the urinary tract.

Blood cells: White blood cells defend the body from microorganisms and play a role in the secretion of antibodies.

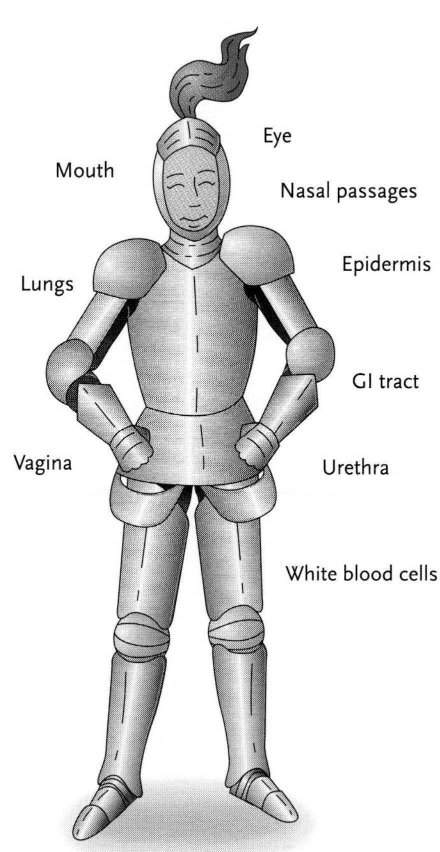

Figure 11-7. **The body's natural "armor."**

Chain Link 6: Susceptible Host

A person turns into a susceptible host when his or her resistance to disease decreases. Some reasons for lowered resistance include existing illnesses, fatigue, and stress. When a pathogen invades the human body, it will start reproducing itself. The pathogen will then try to damage the body in some way. The elderly tend to have lower resistance to pathogens and must be protected from them.

Infection Control Example for Link 6: Staying healthy and protecting the ill from exposure.

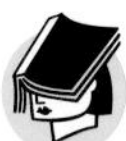

The Amazing Discovery of Edward Jenner

In 18th-century England, smallpox was a very common, horribly disfiguring disease. A doctor at that time, Edward Jenner, 1749-1823, noticed that people who were exposed to cowpox, like milkmaids who milked them, would develop a small sore and then never get smallpox. He then went on to develop a vaccine from the cowpox sores that gives people immunity to smallpox. After he injected the matter from the sore into a boy, James Phipps, he tested the "vaccine" by actually trying to give James the disease more than once. Each time, Jenner found that little James was immune to the disease!

5 Identify when to wash hands.

Wash your hands at these times:

- When you first arrive at your facility
- When you enter a resident's room
- Each time you remove your gloves or if gloves rip or tear
- When you leave a resident's room
- Before entering a "clean" supply room
- Before obtaining clean linen from a linen cart
- Before and after drinking, eating, or smoking
- After handling your hair or applying makeup, lip balm, and before and after inserting contact lenses
- After using the bathroom
- After coughing, sneezing, or blowing your nose
- Immediately after touching anything that may be considered dirty—especially blood or body fluids—such as after changing a tampon or pad.

Handwashing

1. **Stand away from the sink. Push your watch and sleeves up your arm.**
2 **Use a paper towel to turn on the warm water faucet.**
3. **Wet your hands holding fingertips pointing down into sink.**

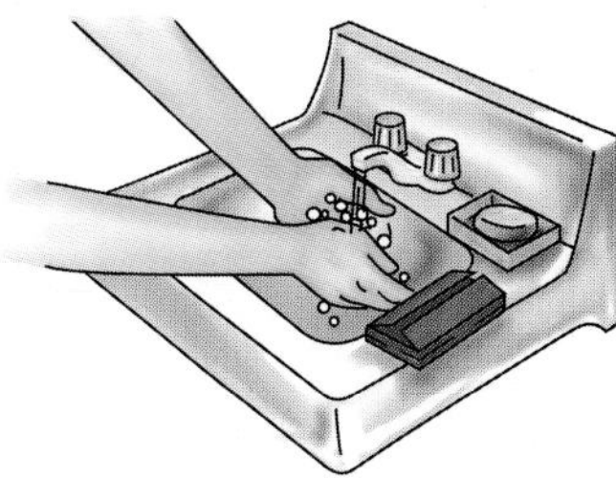

Figure 11-8.

4. **Add soap to your hands and scrub your hands, between your fingers, and wrists.**

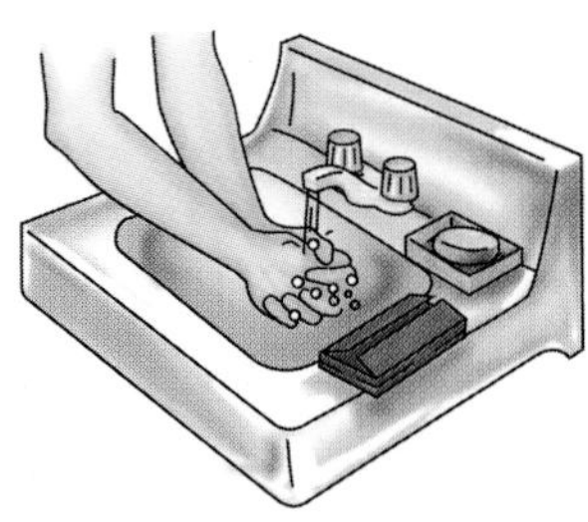

Figure 11-9.

5. **Rub the nails of each hand across your palm to remove dirt under fingernails. Special nail brushes exist; however, bacteria may transfer from brushes to hands. Follow facility's policy regarding brushes.**

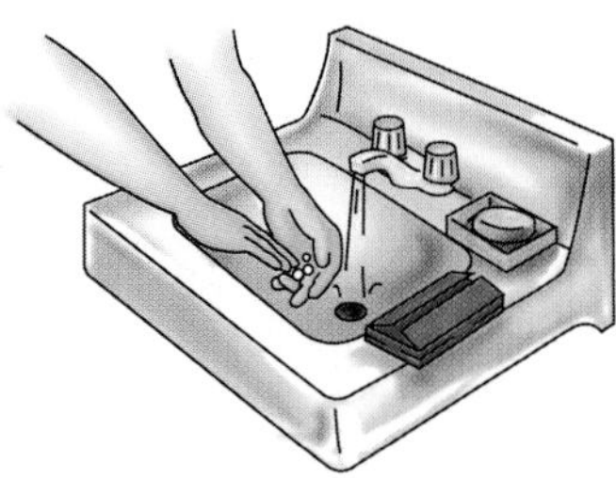

Figure 11-10.

6. **After scrubbing vigorously for at least 15 seconds, rinse hands so water runs downward into sink.**
7. **Dry hands with clean paper towel. Drop paper towel into waste container, being careful not to touch container.**
8. **With a new paper towel, turn off faucet and carefully discard this paper towel. Apply unscented, hypo-allergenic lotion to hands if needed.**

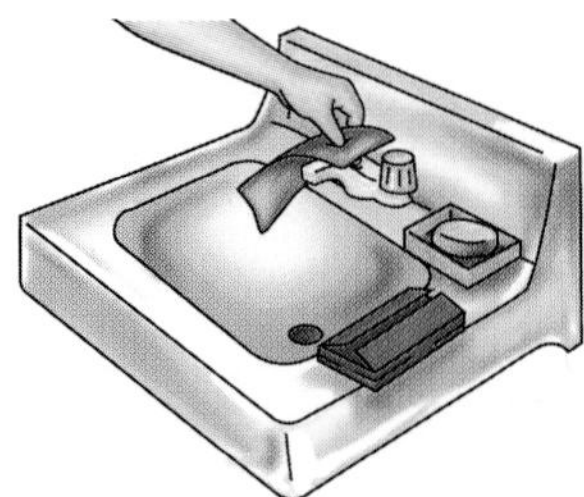

Figure 11-11.

9. **As you leave handwashing area, if a doorknob must be opened, use another paper towel to open door. If no doorknob exists, push door open with your entire body so you do not use your hands.**

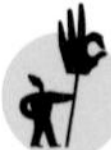

Take the time to properly wash your hands!

Recently, handwashing has often been written about in the press. People are reading about patients who developed serious illnesses due to the lack of handwashing among staff members. One way to make sure you wash your hands for a long enough period of time is to hum or sing a tune to yourself. Here is one example of a song you might try: "This is the way we wash our hands, wash our hands, wash our hands. This is the way we wash our hands so early in the morning." If you say this to yourself two times all the way through, you will wash hands for about 15 to 20 seconds. You must take handwashing very seriously. It could mean the difference between a resident's life and death.

Wash hands before resident care!

As you move from resident room to resident room, you must always wash your hands. Taking care of residents means you will gather many bacteria and other microorganisms on your hands. When nursing assistants do not wash their hands before giving care to a resident, this can be considered abuse.

6 Discuss the basic principles of using PPE in the healthcare facility.

Personal protective equipment **(PPE)** is the **barrier** (a block or obstacle of some kind) between you and a potential infectious disease. PPE is what you wear to prevent dangerous microorganisms from getting on your uniform or inside your body. Applying personal protective equipment the correct way may save your life or the life of another person. The basic categories of PPE are: gloves, gowns, masks, goggles, and face shields.

Non-sterile Gloves

Non-sterile gloves are used for basic care inside a facility. These come in different sizes: XS, S, M, L, and XL. They may be made of different materials, such as latex or vinyl.

Always wear gloves when:

- you may come into contact with body fluids, open wounds, or mucous membranes
- performing or assisting with care of the perineal area (the area between the anus and genitals)
- performing care on a resident who has **non-intact skin**—broken by abrasions, cuts, rashes, acne, pimples, or boils
- you have any cuts or tears in the skin on your hands
- shaving a resident

Gloves must be changed immediately should they become wet, worn, soiled, or torn. Do not touch anything with contaminated gloves that anyone else may touch without wearing gloves. For example, if you are carrying a used bedpan to empty it, you cannot touch the doorknob or open the door with gloved hands.

Applying and Removing Non-Sterile Gloves

If you are allergic to a type of glove, such as latex, your facility should supply you with gloves that you can wear without a reaction. Always report allergies or reactions to gloves.

Collect equipment: gloves

Applying

1. **Wash your hands.**
2. **Gather gloves.**

   A. Choose correct size.

   B. Choose correct style, latex or vinyl.
3. **If you are right-handed, take one glove and slide it on your left hand (reverse if left-handed).**
4. **Pick up second glove with your gloved hand, and slide the other hand into the glove.**
5. **Check for tears, rips, cracks, or funny-looking folds in the gloves.**
6. **Adjust gloves until they are pulled up all the way and fit correctly. If wearing a gown, pull the cuff of each glove over the sleeve of the gown.**

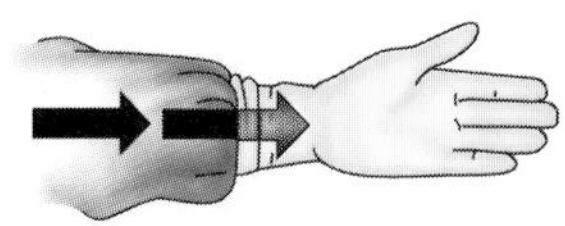

Figure 11-12.

Removing

1. **Touching only the outside of one glove in the palm of the hand, pull the first glove off by pulling downward from the cuff.**
2. **As this first glove comes off, it should be turned inside out.**

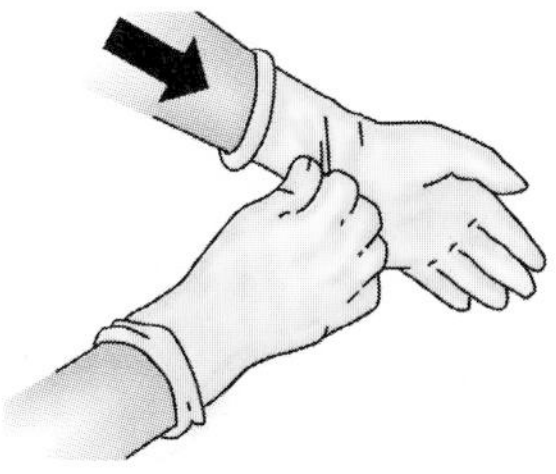

Figure 11-13.

3. **With the fingertips of your gloved hand, continue to hold the glove you just pulled off.**
4. **With your ungloved hand, reach two fingers INSIDE the second glove, being careful not to touch any part of the outside of the glove.**
5. **Pull down, turning this glove inside out and over the first glove as you pull it off.**
6. **You should now be holding one glove from its clean inner side, and the other glove should still be inside it.**

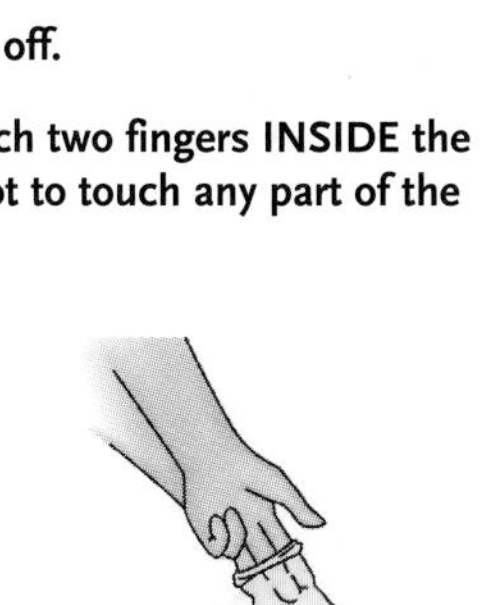

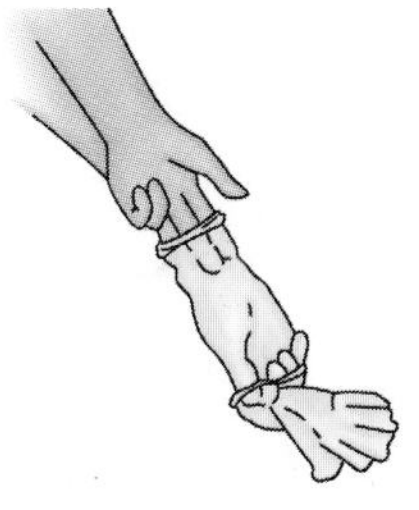

Figure 11-14.

7. **Drop both gloves into the proper container.**
8. **Wash your hands using proper procedure.**

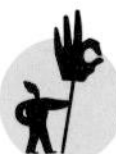

Double-glove to stay safe!

When you have any kind of opening in the skin on your hands, such as a cut, scrape, or rash, you should report this to your supervisor. If your health service or doctor has cleared you to be at work, you may want to double-glove (put two complete sets of gloves on) while working until the openings in your skin have healed.

Fluid-resistant Gowns

Gowns must be worn whenever you feel you may come into contact with blood, body fluids, or tissue that may splash or spray onto your uniform. Gowns usually come in one-size-fits-all. If the gown does not fit you, report this to your supervisor. Do not wear a gown that is too small or too large. Gowns are usually made of a fluid-resistant material; however, they may still become wet or soiled! Gowns must be changed immediately should they become wet or soiled.

Applying and Removing a Gown

Collect equipment: gown

Applying

1. **Wash your hands.**
2. **Gather gown.**
3. **Remove jewelry and wristwatch and place them on a clean paper towel. If wearing long sleeves, push or roll them up.**
4. **Pick up gown. Do not shake gown or touch it to the floor. Slip your arms into the sleeves and pull the gown on.**
5. **Tie the neck ties into a bow so they can be easily untied later. Use tapes to hold together.**

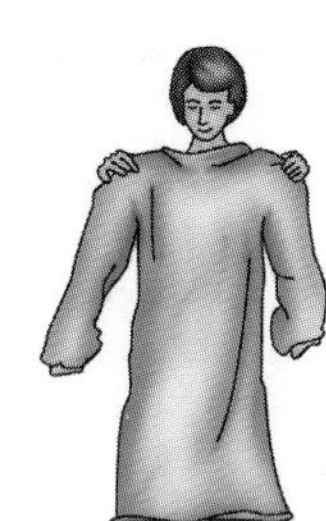

Figure 11-15.

6. **Reaching behind you, pull the gown until it completely covers your clothes and tie the back ties.**

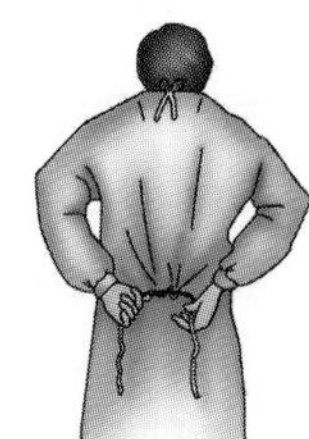

Figure 11-16.

Removing

1. **Remove gloves.**
2. **Wash hands.**
3. **Untie waist or back ties or undo tape at waist/back.**

4. Untie ties or undo tape at neck. Do not touch neck or outside of gown.
5. Grasping the ties/tape at the neck of the gown, loosen at neck and roll gown downward inside out in the direction of the bottom hem of the gown. Make sure you only touch the inside of the gown and hold gown away from your body.
6. After it is rolled up, contaminated side inward, drop into facility-approved container.
7. Wash your hands.

Masks

Masks should be worn when caring for a resident who may cough or sneeze and spread an infection. Masks can prevent you from inhaling some microorganisms through your nose or mouth. Masks that become wet or soiled must be changed immediately!

Applying and Removing a Face Mask

Collect equipment: mask

Applying

1. Wash your hands.
2. Gather mask.
3. Remove jewelry, wristwatch, and eyeglasses and place them on a clean paper towel. If wearing long sleeves, push or roll them up.
4. Pick up the mask by the top strings or the elastic strap. Be careful not to touch the mask where it touches your face.
5. Adjust the mask over your nose and mouth. Tie top strings first, then bottom strings. Never wear a mask hanging from only the bottom strings.
6. Pinch the metal strip at the top of the mask (if part of the mask) tightly around your nose so that it feels snug.
7. Replace eyeglasses, if worn.

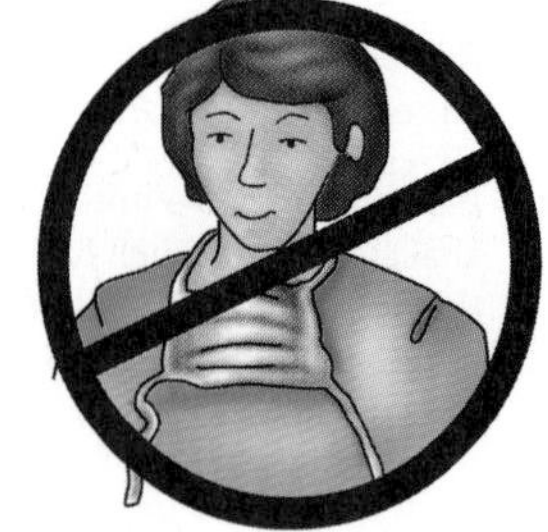

Figure 11-17.

Removing

1. Wash your hands.
2. Untie the lower tie of the mask first.
3. Untie the upper tie of the mask last.
4. Pull off face using only the ties and drop into facility-approved container.
5. Wash your hands.

Certain respiratory diseases such as tuberculosis require that special personal protective equipment be worn by all staff who care for these residents. More information on tuberculosis is in Chapter 29. This equipment helps to safeguard the staff from this disease. Airborne precautions are required. These precautions are discussed later in this chapter. A special private room is provided for the resident. This room has a system in which the air inside of the room is not re-circulated through the ventilation system in the facility. Instead, the air is vented directly outside the facility.

When supervisors determine who will care for tuberculosis residents, they may ask a series of questions regarding your exposure to certain diseases in the past, such as chicken pox. They will tell you if you qualify to take care of the resident.

Everyone who enters the room for any reason must be fitted with a special mask. These masks may have different names at different facilities. A standard-style mask does not protect the caregiver from tuberculosis. One style of mask worn during the care of tuberculosis residents is called the N95 respirator mask. These masks usually come in more than one size. The caregiver must be fitted for this mask by a designated department within the facility. Each time the person puts the mask on, a "fit test" must be done so that no air goes through the mask without passing through the special mask filters. These tests may be done on the unit or at a special site within the facility.

When people care for residents with tuberculosis, they may need to be tested for this disease more often. Your facility will identify this need and coordinate your testing. If you cannot have a standard TB test, a chest x-ray may be required periodically.

Sometimes, people are admitted who are not identified as having tuberculosis. When tuberculosis is diagnosed after admission and certain people have been exposed to the person with the disease, the facility will normally do follow-up testing for tuberculosis. The facility will give you directions should this situation occur.

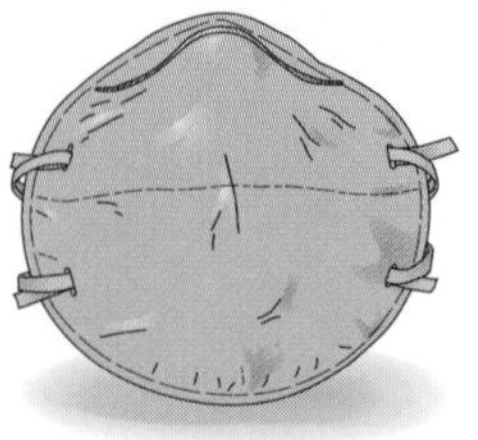

Figure 11-18. **N-95 respirator mask.**

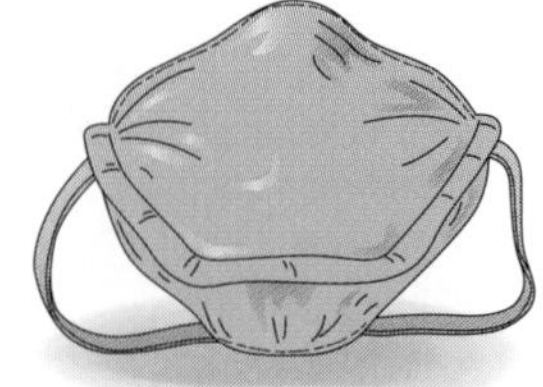

Figure 11-19. **PFR-95 respirator mask.**

Applying an N95 Respirator Mask

Collect equipment: N95 mask

Applying

1. **Wash your hands.**
2. **Gather respirator.**
3. **Hold respirator cupped in your hand with the nosepiece facing toward the tips of your fingers.**
4. **Bring the respirator up to your face, covering your nose with the nosepiece at the top against the nose.**
5. **Pull the top strap over your head and secure it high on the head.**
6. **Pull the bottom strap over your head and secure it below the ears.**

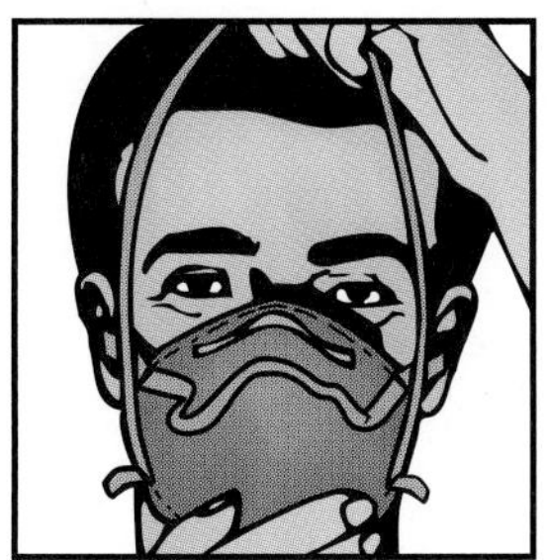

Figure 11-20.

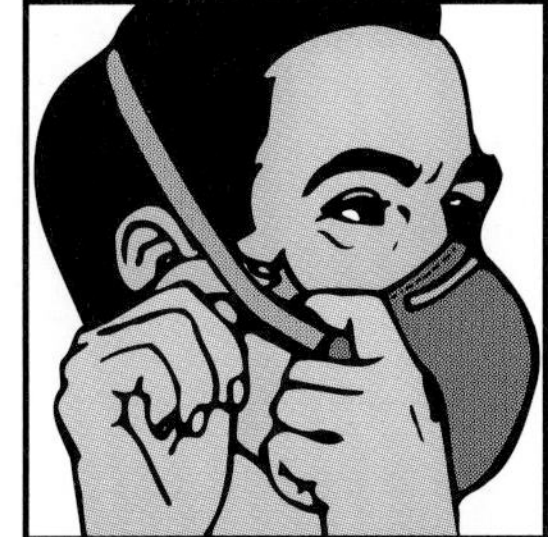

Figure 11-21.

7. **Using both hands, beginning in the center of your nose moving downward on each side, shape the firm part of the nosepiece so that it molds to your nose. The nosepiece should form a complete seal around your nose.**

Figure 11-22.

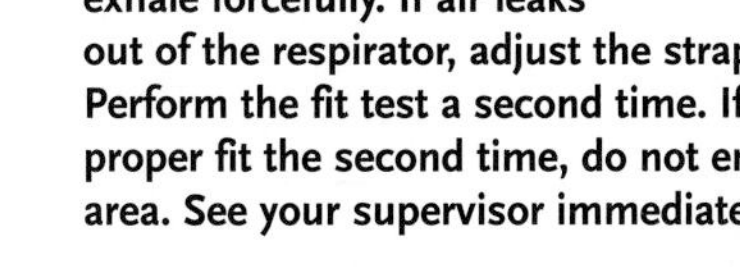

8. **Fit Test: Place both hands over the respirator and exhale forcefully. If air leaks out of the respirator, adjust the straps to obtain a tighter fit. Perform the fit test a second time. If you cannot achieve a proper fit the second time, do not enter the contaminated area. See your supervisor immediately.**

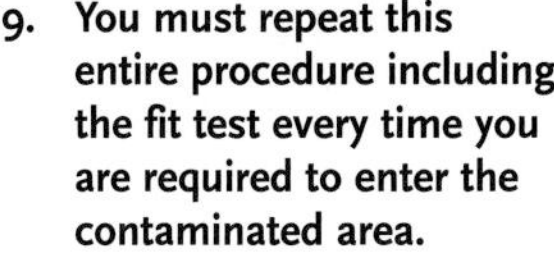

9. **You must repeat this entire procedure including the fit test every time you are required to enter the contaminated area.**

   Once the fit test has determined the proper respirator size, the respirator must be checked for adequate fit each time it is to be used.

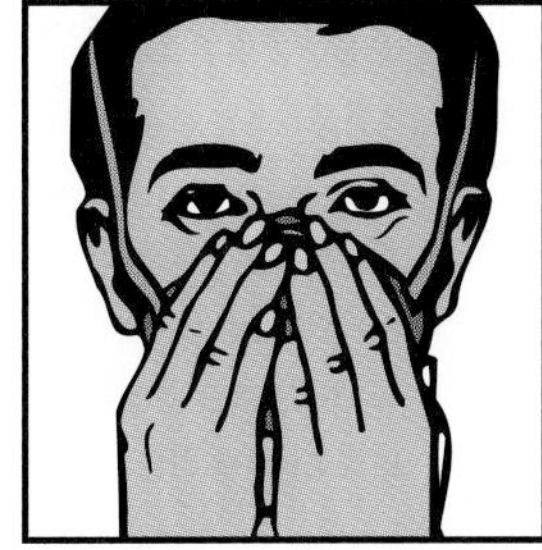

Figure 11-23.

Protective Eyewear

Eyewear, such as goggles or shields, are used whenever blood or body fluids may be splashed or sprayed into your eye area or your eyes. You must wear a mask and eyewear together!

Face Shield

A fairly new style of face shield consists of a plastic shield that also has a covering for the mouth. This combination eye and mouth shield provides an easy-to-use one-piece barrier and streamlines the application of PPE.

Applying and Removing Goggles/Face Shield/Combo Face Shield

Collect equipment: goggles/face shield

Applying

1. **Wash your hands.**
2. **Apply the goggles/face shield/combo shield, adjust, and secure.**
3. **The bottom of the goggles must fit over a mask, if used.**

Removing

1. **Wash your hands.**
2. **Remove goggles/face shield/combo shield by carefully grasping the sides and pulling them away from your face. Do not touch the front of the device with ungloved hands.**
3. **Wash your hands.**

Applying and Removing the Full Set of PPE in Correct Order

Collect equipment: gown, mask, goggles, gloves

Applying a full set of PPE

1. **Wash your hands.**
2. **Remove jewelry, wristwatch, and eyeglasses.**
3. **Apply gown.**
4. **Apply mask. Pinch metal strip over nose, if on mask. May replace eyeglasses now if not wearing goggles/shield.**
5. **Apply goggles or face shield, if needed.**
6. **Apply gloves LAST. Pull gloves completely over cuffs of gown.**
7. **Provide care.**

Removing a full set of PPE

1. Remove gloves first. Discard gloves in facility-approved container.
2. Wash your hands.
3. Remove gown second.
4. Untie waist strings.
5. Wash hands again if it is facility's policy to do so.
6. Untie neck strings. Discard gown in facility-approved container.
7. Remove face shield or goggles if used.
8. Remove your mask.
9. Untie bottom, then top strings of mask. Discard in facility-approved container.
10. Wash your hands.

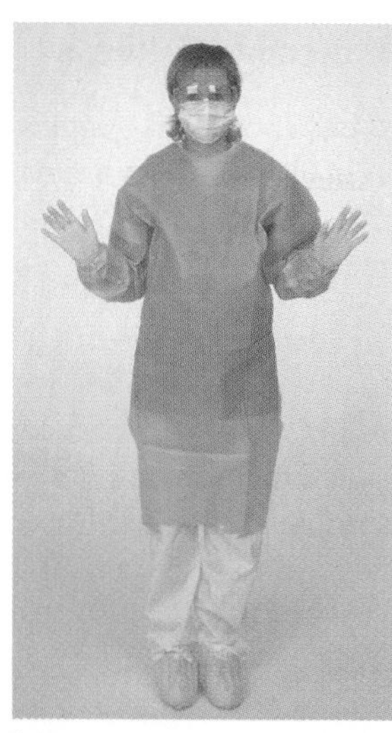

Figure 11-24.

7 Explain OSHA and describe five guidelines OSHA requires that employers follow for the Bloodborne Pathogen Standard.

The **Occupational Safety and Health Administration**, known as **OSHA**, is a government agency that is responsible for the safety of the workers in the United States. OSHA is under the control of the Department of Labor. OSHA conducts workplace inspections to check on worker safety and updates the health and safety standards as needed in the workplace. OSHA also provides training for employers and employees on workplace safety. The employer is responsible for meeting all workplace safety standards and providing a workplace for employees that is free of the hazards identified under OSHA. Employees are responsible for doing their job in such a way that they meet all of the health and safety standards under OSHA.

OSHA has set standards for equipment use along with special techniques to use when working in facilities. One of these standards is the **Bloodborne Pathogen Standard.** This law, passed in 1991, requires that healthcare facilities protect employees and all other people who enter or live in the facility from bloodborne health hazards.

Bloodborne pathogens are microorganisms found in the blood of humans that cause disease in humans when they have contact with blood or body fluids like tears, saliva, respiratory secretions, perspiration (sweat), vomit, urine, feces, vaginal fluid, or semen. Infections from these pathogens can be spread by having accidental contact with contaminated skin, contaminated needles or other sharp objects, or contaminated supplies or equipment. The types of wastes that must be considered infectious are identified below.

Types of Hazardous Infectious Waste — Box 11-7

Contaminant: Blood, body fluids or tissue from a human

Found on: Any object with blood, body fluids or tissue on it

Examples: Any "sharps" (needles or other sharp objects)

Any used instruments or equipment of any kind

Any used supplies of any kind (gloves, dressings, linen)

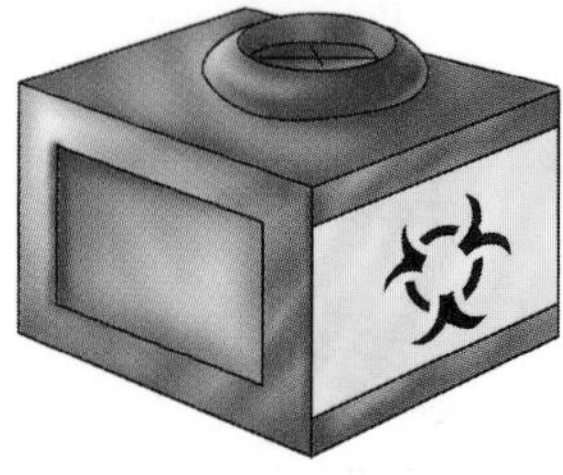

Figure 11-25.

Employers are required by law to follow the Bloodborne Pathogen Standard in order to reduce the risk of employees or other people acquiring an infectious disease in facilities. The Standard guides employers and employees through the steps to follow if exposed to infectious material. Some of the things employers must do to help keep their employees safe include the following guidelines:

1. Employers must provide in-service training on the risks from bloodborne pathogens and updates on any new safety standards. An **exposure incident** is when an employee is exposed to infectious blood or a body fluid.

   After an exposure incident, certain steps must be followed to prevent infection. A spill is when an amount of blood or a body fluid gets spilled on any object or person within the facility, including the floor. After a spill, these steps must be taken:
   - Apply gloves immediately.
   - Wipe up spill immediately.
   - A cleaning solution of one part bleach to 10 parts water can be used to finish cleaning the area. You may have ready-to-use spray bottles already available at your facility.

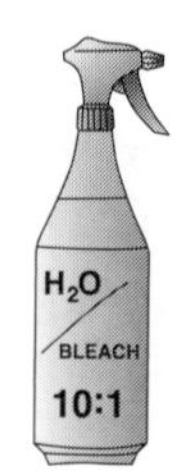

Figure 11-26.

- Be extremely careful if any glass or other sharp objects are within the spill. Get help for picking up and disposing of sharps and other objects. Never pick up glass, even with gloved hands. If you do accidentally cut yourself, follow exposure incident guidelines listed below.
- For large spills, call for the nurse and he will follow your facility's policy for large-spill clean-up. Dispose of gloves and cleaning equipment and supplies according to facility policy.

After an exposure incident, these steps must be taken:

- Immediately follow facility policy regarding spill, splash, or cut. (More information on skin and eye splashes is in Chapter 12.)
- Report an exposure incident immediately to your supervisor.
- Fill out a special exposure report form. Keep a copy for yourself.
- Go to employer's health service department in order to obtain any necessary tests.

Two main reasons for exposure reports are:

- To ensure you get the follow-up care you need after an exposure.
- To investigate ways to prevent exposures from happening again.

2. Employers are also required to provide an **exposure control plan** should an employee accidentally become exposed to any infectious waste. This identifies the step-by-step method of what to do if exposed to infectious material. It is in written form and kept in a particular spot on the unit.

3. Employers have to provide all employees, visitors, and residents with appropriate personal protective equipment to wear when necessary with certain residents. PPE includes such things as gowns, gloves, masks, and eye shields.

4. Employers also must provide **biohazard containers** in each resident room and in other areas in the facility to dispose of equipment and supplies contaminated with infectious waste. Biohazard containers are hard, leakproof containers with clear labels warning of the danger of the contents of the container.

5. Employers are required to provide the hepatitis B vaccine free of charge to all employees within a certain amount of time after the employee is hired. Hepatitis refers to swelling of the liver caused by infection. Liver function can be permanently damaged by hepatitis. Several different viruses can cause hepatitis; the most common are hepatitis A, B, and C. Hepatitis B and C are bloodborne diseases that can cause death. Many more people have hepatitis B (HBV) than HIV.

   HBV poses a serious threat to healthcare workers. If you have never had this three-dose vaccine, you must check with your facility when first hired to set up your appointment to obtain this vaccine. There is no vaccine for hepatitis C.

8 Define the Centers for Disease Control and Prevention (CDC) and explain standard precautions.

The Centers for Disease Control and Prevention (CDC) is a federal government agency in Atlanta, Georgia. This agency is responsible for improving the overall health and safety of the people of the United States. They promote public health and safety through education and try to control and prevent disease. The CDC does extensive research into the control of disease and publishes a weekly guide to keep the country aware and updated regarding diseases.

In 1996, the Centers for Disease Control provided new guidelines to protect healthcare team members and other people within facilities from being exposed to infectious diseases. There are two levels of precautions that facilities must take in order to protect people from these diseases. They are standard precautions and transmission-based precautions.

Standard precautions, the first level of precautions, must be used with each and every resident you will care for. This type of precaution protects people from exposure to:

- Blood and body fluids (except sweat or perspiration): blood, sputum or phlegm from the lungs, vomit, urine, feces, pus or other fluid from a wound, vaginal secretions, or semen
- Open skin areas (non-intact)
- Mucous membranes

Standard precautions are *always* followed because you cannot tell from looking at a person if he or she carries a bloodborne disease. The guidelines for standard precautions are shown below.

Handwashing whenever indicated in "Handwashing Guidelines."

Gloves

- Wear gloves whenever you may contact blood, body fluids, human tissue, open skin, mucous membranes (the inside of the eyes, nose, mouth, vagina, penis, or rectum). Also wear gloves when coming into contact with any equipment or supplies (especially "sharps" of any kind, like razor blades) that may be contaminated with infectious waste.
- Change gloves according to facility policy if they become contaminated during a task.
- Take gloves off after a procedure before touching anything around you.
- Dispose of gloves following your facility policy.
- Wash hands EVERY TIME after removing gloves.

Gowns

- Wear a gown when performing procedures where splashing or spraying of blood or body fluids may occur. Gowns are used ONCE and disposed of.
- Change gown according to facility policy if it becomes wet or soiled.
- Remove gown promptly after care.
- Dispose of gown following your facility policy.
- Wash hands EVERY TIME after removing a gown.

Masks

- Wear a mask along with an eye shield or eye protection when performing a procedure where splashing or spraying of blood or body fluids may occur. Masks are to be used ONCE and disposed of.
- Change mask according to facility policy if it becomes wet or moist.
- Remove mask after procedure according to facility policy.
- Dispose of mask according to facility policy.
- Wash hands EVERY TIME after removing a mask or face shield.

Equipment and Supplies

- Disposable contaminated supplies must be placed into bags supplied by your facility. This waste must be disposed of according to the correct method of disposing of infectious wastes. Special containers are used for disposal.
- Non-disposable contaminated supplies, such as linen and reusable pieces of equipment, must be placed into the appropriate container and sent to the site chosen by your facility for cleaning. This cleaning site may be inside or outside your facility.
- "Sharps" must be placed in biohazard containers.
- Never touch a needle if you find one. Never try to locate a cap for a needle if you find one. You must NEVER recap a needle, for you might stick yourself. Call the nurse who will place the needle immediately into the biohazard container for "sharps."
- Clean all surfaces that may be contaminated with infectious waste according to facility policy. Examples of these areas include: overbed tables, beds, and wheelchairs.
- When assisting a resident in an emergency, you must use a special mouthpiece should you have to perform **mouth-to-mouth resuscitation**. This is also called rescue breathing, when we breathe air into the body of a person who has stopped breathing for some reason.

9 Summarize the current CDC transmission-based precautions.

In 1996, the Centers for Disease Control and Prevention also set forth a second level of precautions to protect people within facilities from acquiring certain types of infectious diseases. These new guidelines, called transmission-based precautions, updated the precautions used for isolation precautions. **Isolation** means to separate a person from others to prevent the spread of infection. Transmission-based precautions include airborne isolation precautions, droplet isolation precautions, and contact isolation precautions.

Airborne Precautions

Airborne precautions prevent the spread of microorganisms that may travel through the air over long distances. An example of an airborne disease is TB, or tuberculosis. Tuberculosis is a disease that is transferred through droplets in the air that can travel a long distance. TB can be fatal if not treated.

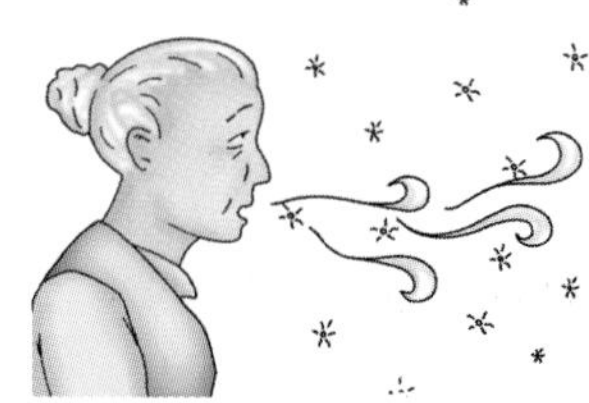

Figure 11-27. Airborne diseases stay suspended in the air.

- Follow all standard precautions.
- Resident room: Resident must be in a private room that has a special flow of air, which causes the resident's exhaled air to be sent out into the outside environment. This prevents the air in the room from mixing with the air in the rest of the facility. The doors and windows to the resident's room must be closed at all times.
- Mask: All individuals entering the room must wear a special mask such as an N95 respirator mask. Each employee must be fitted for this type of a mask. A standard mask is not safe during care of this resident.

- Transporting resident: Should the resident have to leave the room for any reason, he must wear a disposable surgical mask or other type of mask.

Droplet Precautions

Droplet precautions are used when residents have a disease that may be spread by droplets in the air. Droplets normally do not travel further than three feet. Examples of the way a resident may spread this type of disease include talking, singing, sneezing, or coughing. An example of a droplet disease is the mumps.

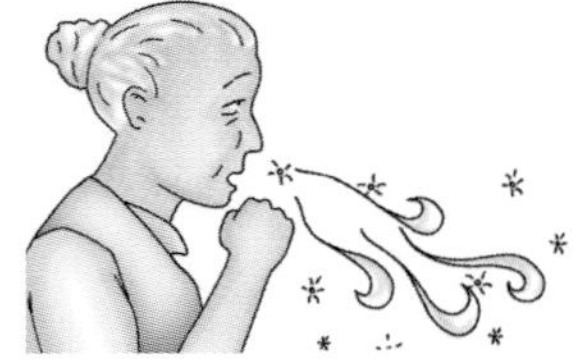

Figure 11-28. **Droplet precautions are followed when the disease causing microorganism does not stay suspended in the air.**

- Follow all standard precautions.
- Resident room: Resident should be placed in a private room.
- Mask: A mask must be worn when working within three feet of the resident.
- Transporting resident: Should the resident have to leave the room for any reason, she must wear a disposable surgical mask.

Contact Precautions

Contact precautions are used when a resident may spread an infection by direct contact with another person. The infection may be spread when a nursing assistant touches a contaminated area on the body of the resident or touches contaminated blood or body fluids of the resident. It may also be spread by touching contaminated personal belongings, linen, equipment, or supplies of a resident. An example of a contact disease is impetigo, a contagious skin disease.

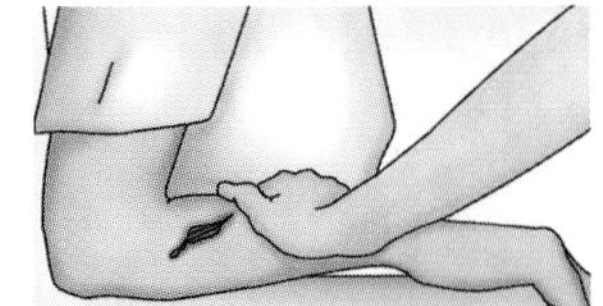

Figure 11-29. **Contact precautions are followed when the client is at risk of transmitting or contracting a microorganism from touching an infected object.**

- Follow all standard precautions.
- Resident room: Resident should be placed in a private room.
- Gloves: Gloves must be put on before entering a resident room. Gloves must be changed if contaminated with infected material. Gloves must be removed before leaving resident room.
- Handwashing: While still inside room, immediately wash hands with an appropriate antimicrobial agent after removing gloves. Leave room without touching ANY surface with your hands.
- Gowns: Gown must be put on before entering a resident room. Remove gown before leaving resident room disposing of properly. Wash hands after removing gown before leaving room. Leave room without touching ANY surface with your uniform.
- Transporting the resident: limit transporting resident, if possible. If you must transport, take precautions to not spread the microorganisms to others or contaminate any other outside objects.
- Equipment: This type of resident's equipment should never be shared with another resident. For any equipment that must be used by more than one resident, the equipment must be completely cleaned and disinfected before being used again.

10 Describe overall care of the resident in an isolation unit.

When a resident is placed in an isolation unit or area, his life changes. Suddenly, he cannot move about freely anymore because he is isolated or separated from everyone else. He may feel as though he is "locked inside a room," even though the door is not really locked. Healthcare team members caring for the resident in isolation must consider how they would feel if they were placed inside an isolation room. Contact with the resident should be as frequent as possible. This provides the required connection with the outside world.

Some tips for caring for the resident in isolation include the following.

1. Spend as much time with the resident as possible throughout your work day. This may reduce the loneliness she will feel because of the separation from others. Listen and encourage the resident to talk about her feelings and concerns. Be certain residents know it is the disease that is being isolated, not them.

2. If allowed visitors, allow as much time for family to visit as possible. Assist family with putting on isolation gear like gowns and masks.

3. Make sure the resident's TV, telephone, and radio are all in working order.

4. Encourage the use of reading material that may be disposed of, like catalogues and magazines. Make sure the resident has access to eyeglasses if needed.

5. Always place the signal light within reach of the resident when leaving the isolation room.

Care of the Resident in Isolation

When a resident is in isolation, she is separated from everyone else. Imagine how this would make you feel. A resident in isolation needs more of our attention so that she has as much contact with other people as possible. This may help reduce her feelings of loneliness. It may also help decrease her sense of being "contagious." When staff members purposefully avoid residents placed in isolation, this is considered a form of abuse—both psychological abuse and neglect. Nursing assistants need to make sure all residents in isolation have contact with others.

11 Define the terms "MRSA" and "VRE."

Methicillin-Resistant Staphylococcus Aureus (**MRSA**) is an infectious disease caused by a pathogen that is resistant to many antibiotics. MRSA can develop when people do not take all of the medication prescribed to them. When the full course of medication is not taken, the "strongest" bacteria survive and may develop an immunity to the antibiotics.

MRSA is spread by direct contact with an infected person or indirect contact with contaminated equipment or supplies.

Vancomycin-resistant Enterococcus (**VRE**): **enterococci** that are resistant to Vancomycin, a powerful antibiotic designed to prevent or kill bacterial infections. VRE can develop when people do not take all of the Vancomycin prescribed to them. When the full course of medication is not taken, the "strongest" bacteria survive and may develop an immunity to the antibiotics.

Remember to practice standard precautions and follow the guidelines very carefully for a resident with MRSA or VRE.

Residents with MRSA may be placed in contact or droplet isolation depending upon the site of the infection. Residents with VRE may be placed in contact isolation.

New guidelines for the care of MRSA and VRE residents may be introduced in your facility. Attend all MRSA and VRE in-services and carefully follow any new guidelines.

As with VRE and MRSA, tuberculosis can become resistant to available treatments. This is called multidrug resistant tuberculosis. Risk of MDR-TB increases when people do not complete their prescribed course of medications.

Summary

Infection control saves lives. It is as simple as that. If you follow the infection control methods and techniques in this chapter, along with any new or updated methods you learn at your facility, you will be at less risk and so will everyone around you. This means everyone. This is not limited to your residents. Take infection control very seriously. The world is a safer place when people follow proper infection control standards.

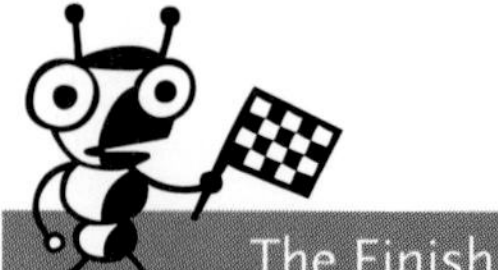

The Finish Line

What's Wrong With This Picture?

1. Nursing assistant Anne Anderson opens the drawer in the overbed table and pulls out the razor inside. Resident Emilio Chavez says, "No, that's not my razor." Anne believes he is confused and uses the razor anyway. What is wrong with this picture?
2. Nursing assistant Jennifer Lee is in a hurry. She has two more residents to help feed before she is done with her shift. She enters resident Yvonne Otero's room and realizes she has not washed her hands since she helped her last resident eat. Jennifer reasons that she doesn't need to stop and wash her hands because neither she nor Yvonne Otero are sick. What is wrong with this picture?

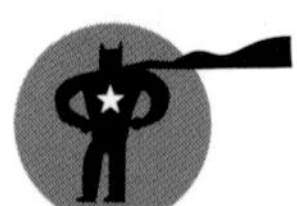

Star Student Central

1. Arrange for a visit to your local health department. During the visit, gather educational pamphlets to bring back and share with your class and/or your family. When gathering information, pay special attention to anything you may find about diseases like tuberculosis, AIDS, and all forms of hepatitis.

2. Pay a visit to your local school nurse or health clerk, AIDS awareness center, or poison control center. During the appointment, ask for any educational pamphlets they may have available. Bring these back and share with your class and/or your family.

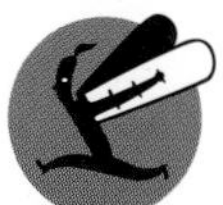

You Can Do It Corner!

1. How do localized and systemic infections differ? (LO 2)
2. List when handwashing should be performed. (LO 5)
3. List when PPE should be worn. (LO 6)
4. Describe when airborne, droplet, and contact precautions are used. (LO 9)
5. List each link in the chain of infection and one way to break each. (LO 4)
6. List eight examples of the body's natural armor against infection. (LO 4)
7. Identify the main difference between disinfection and sterilization. (LO 3)
8. Explain why standard precautions are always followed. (LO 8)
9. List the best way to prevent nosocomial infections. (LO 2)
10. Describe five tips for caring for a resident in an isolation unit. (LO 10)
11. List three types of hazardous infectious waste. (LO 7)
12. Explain the two main reasons for exposure reports. (LO 7)
13. Describe the terms "clean" and "dirty" as they relate to infection control. (LO 3)
14. List five guidelines required by OSHA that employers must follow for the Bloodborne Pathogen Standard. (LO 7)

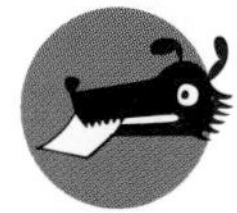

Star Student's Chapter Checklist

1. I have read my textbook chapter.
2. I have reviewed my own "Pocketful of Terms."
3. I have listened to my tutor tape.
4. I have reviewed and highlighted my class notes.
5. I have read and completed any handouts from this chapter.
6. I have completed "The Finish Line."
7. Star Time! Choose your reward!

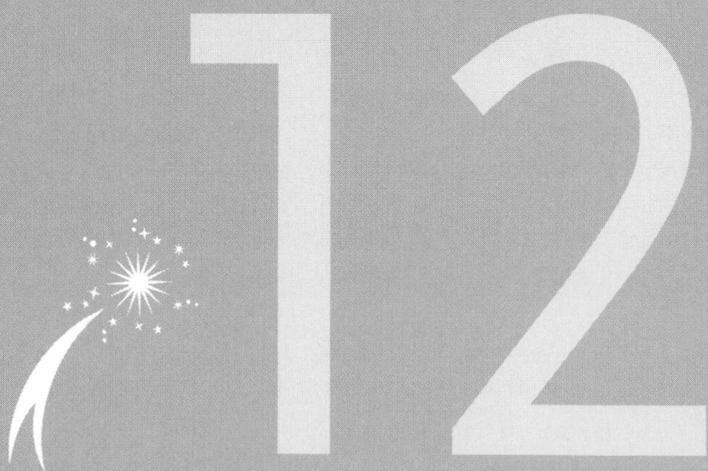

Your Safety Review: Preventing Accidents and Injuries

Look Like a Star!

Look at the Learning Objectives and The Finish Line before you begin reading this chapter.

Look at your pocket calendar. With your pencil, put a bracket ( ) around a study period every single day.

Look at your homework for this chapter. Plug each piece of homework into a certain time slot.

Look at the Star Student's Chapter Checklist at the end of this chapter. Check off each item as it is completed.

"The biggest problem in the world could have been solved when it was small."

Witter Bynner, 1881-1968, ***The Way of Life According to Laotzu***

"When you see a rattlesnake poised to strike, you do not wait until he has struck before you crush him."

Franklin Delano Roosevelt, 1882-1945

The Great Chicago Fire and "Daisy" the Cow

Legend has it that a cow named Daisy kicked over a lantern and started the Great Chicago Fire of October 8, 1871. That fire killed more than 300 people and left 100,000 more homeless, including patients at Passavant Hospital, who were forced to flee for their lives as the fires burned out of control.

At the time of the fire, the hospital was known as the Deaconess Hospital of Chicago; it became Passavant Memorial Hospital in 1895 following the death of the founder.

Two weeks after the fire, Reverend Passavant arrived in Chicago to survey the damage and assist the homeless and destitute. He observed that "ruin reigns supreme." In fact, the remains of Passavant Hospital were sold for the pathetic sum of $8.50.

If the story of Daisy the Cow is true, then the fire that devastated the nation's fourth-largest city in 1871 didn't have to happen. It could have been prevented with a little care and caution.

(Adapted from "To Be a Nurse" by Susan M. Sacharski, © 1990.)

Learning Objectives

1. **Spell and define all STAR words.**
2. **Discuss the three most common reasons for accidents and injuries.**
3. **List six common accidents that occur in long-term care facilities and guidelines to prevent them.**
4. **List five common injuries that may happen to you and guidelines to prevent them.**
5. **Explain the Material Safety Data Sheet (MSDS).**
6. **Explain the principles of body mechanics and apply them to daily activities.**
7. **Explain the importance of writing an incident report and show the correct method.**
8. **List six safety guidelines with residents using oxygen.**
9. **Identify safety and observation guidelines used with intravenous lines.**
10. **Describe the guidelines in the safe use of sharps and biohazard containers.**
11. **Identify the two categories of restraints and discuss restraint alternatives.**
12. **Demonstrate the acceptable use of the wheelchair positioner cushion.**
13. **Describe how this text begins and ends care procedures and how it treats other important procedural elements.**
14. **Identify and discuss the ten primary safety standards for using physical restraints.**
15. **Discuss fire safety and explain the RACE and PASS acronyms.**
16. **List the steps you can take to protect yourself and your residents from danger inside or outside of a facility.**

Successfully perform these Practical Procedures

The Safe Application of a Physical Tie Restraint

1 Spell and define all STAR words.

ABC extinguisher: an extinguisher suitable for use on all types of fires.

body mechanics: the way the parts of the body work together whenever you move.

chemical restraint: a medication that reduces a person's ability to move freely.

cyanosis: bluish tinge or color of the skin when a resident has a decreased oxygen level in the blood.

eye splash: splashing a substance into the eyes.

incident report: a report completed whenever an accident or injury occurs to a resident, staff member, or a visitor that documents the incident along with the response to the incident.

MSDS (Material Safety Data Sheet): sheets that provide information on the safe use, hazards, and emergency steps to take when using chemicals.

name alert: when two residents have similar names or the same name.

occurrence report: incident report; a report completed whenever an accident or injury occurs to a resident, staff member, or a visitor that documents the incident along with the response to the incident.

PASS: acronym for use of a fire extinguisher, which stands for Pull-Aim-Squeeze-Sweep.

physical restraint: a restraint that is attached to the resident in a way that makes the resident unable to remove the restraint alone.

point of care: place where care is being performed.

postural support: device that maintains good posture or body alignment; can also be a restraint.

protective device: another word for a physical restraint or postural support.

RACE: acronym for steps taken during a fire—Remove-Activate alarm-Contain-Extinguish.

restraint: a physical or chemical agent that is designed to restrict voluntary movement.

restraint alternatives: measures that may be used instead of physical or chemical restraints.

resuscitate: to perform life-saving measures like cardiopulmonary resuscitation (CPR).

sentinel event: an unexpected occurrence involving death or serious physical or psychological injury (or the risk of it).

skin splash: splashing a substance onto the skin.

slip knot: a special quick-release knot used to tie restraints.

synthetic: artificial or man-made.

wheelchair positioner cushion: restraint alternative used in a wheelchair or chair that is not physically tied to the resident.

2 Discuss the three most common reasons for accidents and injuries.

Every day, the decisions we make determine whether we will reach the end of our day safely. Many, if not most, accidents and injuries are due to carelessness, laziness, risk-taking, or more than one of these mixed up together. Consider for a moment the things you did today:

Did you take any unnecessary risks?
Did you act carelessly, causing any problem?
Were you lazy and did something bad happen?

Minute by minute, we all have to make quick decisions that sometimes make the difference between our safety and the safety of people and many other things around us.

Look at the following examples:

1. A nursing assistant on her way to work answers a cell phone call from a friend while driving at 60 m.p.h. She accidentally drives into the next lane, hits a car in that lane, then runs off the road and flips her car twice, resulting in a concussion.
2. A mother decides to use some milk for breakfast one morning before school, even though it is past the expiration date on the container. Shortly after arriving at school, her children become ill and she has to go pick them up.
3. A young female decides to walk home from her girlfriend's home at 12:30 in the morning. She is chased and almost grabbed by three young men and barely escapes.
4. A yard worker at a facility finishes raking the backyard and leaves the rake flat on the ground

with the sharp end facing up. He forgets to pick it up. A resident decides to take a walk in the yard and steps on the rake, causing it to fly up and hit her in the head.

If everyone were careful, responsible, and took less risks every day, we would have fewer accidents and injuries. Some accidents are bound to happen and cannot really be prevented. However, those caused by carelessness, laziness, or risk-taking might decrease in number.

3 List six common accidents that occur in long-term care facilities and guidelines to prevent them.

A healthcare facility has been described as "an accident waiting to happen." There are many accidents and injuries that may occur within a long-term care facility. You must always be on your guard during your workday to try to keep your residents, your fellow team members, visitors, and yourself safe. Being proactive—trying to *prevent* an accident from occurring in the first place—is much better than being reactive. Reacting or responding to an accident means that it has already taken place. You can change policy, but you cannot change the fact that an accident happened after it has occurred.

Some common resident accidents and injuries include the following:

- falls
- performing a procedure on the wrong resident
- burns
- poisoning
- choking
- cuts

Step 1. Fall Prevention

The majority of accidents within a facility are related to falls. There are many potential causes for falls in a facility. Following these guidelines can help prevent falls.

1. Respond to signal or call lights promptly. Never wait to respond.
2. Report wet floors immediately!

★ *"Don't Delay. Report Right Away!"*

3. Allow room for moving about in resident rooms and bathrooms. Remove clutter and pick up anything that has fallen on the floor promptly.
4. Get enough help when moving a resident from place to place. Make sure the residents have their canes or walkers handy. Be sure your residents have proper support. Never assume you can handle it alone. When in doubt, ask for help.
5. Make sure that a resident's bed or chair wheels are locked when you leave.
6. If side rails are ordered for your resident, check before leaving room to make sure they are all raised. Return beds to their lowest position when you're done with care. You will learn a quick-memory tip to help you enter and leave a resident's room safely later in this chapter.
7. Residents should wear clothing that fits properly. Residents must be wearing safe, non-slippery footwear at all times when out of bed. Always report the need for safer shoes. Non-skid mats or rugs should be used to prevent slipping. Always report any rugs that slip.

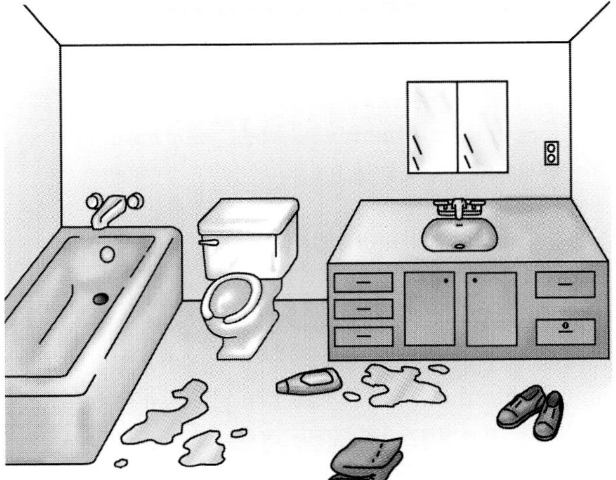

Figure 12-1. **An unsafe bathroom with many risks for falls.**

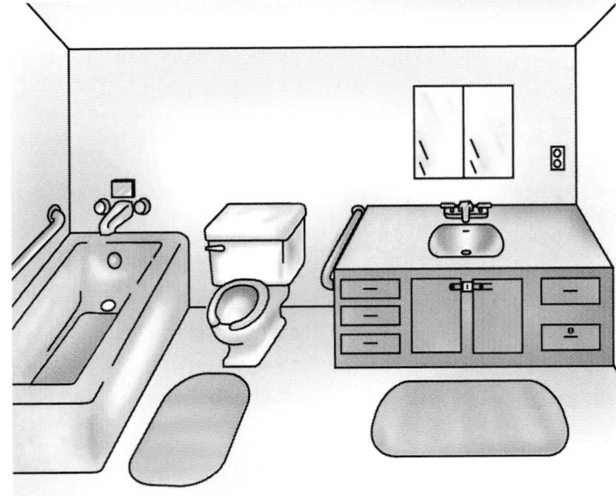

Figure 12-2. **A safe bathroom which reduces falling hazards.**

8. Non-skid mats must be used in a bathtub or shower each time a resident bathes. If allowed or ordered, stay with a resident the entire time he is showering or tub-bathing for safety reasons.
9. Keep everything within reach at the bedside or by the chair in a room, especially call lights.

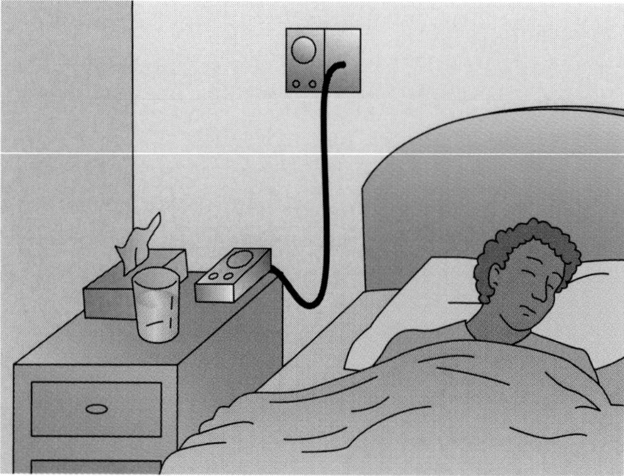

Figure 12-3.

10. Keep walkers and canes close by residents. Allow residents to sit for short periods before getting up to prevent lightheadedness.
11. Offer trips to the bathroom often. Respond to residents' requests promptly.

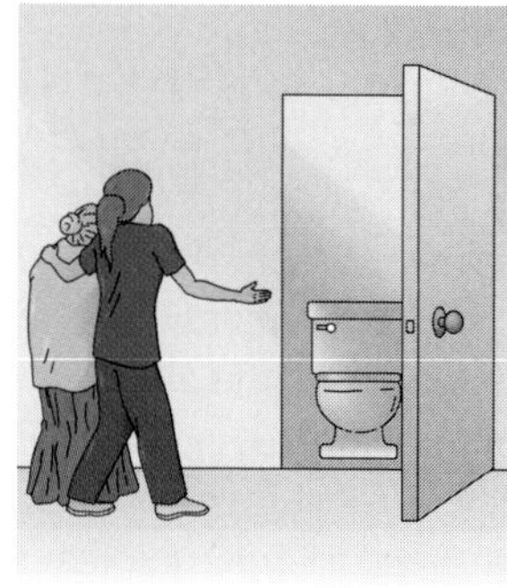

Figure 12-4.

12. Keep night light on in room if approved by facility and resident. Keep halls and other areas well-lit. Make sure resident has eyewear within reach.

Step 2. Resident and Staff Identification

Most people are used to seeing armbands on patients in hospitals. However, residents living in a long-term care facility may not wear name bracelets or identification armbands. Sometimes, photos are placed above the bed or just outside the door to serve as a way to identify the residents. See Figure 12-5. The photo should be very recent and must be updated periodically, especially if the resident's appearance changes. Following these identification guidelines can help prevent problems.

1. If used, make sure that a name bracelet is on the resident at all times. If it comes off, it must be replaced. Name bracelets often have important information on them, such as if a "code" should be called. Quick access to this information prevents staff from performing procedures the resident does not want done, such as resuscitation. To **resuscitate** a person means to perform life-saving measures like CPR.

   Robert Castro

   Figure 12-5.

   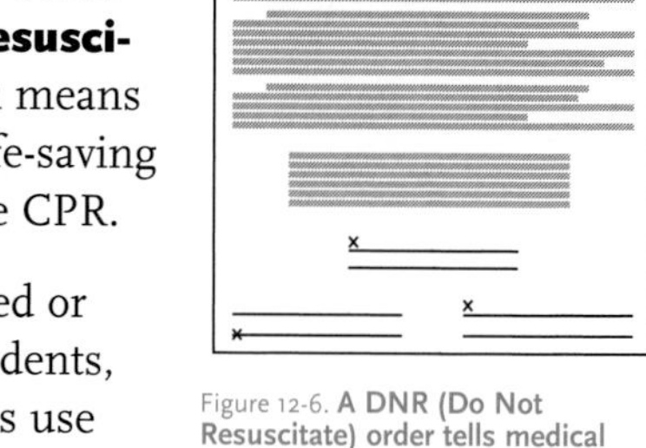

   Do Not Resuscitate Order

   Figure 12-6. A DNR (Do Not Resuscitate) order tells medical professionals not to perform CPR.

   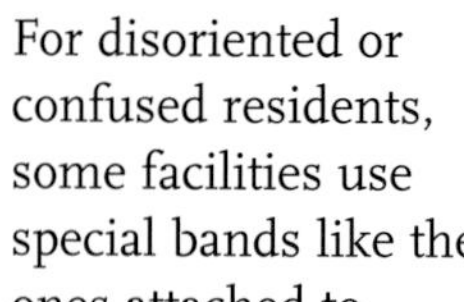

   For disoriented or confused residents, some facilities use special bands like the ones attached to clothing in stores. An alarm will sound when a resident who wanders tries to leave the facility. Respond promptly to an alarm.
2. Identify each resident before starting any procedure or giving any care. There is never an excuse for not checking ID. Do it each time you see a resident before providing care.

   Residents who have similar names may be living in the same unit. These people may be identified in the Kardex as a "name alert." **Name alert** means that proper identification of the resident is necessary for each **point of care**.
3. Identify yourself to all unknown residents, visitors and staff members. Wear your name badge every day in a spot that can be easily seen.

Step 3. Burn Prevention

Burns are a common safety concern in facilities. Burns are extremely painful. They may also cause a resident's condition to deteriorate rapidly, depending on whether they had a weakened physical state prior to the burn. Burns are costly because they require a great deal of care. Following these guidelines can help prevent burns:

1. Check the temperature of water before giving a resident a bath or shower. Temperature should not be over 110 degrees.
2. Check for proper temperature of hot water applications, such as hot packs. A resident's skin is fragile. Hot or cold water applications may only be applied for 20 minutes at a time. (See Chapter 24. This chapter will provide more details on hot and cold applications, such as hot water soaks and ice packs.)
3. Wrap electric heating pads inside approved covers before using them on residents. Check heating pads first for hazards.

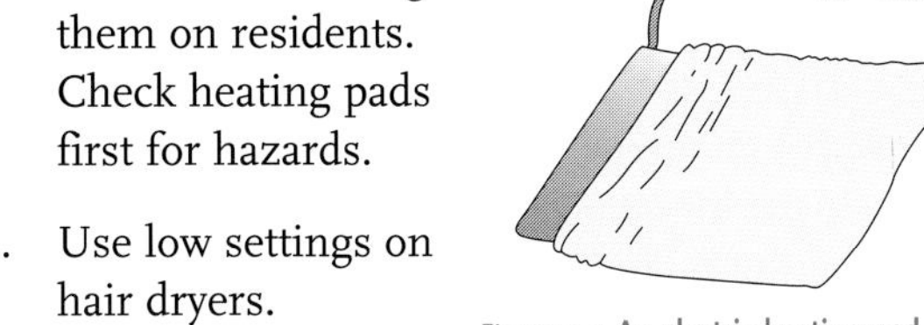

Figure 12-7. **An electric heating pad should have an approved cover on it.**

4. Use low settings on hair dryers.
5. Check space heaters frequently, and never leave them near anything flammable.
6. Do not leave a resident near a radiator or furnace. Furnaces should be checked often by the facility for safety.
7. Watch a resident who is near a stove or an oven. Never leave the resident alone.
8. Be very careful when serving hot beverages. Spills can cause burns. Residents may spill drinks on themselves if they are unsteady. Drinking hot beverages can also cause burns. Make sure the drink has cooled enough before encouraging the resident to drink.
9. Residents can be burned by reaching into a toaster with their fingers. Nothing should ever be inserted into a toaster to remove any food. There is a risk of being electrocuted.

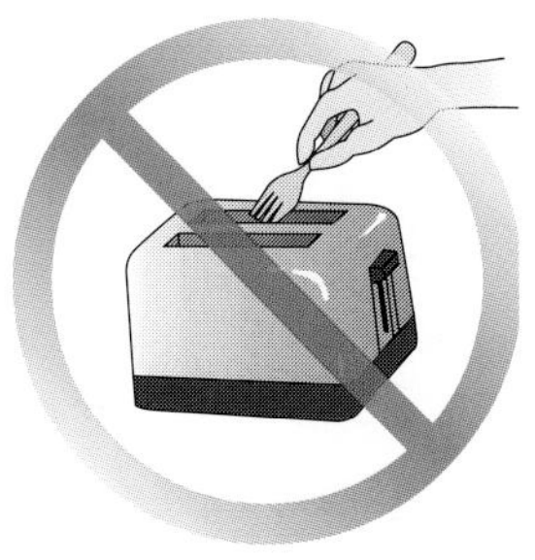

Figure 12-8.

10. Always make sure anything that was left in the sun, such as a car or a wheelchair, has cooled off completely before allowing a resident to sit in it or touch it. Residents themselves should not be left out in the sun too long.
11. Inform residents about smoking precautions. Smoking may be allowed in a specific area of the facility. Serious burns can occur if a resident falls asleep with a cigarette or cigar burning.

Step 4. Poison Prevention

Containers of any kind may be opened by residents, no matter how resident-proof you might think they are. Items you know would not interest or be consumed by an oriented person can be very dangerous for a confused resident. Following these guidelines can help prevent poisoning:

1. Keep fresh flowers or plants sent by friends or family away from disoriented resident. Items like nail polish remover, special soaps and body washes, perfumes, or hair-care products may also be eaten by a disoriented person.
2. Always check dates of foods to ensure that they are fresh.
3. Residents can be overcome by fumes when using chemical products. Make sure you always have adequate ventilation. Always report to the nurse any situation that you believe to be risky.

Step 5. Preventing Choking

Residents must be constantly monitored during meals to watch for signs of choking. Following these guidelines can help prevent choking:

1. Residents should be sitting up straight whether in bed or a chair while eating.
2. Assist with feeding slowly. Never rush a resident during a meal!
3. Cut food into small pieces.
4. If you believe a resident would be helped by a softer diet, report this to the nurse.

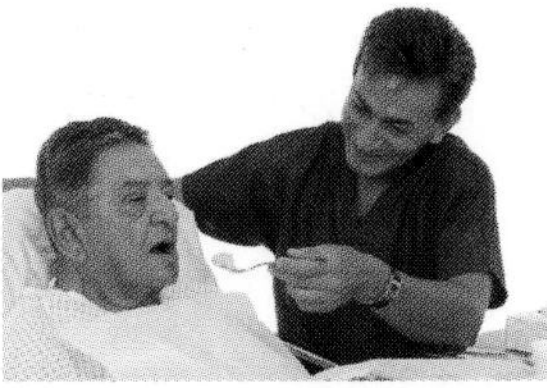

Figure 12-9. **Residents should be sitting up straight while eating. Do not rush a resident who is eating.**

5. Make sure dentures are in place and fit properly.
6. Be informed about any specific swallowing precautions a resident has.

Step 6. Preventing Cuts, Bruises, and Other Injuries

Cuts and scrapes can happen quickly. There are

many things that cause injuries of which you may not have been aware. Following these guidelines can help prevent injuries:

1. Never leave any sharp objects in reach of any resident. Resident supplies, like razors, must be carefully put away after use.

2. When you are moving through doors, look on the other side of the door before opening if there is a window in the door.

   If there is no window, open slowly. You can knock a resident to the floor by not looking first.

3. When moving a resident in a wheelchair or a stretcher, protect her arms and legs. Hands and feet are sometimes hit or bumped into walls or doors. Fingers may be caught in a wheelchair.

4. When moving a resident in an elevator, be careful moving him in or out. Do not catch arms or legs in the door. Fingers can be caught in elevators, too. Fingers may be caught in any door in the facility. Be careful when opening or closing doors.

4 List five common injuries that may happen to you and guidelines to prevent them.

Some examples of accidents that may happen to you include:
- falling
- getting cut by a sharp object, such as glass or a needle
- hurting your back, neck, arms, legs, or abdominal muscles when lifting
- getting hit, kicked, or scratched by a resident
- having something splashed on your skin or in your eyes

Step 1. Fall Prevention

Try not to run in a facility if you can avoid it. If you have to run in an emergency, be careful. Pay attention when you are walking down the halls. Look for wet areas or things that you or someone else may trip over.

Step 2. Preventing Cuts

Never stick your hand into a bed or anywhere else without looking first! Always be on the lookout for sharp objects or needles. They can hide in the most unexpected places.

Step 3. Lifting Safety

Ask for help any time you feel you might need assistance lifting or assisting a resident. If your facility has guidelines such as "one staff member for every 50 to 75 pounds lifted," follow the guidelines! Never take risks with yourself or your residents. Use proper equipment provided for lifting. Learning Objective 6 contains information on body mechanics.

Step 4. Combative Residents

Become familiar with your residents and watch them closely. Have a person with you in a room with a resident who sometimes tries to hit or injure others. Learn the triggers of this behavior. If a resident tries to strike you, protect yourself with your arm or step out of the way. Never strike back at the resident.

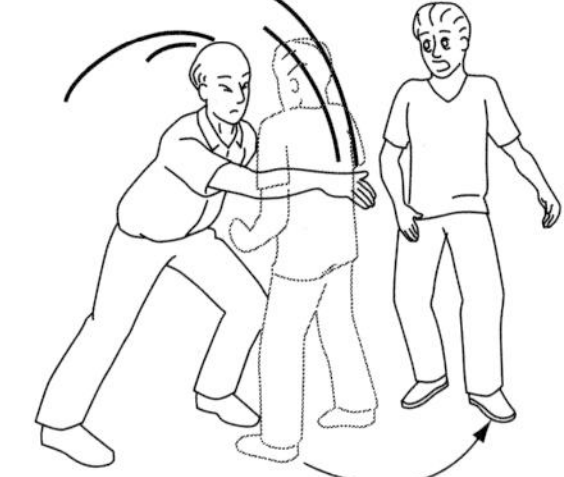

Figure 12-10. **Never strike back at an angry or combative resident.**

Step 5. Splashes

If a **skin splash** occurs, review the guidelines for each type of splash and know where to locate information about what to do when skin gets splashed by a chemical. Immediately rinse with large amounts of water at a sink or follow your facility policy.

If an **eye splash** occurs, follow facility policy regarding steps to take. Immediately rinse with large amounts of water at a sink, if no eye wash station is available. If an eye wash station is available at your facility, follow directions shown at your eye wash station.

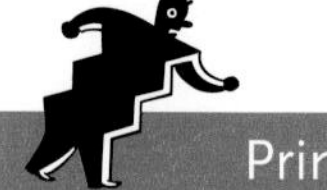

Principal Steps

Use of the Emergency Eye Wash

1. *Flip cup lid open*
2. *Open eyelid with thumb and index finger.*
3. *Press cup against eye and squeeze bottle repeatedly.*
4. *See a physician as soon as possible.*

5 Explain the Material Safety Data Sheet (MSDS).

The Occupational Safety and Health Administration (OSHA - see Chapter 11) is responsible for the overall safety of employees in their workplaces. OSHA requires that all dangerous chemicals come from their manufacturer with something called an **MSDS** (Material Safety Data Sheet). These sheets are placed in certain places in the facility so that all staff may have access to the sheets in an emergency.

The important types of information the MSDS will provide to staff include:

- What to wear when using certain chemicals
- The correct method of using and cleaning up a chemical
- What first aid measures are required when a chemical is splashed, sprayed, or accidentally eaten or drunk by a person
- Other known hazards of using the product

Material Safety Data Sheet
May be used to comply with
OSHA's Hazard Communication Standard.
29 CFR 1910.1200. Standard must be
consulted for specific requirements.

U.S. Department of Labor
Occupational Safety and Health Administration
(Non-Mandatory Form)
Form Approved
OMB No. 1218-0072

IDENTITY *(As Used on Label and List)*	*Note: Blank spaces are not permitted. If any item is not applicable, or no information is available, the space must be marked to indicate that.*

Section I

Manufacturer's Name	Emergency Telephone Number
Address *(Number, Street, City, State, and ZIP Code)*	Telephone Number for information
	Date Prepared
	Signature of Preparer *(optional)*

Section II — Hazardous Ingredients/Identity Information

Hazardous Components (Specific Chemical Identity; Common Name(s))	OSHA PEL	ACGIH TLV	Other Limits Recommended	% *(optional)*

Section III — Physical/Chemical Characteristics

Boiling Point		Specific Gravity (H_2O = 1)	
Vapor Pressure (mm Hg.)		Melting Point	
Vapor Density (AIR = 1)		Evaporation Rate (Butyl Acetate = 1)	

Solubility in Water

Appearance and Odor

Section IV —Fire and Explosion Hazard Data

Flash Point (Method Used)	Flammable Limits	LEL	UEL

Extinguishing Media

Special Fire Fighting Procedures

Unusual Fire and Explosion Hazards

OSHA 174, Sept. 1985

Figure 12-11. **A Material Safety Data Sheet.**

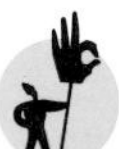

Do you know the location and use of the MSDS in your facility?

As an employee, you are responsible for certain things regarding the MSDS. To find out what these responsibilities are within your facility, attend the MSDS in-service that may be held annually. The nursing assistant's primary responsibility is to know the exact location of the MSDS in your area and how to use the MSDS when anyone has eaten or been exposed to a dangerous substance.

6 Explain the principles of body mechanics and apply them to daily activities.

Body mechanics is the way the parts of the body work together whenever you move. Good body mechanics helps save energy and prevents injuries and muscle strain. When muscles are used in the correct fashion to move and lift, you reduce the risk to you and also help decrease the possible risk to your residents. Understanding some basic principles will help you develop good body mechanics.

Alignment: The concept of alignment is based on the word "line." When you stand up straight, a vertical line could be drawn right through the center of your body and your center of gravity. When the line is straight, we say that the body is in alignment. This means that the two sides of the body are mirror images of each other, with body parts lined up naturally and properly supported.

Base of Support: The base of support is the foundation that supports an object. Something that has a wide base of support is more stable than something with a narrow base of support. Feet are the body's base of support. A person who is standing with the feet and legs apart has a greater base of support and is more stable than someone standing with the feet and legs close together. For a good, wide stance, the feet should be about shoulder-width apart.

Center of Gravity: The center of gravity in the human body is the point where the most weight is concentrated. This point will depend on the position of the body. When you stand, your weight is centered in your pelvis. A low center of gravity provides a more stable base of support. Bending your knees when lifting an object lowers your pelvis and your center of gravity. This gives you more stability and makes you less likely to fall. If you are moving or transferring a resident, the center of gravity includes the resident and still needs to be maintained close to your base of support. Remember that when you are transferring a resident, the resident needs to be as close to your body as possible.

Consider all of the activities that require moving or lifting something:

- Lifting a resident
- Picking up a resident's heavy bag of laundry
- Carrying a new resident's luggage
- Taking heavy trash bags to the appropriate site
- Cleaning a floor
- Moving a resident's bed into another room

Each one of these tasks could cause serious injury if done incorrectly without using proper body mechanics. Even the simple task of picking up a pencil from the floor, if you bend the wrong way, could cause a permanent injury to your back. Common tasks we must do every day with comparisons of the correct and incorrect methods to complete the tasks are listed below:

Incorrect Method	Correct Method
1. Lifting a resident	• Get help, if needed. Use lifting equipment.
2. Picking up a resident's heavy bag of laundry	• Reduce weight per bag.
3. Carrying a new resident's luggage	• Use a cart or make more than one trip.
4. Taking heavy trash bags to the appropriate site	• Ask for help.
5. Carrying heavy bags of groceries	• Ask checker to reduce weight of bags.
6. Moving a resident's bed	• Ask for help.

Using good body mechanics in a facility means understanding the importance of the following:

- Get help from a co-worker if needed.
- Raise the bed to a good height for your size to protect your back.
- Stand close to the object.
- Stand with a wide base of support.
- Use largest muscles of your upper arms and upper thighs to lift.
- Bend at your knees (squat) instead of at your waist.
- Never try to lift with just one hand.
- Hold objects close to your body.
- Push or pull objects, if possible, instead of lifting them.
- Avoid twisting or choppy movements; keep movements smooth.

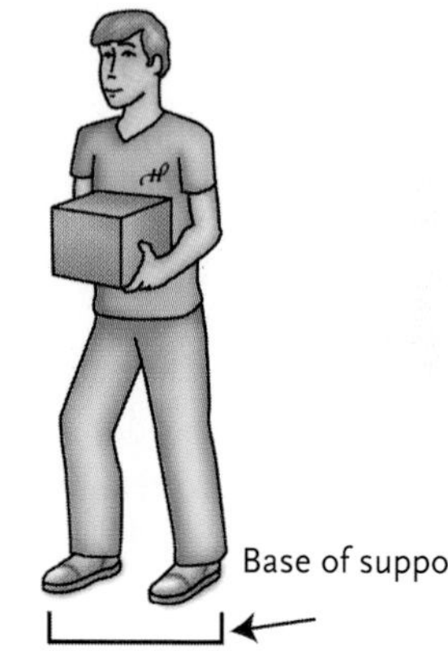

Figure 12-12.

Back injuries are often the result of performing a task incorrectly over many months or years. The importance of good body mechanics will become clearer to you as you spend more time within the facility. Using your body correctly can ensure that you will be a valued employee for many years to come. Don't let an injury happen to you; work smart!

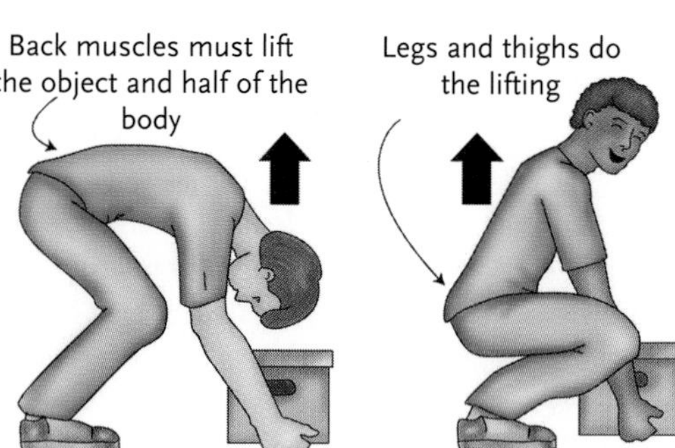

Figure 12-13. Lifting from a squat, with the back straight, allows the stronger muscles of the legs and thighs to do the lifting. In this illustration, which person is lifting correctly?

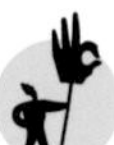

Bend your knees for ease!

When preparing to move or position a resident in bed, always bend your knees and be able to feel the bed with your knees before you begin the procedure. If you can't "FEEL THAT BED," STOP and BEND YOUR KNEES! If you don't bend your knees properly, you might seriously injure your back!

7 Explain the importance of writing an incident report and show the correct method.

Incident reports, or occurrence reports, are vital to the safety of the staff and the residents within facilities. An **incident report** or an **occurrence report** is a written report documenting and outlining the incident and listing the response to the incident. You must always fill out an incident report if you are injured in any way, no matter how slight, while on the job. This protects you and identifies the fact that the injury occurred on the job and not at home or anywhere else. Nurses may sign and add information to a staff incident report. The nurse will complete incident reports for any accident or injury that may occur to a resident or a visitor. You may be asked to add information to an incident report regarding a resident or a visitor. It is important that you write exactly what you saw. Do not write anything but truthful facts on an incident report.

A **sentinel event** is an unexpected occurrence involving death or serious physical or psychological injury (or the risk of it). Events are called "sentinel" because they signal the need for an immediate investigation and response. An example of this type of event is the death of a resident due to restraints.

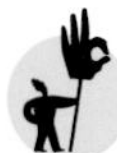

Incident or Occurrence Reports

Nursing assistants must never let ANYONE try to talk them out of filling out an incident report when they have been in an accident while on the job. It may be extremely important to have that incident report on file someday. You must take the time to complete it THE SAME DAY the incident occurs. In addition, you must KEEP A COPY of the incident report for yourself at home or in a safe place. This will protect you should the report be filed in the wrong place or lost by the facility.

8 List six safety guidelines with residents using oxygen.

When dealing with oxygen, nursing assistants need to fully understand the risks involved. For example, residents using oxygen sometimes want to smoke a cigarette or a cigar. This is very dangerous to the resident along with everyone else in the facility! Oxygen is a gas that can make any fire worse. A simple spark from an electrical appliance can turn into a serious fire near oxygen. Any flame may increase in size if it is close to oxygen. There are strict safety guidelines when using oxygen with residents.

Watch for flammables!

Do you know anyone who smokes at the same time they apply nail polish or use nail polish remover? If so, advise them to stop this practice before they injure themselves or someone else nearby. Products like nail polish and nail polish remover are flammable and dangerous when around sparks or flames. Lighting a cigarette or any other smoking material, or smoking a cigarette near one of these flammable products might cause the product to explode, possibly injuring someone and/or starting a fire.

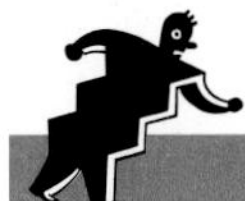

Principal Steps

Safety Guidelines with Oxygen Use

1. *SMOKING: A "No-Smoking" sign stating that oxygen is being used must be posted on each door and over the resident's bed. If you ever find any smoking materials in a resident's room or on the resident, you must promptly notify your supervisor.*

   ★ *"Don't Delay. Report Right Away!"*

2. *ELECTRICAL EQUIPMENT: Never allow the use of any electrical equipment such as electric razors, hair dryers, or radios. Ask your supervisor regarding the use of television sets and the signal light or call signal.*
3. *FLAMMABLE LIQUIDS: Never allow the use of any liquids like alcohol or nail polish remover. READ THE LABEL! If it says "Flammable" this means there is a high risk of fire.*
4. *OPEN FLAMES: never allow a resident near any kind of flame like a gas stove, candle, lighter, or match.*
5. *CLOTHING: Residents using oxygen must not use any wool or nylon or any other* ***synthetic*** *clothing or bedcovers. Synthetic means artificial or man-made fabric. Staff members must never wear wool clothing or sweaters near a resident with oxygen.*
6. *Oxygen tanks should be secured in an appropriate holder. When a tank holder is not available, some states require securing the tank with a chain. Follow facility policy regarding securing oxygen tanks.*

9 Identify safety and observation guidelines used with intravenous lines.

IV stands for "intravenous," or into a vein. A resident with an IV is receiving medication, nutrition, or fluids through a vein. A heparin lock is an IV that is kept open with a flush of heparin several times a day and hooked up to IV tubing only when medication is needed. Caring for residents with IVs can be a challenge.

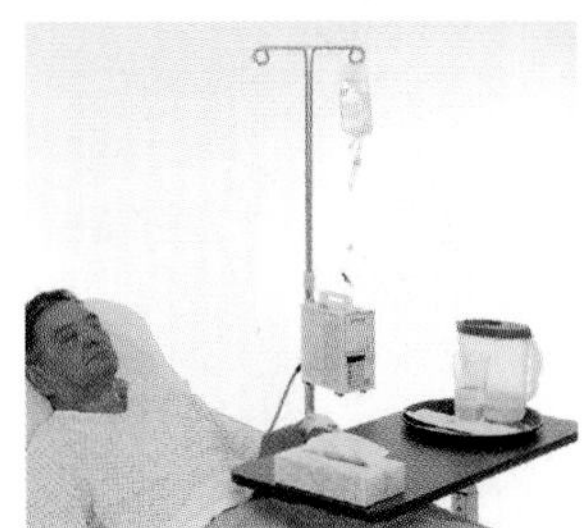

Figure 12-14. **A resident with an IV.**

Nursing assistants must follow the Principal Steps when caring for a resident with an intravenous line.

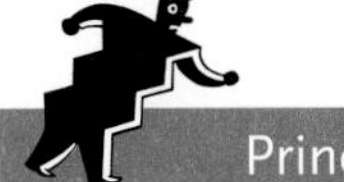

Principal Steps

Safety Guidelines with IVs

1. ★ *"Don't Delay. Report Right Away!"*

   A. The needle or catheter has fallen out.

   B. The tubing is disconnected.

   C. Blood appears in the tubing.

D. The IV fluid in the bag or container is gone or almost gone.

E. The IV fluid is not dripping, is leaking, or the bag breaks.

F. The special IV pump is beeping.

G. The area around the IV or heparin lock is wet, bleeding, swollen, red, or hot to the touch.

H. The resident complains of pain or has difficulty breathing.

2. *Never do any of the following when caring for a resident with an IV:*

   A. Take a blood pressure in an arm with an IV.

   B. Get the IV site wet.

   C. Pull on or catch the tubing in anything, such as clothing.

   D. Leave the tubing with a kink in it.

   E. Lower the IV bag below the IV site.

   F. Touch the clamp.

   G. Disconnect IV from pump or turn off alarm.

3. *ALWAYS WEAR GLOVES if you have to touch the IV area for any reason.*

10 Describe the guidelines in the safe use of sharps and biohazard containers.

Sharps and biohazard containers are the containers into which we place sharp objects and infectious waste. There are guidelines for using sharps and biohazard containers that you must follow in order to keep yourself safe.

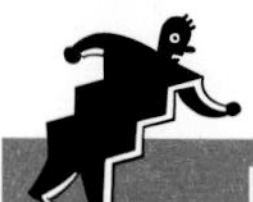

Principal Steps

Safety Using Biohazard and Sharps Containers

SHARPS CONTAINERS

1. *Never touch the sharps container without wearing gloves.*
2. *When dropping a sharp object into the container, KEEP YOUR FINGERS ABOVE THE OPENING at the top!*
3. *When touching the sharps container, TOUCH THE CONTAINER AT THE BOTTOM ONLY! Never place your fingers near the TOP OPENING!*
4. *Replace the sharps container when it is ¾ full (or follow your facility policy). Ask your supervisor for information on your facility's guidelines for replacing sharps containers.*
5. *If you must carry the container, carry it by the BOTTOM and be sure it is closed.*
6. *Wash your hands after throwing anything into the sharps container.*

BIOHAZARD CONTAINERS

1. *Drop anything contaminated with infectious waste (blood, body fluids, or human tissue) into the biohazard container, except anything SHARP!*
2. *Always wear gloves when disposing of infectious waste.*
3. *When dropping an object into the biohazard container, KEEP YOUR HANDS ABOVE THE OPENING at the top!*
4. *Wash your hands after throwing anything into the biohazard container.*

11 Identify the two categories of restraints and discuss restraint alternatives.

A **restraint** is a physical or chemical agent that is designed to restrict voluntary movement. A doctor's order is required for the use of any physical or chemical restraint. Restraints cannot be applied for the convenience of the staff or to discipline a resident. Residents who are restrained must be continually monitored. This is important. Residents have died due to improper restraint use and lack of monitoring. Restraints must be removed periodically, and the resident must be offered fluids and a trip to the bathroom and made comfortable.

Physical restraints are also known as **postural supports** or **protective devices**. There are many different styles of **physical restraints**. The most common restraints are the vest restraint, belt restraint, wrist/ankle restraint, and mitt restraint. Side rails and special chairs, like geri-chairs, are also considered physical restraints.

There are many potential hazards and complications of restraint use. Some of these, separated by body system, are listed below:

- Integumentary: bruises, cuts, pressure sores
- Respiratory: pneumonia due to a decreased ability to move

- Circulatory: reduced blood circulation
- Urinary: incontinence
- Muscular and Skeletal: wasting of muscle and bone
- Gastrointestinal: malnutrition
- Nervous: depression, sleep disorders, anxiety, loss of independence

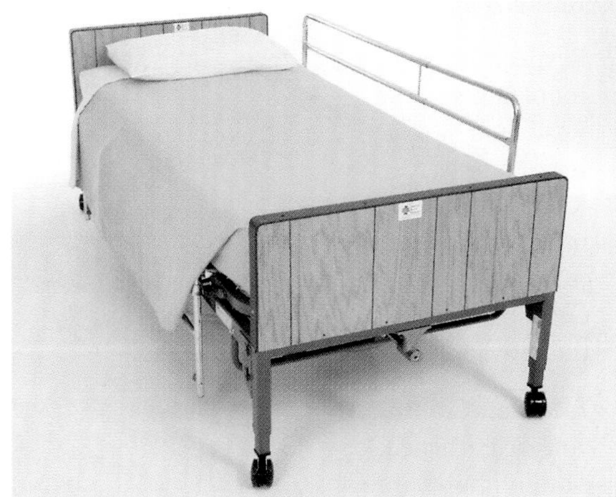

Figure 12-15. **Side rails.**

Chemical restraints are medications that may be given by a nurse or doctor to calm a resident. The overuse of chemical restraints has been a common problem in many facilities. In the past, residents were routinely restrained at most facilities. Today, the use of both physical and chemical restraints in facilities has greatly decreased due to the introduction of new types of safety devices and new laws.

Relatively new and creative ideas to help avoid restraints called **restraint alternatives**, are now being widely used. Residents tend to respond better to the use of creative ways to reduce tension, pulling at tubes, wandering, and boredom. Residents who are aggressive enough to try to hurt others or themselves may have to be restrained. Other types of restraints are used for the residents' safety. For example, side rails may be used to keep a resident from rolling out of bed. If you believe there is a better way than tying down a particular resident, offer your ideas to the nurses and doctors. The nurses may suggest that the doctor have the resident assessed for the use of physical restraint alternatives. Some restraint alternatives are outlined below:

Methods of Reducing Tension in Residents without using Physical Restraints

CALL SIGNALS: Answer call lights or signals immediately! A resident may try to get up by herself if no one answers the light, resulting in a fall.

VOLUNTEERS: The nurse may ask volunteers to stay with residents who need to be watched more closely. The nurse may ask the volunteer to ring for the staff promptly if the resident needs anything.

ACTIVITIES: The nurse may have the resident assessed by the activities department to see what activities may calm the resident while also keeping him busy.

FAMILY: Get the family involved as much as possible. Family members may decrease the tension in residents just by being there with them.

WANDERING AREA: If available, bring the resident to a covered, specified "wandering area." This area MUST be completely secure with no chance of the resident escaping the area.

MUSIC: Certain types of music have been shown to provide a calming effect on some people. This may provide a quieter, calmer environment for residents.

Music soothes.

"Music that gentlier on the spirit lies,
Than tir'd eyelids upon tir'd eyes;
Music that brings sweet sleep down
from the blissful skies."
Alfred Lord Tennyson (1809-1892), The Lotus Eaters

Some people use music to relax. Nursing home residents may also respond to music in a positive manner. Some may prefer classical, while others might like reggae, country and western, jazz, or rock and roll. When new residents are admitted, asking them the type of music they prefer might help guide the staff in choosing soothing music. Music may be just the right "medicine"!

There are several types of pads, wheelchair inserts, special chairs, and alarms that may be used instead of restraints. They are listed in Box 12-1.

Restraint Alternatives At-a-Glance (Box 12-1)

- Saddle cushion
- Wedge cushion
- Self-releasing belt
- Lap pillow
- Lap tray
- Foam body support
- Safety sensors
- Wheelchair positioner cushion

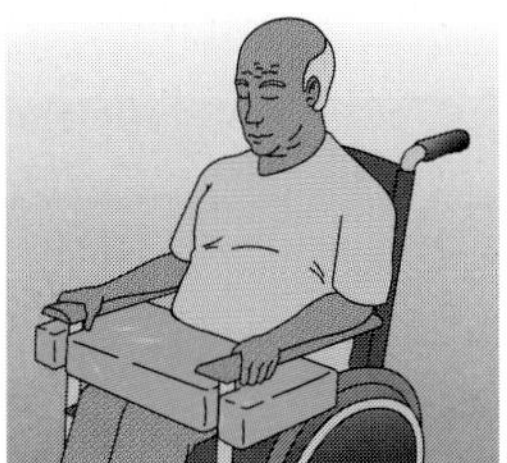

Figure 12-16. **Wheelchair positioner cushion.**

12 Demonstrate the acceptable use of the wheelchair positioner cushion.

One commonly-used type of restraint alternative is the **wheelchair positioner cushion**. It is a specially-made cushion that slides into position on the wheelchair. It encourages correct posture and good body alignment. The device may prevent the resident from falling or leaning forward in the chair.

The wheelchair positioner cushion reminds a resident that he has a support in front of him, and yet the resident understands that he may remove it on his own at any time. If the resident cannot remove the wheelchair positioner cushion, it is no longer a restraint alternative. It would become a restraint and would then require a doctor's order. All of the regulations regarding restraints would then apply.

13 Describe how this text begins and ends care procedures and how it treats other important procedural elements.

At the beginning of this book, in the "Using Your Textbook for Success" section, we showed you the following box:

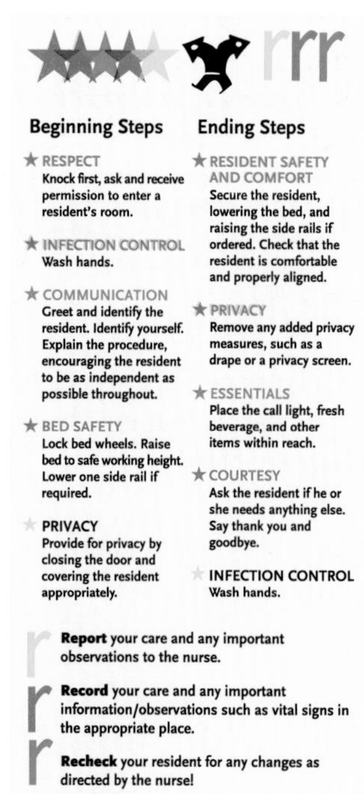

Beginning Steps	Ending Steps
★ RESPECT Knock first, ask and receive permission to enter a resident's room.	★ RESIDENT SAFETY AND COMFORT Secure the resident, lowering the bed, and raising the side rails if ordered. Check that the resident is comfortable and properly aligned.
★ INFECTION CONTROL Wash hands.	★ PRIVACY Remove any added privacy measures, such as a drape or a privacy screen.
★ COMMUNICATION Greet and identify the resident. Identify yourself. Explain the procedure, encouraging the resident to be as independent as possible throughout.	★ ESSENTIALS Place the call light, fresh beverage, and other items within reach.
★ BED SAFETY Lock bed wheels. Raise bed to safe working height. Lower one side rail if required.	★ COURTESY Ask the resident if he or she needs anything else. Say thank you and goodbye.
★ PRIVACY Provide for privacy by closing the door and covering the resident appropriately.	★ INFECTION CONTROL Wash hands.

r **Report** your care and any important observations to the nurse.

r **Record** your care and any important information/observations such as vital signs in the appropriate place.

r **Recheck** your resident for any changes as directed by the nurse!

This book will remind you of these steps once in most chapters. However, within each procedure, the following icons will be used to represent these steps as well as three additional reminders:

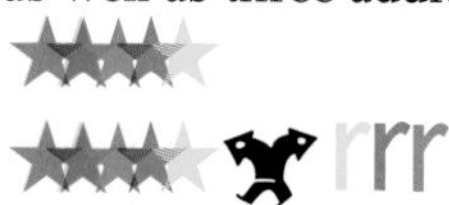

Understanding why each step is important will help you remember to perform each step every time care is provided.

Beginning steps

1. **Respect:** A resident's room is his home. Residents have a right to privacy. Knocking and waiting to receive permission before entering respects this privacy.

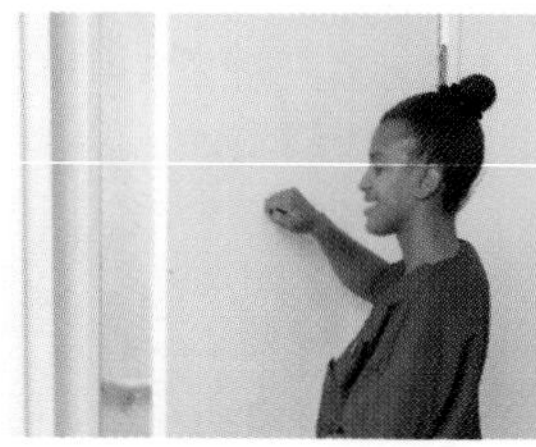

Figure 12-17.

2. **Infection Control:** As you have learned, nothing fights infection in facilities like consistent, proper hand washing.

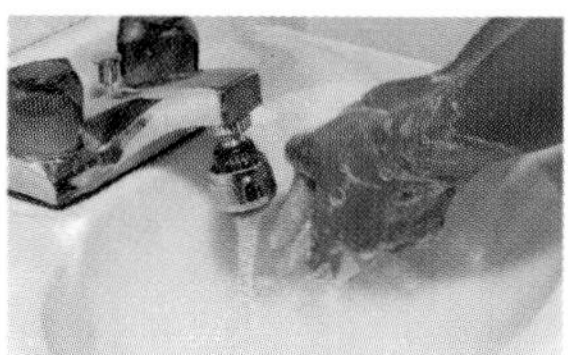

Figure 12-18.

3. **Communication:** Residents must know who is providing their care. Greeting residents shows courtesy and respect. Being careful to identify residents prevents care from being performed on the wrong person. Residents have a right to know exactly what care you will provide. Finally, encouraging residents' independence is important, and residents are more able to do for themselves if they know what needs to happen.

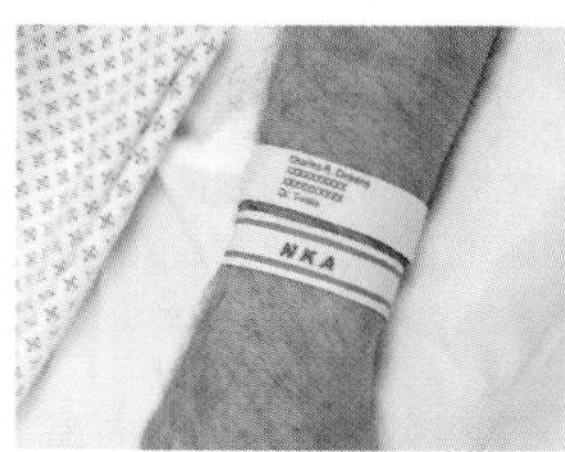

Figure 12-19.

4. **Bed Safety:** Locking the bed wheels is an important safety measure. It ensures that the bed will not move as you are performing care. Raising the bed helps you to remember to use the principles of good body mechanics. Remember that side rails are considered restraints, and side rails should only be used

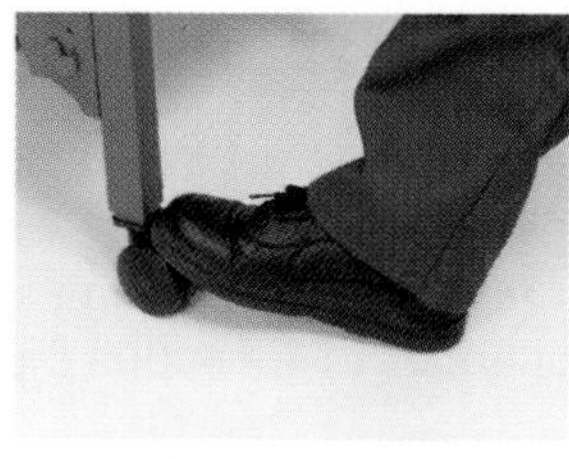

Figure 12-20.

when specifically ordered or when you are raising the bed for care.

5. **Privacy:** Remember the learning objective on residents' rights? Providing for privacy in a facility is not simply a courtesy; it is a legal right.

Ending steps

1. **Resident Safety and Comfort:** Securing the resident after you perform care prevents injury. Proper alignment promotes resident comfort and health after you leave the room.

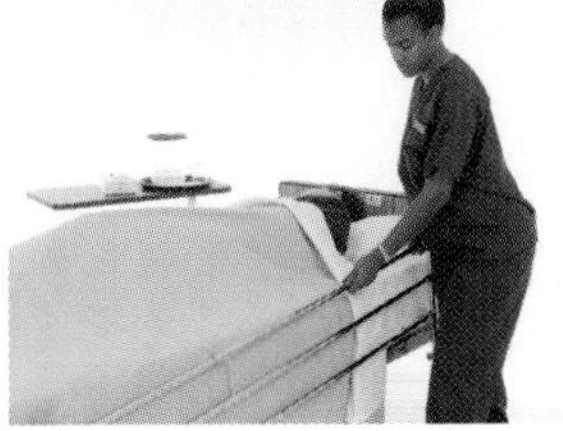

Figure 12-21.

2. **Privacy:** Remove any extra privacy measures added during the procedure. This includes anything you may have draped over and around residents, as well as privacy screens.

3. **Essentials:** A call light ensures that residents can reach a staff member whenever a problem or a need arises. Remember that the decision not to respond to a call light is considered neglect. Dehydration is a serious problem, especially with the elderly. Keeping beverages close by encourages residents to drink more often. You should also encourage residents to drink every time you see them, as long as they are not NPO (nothing by mouth). Make sure that the pitcher and cup are light enough for residents to lift.

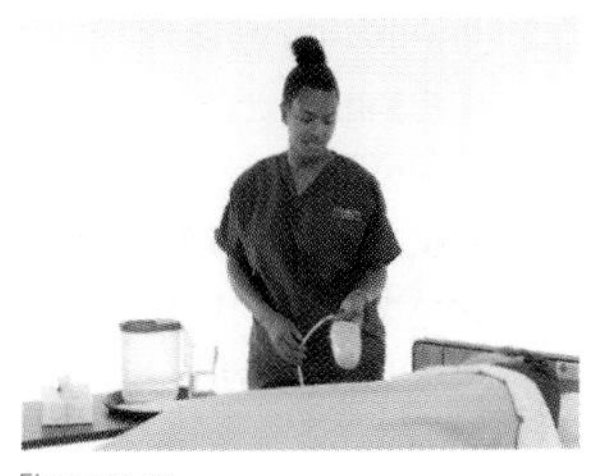

Figure 12-22.

4. **Courtesy:** Saying "Thank you" for the service you provided is polite and the proper thing to do. Letting residents know you are leaving promotes respect.

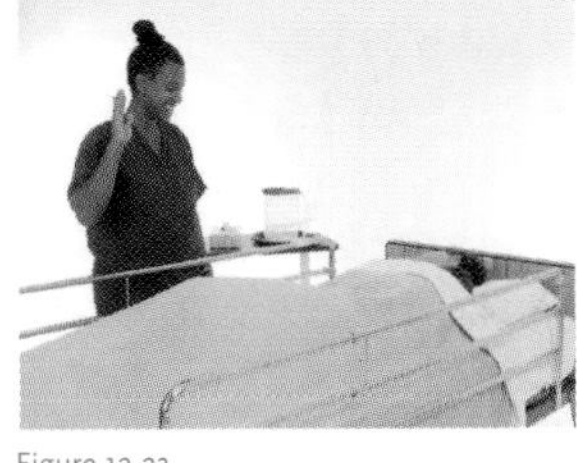

Figure 12-23.

5. **Infection Control:** Again, handwashing is important in preventing the spread of infection.

The 3Rs

The 3Rs are a helpful tool reminding you to do the most important things after a procedure: report, record, and recheck. You will often be the person who spends the most time with a resident. So, you are in the best position to note any changes in a resident's condition. Every time you provide care, observe the resident's physical and mental capabilities, as well the body's condition. For example, a change in a resident's ability to perform activities of daily living (ADLs)-grooming and hygiene activities, dressing, and eating-may signal a greater problem. After you have finished providing care, you must:

1. **Report** your care and observations to the nurse.
2. **Record** the care you have given and any additional information in the appropriate place.
3. **Recheck** the resident as directed by the nurse.

In most procedures you will see these statements:
Follow all standard and/or transmission-based precautions.
Follow all rules for body mechanics.

The first statement reminds you to use your judgment based on what you have learned regarding infection control. While a procedure in this book may not include wearing gloves, masks, or other personal protective equipment, there are circumstances when PPE may be appropriate. For example, the procedure in this text that teaches giving a resident a backrub will not include gloves because gloves are generally not required. However, if the resident has non-intact skin or open sores, gloves are necessary. Wearing gloves or other PPE when they are not required may be considered abuse. Not wearing gloves when a risk of contact with body fluids exists is dangerous for you.

The second reminder is for your safety and the safety of your resident. While the procedures will describe the correct way to perform the task, remembering those basic rules of body mechanics during each step is up to you. Those basic rules help prevent injury to you and to your residents.

14 Identify and discuss the ten primary safety standards for using physical restraints.

The OBRA law sets specific guidelines for the use of restraints. You must remember that restraints are used only when everything else has been ruled out for the resident. They cannot be the first choice or used for the purpose of convenience or discipline. When restraints have been ordered, there are certain safety standards that must be followed.

10 Safety Standards when using Physical Tie Restraints

Know your state's laws and facility rules regarding a nursing assistant's role in applying restraints. Before applying a restraint, check with the nurse to make sure there is a written doctor's order.

1. Use the correct size and style of restraint. Ask the nurse for help if needed.
2. Always use a **slip knot**. Never tie to side rails; only tie to the movable part of a bed frame.
3. Keep scissors in your pocket in case you must remove a tie restraint suddenly and have trouble removing the tie.
4. Check to make sure the restraint is not too tight.
5. Apply the restraint over clothing if vest or belt style. Use a hand roll with some styles of mitt restraints.
6. Be careful not to catch the resident's breasts in the restraint.
7. Place the call light in reach of the person at all times. Residents with mitt restraints will not be able to press the call light. Because of this, they MUST be checked every five minutes!
8. Check the resident every 15 minutes (every five minutes for a mitt restraint) for safety. If wrist/ankle or mitt restraint is used, check the wrist/ankle pulse each time (see Chapter 16). Look at the skin around the restraint to check for blue-tinged skin, or **cyanosis**, which could mean lack of blood circulation (oxygen) to the area. Check for redness or swelling of the body part.
9. Remove the restraints every two hours, or more often if needed, for at least 15 minutes, and provide personal care. Take resident to the bathroom or change incontinent brief, exercise the resident, and provide anything else the resident needs.
10. Document the following regarding restraint use:
    a. Type of restraint and time applied
    b. Each time of removal
    c. Care given when released
    d. Any circulation, skin, or other problems

The Safe Application of a Physical Tie Restraint

Follow all standard and/or transmission-based precautions. Follow all rules for body mechanics.

Collect equipment: The correct size and type of restraint.

1. **Perform the "5 Stars."**

2. **Have the correct size and type of restraint ready per doctor's order.**
3. **Apply the restraint carefully following manufacturer's directions or facility policy. For each type of restraint, make sure that it is never too tight.**

   ALL CHEST or BELT-STYLE RESTRAINTS: Make sure you don't catch breasts or skin in the restraints. Double-check before actually tying together or attaching buckle.

   VEST: The criss-cross in the vest restraint must be placed on the front of the body.

   MITT: Remember to use a hand roll with certain styles of mitt restraints.

   WRIST/ANKLE: Make sure the restraint will not slide off of the wrist or ankle.
4. **Use a single-tie or double-tie slip knot to tie the restraint. Make sure it is not too tight!**

   It must be tied to the movable part of the bed frame, if used in bed, not the side rail!
5. **Perform the "5 Stars and 3 Rs."**

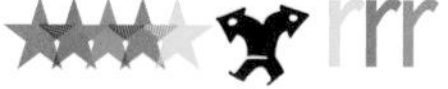

   a. Check resident every 15 minutes. (Residents with mitt restraints must be checked every five minutes because they are unable to use the call light.)

   b. Release the restraint(s) every two hours for at least 15 minutes and provide all care, such as giving fluids, toileting, walking (if ambulatory), or range of motion.

15 Discuss fire safety and explain the RACE and PASS acronyms.

There are many causes of fire. For a fire to occur, it must have these three things:

Heat	what makes the flame
Fuel	what will burn
Oxygen	what will keep the fire burning

There are many potential causes of a fire in facilities. Some examples are listed on the next page:

- resident with poor hand control, or is unsteady
- careless smoking
- frayed or damaged electrical cords
- electrical equipment in need of repair
- space heaters
- overloaded electrical plugs
- oxygen use
- careless cooking
- flammable liquids or rags with special oils on them
- stacks of newspapers or other clutter
- extension cords

When a fire occurs, make sure you know the location of alarms. Also, two acronyms will help you remember what to do. The first is the **RACE** acronym, which outlines what to do in case of a fire.

RACE

Remove residents, visitors, and staff nearest to the fire.

Activate the alarm.

Contain the fire and smoke by closing all doors and windows in the area.

Extinguish the fire, or fire department will extinguish.

Usually the type of fire extinguisher at most facilities is the **ABC extinguisher**, suitable for use on all types of fires. Using a fire extinguisher is handled by following the acronym **PASS**.

PASS

Pull the pin.

Aim at the base of the fire when spraying.

Squeeze the handle.

Sweep back and forth at the base of the fire.

Other fire safety measures:

- Stay low in a room when trying to escape a fire.
- Block doorways to prevent smoke from entering a room.
- Use a covering over the face to reduce smoke inhalation.
- If clothing is on fire, remember to **stop**, **drop**, and **roll** to put out fire.

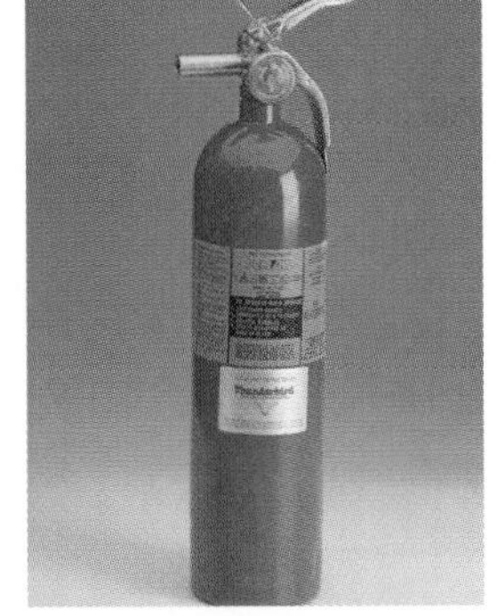

Figure 12-24. **Know where the extinguisher is stored in your facility and how to operate it.**

- If a door is closed, always check for heat coming from a door before opening it.
- Never get into an elevator during a fire.

Smoke Alarms, Carbon Monoxide Detectors, and Fire Extinguishers

Have you checked your smoke alarm, carbon monoxide detector, and fire extinguisher lately? Make sure the smoke alarm and carbon monoxide detector are in working order and have new batteries, if battery-operated. Your fire extinguisher will not be any good in a fire if it is not charged. To see if your fire extinguisher needs a recharge, you might want to take it to a local fire department to have it checked.

When holidays or birthdays come, why not consider buying something that may someday save someone's life? Carbon monoxide detectors or a combination carbon monoxide/smoke detector can alert your loved ones to the presence of the dangerous odorless gas called carbon monoxide along with alarming if there is a fire. This alarm might someday be the only thing between your loved ones and possible death.

Evacuation carries save lives!

If an evacuation is required, you must be familiar with the different types of evacuation carries. Contact your local fire department for information and/or training.

16 List the steps you can take to protect yourself and your residents from danger inside or outside of a facility.

Living, visiting, or working in a facility may occasionally put a person at risk of crime. Many people may go in and out of a facility during a single day. Delivery people, visitors, clergy, temporary workers, and others come to a facility for specific reasons. Unfortunately, not everyone is as honest and trustworthy as we would like them to be. So, it is best to be on guard at all times for any suspicious behavior.

★ *"Don't Delay. Report Right Away!"*

Never believe someone else will report the situation. Never think reporting it is not necessary. It is better to be safe. Report suspicious behavior to the charge nurse or security; follow facility policy regarding reporting. The following list outlines some of the dangers that may exist in a facility:

1. Theft of your belongings or your residents' belongings may occur.
2. You or your residents may be at risk of being attacked by someone.

3. Vandalism may occur to your residents' belongings or your car.
4. Someone may try to follow you or a visitor home.
5. Someone may gain access to your telephone number, address, or e-mail address.

These are just a few of the criminal dangers that exist within a facility. Some suggestions for keeping you, your residents, and visitors safe from crime are listed below:

Eleven Tips to Stay Safe from Crime

1. Take a self-defense course or a rape self-defense class from a local organization.
2. Buy a hand-held emergency alarming device that you can press if necessary when walking to your car or to the bus. A flashlight can also be used as a weapon to temporarily blind a person trying to attack you.
3. Always ask for an escort to walk you to your car or bus, if available. When walking, keep your head up at all times and stay alert. Scan your surroundings.
4. Always hold your house key or car key in your hand ready to be used right away. Keys can be used as a weapon if needed. Be prepared.

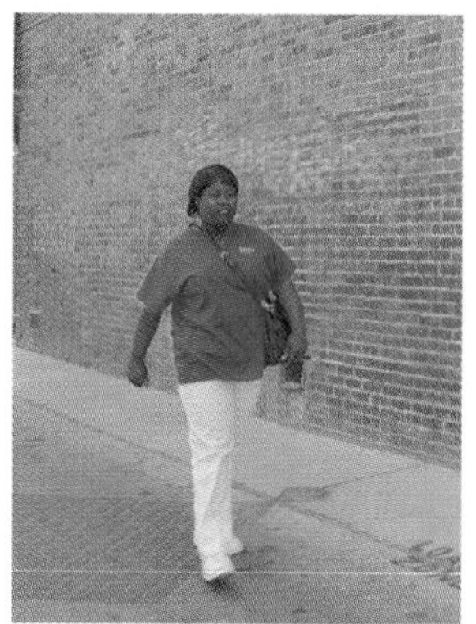

Figure 12-25. **Be alert and check your surroundings as you walk.**

5. Look into the vehicle before you get in to check for anyone hiding in it.
6. Get inside the car or bus right away, if possible. Close the door and lock the car immediately. Keep the windows up.
7. Keep enough gas in your car at all times so you never run out.
8. Always keep emergency bus fare handy. If you're not on a bus line, walk with someone to the bus stop. Do not walk alone, especially at night.
9. You may want to leave your purse at home. Carry only what is absolutely necessary.
10. Go straight to a well-lit area if you think you are being followed. Never go straight home! You may also go to a fire or police station, if one is nearby.
11. Leave only your car key. Whenever you have to leave your car key with anyone, such as for an oil change or for valet parking, never leave your house keys. This prevents the person from making a copy of your other keys.

Keeping Residents and Staff Safe in a Facility

1. Stay on guard and be watchful at all times before, during, and after your shift.
2. Ask the nurse to lock up valuable resident belongings.
3. Never leave a resident alone with someone if you are uneasy about the person.
4. Follow the guidelines about the number of visitors allowed at one time in a resident room.
5. Keep your personal information private and do not share numbers, etc. Ask the staff to never post your phone number or address!

Summary

Focusing on safety in the workplace means that you, your residents, fellow staff members, and visitors are able to complete another day without any type of injury. Countless hazards exist within a facility and many more are lurking on the trip to or from a facility. When nursing assistants are constantly watchful and cautious both inside and outside of the facility, they will be safer and able to care for their special residents for many quality years.

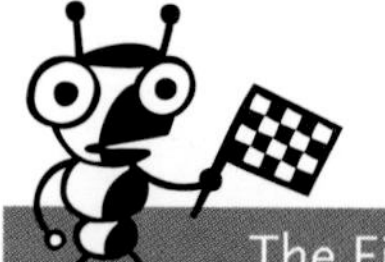

The Finish Line

What's Wrong With This Picture?

1. List the one missing step about documenting restraint use.

   Document the following regarding restraint use:

a. Type of restraint and time applied

b. Care given when released

c. Any circulation, skin, or other problems

2. List two additional fire safety measures not included in the list below.
   - Block doorways to prevent smoke from entering a room.
   - Use a covering over the face to reduce smoke inhalation.
   - If a door is closed, always check for heat coming from a door before opening it.
   - Never get into an elevator during a fire.

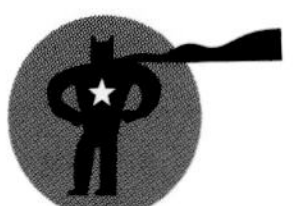

Star Student Central

1. Contact a local safety specialist or OSHA office in ergonomics (methods used to prevent work-related injuries) and ask for information to share with your class.

2. Contact your local fire department and ask for fire safety pamphlets and other information to share with your class.

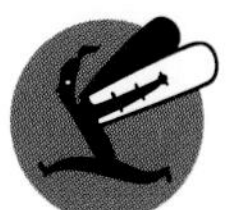

You Can Do It Corner!

1. Write out the "5 Stars" and the "3 Rs" (using a marker or on your computer) on two sheets of paper and put them in two spots in your home where you will see them all of the time. Practice and memorize the "5 Stars" and the "3 Rs." Be able to repeat both of them. (LO 13)

2. Identify the parts to the acronyms RACE and PASS. (LO 15)

3. What is an MSDS and what do you need to know about it? (LO 5)

4. What is a name alert and how do we prevent accidents from occurring regarding this situation? (LO 3)

5. What items should not be in a room where oxygen is in use? (LO 8)

6. Name at least three things you should not do for a resident who has an IV. (LO 9)

7. Name and explain three restraint alternatives and when it is appropriate to use them. (LO 11)

8. What does a restraint do? (LO 11)

9. What object must you have with you at all times when using physical tie restraints? (LO 14)

10. List the three most common reasons for accidents and injuries. (LO 2)

11. Why is a resident with a mitt restraint at additional risk? (LO 14)

12. Review the safety steps to take when getting into your vehicle. (LO 16)

13. Explain the steps you should take if you think someone is following you. (LO 16)

14. List six common resident accidents that occur in long-term care facilities. (LO 3)

15. What are some things you can do to make sure you lift safely? (LO 4)

16. Explain why it is vitally important for you to fill out an incident report as soon as possible after a workplace injury. Why should you always ask for a copy of the incident report? (LO 7)

17. Describe three basic principles of body mechanics. (LO 6)

18. Explain how to carry a sharps container. (LO 10)

19. When does a wheelchair positioner cushion become a restraint rather than a restraint alternative? (LO 12)

Star Student's Chapter Checklist

1. I have read my textbook chapter.

2. I have reviewed my own "Pocketful of Terms."

3. I have listened to my tutor tape.

4. I have reviewed and highlighted my class notes.

5. I have read and completed any handouts from this chapter.

6. I have completed "The Finish Line."

7. Star Time! Choose your reward!

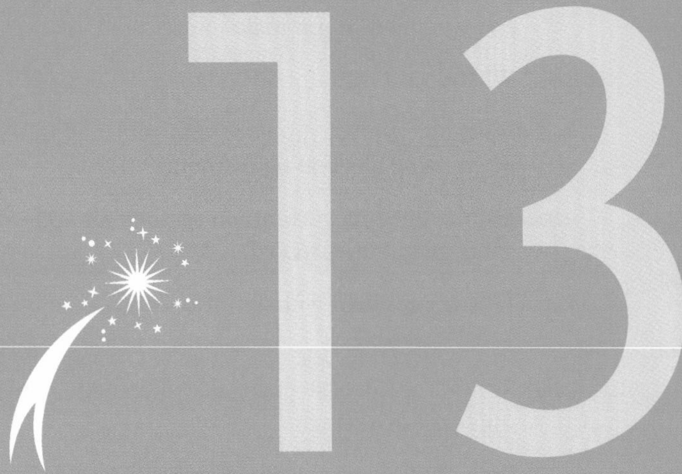

Your Introduction: Emergency Care, Disasters, and First Aid

Look Like a Star!

Look at the Learning Objectives and The Finish Line before you begin reading this chapter.

Look at your pocket calendar.
With your pencil, put a bracket ( ) around a study period every single day.

Look at your homework for this chapter.
Plug each piece of homework into a certain time slot.

Look at the Star Student's Chapter Checklist at the end of this chapter. Check off each item as it is completed.

Learning Objectives

1. Spell and define all STAR words.
2. Explain the difference between a cardiac arrest and a respiratory arrest.
3. Name the two types of PPE that you should always have with you in case of an emergency.
4. Identify the acronym that may be used when confronted with an emergency situation requiring first aid.
5. Explain the role of the nursing assistant on a facility code team.
6. Describe a standard disaster response at a facility and explain the nursing assistant's role in disasters.
7. Describe how to assess a person involved in a medical emergency.
8. Identify the correct first aid procedures for each of these emergency situations:
    - an obstructed airway in a child or adult
    - shock
    - bleeding
    - poisoning
    - burns
    - fainting (syncope)
    - nosebleed
    - myocardial infarction or heart attack
    - insulin shock and diabetic coma
    - seizure
    - CVA or stroke

"It is by presence of mind in untried emergencies that the native metal of a man is tested."

James Russell Lowell, 1819-1891

"... the truly noble and resolved spirit raises itself, and becomes more conspicuous in times of disaster and ill fortune."

Plutarch, A.D. 46-120

Emergency Transfer of Victims During the 1500s

The rescue of a traveler during an emergency has come a long way from the treatment one poor man had to suffer in the 1500s. Consider the care and caution most rescue squads now take when helping an injured person. What a difference!

"The misfortune befell me in the manner which follows: wishing to pass across the water and trying to make my hackney enter a boat, I struck [the horse]. . .with a riding crop [and] the animal gave me such a kick that she broke entirely the two bones of my left leg. . .I was quickly carried into the boat to cross to the other side in order to have me treated. But its shaking almost made me die, because the ends of the broken bones rubbed against the flesh, and those who were carrying me could not give it fit posture.

From the boat, I was carried into a house of the village with greater pain than I had endured in the boat. . .Finally, however, they placed me on a bed to regain my breath a little. . .while my dressing was being made. . ."

Ambroise Paré, 1510-1590, from *Ten Books of Surgery*

1 Spell and define all **STAR** words.

aphasia: loss of ability to speak or recognize words.

Automated External Defibrillators (AED): portable defibrillator that gives the heart an electric shock to try to restore a normal heartbeat after the heart stops suddenly.

cardiac arrest: when the heart stops.

code team: group of people chosen for a particular shift that respond in case of a resident emergency.

CPR: cardiopulmonary resuscitation; medical procedures used to restart a person's heart and breathing when that person suffers sudden cardiac or respiratory arrest.

fainting: syncope, loss of consciousness.

first aid: care given by the first people to respond to an emergency.

Heimlich maneuver: method of attempting to remove an object from the airway of a person who is choking.

hemiplegia: paralysis of one-half of the body.

hemorrhage: severe bleeding.

pocket mask: small mask or barrier device providing protection in situations where rescue breathing is needed.

respiratory arrest: when breathing stops.

shock: decreased blood flow to organs and tissues.

syncope: fainting.

xiphoid: sword-shaped lowest part of sternum; can be accidentally cracked while giving CPR.

2 Explain the difference between a cardiac arrest and a respiratory arrest.

When a person is involved in a serious accident, such as drowning or choking on an object, the first thing that happens to the person is respiratory arrest. **Respiratory arrest** means that breathing stops. If the person is not helped quickly, cardiac arrest may soon follow. **Cardiac arrest** is when the heart stops. During respiratory arrest, rescue breathing may bring the victim out of the arrest and help the person to resume breathing. Rescue breathing means breathing into the victim's mouth, following accepted guidelines. Cardiopulmonary resuscitation (**CPR**) may bring a victim of cardiac arrest back and restore life. This textbook is not a CPR course, so it contains only basic first aid for emergencies. If your facility does not arrange for you to be trained in CPR and rescue breathing, the American Heart Association and the American Red Cross, among others, offer courses in CPR. Keep your CPR certification current and consider taking a separate first aid course to stay up-to-date on first aid and life-saving methods. These methods change periodically, and staying up-to-date will prevent you from using an outdated procedure.

First aid *is defined as the care given by the first people to respond to an emergency. The first few minutes of any emergency may determine the victim's ability to survive the accident. Sometimes, doing the wrong thing may make a situation worse. Understanding the first steps to take in many emergencies may help prevent additional injury and ensure the recovery of the victims.*

In an emergency situation, it is best to remember to provide the type of care you are familiar with, and never try to do anything that is beyond your ability or training. Performing CPR incorrectly can further injure a person. Give basic first aid until the emergency medical team is able to respond and begin their care.

3 Name the two types of PPE that you should always have with you in case of an emergency.

There are many dangerous diseases that people may come into contact with when they respond to an emergency situation or a disaster. The best thing for all people to do is to make sure they have adequate protection in case they come upon an emergency. To do this you must gather the following and keep it with you at all times:

- two sets of gloves
- a **pocket mask** or barrier

A pocket mask is a small mask or barrier device that can protect you in situations where you give rescue breathing. Keep two sets of gloves in every vehicle you own, your purse or bag, or your pocket at all facilities. Look at the gloves periodically and check to see if they have dried out. Dried-out gloves may tear easily and should be replaced with new gloves. You should carry two sets in case one glove tears or if you have to replace your gloves with clean gloves. Some facilities have pocket masks and barriers available for purchase through a central supply department. There are places that sell tiny key chain sets with a pair of gloves and a barrier mask inside. This can be carried as a key chain or hung on a belt.

"Flying Ambulances"

Napoleon invaded Italy in 1796. During that invasion, Dominique Jean Larrey (1766-1842) developed "flying ambulances." These were horse-drawn vehicles that were able to quickly remove the wounded from the front lines for treatment. During the American Civil War, around 1863, "ambulance trains" similar to the legendary wagon trains of western lore appeared.

4 Identify the acronym that may be used when confronted with an emergency situation requiring first aid.

First aid may be necessary when you least expect it. Residents may require first aid inside or outside a facility. Some examples of potential first aid situations in facilities include:

A resident may:
- fall during a short trip in a van
- become injured at night when few staff are present to respond quickly
- choke on food, drink, or another object
- receive a serious wound
- get hit and lose a tooth
- have a diabetic emergency
- become poisoned due to eating something
- have a heart attack or a stroke
- be overcome with smoke or fumes

These situations could also happen to anyone. Performing first aid is something for which many people are not prepared. It is important to consider the steps to take in an emergency situation that requires first aid. If you ever have to perform first aid, try to remember the following acronym:

PPE SCC

PPE: Grab and apply **P**ersonal **P**rotective **E**quipment!

Safety first!

Call for help or point to person and say: "YOU, CALL 911 NOW!"

Care for victims.

As you are preparing to enter the emergency scene, take your glove/barrier kit or your gloves and pocket mask and look around you to make sure the area is safe. Make sure you are safe before providing necessary care. At the same time, if you have access to a phone, you can call 911 or point to someone and tell that person to call 911. If another person calls 911, have her return after making the call so that you know the call was placed. Finally, once you have your gloves on, you may provide care for the victims.

5 Explain the role of the nursing assistant on a facility code team.

When staff members are given their assignments at the beginning of the shift, some facilities also assign positions on the "code team." The **code team** is the team chosen for that shift to respond in case of a resident emergency. People assigned to the code team may be asked to obtain the "crash cart" or "code cart" or any other emergency equipment, such as a suction machine, CPR equipment, CPR clipboard, oxygen, or other items. Although nursing assistants will not do many of the code team procedures, such as giving medications, they may be asked to do chest compressions during CPR. If it is your facility policy to place nursing assistants on the code team, it is important to note whether you have been placed on the code team at the start of your shift. Should a code be called during your shift that day, you normally must respond from wherever you are within the facility. This means if you hear a code called while caring for a resident, it is your responsibility to get another person to take over the care so that you can respond to the code. You must make sure that the resident is secured before leaving the room to respond to the code. Follow your facility's policy regarding nursing assistants on code teams and the correct response when a code is called. Annual or periodic in-services may be held to update the correct response to codes in your facility.

Remove those roommates during a code!

When a code is called on a resident, it can be very difficult emotionally for staff members to deal with, in addition to residents and visitors. When a code occurs, the staff's primary concern is the survival of the victim. Sometimes, staff does not consider the impact of a code on the other people within a facility. It is a good idea for staff members who are not on the code team to be aware of all of the people closest to the code. Staff members can then move people to another area of the facility away from the emergency until the problem has been resolved.

Never leave a resident inside a room during a code or close to an area where a code is occurring. Remember, even a resident who seems to be unconscious may be aware of every event that is happening within a room or area. Unconscious residents need reassurance, too, during emergency situations.

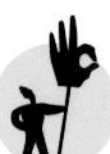

"Code Watchers"

As outlined on the previous page, when a code occurs, other residents, visitors, and even staff may become very emotional. It may be helpful for a charge nurse to establish a "Code Watcher" team to immediately respond to a code and deal only with the emotional concerns of residents, staff, and visitors. This team may be made up of different representatives from the facility. Because extra nursing staff may not be available, some examples of possible personnel who could be utilized are a member from pastoral care, if present in the facility, a social worker, any specially-trained volunteers, representatives from administration, and specially-trained unit clerks from the desk.

6 Describe a standard disaster response at a facility and explain the nursing assistant's role in disasters.

When any kind of a disaster occurs, it may be the responsibility of the staff members to return to the facility, if called in from home. When disasters occur, all available healthcare personnel should try to be available so that disaster victims receive proper care. Annual in-services and disaster drills are held at facilities so that staff may "practice" for a disaster ahead of time. Take advantage of these sessions and pay close attention to the instructions during the presentation.

When a local disaster is called, one of the first steps a facility takes is to activate the disaster call list. This is a list of all staff. You may someday be asked to contact staff members on the disaster call list. If you are placed in this position, remember to follow the rules of telephone etiquette found in Chapter 6. As you move down the list, check off the people that you have called so that you do not call a second time. When calling a large number of people, it is easy to lose your place on the list.

Emergency Disaster Kit — Box 13-1

Everyone should be prepared for the possibility of a disaster or emergency someday. Understanding the importance of having an emergency disaster kit is the first step in being prepared for any disaster. Following is a list of materials necessary for an emergency disaster kit that may last for at least three days. Disaster kits may vary from facility to facility, but here are some general items you may expect to see in a kit:

Food and water:

- Sealed water jugs (one gallon per person per day). Check and replace water every six months.
- Non-perishable food and a simple non-electric can opener
- Clothing and sleeping materials
- Clothing, rain gear, and shoes for each family member
- One blanket and one sleeping bag for each person

Safety Equipment:

- First aid kit
- Radio and flashlights for each person, extra batteries

Extra sets of:

- Regular medication (make sure all medication is carefully stored when around confused adults or children).
- Eyeglasses
- Car keys

Lists of:

- All doctors, dentists, and phone numbers
- Lists of all insurance agents, account and phone numbers
- Important family information such as allergies, medical conditions, medications, and medical devices that have been inserted inside the body of family members, like heart stents and pacemakers

Miscellaneous items:

- Portable equipment (cellular phones, pagers, and shortwave radio if your facility permits this)

7 Describe how to assess a person involved in a medical emergency.

The most serious medical emergencies involve one or more of the following:

- person is unconscious
- person is not breathing
- person has no pulse
- person is bleeding severely

To determine whether a person is conscious, tap the person and ask if she is all right. Speak loudly, and use the person's name if you know it. If the person does not respond, she is probably unconscious. Call for help right away, or send someone else to call for help. After calling for help or having someone else do it, return to the person and check for breathing, pulse, or severe bleeding, following these steps:

1. Check for breathing. Look for the chest to rise and fall, listen for sounds of breathing, and feel for the person's breath on your cheek.
2. Check the person's airway. Tilt the head back slightly to open the airway. See Figure 13-1. Check for breathing again. If the person still is not breathing, give two rescue breaths (rescue

breathing is discussed in the next learning objective) before checking the pulse. If the person is breathing, she also has a pulse.

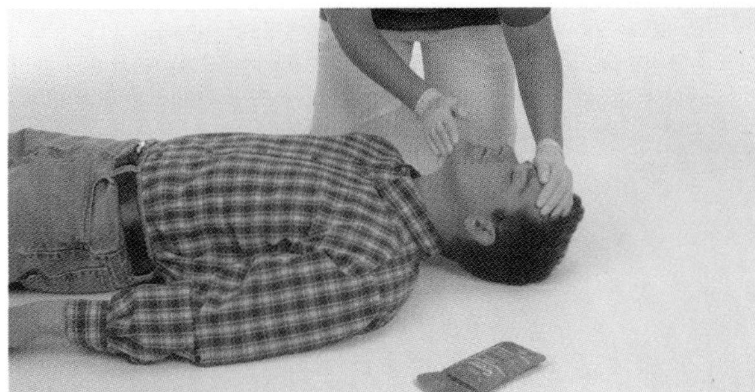

Figure 13-1. **Check the person's airway.**

3. Check for pulse by feeling the carotid artery in the neck. Determine if there is a pulse. If there is no pulse, make sure help is on its way. Initiate cardiopulmonary resuscitation (CPR) if you are trained and authorized to do so.

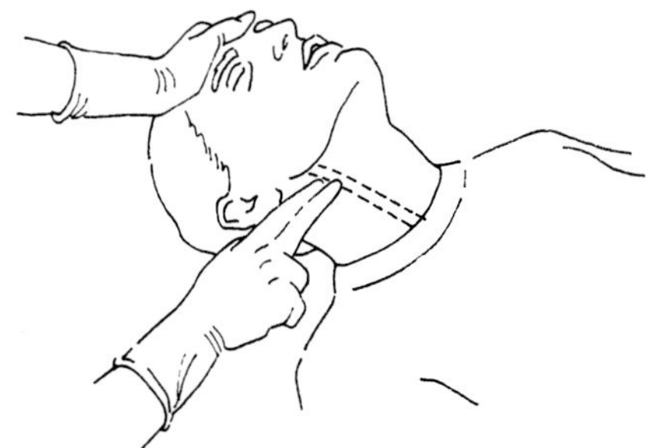

Figure 13-2. **Check the pulse by feeling the carotid artery in the neck.**

4. If the person has a pulse but is still not breathing, she may have inhaled or choked on something. If this has happened, the airway may be blocked, preventing breathing. Clearing an obstructed airway is discussed in the next learning objective.
5. Check for severe bleeding. Look up and down the person's body. If you see blood spurting or running from any part of the body, or if you see a significant amount of blood on the person's clothes or on the ground, make sure help is on its way and then take steps to control bleeding. Controlling bleeding is discussed in the next learning objective.

If a person is conscious and able to speak to you, she is breathing and has a pulse. Talk with the resident about what happened, and check the person for injury. Symptoms to look for include severe bleeding, changes in consciousness, irregular breathing, unusual color or feel to the skin, odd bumps or depressions on the body, medical alert tags, and anything the resident says is painful. If one of these conditions exists, you may need professional medical help. Follow your facility's policies about whom to call in different situations.

8 Identify the correct first aid procedures for each of these emergency situations:

- an obstructed airway in a child or adult
- shock
- bleeding
- poisoning
- burns
- fainting (syncope)
- nosebleed
- myocardial infarction or heart attack
- insulin shock and diabetic coma
- seizure
- CVA or stroke

FIRST AID — Box 13-2

Clearing an obstructed airway in an adult or child, performing the Heimlich maneuver, and rescue breathing

Residents who have difficulty chewing or swallowing, are confused, or have poor vision may be at risk of choking. An obstructed airway means the person cannot breathe normally because something is blocking the trachea, the tube through which air enters the lungs. When people are choking, they usually put their hands to their throats and cough. As long as the person can speak, cough, or breathe, do nothing. Encourage him to cough as forcefully as possible to get the object out. Stay with the person at all times, until he stops choking or can no longer speak, cough, or breathe.

If a person can no longer speak, cough, or breathe, you should call for help immediately, or have someone else do it. After calling for help return to the person. If he is still conscious, begin giving abdominal thrusts:

1. Ask the person if he is choking. You must make sure he needs help before starting abdominal thrusts. If the person needs help, continue.
2. Stand behind the person and wrap your arms around his waist.
3. With one hand, make a fist. Place the flat, thumb side of the fist against the person's mid-abdomen, slightly above the navel and below the breastbone, avoiding the **xiphoid**. See Figure 13-3.
4. Grasp the fist with your other hand and pull both hands toward you and up, quickly and forcefully.

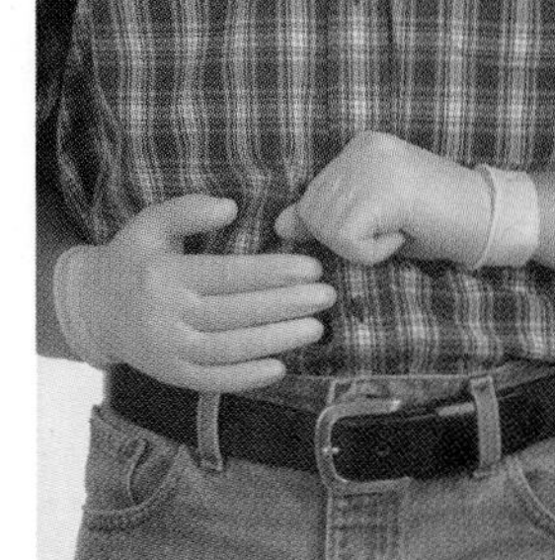

Figure 13-3.

5. Repeat until the object is expelled and removed, the airway

is cleared, and person breathes successfully on his own, or the person becomes responsive, or until help arrives.

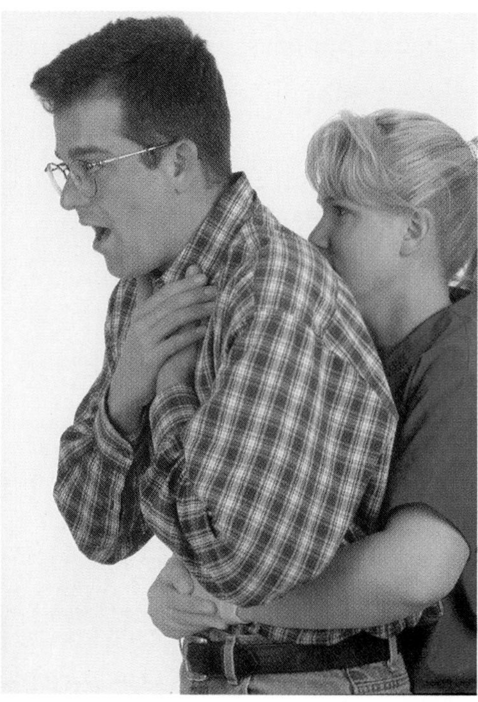

Figure 13-4. **A caregiver performing abdominal thrusts on a person in the upright position.**

If the person becomes unresponsive, help him or her to the floor gently into a supine position, or lying on the back with the face up. Make sure help is on its way. A person who has become unconscious while choking probably has a completely blocked airway. He needs professional medical help immediately. While you wait for help to arrive, stay with the person and check for breathing as you learned to earlier in this chapter.

If the person is not breathing and you are trained to perform rescue breathing, begin to do so immediately. To protect yourself from infectious diseases, you should use a face shield or mask when performing rescue breathing. To perform rescue breathing, follow these guidelines:

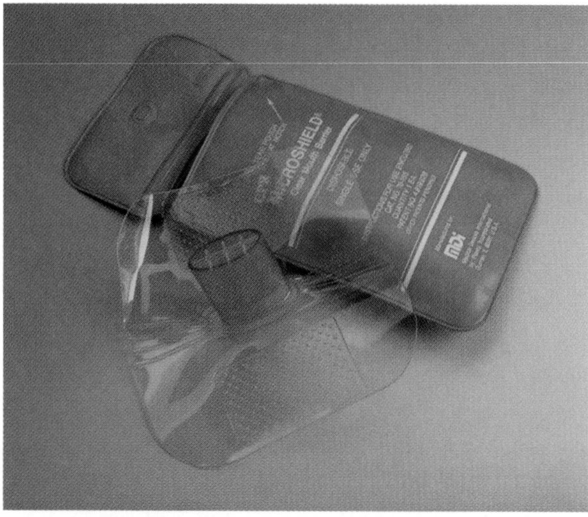

Figure 13-5. **Face shields or face masks protect your and the person you are helping from contact with body fluids.**

6. Keep airway open. Pinch the person's nose tightly closed with your thumb and index finger. Take a deep breath. Form an airtight seal with the face mask, shield, or your mouth over his mouth.

7. Breathe slowly into the face mask, shield, or the person's mouth for about 2 seconds, watching for the chest to rise. If the chest rises, air is going in. Continue following these steps. If the chest does not rise, air is not getting in the person's lungs. Skip to step 11 below.

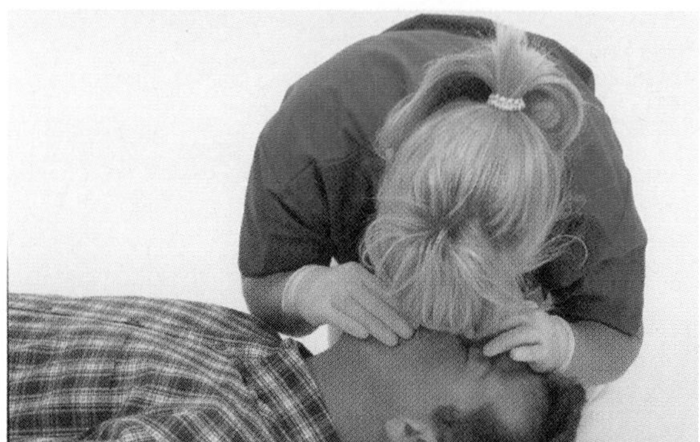

Figure 13-6. **Breathe slowly into the face mask, shield, or person's mouth, watching for the chest to rise. If the chest rises, air is going in.**

8. Pause to let the air come back out, then give another breath.

9. Check for a pulse.

10. If a pulse is present but the person still is not breathing, give a slow breath about every 5 seconds, with each breath lasting about 2 seconds. Check for pulse once a minute until the person starts breathing on his own or help arrives. If at any time no pulse is present, begin CPR if you are trained to do so, or wait for help to arrive.

If your breath will not go into the person's lungs, you need to check the person's airway and try to remove any obstructions.

11. Open airway and do a finger sweep. Look in the mouth for any foreign objects. If you see an object, carefully remove it using your finger. Reach in with your finger and sweep the object forward, out of the person's mouth. (Figure 13-7) Never place fingers inside the mouth of a person who is having a seizure.

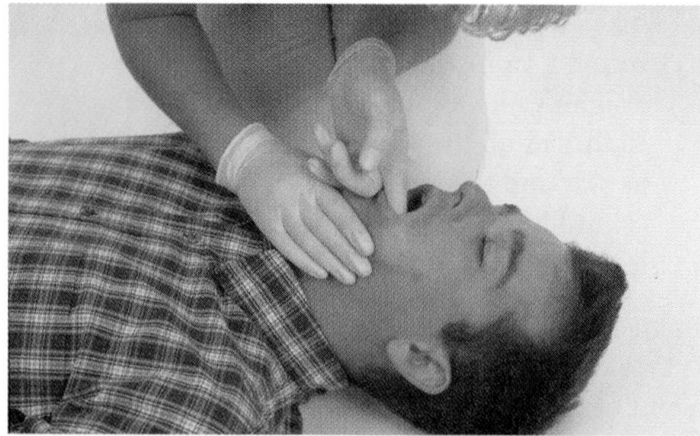

Figure 13-7.

If unable to see object, open the airway using head tilt, chin lift or jaw thrust if you suspect a head, neck, back, or spinal injury.

12. If chest still does not rise, with person still supine, straddle the person's thighs, facing his head, and give up to 5 quick inward and upward abdominal thrusts. Place heel of one hand on abdomen, slightly above navel and below breastbone, avoiding the xiphoid.
13. Interlace the fingers of both hands.
14. Using both hands, press quickly and forcefully into abdomen, using inward and upward thrusts in middle of the abdomen. Avoid pressing into left or right side of abdomen. Repeat up to five times. If the person vomits, roll him as a unit (in case of head, neck, back, or spinal injury) onto his side. Clear the vomit from his mouth, and resume abdominal thrusts.
15. Repeat steps 6 to 14 until the object is expelled and removed, the airway is cleared, and person breathes successfully on his own, or the person becomes responsive, or until help arrives. If person breathes successfully and has no suspected head, neck, back, or spinal injury, carefully turn to one side into recovery position. Keep airway open, and monitor closely until help arrives.

For a child who is choking, follow the same basic procedure as for an adult, with the following changes:

- Stand or kneel behind child and wrap your arms around child's chest directly underneath child's axilla (underarm).
- If the child is small enough and there are no head, neck, or spine injuries, you can carry her to the phone and continue to give first aid while calling for help.
- The force of abdominal thrusts should be adjusted for the child's size.
- If you must give rescue breathing, give one breath every 3 seconds instead of every 5 seconds.

For an infant who is choking, you will need to give back blows and chest thrusts:

1. Sit or kneel with infant on her stomach on your lap. Hold face down with infant's head slightly lower than chest, supporting head by firmly supporting the jaw. Do not press on an infant's throat. Rest your forearm on your thigh to support infant.
2. Using heel of one hand, give 5 back blows forcefully in the middle of the back between infant's shoulder blades.
3. After 5 back blows, place your free hand on infant's back, supporting the back of the head with the palm of your hand.
4. Turn infant as a unit while carefully supporting her head and neck. Hold infant in supine position with forearm resting on your thigh. Keep infant's head lower than trunk.
5. Place 2 or 3 fingers on lower third of sternum, about one finger's width below nipple line. Give 5 quick downward chest thrusts. Give one chest thrust per second.
6. Repeat steps 1 thru 5 until object is expelled and removed, the airway is cleared, and the infant breathing successfully on her own, or the infant becomes unresponsive, or until help arrives.
7. If infant becomes unresponsive, get a second person to call 911.

If infant becomes unresponsive:

8. Lie infant on back.
9. Open airway. If you see an object, carefully remove it using finger sweep. Do not do a finger sweep if you are unable to see an object. Do not place fingers inside mouth of infant having a seizure.
10. If unable to see the object, open airway using head tilt, chin lift or jaw thrust if you suspect head, neck, back or spinal injury.
11. Attempt rescue breathing giving two slow, shallow (small) rescue breaths. Each breath should last about 1.5 seconds. If chest does not rise, reopen airway by repositioning head and chin and give two more slow rescue breaths.
12. If chest does not rise, complete a series of up to 5 back blows and up to 5 chest thrusts.
13. Repeat steps starting with infant lying on her back until the object is expelled and removed, the airway is cleared, and infant breathes successfully on her own for about one minute, or the infant becomes responsive, or until help arrives. If infant breathes successfully on her own for about one minute, and she has no suspected head, neck, back, or spinal injury, carefully turn to one side into recovery position. Keep airway open and monitor closely until help arrives.

FIRST AID — Box 13-3

Shock

Shock occurs when organs and tissues in the body do not receive an adequate blood supply. Bleeding, heart attack, severe infection, and conditions that cause the blood pressure to fall can lead to shock. Shock can become worse when the person is extremely frightened or in severe pain.

Shock is a dangerous, life-threatening situation. Signs of shock include pale or cyanotic skin, staring, increased pulse and respiration rates, decreased blood pressure, and extreme thirst. Always call for emergency help if you suspect a person is experiencing shock. To prevent or treat shock, do the following:

1. Have the person lie down in a supine position. If the person is bleeding from the mouth or vomiting, place her on her side unless you suspect a head, neck, back, or spinal injury.

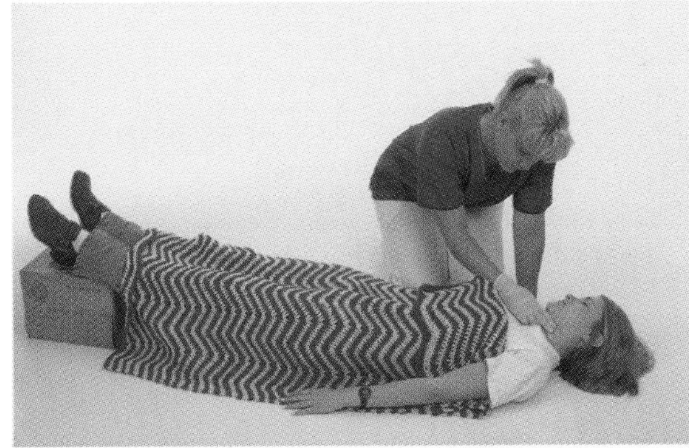

Figure 13-8. **If a person appears to be in shock, keep her as quiet as possible, with her legs elevated about 12 inches.**

2. Control bleeding. Box 13-4 describes how to do this.
3. Check pulse and respirations if possible. You will learn how to do this in Chapter 16.
4. Keep the person as calm and comfortable as possible.
5. Maintain normal body temperature. If the weather is cold, place a blanket around the person. If the weather is hot, provide shade.
6. If no head, neck, abdominal, or back injuries or breathing difficulties exist, you may place in the shock position with feet elevated about 12 inches (Figure 13-8). If unsure, leave flat on back. Lower person's feet if breathing becomes difficult. Elevate the head and shoulders if a head wound or breathing difficulties are present. Never elevate a body part if a broken bone exists.
7. Do not give the person anything to eat or drink.
8. Call for emergency help. Victims of shock should always receive medical care as soon as possible.

FIRST AID — Box 13-4

Controlling Bleeding

Severe bleeding can cause death quickly and must be controlled. Call for help immediately, then follow these steps to control bleeding:

1. Put on gloves.
2. Hold a thick sterile pad, a clean pad, or a clean cloth such as a handkerchief, towel, or clean sanitary napkin against the wound. Have the injured person use his bare hand until you can get a clean pad. Also have the resident hold the pad if he is able until you can put on gloves.
3. Press down hard directly on the bleeding wound until help arrives. Do not decrease pressure. Put additional pads over the first pad if blood seeps through. Do not remove the first pad.

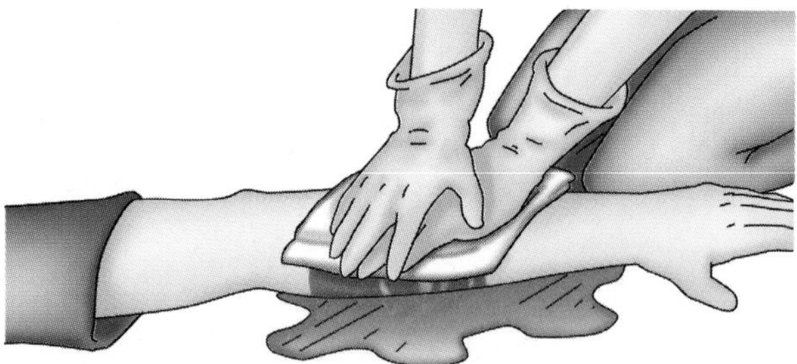

Figure 13-9.

4. Raise the wound above the heart to slow down the bleeding. If the wound is on an arm, leg, hand, or foot, and there are no broken bones, prop up the limb on towels, blankets, coats, or other absorbent material.
5. If you cannot stop excessive bleeding, pressure points can be used as a last resort. Press the artery against the bone just above the wound. Do not use a pressure point for more than five minutes.

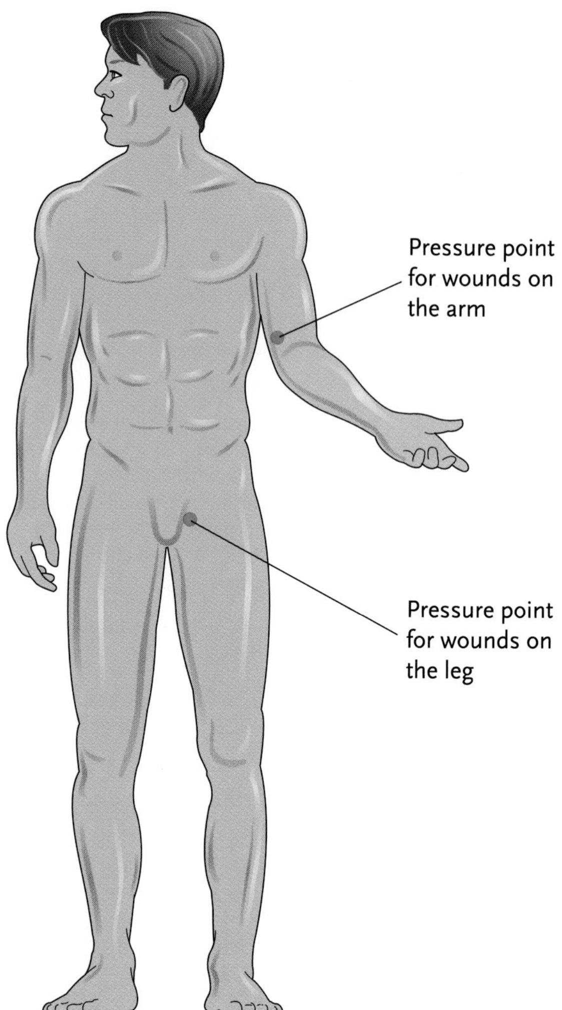

Figure 13-10. **Pressure points can be used if you are unable to control bleeding with direct pressure on the wound.**

6. When bleeding is under control, secure the dressing to keep it in place and check the person for symptoms of shock (pale skin, increased pulse and respiration rates, decreased blood pressure, and extreme thirst). Stay with the person until medical help arrives.
7. Wash hands thoroughly when finished.

FIRST AID — Box 13-5

Poisoning

Always have the Poison Control Center phone number available. Suspect poisoning when a resident suddenly collapses, vomits, and has heavy, labored breathing. If you suspect poisoning, take the following steps:

1. Call the local or state Poison Control Center immediately. Follow instructions from poison control.
2. Look for a container that will help you determine what the client has taken or eaten. Check the mouth for chemical burns and note the breath odor.
3. Notify your supervisor.

FIRST AID — Box 13-6

Burns

The severity of a burn depends on its depth, size, and location. There are three types of burns: 1st, 2nd, and 3rd degree. You will learn more about burns in Chapter 24.

Call for emergency help in any of the following situations:

- An infant or child, or an elderly, ill or weak person has been burned, unless burn is very minor.
- The burn occurs on the head, neck, hands, feet, face, or genitals, or burns cover more than one body part.
- Person who has been burned is having trouble breathing.
- The burn was caused by chemicals, electricity, or explosion.

To treat a minor burn:

1. Use cool, clean water (not ice) to decrease the skin temperature and prevent further injury. Ice will cause further skin damage. Dampen a clean cloth and place it over the burn See Figure 13-11.

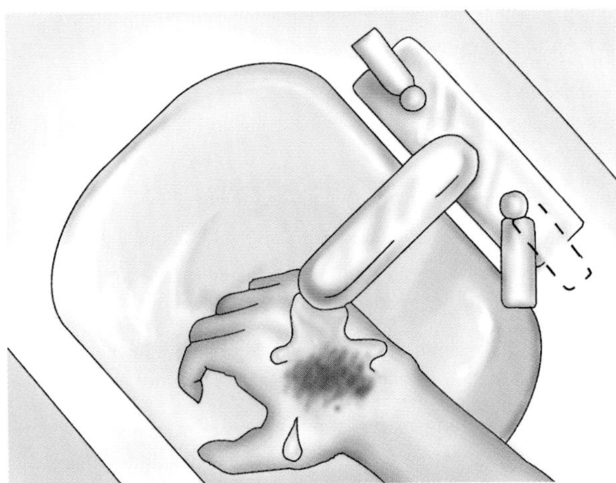

Figure 13-11.

2. Once the pain has eased, you may cover the area with a dry, sterile gauze.
3. Never use any kind of ointment, salve, or grease on a burn.

For more serious burns:

1. Remove the person from the source of the burn. If clothing has caught fire, smother it with a blanket or towel to extinguish flames or STOP, DROP and ROLL. Stop any burning with cool (not icy) water. Protect yourself from the source of the burn.
2. Check for breathing, pulse, and severe bleeding.
3. Call for emergency help.
4. Remove as much of the person's clothing around the burned area as possible, but do not try to pull away clothing that sticks to the burn. Cover the burn with a thick, dry, sterile gauze if available, or a clean cloth. A dry, insulated cool pack may be used over the dressing. Again, never use any kind of ointment, salve, or grease on a burn.
5. Ask the person to lie down and elevate the affected part if this does not cause greater pain.
6. If the burn covers a larger area, wrap the person or the extremity in several thicknesses of a dry, clean sheet and apply a cool compress if possible. Take care not to rub the skin or break any blisters.
7. Wait for emergency medical help.

FIRST AID — Box 13-7

Fainting (Syncope)

Fainting occurs when the blood supply to the brain suddenly becomes insufficient, resulting in a sudden loss of consciousness. Fainting may be the result of hunger, fear, pain, fatigue, standing for a long time, poor ventilation, or overheating.

Signs and symptoms of fainting include dizziness, perspiration, pale skin, weak pulse, shallow respirations, and blackness in the visual field. If someone appears likely to faint, follow these steps:

1. Have the person lie down or sit down before fainting occurs.
2. If the person is in a sitting position, have her bend forward and place her head between her knees. If the person is in a supine position, elevate the legs. See Figure 13-12.

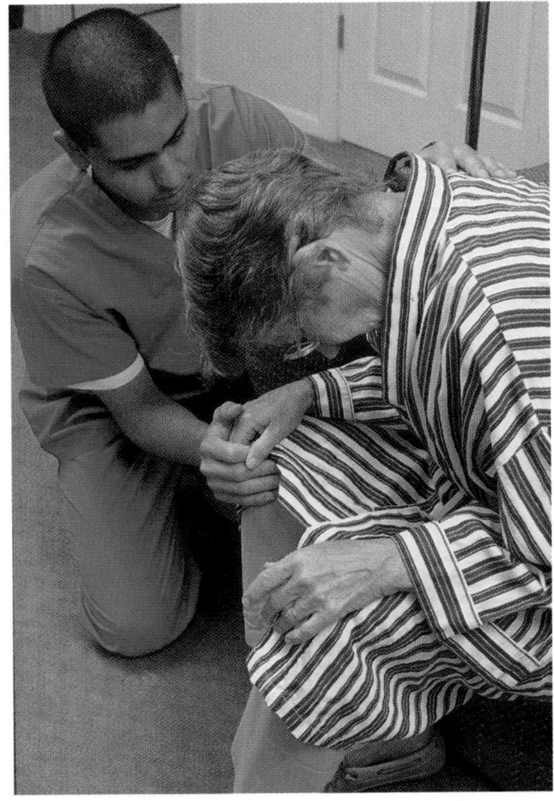

Figure 13-12.

3. Loosen any tight clothing.
4. Have the person stay in position for at least five minutes after symptoms disappear.

5. Help the person get up slowly and continue to observe her for symptoms of fainting.

6. Report the incident to the nurse.

If a person does faint, lower her to the floor or other flat surface and position her on her back. If she has no head, neck, back or spinal injury, place in the shock position with feet and legs elevated 12 inches. If unsure, leave flat on back. Loosen any tight clothing. Check to make sure the person is breathing. She should recover quickly, but keep her lying down for several minutes. Report the incident to the nurse immediately. Fainting may be a sign of a more serious medical condition.

FIRST AID — Box 13-8

Nosebleed

A nosebleed can occur spontaneously, when the air is dry, or when injury has occurred. If a resident has a nosebleed, take the following steps:

1. Elevate the head of the bed or tell the resident to remain upright. Offer tissues or a clean cloth to catch the blood. Do not touch blood or bloody clothes, tissues or cloths without gloves.

2. If the resident is able, have her apply firm pressure over the bridge of the nose by squeezing the bridge of the nose with her thumb and forefinger. If the resident is unable to do this, you must perform this step. Put on gloves first! (Figure 13-13)

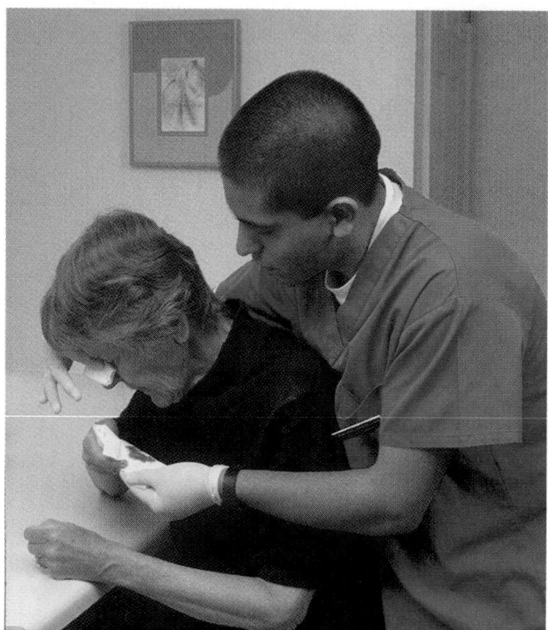

Figure 13-13.

3. The pressure must be applied consistently until the bleeding stops.

4. Use a cool cloth or ice wrapped in a cloth on the back of the neck, the forehead, or the upper lip to slow the flow of blood. Never apply ice directly to skin.

5. If this does not stop the bleeding, get help. Keep person still and calm until help arrives.

FIRST AID — Box 13-9

Myocardial Infarction or Heart Attack

When blood flow to the heart muscle is completely blocked, oxygen and important nutrients fail to reach the cells in that region. Waste products are not removed and the muscle cell dies. This is called a myocardial infarction (MI) or heart attack. The area of dead tissue may be large or small, depending on the artery involved. See Chapter 28 for more information.

A myocardial infarction is an emergency that can result in serious heart damage or death. The following are signs and symptoms of MI:

- sudden, severe pain in the chest, usually on the left side or in the center behind the sternum
- a feeling of indigestion or heartburn
- nausea and vomiting
- dyspnea (DISP-nee-a) or difficulty breathing
- dizziness
- discoloration of the skin; it may be pale, gray, or cyanotic
- perspiration
- cold and clammy skin
- weak and irregular pulse rate
- low blood pressure
- anxiety and a sense of impending doom
- denial

You must take immediate action if a resident experiences any of these symptoms. Follow these steps:

1. Place the resident in a comfortable position. Encourage him to rest, and reassure him that you will not leave him.

2. Loosen clothing around the neck.

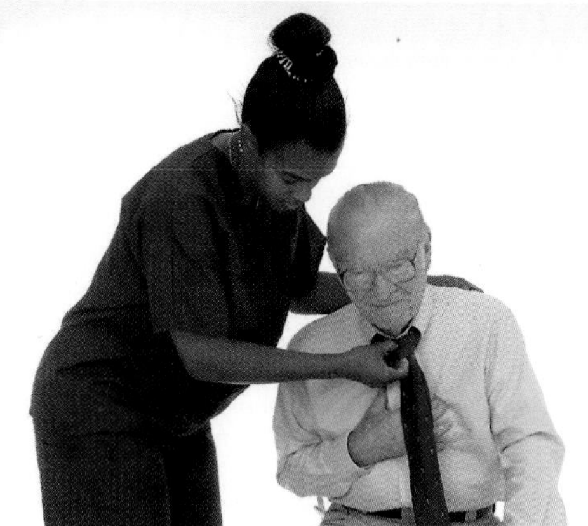

Figure 13-14.

3. Call or have someone call emergency services.

4. Do not give the resident liquids or food.

5. If the resident takes heart medication, such as nitroglycerin, find the medication and offer it to the resident. Never place medication in someone's mouth.

6. Monitor the resident's breathing and pulse. If the resident stops breathing or has no pulse, perform rescue breathing or CPR if you are trained to do so.
7. Once help has arrived, notify the nurse.

FIRST AID Box 13-10

Insulin Shock and Diabetic Coma

Insulin shock and diabetic coma are complications of diabetes that can be life-threatening. Much more information on diabetes can be found in Chapter 33. Insulin shock, or hypoglycemia, can result from either too much insulin or too little food. It frequently occurs when a dose of insulin is administered and the person with the illness skips a meal or does not eat all the food required. Even when a regular amount of food is eaten, excessive physical activity may rapidly metabolize the food so that the amount of insulin in the body is excessive. Vomiting and diarrhea may also lead to insulin shock in people with diabetes.

The first signs of insulin shock include feeling weak or different, nervousness, dizziness, and perspiration (see list below for further signs). These are signals that the resident needs food in a form that can be rapidly absorbed. A lump of sugar, a hard candy, or a glass of orange juice should be consumed right away. The resident who is diabetic should always have a quick source of sugar handy. Contact the nurse if the resident has shown early signs of insulin shock.

The following are signs and symptoms of insulin shock:

- hunger
- weakness
- rapid pulse
- headache
- low blood pressure
- perspiration
- cold, clammy skin
- confusion
- trembling
- nervousness
- blurred vision
- numbness of the lips and tongue
- unconsciousness

Diabetic coma, also known as acidosis or hyperglycemia, is caused by having too little insulin. It can result from undiagnosed diabetes, going without insulin or not taking enough, eating too much food, not getting enough exercise, and physical or emotional stress.

The signs of diabetic coma include increased thirst or urination, abdominal pain, deep or labored breathing, and breath that smells sweet or fruity (see complete list of symptoms at right). Notify the nurse immediately if you suspect your resident is experiencing a diabetic coma.

Other signs and symptoms of diabetic coma include:

- hunger
- weakness
- rapid, weak pulse
- headache
- low blood pressure
- dry skin
- flushed cheeks
- drowsiness
- slow, deep, and labored breathing
- nausea and vomiting
- abdominal pain
- sweet, fruity breath odor
- air hunger, or person gasping for air and being unable to catch his breath
- unconsciousness

FIRST AID Box 13-11

Seizures

Seizures or convulsions are involuntary, often violent, contractions of muscles. They can involve a small area or the entire body. Seizures are caused by an abnormality in the brain. They can occur in young children who have a high fever. Older children and adults who have a serious illness, fever, head injury, or epilepsy may also have convulsions.

The primary goal of a caregiver during a seizure is to make sure the resident is safe. During a seizure, a person may shake severely, thrust arms and legs uncontrollably, clench his jaw, drool, and be unable to swallow. The following emergency measures should be taken if a client has a seizure:

1. Lower the person to the floor.
2. Have someone call for emergency medical help if needed. Do not leave the person during the seizure unless you must do so to get medical help. Note the time.
3. During seizure, turn head or entire body to left side, especially if person is vomiting or drooling, and cradle and protect head by placing a blanket or folded linen under head until seizure ends.
4. Move furniture away to prevent injury.
5. Do not try to stop the seizure or hold the person down in any way.
6. Do not force anything between the person's teeth and do not place your hands in the person's mouth for any reason. You could be severely bitten.
7. Do not give liquids or food.
8. When the seizure is over, check breathing. Note the time.
9. Call the nurse. Report the length of the convulsion and your observations.

FIRST AID Fig 13-12

CVA or Stroke

A cerebrovascular accident (CVA), or stroke, is caused when blood supply to the brain is suddenly cut off by a clot or a ruptured blood vessel. A stroke may be preceded by symptoms that signal the oncoming **hemorrhage** or blockage. These symptoms may include dizziness, ringing in the ears, headache, nausea, vomiting, slurring of words, and loss of memory. These symptoms should be reported immediately.

A transient ischemic attack, or TIA, is a warning sign of a CVA. It is the result of a temporary lack of oxygen in the brain and may last several days, weeks, or months. Symptoms include tingling, weakness, or some loss of movement in an extremity. These symptoms should not be ignored. Report any of these symptoms to the nurse immediately. More information on CVAs and TIAs can be found in Chapter 27.

Signs that a stroke is occurring include any of the following:

- loss of consciousness
- redness in the face
- noisy breathing
- seizures
- loss of bowel and bladder control
- **hemiplegia**
- **aphasia**
- use of inappropriate words
- elevated blood pressure
- slow pulse rate

The AED: Coming to a Home or Store Near You

Automated external defibrillators, or AEDs, are everywhere, from airplanes to your local discount store. Training in the use of portable defibrillators is being given to flight attendants and employees of local department stores and offices. The cost of these devices is falling rapidly and may soon be low enough for the average person to purchase one. The device may be about the size of your toaster. An electric shock is used to bring back a normal heartbeat when the heart suddenly stops. A clear computerized voice inside the defibrillator takes the user through each step. Many agencies have added AED training to their CPR courses. Studies are being done to determine whether the overall survival rate is better using the AED or CPR alone. Keep current on the use of the AED by reading your local newspaper, keeping your CPR certification current, and attending any AED in-services that might be held at your facility. AEDs may become so common that many families will have one in their home. If you choose to have one in your home, make sure that every person in your home is completely trained in the use of the AED. Someday, even your youngest family member could save a life.

Summary

Emergencies are times when the inner strength of a person can be tested. In order to deal effectively with any possible emergency, you must simply arm yourself with the following:

- The safety equipment you may need
- The first steps to take
- The correct knowledge of first aid to use when dealing with each emergency

Keeping up-to-date on your CPR certification and obtaining a first aid certificate may help you feel more prepared for anything that happens; you may have the chance to save a person's life someday.

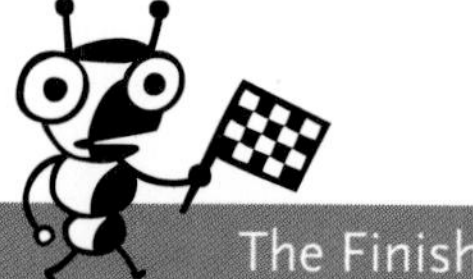

The Finish Line

What's Wrong With This Picture?

All of the specific items under each category are missing for the emergency disaster kit. List the missing items.

Food and water:
Extra sets of:
Lists of:
Miscellaneous items:

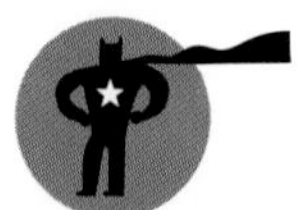

Star Student Central

1. Contact your local fire department or rescue squad, and identify yourself as a nursing assistant student. Ask whether you may set up a time to talk to members of the department or squad for a brief period of time to ask for tips on dealing with emergencies.

2 Put together an emergency disaster kit for your home. This should include items from this chapter. Store smaller items on the list in an easy-to-carry bag like a backpack.

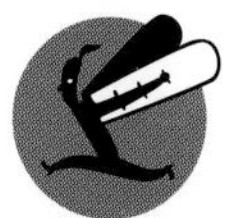

You Can Do It Corner!

1. List the acronym identified to help you in an emergency situation. What does each letter mean? (LO 4)
2. What is the difference between a respiratory and cardiac arrest? (LO 2)
3. List two types of PPE you should always have with you in case of an emergency. (LO 3)
4. What is one of the first steps a facility takes in a disaster? (LO 6)
5. What are the steps you should take in a medical emergency after calling for help? (LO 7)
6. What types of things may people on a code team be asked to obtain? (LO 5)
7. What are two things you must never do during a seizure? (LO 8)
8. If a person faints and has no head, neck, back, or spinal injury, in what position should she be placed? (LO 8)
9. List the signs and symptoms of each of the following: MI, insulin shock, diabetic coma, and CVA. (LO 8)
10. What position should a person be placed if he is in shock? (LO 8)
11. What is the first step to take if you suspect a resident has been poisoned? (LO 8)
12. Before turning an adult who is choking into the recovery position, what has to happen? (LO 8)
13. Where may you apply a cool cloth to stop the flow of blood during a nosebleed? (LO 8)
14. How should the wound be positioned when a person is bleeding? (LO 8)
15. What should never be applied to a burn? (LO 8)

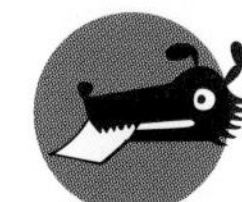

Star Student's Chapter Checklist

1. I have read my textbook chapter.
2. I have reviewed my own "Pocketful of Terms."
3. I have listened to my tutor tape.
4. I have reviewed and highlighted my class notes.
5. I have read and completed any handouts from this chapter.
6. I have completed "The Finish Line."
7. Star Time! Choose your reward!

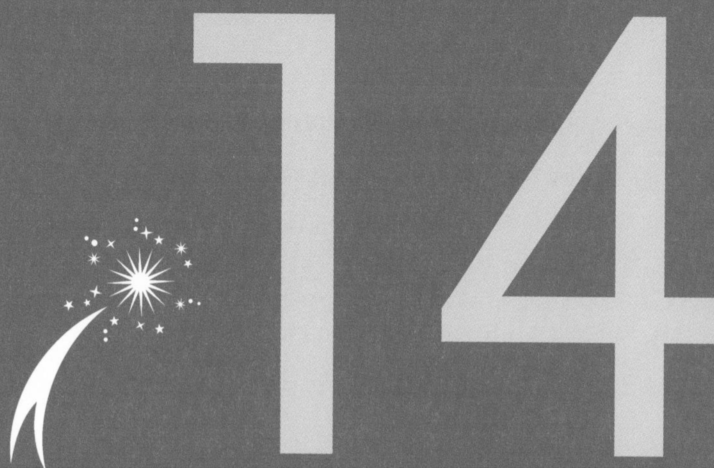

14

Your Responsibilities: Admission, Transfer, Discharge, and Physical Exams

Look Like a Star!

Look at the Learning Objectives and The Finish Line before you begin reading this chapter.

Look at your pocket calendar. With your pencil, put a bracket ( ) around a study period every single day.

Look at your homework for this chapter. Plug each piece of homework into a certain time slot.

Look at the Star Student's Chapter Checklist at the end of this chapter. Check off each item as it is completed.

"Where we love is home, Home that our feet may leave, but not our hearts."

Oliver Wendell Holmes, 1809-1894

"The best thing we can do is to make wherever we're in look as much like home as we can."

Christopher Fry, 1907-present

Learning Objectives

1. **Spell and define all STAR words.**
2. **List fourteen questions family members may ask when choosing a facility.**
3. **Explain the nursing assistant's role in the emotional adjustment of a new resident.**
4. **Describe the role of the nursing assistant during the admission process.**
5. **Describe six nursing assistant responsibilities during a physical exam.**
6. **Demonstrate eight bed positions and discuss the Trendelenburg and Reverse Trendelenburg positions.**
7. **Explain the nursing assistant's responsibilities during the in-house transfer of a resident.**
8. **Explain the nursing assistant's role in discharge planning.**
9. **Describe the nursing assistant's role in discharge of a resident.**
10. **Explain the proper response if a resident wants to leave the facility against medical advice (AMA).**

Successfully perform these Practical Procedures

Admitting a Resident to a Facility

Measuring Height and Weight on an Upright Scale

Measuring Weight on a Wheelchair Scale

Measuring Weight of a Bedridden Resident

Measuring Height of a Bedridden Resident

Measuring Abdominal Girth

Measuring Thigh, Calf, and Inseam for Special Stockings

Assisting with the Physical Exam

Transferring a Resident

Discharging a Resident

"A Walk Through a Ward of the Eighteenth Century"

by Grace Goldin

The old ward of St. John's Hospital, Bruges, housed patients continuously from the 12th century, when its first section was built, until the 20th. . . .A division was customary in medieval times. . . forming two wards side by side with separate entrances; or two wards built one above the other to separate the sexes. . . .The . . . hospital of the 18th century was a dangerous place, mortality there was higher than among patients nursed at home, and therefore it catered only to wretches with no alternative; but among these, many got better. The bonneted beldame at the rear of the center aisle, being shown out the door with a pat on the shoulder, is very likely being discharged "cured."

1 Spell and define all STAR words.

abdominal girth: a measurement of the circumference around the abdomen at the umbilicus (navel).

admission: first entry of a resident into a facility or unit.

admission pack: personal care items supplied upon admission.

AMA: against medical advice.

baseline: initial value that can be compared to future measurements.

bedridden: confined to bed.

discharge: when a resident leaves a facility or unit.

dorsal recumbent: position with resident flat on back with knees flexed and slightly separated; feet are flat on bed.

Fowler's: positioned on back with the head of bed (HOB) elevated about 60 degrees.

kilogram: 1000 grams; 1 kilogram = 2.2 pounds.

knee-chest: position with the resident on abdomen with knees pulled up towards the abdomen and with legs separated; arms are pulled up and flexed to either side the head; the head is turned to one side.

lateral: position with a resident lying on his or her side.

lithotomy: position with the resident on the back with legs flexed and feet placed in the stirrups.

metric: system of weights and measures based upon the meter.

pound: measurement of weight equal to 16 ounces.

prone: position with a resident lying on the abdomen with legs extended and arms flexed.

Reverse Trendelenburg: position with the resident on the back with the head of the bed (HOB) up and the foot of the bed (FOB) lowered or down.

Sims': position with the resident on the left side with the right knee bent toward the chest.

supine: position with the resident on the back with the face upward.

transfer: moving a resident from one location to another within the organization.

Trendelenburg: position with the resident on the back with the head of the bed (HOB) down and the foot of the bed (FOB) up.

2 List fourteen questions family members may ask when choosing a facility.

Choosing a warm and secure facility for a family member is a challenging process. One of the first steps in the process is to personally visit each facility unannounced and take a tour of the facility. This means family members visit more than once to make an assessment of the facility. Sometimes one visit gives a family a great deal of important information. For example, if there is a strong smell of urine in the facility during a visit, they may not even return a second time to make sure it was not an isolated incident. If they do visit again and the smell is still present, they may look carefully at other options before returning.

Some questions families may ask themselves, as well as staff members, during a visit to a facility include the following:

- Does the staff seem courteous and friendly?
- Does most of the staff speak enough of the resident's native language so that the resident can easily understand them?
- Is the facility adequately staffed? What is the ratio of nurses and nursing assistants to residents?
- Is there a strong smell of urine or other foul odors in the facility?
- What is the food like at the facility?
- Are the residents up and dressed early in the morning and ready to "meet the day?"
- Do the staff interact with residents in a positive way?
- Do residents look groomed, taken care of, and happy?
- Is the facility licensed?
- How has it done on previous inspections?
- Does the facility provide assistance with Activities of Daily Living (ADLs)? If so, how are they provided and what are the associated fees?
- Does the facility provide the level of care the resident needs? What about future needs?
- Is the environment safe, functional, and homelike?
- What are the "move-out" criteria?

These are only some of the things families watch for when choosing a facility for a loved one.

3 Explain the nursing assistant's role in the emotional adjustment of a new resident.

New residents to a facility may have been independent for a long time or may be moving from a family member's home. Either way, there is a tremendous emotional adjustment to be made when moving belongings into an unfamiliar place full of strangers. The difference between a smooth transition into a facility and a "bumpy" one may very well be YOU. You, the person on the front-line of care, will be the team member most involved with the resident.

Think about some of the life-altering changes residents have had to make. The move into a long-term care facility may have been a sudden event due to health reasons. They may have had to sell their home, vehicles, and other personal belongings. They also may have had to get rid of a beloved pet. Because of all these things, they may be experiencing fear, loss, and uncertainty, along with a decline in health and independence.

When nursing assistants fully understand some of the massive changes new residents may be going through, they can have more empathy for residents. This understanding will help you provide compassionate care. Your residents will need it during those early days and weeks in their new home.

In order to learn how to assist residents emotionally during their transition to a facility, first, we will review the acronym **CATCH ME UP**.

CATCH ME UP

Communication skills and **C**ommon sense.

Attitude of a STAR!

Tact dealing with others.

Confidentiality with resident and staff information.

Honest and trustworthy "to a fault."

Managing mistakes responsibly.

Empathy for resident and staff problems.

Understanding and caring toward everyone.

Patience.

On The Star Path To Success!

Your ability to help the new resident adjust to new surroundings will depend upon a few important things found in this acronym. Communication will be of primary importance to the resident's early adjustment to the new home. A simple reminder to the resident of the correct meal times helps the resident feel more connected.

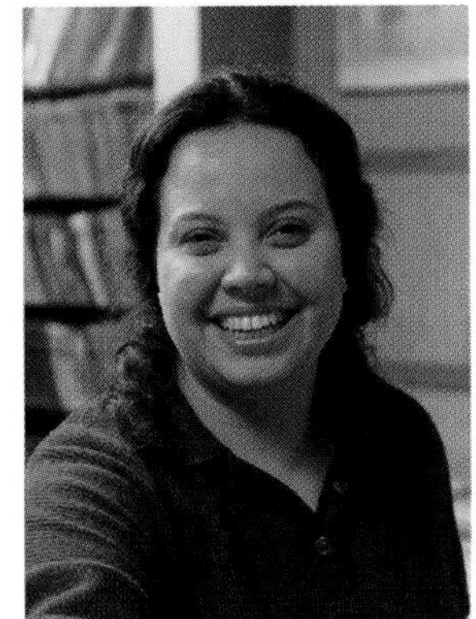

Figure 14-1. **It is important to have a good attitude when working in a long-term care facility.**

Attitude is everything! A new resident will be uncomfortable around a nursing assistant with a negative attitude. Everyone has a bad day now and then. However, the bad days should not be every day. People want to be near nice, pleasant people. Don't you? Residents want to feel comfortable around the staff that provides their care. Residents should never feel as though they are a burden to the nursing assistant or that the team member is doing them a favor by providing care.

The ability to be tactful, especially with a new resident, is very important. Residents do not want to be offended or have their feelings hurt by anyone, especially the person responsible for their care.

New residents want their personal information protected and kept confidential. Remember, a new resident who has always lived in a private home may never have had personal information passed on to large groups of people. Think for a moment about the number of people within a facility who have access to personal information about the new resident. This may be very unsettling for the resident. It is important never to pass along any confidential information or to speak about a resident in the hallways, elevators, restrooms, locker rooms, parking lots, or lunch- or breakrooms.

New residents may be very frightened of their new surroundings. They may feel afraid of everyone and be very protective of their belongings. Remember to be respectful of residents' belongings and their feelings of apprehension. Showing honesty and trustworthiness right from the start will help make the feelings of fear and mistrust disappear.

If you make a mistake involving resident care during the early days or weeks of the resident's stay, assume responsibility and report this to your immediate supervisor. People respect and trust you more when you admit mistakes. It's also important to keep your word. Forgetting if you promised to visit or read a resident's mail should also be admitted. When you tell residents you are coming, they will look for you. If you forget, apologize to the resident and reschedule the visit as soon as possible.

The ability to empathize with a new resident is important. Residents can experience great loss upon entering a long-term care facility. They may be dealing with the loss of health, mobility, independence, family, friends, pets, plants, and personal possessions. Imagine it was you having to give up your dog, cat, or bird. What about your friends? Will they ever come to see you? Are they able to come to see you? Think about this whenever a new resident gets teary-eyed. She may be thinking about a lost pet or friend. Families or friends are experiencing a loss too. They may also need to express their feelings. Make time to listen.

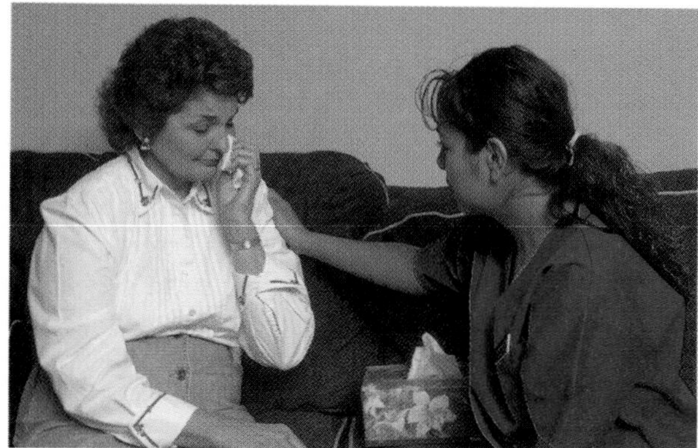

Figure 14-2. **Listening to residents and their families and friends is sometimes the best way to provide emotional support.**

Understanding a resident's feelings about a move into a facility is also very important. For example, if a resident seems to genuinely want to be alone instead of joining other residents for a special activity, a nursing assistant might say, "Maybe next time," and allow him his privacy. Privacy is important, especially when residents are first admitted. They may be used to being very independent. They have the right to freedom of choice, and if they choose to be alone, staff have to honor this decision as long as residents are safe. Once the resident has adjusted a bit, the nursing assistant might encourage the resident to join in more often.

Kindness and patience are priceless qualities. The new resident might have a good day followed by a not-so-good day. Nursing assistants need to allow residents to adapt to the new environment at their pace, not the pace the staff would choose for them. Everyone is different, and the process of getting used to their new home may take quite some time. Dealing with multiple losses is like a grieving process for some residents. They are grieving that they have lost their home, their pets, their plants, perhaps their friends, and maybe even some of their family members. Have you ever read about the number of residents within facilities who never get any visitors? Residents know these facts, too, and may be afraid they'll experience the same situation.

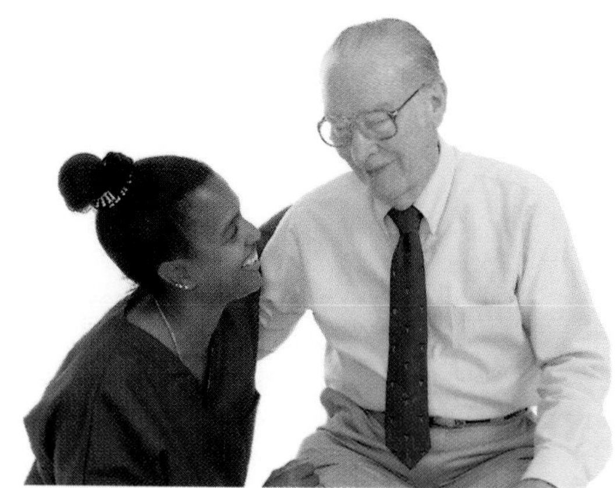

Figure 14-3. **You can help your residents make the adjustment to move to a long-term care facility.**

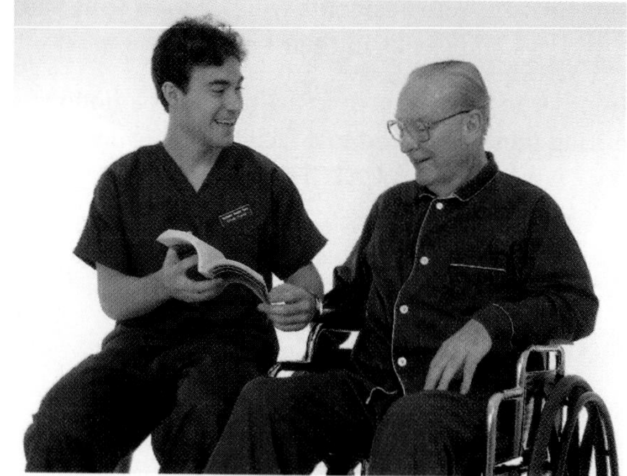

Figure 14-4. **Spending quality time with new residents may help reduce their anxiety.**

The Welcome Committee

To assist new residents with the transition into a facility, a "Welcome Committee" is helpful. Team members from each department can be chosen to greet the new resident. Each department can have a special cards made on a computer or ordered from a supplier. The special card can be brought to the resident's new room either as a group or one at a time. This idea can be expanded to include other little niceties like having a carnation for a resident waiting in her new room. Sometimes little things can make all of the difference for a new resident.

4 Describe the role of the nursing assistant during the admission process.

When a new resident is coming to a facility, a supervisor may give the unit staff the approximate time that the new resident will arrive. The manager of the unit will then inform the nursing assistant assigned to that area that the room must be set up for the new resident. The nursing assistant must wash her hands before gathering equipment and supplies which include the following:

- An **admission pack**, also known as a unit or a resident pack, consists of personal care items supplied upon **admission**. This generally includes a wash basin, bedpan, urinal (male residents), pitcher and cup, and possibly a soap dish. In some facilities other items are included within a pack, such as special lotions, powders, or soaps.
- A stethoscope and a sphygmomanometer to take the new resident's blood pressure
- A thermometer to take the new resident's temperature
- An IV pole if a resident has an IV line
- A facility gown or pajamas, depending upon the resident

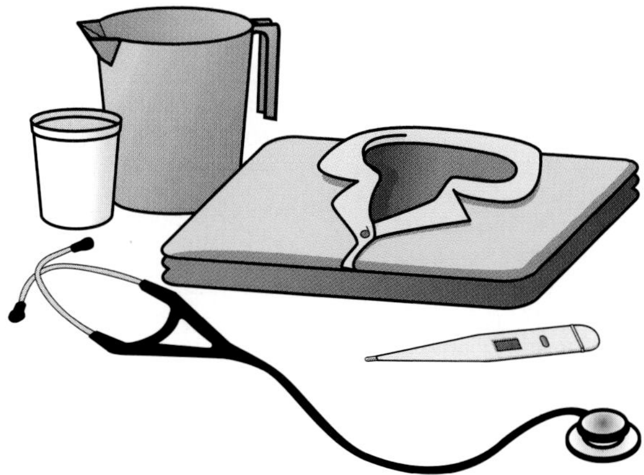

Figure 14-5. Nursing assistants may need to gather supplies for a newly-admitted resident.

The nursing assistant must take all of the equipment to the new resident's room so that the admission moves along smoothly. When the nursing assistant has set up the equipment in the new resident's room, he must then prepare the bed and the room itself. The following steps may be taken to prepare the room:

The Bed

1. If the new resident is ambulatory (walking) or in a wheelchair, the bed must be in its lowest position. Make sure handles on manual beds are returned to the "in" position so that a new resident or family member does not trip over them. The bed may be turned down for the resident or left made, depending upon the nurse's orders.
2. If the resident will arrive by stretcher, a surgical bed must be made (See Chapter 15). The bed must be left elevated to allow for the transfer of the resident from the stretcher (See Chapter 17).

The Room

1. If the resident is coming during the day, the blinds or curtains may be opened to add some light to the room.
2. If the room is a semi-private room and a roommate is present, notify the resident already in the room of the new arrival.

Orientation of the New Resident and Family

When the resident arrives, welcome him using his last name in a friendly manner. Introduce yourself to the resident and all family members. When speaking to family, address them by their last names as well, unless they specifically ask you to call them by their first names. Remember to get information on personal preferences, history, rituals, and routines from the resident, as well as from family and friends before they depart. Family members are great sources of information about the resident. Take time to ask them questions. Orient them to the following:

1. **The roommate and neighbors.** Introducing the new resident and family to roommates and neighbors in the rooms on either side and across the hall is a good thing to do. This helps the resident feel more comfortable and adapt more quickly to his new surroundings. It may also help the family feel better.

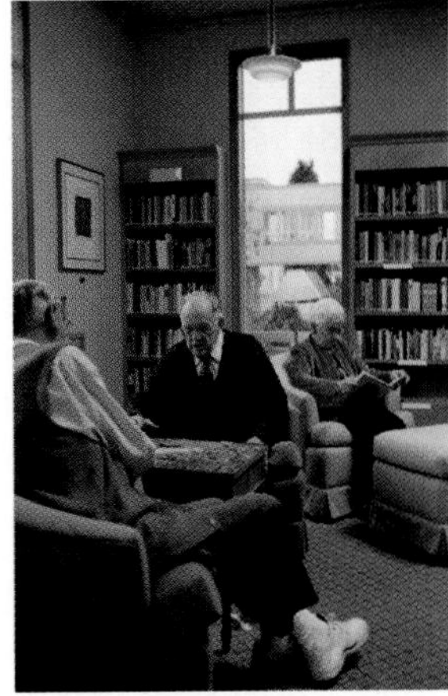

Figure 14-6. Always introduce new residents to other residents.

2. **The resident's new bed.** Show the new resident how to work the new bed controls.

3. **The signal cord or call light.** Make sure the call light is attached to the bed and that the new resident understands how to use it.

4. **The television and telephone.** Familiarize the resident with the use of the television and telephone, if available.

5. **The facility tour.** Take the resident and family members around the facility, if possible, to see the dining room, chapel, and all other important areas, such as the activity room. Activity schedules may be shared at this time, along with information about menus and the dining room. If facility policy, point out special signs, fire alarms, smoke alarms, and fire extinguishers. During the tour, residents should be introduced to all staff members they meet.

6. **Care of belongings including valuables.** Handle all of the resident's belongings with respect and care. Assist the resident in the process of unpacking all of his belongings. Some facilities require that a complete list of all belongings be made as they are put away. For your safety, more than one nursing assistant should complete a belongings list. It is very important to follow the facility policy regarding residents' belongings, whatever it may be. An inventory of valuables might need to be taken. This is usually done by the nurse. The nurse might have a second nurse co-sign the valuables list for safety.

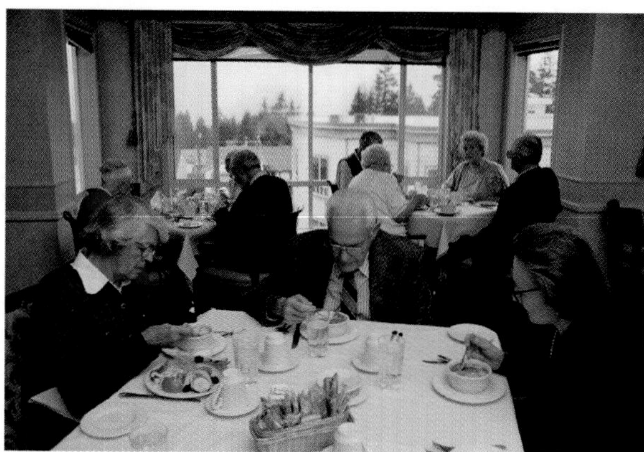

Figure 14-7. When you take a new resident around a facility, point out as much as you can.

7. **Vital signs, height, and weight.** Most facilities require a **baseline** height, weight, and vital signs measurement. Baseline measurements are initial values that can then be compared to future measurements. Weight will be measured using **pounds** or **kilograms** and will sometimes be performed on **bedridden** residents. Kilograms are units of **metric** measurement. Some residents require the measurement of **abdominal girth**, thigh/calf circumference and inseam for special stockings. Abdominal girth is a measurement of the circumference around the abdomen at the umbilicus (navel). These are taken and noted on an admission checklist form. If any vital sign is abnormal in any way, immediately notify the nurse (See Chapter 16).

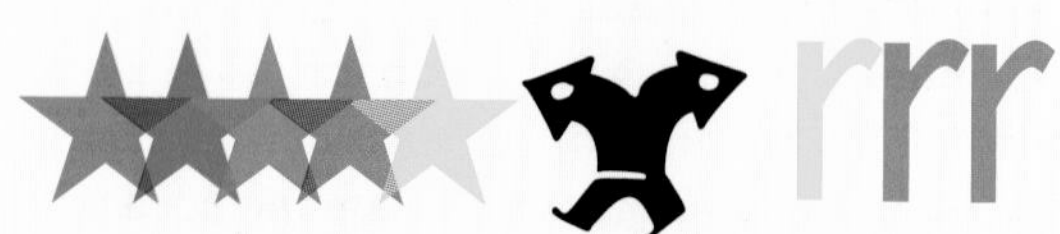

Beginning Steps

★ RESPECT
Knock first, ask and receive permission to enter a resident's room.

★ INFECTION CONTROL
Wash hands.

★ COMMUNICATION
Greet and identify the resident. Identify yourself. Explain the procedure, encouraging the resident to be as independent as possible throughout.

★ BED SAFETY
Lock bed wheels. Raise bed to safe working height. Lower one side rail if required.

★ PRIVACY
Provide for privacy by closing the door and covering the resident appropriately.

Ending Steps

★ RESIDENT SAFETY AND COMFORT
Secure the resident, lowering the bed, and raising the side rails if ordered. Check that the resident is comfortable and properly aligned.

★ PRIVACY
Remove any added privacy measures, such as a drape or a privacy screen.

★ ESSENTIALS
Place the call light, fresh beverage, and other items within reach.

★ COURTESY
Ask the resident if he or she needs anything else. Say thank you and goodbye.

★ INFECTION CONTROL
Wash hands.

Report your care and any important observations to the nurse.

Record your care and any important information/observations such as vital signs in the appropriate place.

Recheck your resident for any changes as directed by the nurse!

Admitting a Resident to a Facility

Follow all standard and/or transmission-based precautions. Follow all rules for body mechanics.

Collect equipment:
- thermometer (check for covers/sheaths)
- sphygmomanometer and blood pressure cuff
- scale • admission pack (unit or resident pack)
- clean gown or pajamas • IV pole (if needed)
- watch with second hand or second counter
- towels and washcloth • pen and pad

ROOM PREPARATION

1. Wash hands.
2. Notify roommate of new resident.
3. Open curtains.
4. Adjust bed up or leave down for new admission, depending upon method of arrival.
5. Make decision regarding how to arrange the bedcovers on the bed per facility policy and resident needs.
6. Put away the clean towels and pajamas or gown.

WELCOME

7. Welcome the resident and the family or other visitors to the new room.
8. Introduce yourself, roommates, staff, and neighbors to the new resident and family or friends.
9. Encourage the resident and the family to sit down and relax for a few minutes. Secure additional chairs, if necessary. Answer any initial questions at this time if possible, or get the nurse.
10. The resident may want to be alone with the family for a time. If this is acceptable with the nurse, allow for some privacy. Tell them you will return in (list minutes) to complete the admission. Make sure the resident is secure before you leave the room.
11. If returning to the room, wash hands and explain what you will do next.

ROOM ORIENTATION and CARE OF BELONGINGS

12. Begin the process of orienting the resident to the following:
    a. The bed controls, including the call light or signal cord
    b. Lights in the room
    c. The television and radio controls
    d. The telephone
    e. The bathroom
    f. The closet and dressers/cabinets
    g. Information regarding the dining room, dinner times, and activity schedules
    h. Where the chapel is located, along with other facility areas the resident may wish to visit, such as a gift shop
13. Carefully unpack all of the resident's belongings and complete the admission belongings checklist as each item is unpacked. Labeling of each item may take place at this time, as well. Laundry markers may be used to label the items; care should be taken to mark on available neck tags so as to not mark clothing needlessly.
14. Valuables may be handled by the nurses. Two staff members should handle valuables and sign off the valuables checklist for safety.
15. Allow resident to change clothes, if desired.

VITAL SIGNS, HEIGHT, and WEIGHT

16. Perform all vital signs procedures and document on admission form and elsewhere per facility policy.
17. Perform height and weight procedures and document on admission form and per facility policy.

WATER PITCHER

18. Follow the instructions of the nurse regarding filling the water pitcher.
19. If resident is NPO (nothing by mouth), explain the reason why and follow facility policy regarding water pitcher and cup. Some facilities remove the pitcher and cup from the room.

LEAVING THE NEW RESIDENT

20. When you have completed the admission process, explain to the resident that you have to leave for the time being.
21. Ask the resident if he needs anything before you leave the room.
22. Perform the "5 Stars and 3 Rs."

Measuring Height and Weight on an Upright Scale

Follow all standard and/or transmission-based precautions. Follow all rules for body mechanics.

Collect equipment:
- pad and pen
- scale

PREPARE:

1. Perform the "5 Stars."

2. Bring the scale as close to the resident as the facility policy allows.
3. Walk the resident to the scale.
4. Some facilities place paper towels on the scale before allowing residents to step on the scale. Other facilities may feel paper towels are a hazard and may cause a resident to slip. Follow facility policy and be careful when using paper towels under the feet.
5. The scale must be balanced. There are many types of scales. If you do not know how to balance your particular scale, ask the nurse before using the scale.

PERFORM:

6. Help the resident remove shoes and step up on the scale. The resident should be facing the scale. Once on the scale, do not allow the resident to hang onto you or the scale. His arms must hang free.

7. Move the heavy weight at the bottom to the right to the weight closest to the resident's prior weight.
8. Move the lighter weight at the top to the right until the bar at the right hangs free.
9. Read the two numbers at the point where each weight has settled and add these two numbers together. This is the resident's weight.
10. Have the resident carefully turn around to face away from the scale. Slide the height bar up so that you can pull out the metal bar. BE CAREFUL NOT TO HIT THE RESIDENT OR YOURSELF WITH THE METAL MEASURE BAR.

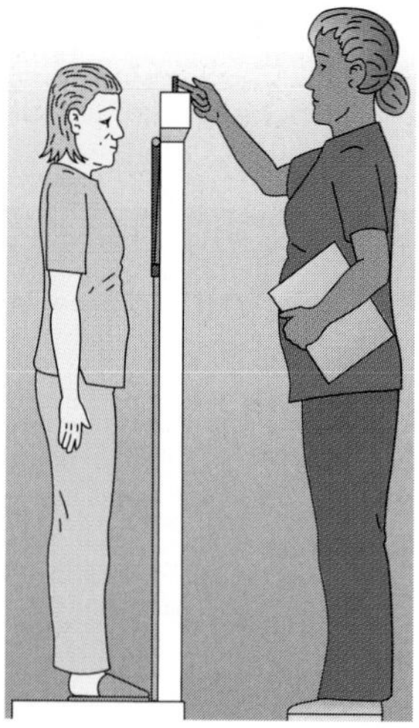

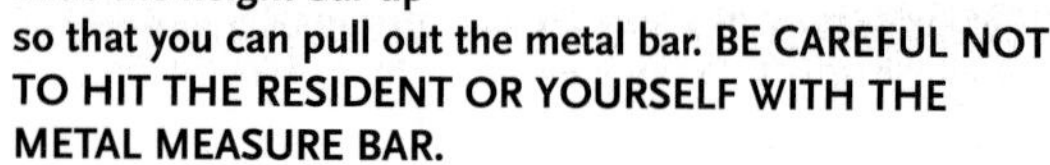

Figure 14-8.

11. Now slide the metal measure bar down so that it lightly touches the top of the resident's head.
12. Read the number at the point where the two bars come together. This is the height. The number will be in inches or centimeters.
13. HOLD THE METAL BAR securely in your hand, and help the resident step down from the scale. DO NOT HIT THE HEAD OF THE RESIDENT WITH THE METAL BAR.

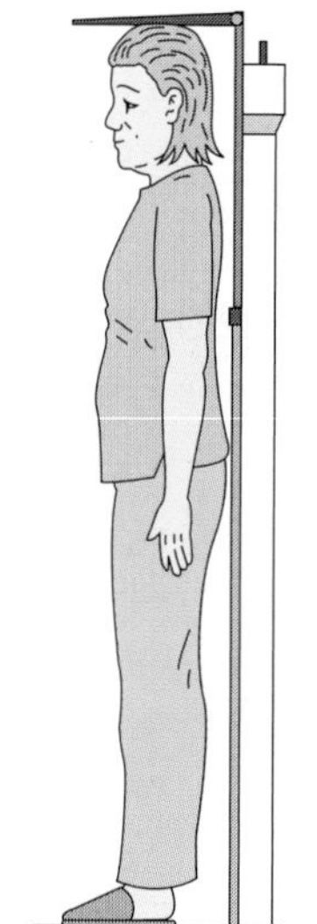

Figure 14-9.

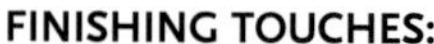

FINISHING TOUCHES:

14. Assist the resident in putting slippers or shoes back on and return resident to room.
15. Note the height and weight on your notepad.
16. Perform the "5 Stars and 3 Rs."

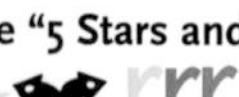

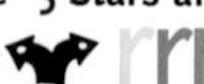

Measuring Weight on a Wheelchair Scale

Follow all standard and/or transmission-based precautions. Follow all rules for body mechanics.

Collect equipment:
- pad and pen
- scale

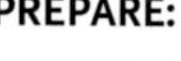

PREPARE:

1. Perform the "5 Stars."

2. Bring the scale as close to the resident as the facility policy allows.
3. Wheel the resident to the scale.
4. Balance the scale. There are many types of scales. If you do not know how to balance your particular scale, ask the nurse before using the scale.

PERFORM:

5. Help the resident remove shoes and wheel resident up onto the scale. Lock wheelchair.
6. Move the heavy weight at the bottom toward the right to the weight closest to the resident's prior weight.
7. Move the lighter weight at the top toward the right until the bar at the right hangs free.
8. Read the two numbers at the point where each weight has settled and add these two numbers together. This is the resident's weight.
9. Unlock wheelchair. Wheel resident off the wheelchair scale.
10. Note the weight. With some wheelchair scales, you must then subtract the weight of the wheelchair from the total weight. To find out the weight of the wheelchair, look on the chair or ask the nurse. Some scales automatically figure the weight.

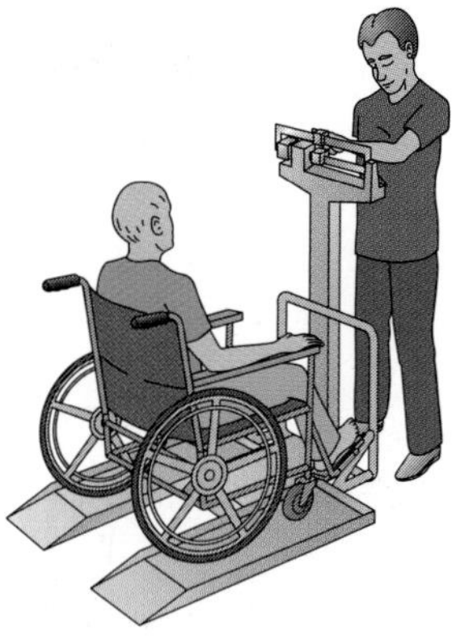

Figure 14-10.

FINISHING TOUCHES:

11. Assist the resident in putting slippers or shoes back on and return resident to room.
12. Perform the "5 Stars and 3 Rs."

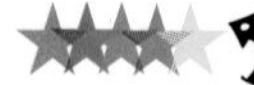
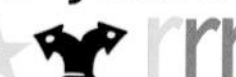

Measuring Weight of a Bedridden Resident

Follow all standard and/or transmission-based precautions. Follow all rules for body mechanics.

Collect equipment:
- pad and pen
- scale

PREPARE:

1. Bring the scale to the resident's room. Have another staff member come with you to assist, if possible.
2. Perform the "5 Stars."

3. The scale must be balanced. There are many types of scales. If you do not know how to balance your particular scale, ask the nurse before using the scale.
4. Examine the sling, straps, chains, and/or pad for any damage or weakness.
5. Turn linen down so that it is off the resident.
6. Turn resident to one side away from you OR if flat pad scale is used, slide resident onto pad using a helper. If sling is used, remove from the scale and place underneath resident without wrinkling.
7. With a sling, turn the resident back to the supine (back) position and straighten sling.

PERFORM:

8. Attach the sling to the scale OR if using a flat pad scale, position resident securely on the pad.
9. DOUBLE-CHECK the straps or other connectors, and raise the sling or the pad until the resident is clear of the bed. With some scales, it is possible to keep the resident directly over the bed while weighing the resident. With others, you may have to move the scale away from the bed. Either way, SECURE THE RESIDENT before moving the resident on the scale.

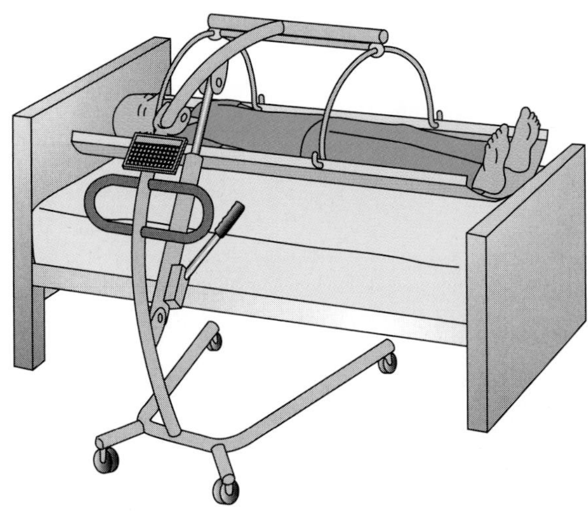

Figure 14-11.

10. Balance the scale following the guidelines for the type of scale being used.
11. With digital scales, turn on and note reading. With other types of scales, move the weights until you get a reading. Note the weight.
12. Lower the resident back down on the bed. If using a sling, turn resident to both sides to remove the sling. If using a pad scale, carefully slide the resident back onto the bed.

FINISHING TOUCHES:

13. Position the resident comfortably and replace linen over the resident.
14. Perform the "5 Stars and 3 Rs."

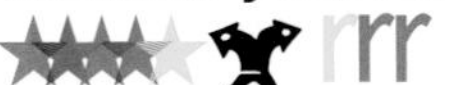

Measuring Height of a Bedridden Resident

Follow all standard and/or transmission-based precautions. Follow all rules for body mechanics.

Collect equipment: • pad and pen • measuring tape • scale

PREPARE:

1. Perform the "5 Stars."

2. Turn linen down so it is off the resident.
3. Position resident comfortably in the supine (back) position.

PERFORM:

4. Using a pencil, make a small mark on the bottom sheet at the top of the resident's head.
5. Go to the FOB and make another small pencil mark at the resident's heels.
6. Using the tape measure, measure the area between the pencil marks. This is the height of the resident.

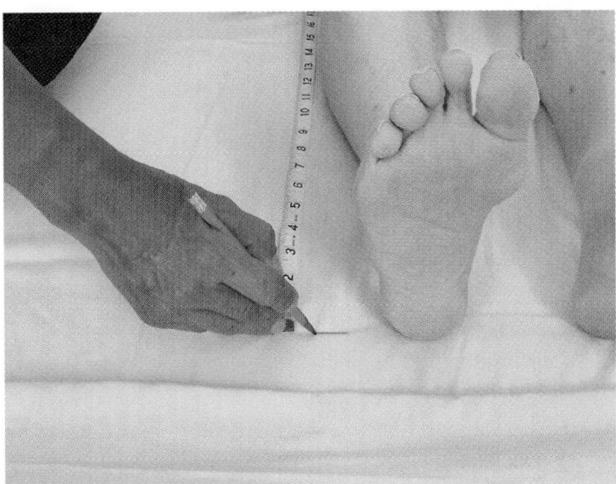

Figure 14-12.

7. Note this number on your pad.

FINISHING TOUCHES:

8. Position the resident comfortably and replace linen over the resident.
9. Perform the "5 Stars and 3 Rs."

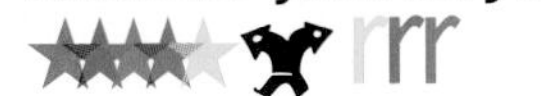

Measuring Abdominal Girth

Follow all standard and/or transmission-based precautions. Follow all rules for body mechanics.

Collect equipment:
- tape measure
- pad and pen

PREPARE:

1. Perform the "5 Stars."

2. Turn linen down and raise resident gown or pajamas just enough so that abdomen can be measured. Keep all areas covered that do not need to be exposed. Promote your resident's dignity.

PERFORM:

3. Carefully wrap measuring tape around the resident's abdomen at the level of the navel (umbilicus).
4. Read the number where the ends of the tape meet.

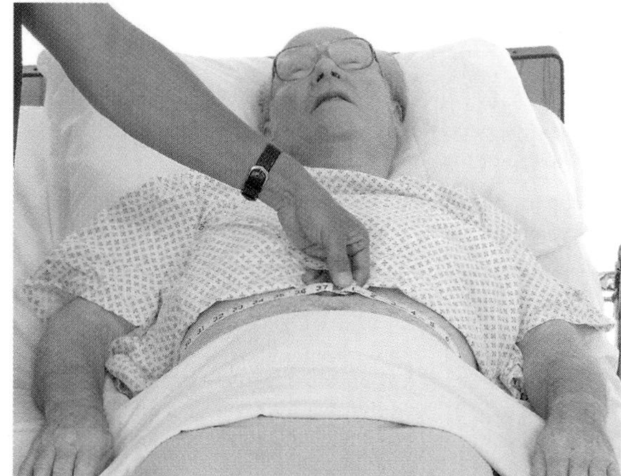

Figure 14-13.

5. Carefully remove the tape measure. Write down the abdominal girth measurement on your notepad.

FINISHING TOUCHES:

6. Replace resident clothing and position comfortably.
7. Perform the "5 Stars and 3 Rs."

 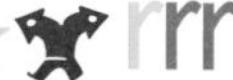

Measuring Thigh, Calf, and Inseam for Special Stockings

Follow all standard and/or transmission-based precautions. Follow all rules for body mechanics.

Collect equipment:

- tape measure
- measuring guidelines for either thigh- or knee-high stockings

PREPARE:

1. Perform the "5 Stars."

2. Turn linen down and raise resident gown or lower pajamas so that thigh and/or calf can be measured. Keep all areas covered that do not need to be exposed. Promote your residents' dignity.

PERFORM:

3. Carefully wrap measuring tape around the resident's thigh OR calf at the largest part of the thigh or calf.

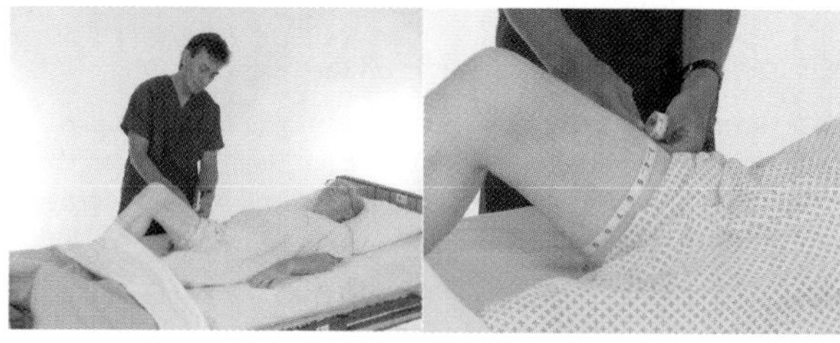

Figure 14-14.

4. Read the number where the ends of the tape meet.
5. Carefully remove the tape measure. Write down the thigh OR calf circumference on your notepad.
6. Measure the distance from the bend of the knee or the spot where the thigh attaches to the body at the hip to the bottom of the heel to obtain length of the stockings.

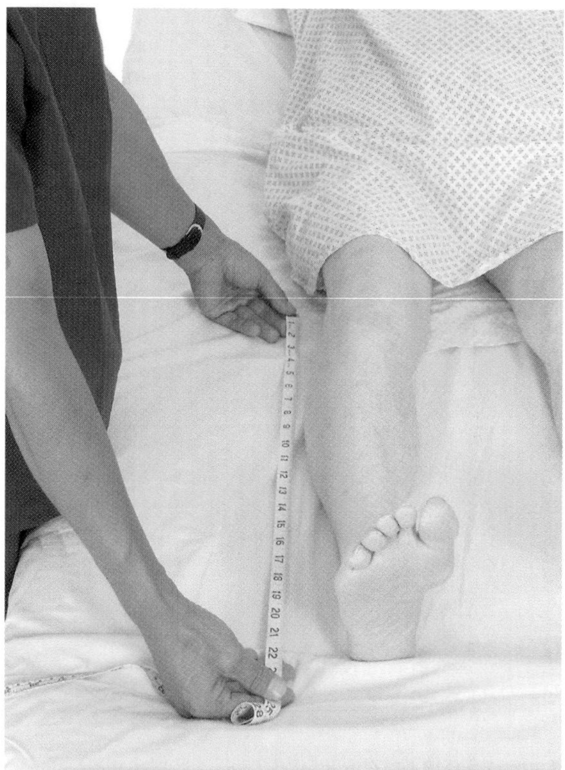

Figure 14-15.

FINISHING TOUCHES:

7. Replace resident clothing and position resident comfortably.
8. Perform the "5 Stars and 3 Rs."

 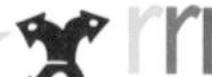

5 Describe six nursing assistant responsibilities during a physical exam.

Some residents may require a physical exam upon arriving at a facility. Others might need a physical exam after they have been at a facility for a while. It is important to become familiar with your role during a physical exam so the process runs smoothly. Sometimes, nurses do all or part of the physical assessment and the examination. In other cases, doctors do all or part of the exam. The nursing assistant might be asked to assist with a physical examination or assessment of a new or existing resident. Some of the responsibilities of the nursing assistant during an exam include the following:

- Help residents with their emotional needs by being there for them. This can include listening to them, talking to them, or even holding their hand.
- Gather equipment for the nurse or doctor.
- Place the resident in the appropriate position and stay with the resident as needed.
- Provide a drape for the resident and other privacy measures, such as closing the privacy screen or curtain and closing the door to the room.
- Provide enough light for the doctor or nurse.
- Gather and label specimens as needed.

Assisting with the Physical Exam

Follow all standard and/or transmission-based precautions. Follow all rules for body mechanics.

Collect equipment:
- two pairs of disposable gloves • gown for resident
- draping linen • disposable bed protector • towel
- waste basket • tissues • clean gown or pajamas
- glass slides and fixative spray • stethoscope
- sphygmomanometer • thermometer
- eye chart • tuning fork • reflex hammer • otoscope
- ophthalmoscope • cotton balls • tongue depressors
- watch with second hand or second counter
- tape measure • flashlight • alcohol wipes
- specimen containers as needed • lubricant
- marking pen for slides • Hemoccult card
- vaginal speculum for females

PREPARE:

1. Perform the "5 Stars."

2. Apply gloves.
3. The resident may need to urinate before the physical examination. Make sure that you collect any urine needed for a specimen at this time (See Chapter 23). Remove gloves after collecting a sample and wash hands.
4. Either bring resident to the examination room or prepare the resident's room for the examination.
5. If resident has to transfer to the examination table, carefully assist the resident to the table and STAY CLOSE to the resident until the examiner arrives, as these tables tend to be very high. Have the drape ready to use.
6. If resident is to be examined in the bed, prepare the bed for draping the resident.

PERFORM:

7. When the examiner has arrived, do the following:
   a. Follow the directions of the examiner.
   b. Hand instruments to the examiner as needed.
   c. Position and reposition the resident as requested.

FINISHING TOUCHES:

8. When the examination is over, assist the resident in cleaning up and putting on clothing or robe. Transport the resident back to the room if needed, and position the resident comfortably in the bed.
9. Dispose of any trash and disposable equipment, as needed.
10. Perform the "5 Stars and 3 Rs."

11. Label and bring any specimens to the desk for transport to the lab. Bring all reusable examination equipment to the appropriate cleaning room. Apply second set of gloves in cleaning room, clean equipment, and store appropriately. Remove second pair of gloves and wash hands again.

6 Demonstrate eight bed positions and discuss the Trendelenburg and Reverse Trendelenburg positions.

The way a resident is positioned can be very important during a physical examination. Draping of the resident is also very important in order to provide privacy during the exam. The following positions may be necessary during a physical examination. Each position should have careful draping for privacy. However, draping is not shown so that you can have a clearer view of the position.

- **supine** position
- **lateral** position
- **dorsal recumbent** position
- **knee-chest** position
- **prone** position
- **Sims'** position
- **Fowler's** position
- dorsal lithotomy or **lithotomy** position

The **Trendelenburg** and **Reverse Trendelenburg** are two positions used with residents with special needs. These positions always require a doctor's order. Trendelenburg is used for residents with special problems, such as a person who has gone into shock and has an inadequate blood flow. Reverse Trendelenburg might be used for residents who need faster emptying of the stomach due to certain problems with the digestive tract. Some electric beds have special buttons or levers that automatically place the bed in these two positions. Remember, these positions are only used with a doctor's order.

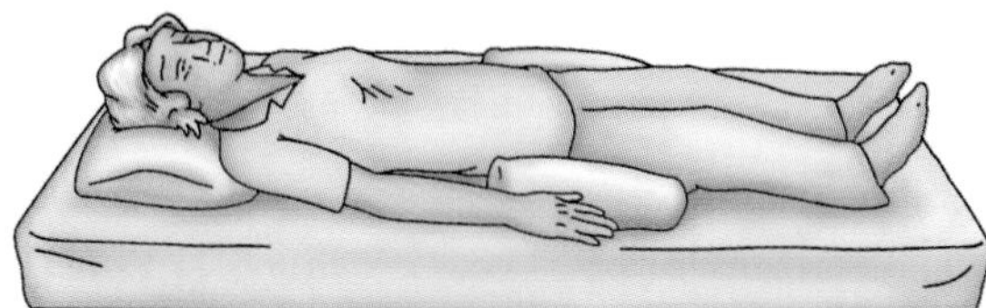

Figure 14-16. **A person in the supine position is lying flat on his or her back.**

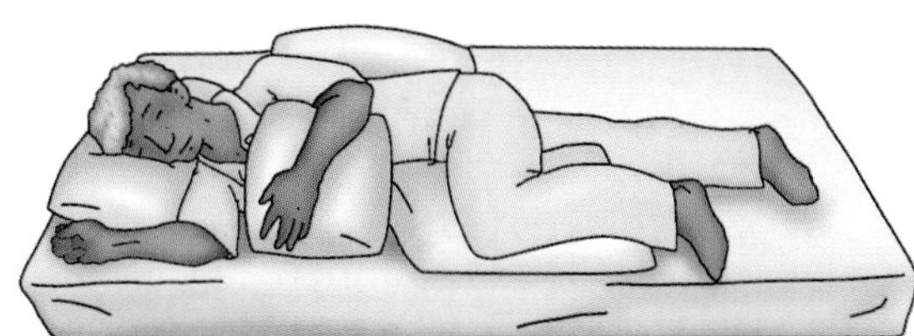

Figure 14-17. **A person in the lateral position is lying on his or her side.**

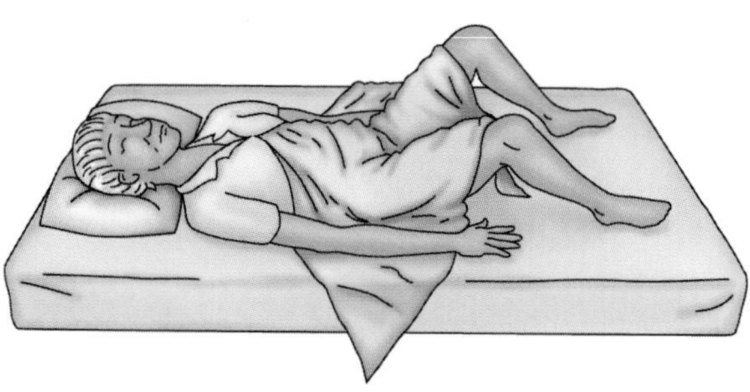

Figure 14-18. **A person in the dorsal recumbent position is flat on his or her back with knees flexed and feet flat on the bed.**

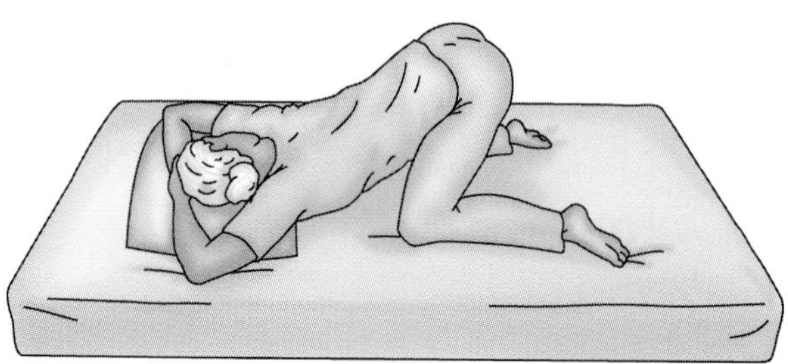

Figure 14-19. **A person in the knee-chest position is lying on his or her abdomen with knees pulled towards the abdomen and legs separated. Arms are pulled up and flexed and head is turned to one side.**

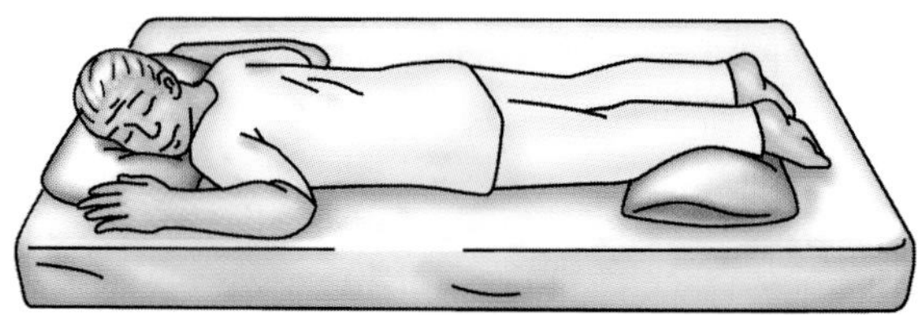

Figure 14-20. **A person in the prone position is lying on his or her stomach.**

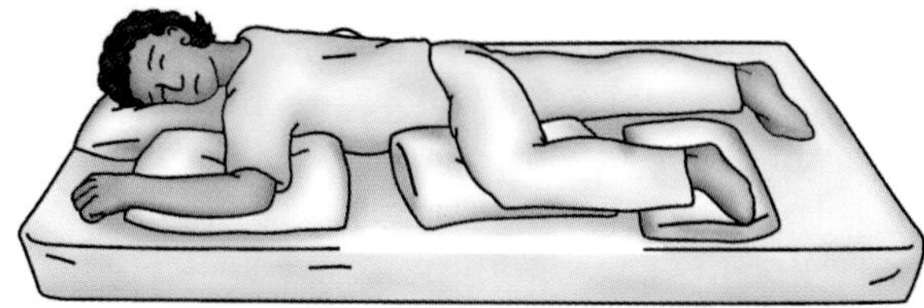

Figure 14-21. **A person in the Sims' position is lying on his or her side with one leg drawn up.**

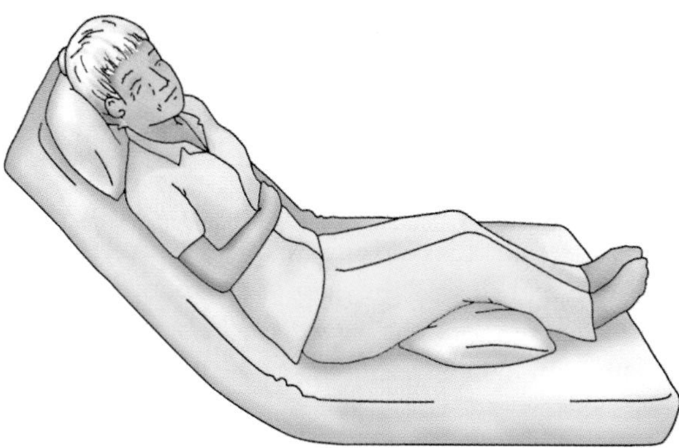

Figure 14-22. **A person in the Fowler's position is partially reclined, with the head of the bed elevated about 60 degrees. In a Semi-Fowler's position, the head of the bed is elevated about 30 degrees.**

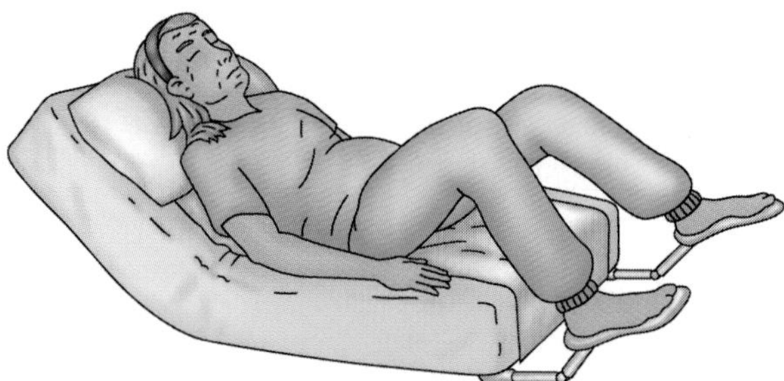

Figure 14-23. **A person in the lithotomy position is lying on his or her back with legs flexed and feet in stirrups.**

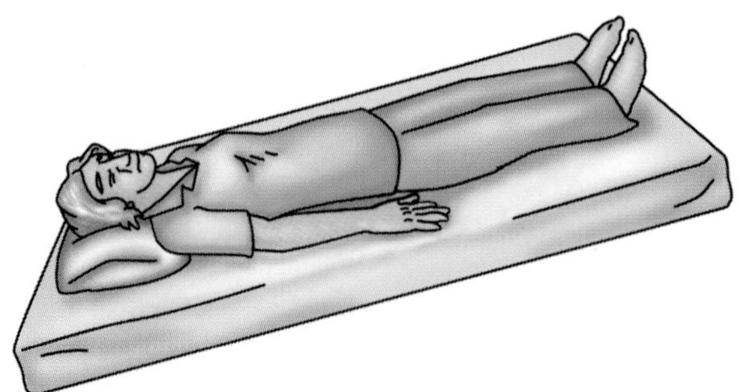

Figure 14-24. **The Reverse Trendelenburg position always requires a doctor's order.**

7 Explain the nursing assistant's responsibilities during the in-house transfer of a resident.

Sometimes residents need to be transferred to another room within a facility. A resident might need to change to a different unit that offers more intensive care. The doctor may make that decision along with the nursing staff and the family. The resident and/or the family of the resident might request a different room. A resident could want another room if he is not getting along with a roommate. When this occurs, the nursing assistant is usually responsible for packing all of the belongings and preparing the resident for the **transfer**. The resident may be transferred in a bed, in a stretcher, or in a wheelchair. You need to find out the method of transfer from the nurse so that you can plan the move. Packing up all of the belongings may take some time, especially if the resident has many cards and personal objects within the room. You must take great care to pack all of the belongings carefully so that nothing breaks, is damaged in any way, or is lost.

When you arrive at the new unit with the resident, one of the first things you should do is to introduce the resident to the new unit staff and the new roommate, if in a semi-private room. Make sure you remember to bring all of the resident's belongings with you. The nurse may bring the valuables envelope, medication, and the resident chart. Some facilities allow the nursing assistant to transfer the resident chart.

If you will be unpacking the resident's belongings, do so very carefully and try to re-create the way the belongings were set up in the former room. When you leave the resident, follow the "5 Stars and the 3 Rs". It is a good idea, along with being a very nice gesture, for you to recheck a resident later in the day or the next day to make sure he is settled into the new room. After that, it is nice to periodically check in with the resident to say hello. This helps him stay connected to you.

When you leave the resident's room, go straight to the nurse-in-charge of that resident. Report that the resident is settled in the new room and that you are leaving to return to your unit. That way, you have formally transferred responsibility to the new unit. It is usually not enough to report to the nursing assistant assigned to that room.

Transferring a Resident

Follow all standard and/or transmission-based precautions. Follow all rules for body mechanics.

Collect equipment:
- **cart for belongings**
- **wheelchair or stretcher**
- **resident chart**

1. **Double-check with the nurse that the room is ready for the new resident.**
2. **Perform the "5 Stars."**

PREPARE:

3. **Carefully pack up all of the resident's belongings on the cart. Get another staff member to help move the belongings on the cart.**
4. **Allow the resident to say goodbye to a roommate and the unit staff.**

PERFORM:

5. **Carefully move the resident to the new unit by bed, wheelchair, or stretcher.**
6. **Introduce the resident to the new unit staff and the new roommate. When going by the nurse's station, you may leave the chart with the nurse. (The nurses usually transfer the medications, treatment supplies, and the valuables envelope.)**
7. **Transfer the resident to the new bed, if necessary, with assistance if using a stretcher.**
8. **Unpack all belongings. Make sure the resident is comfortable and secure before leaving the new room.**

FINISHING TOUCHES:

9. **Say goodbye to the resident.**
10. **Perform the "5 Stars and 3 Rs."**

It is a nice gesture to return to the unit to visit the resident whenever you can. Report to the nurse on the new unit that the resident is settled and secure. Report to your original unit nurse that you have returned and the transfer is complete.

11. **Perform Principal Steps: Unit Cleaning per facility policy. (See Chapter 15)**

8 Explain the nursing assistant's role in discharge planning.

A **discharge** to another facility must be planned carefully. When the process is organized, the discharge will run more smoothly. The nurse or social worker usually plans the discharge. This includes making the arrangements for the following:

- the move to the resident's home or center
- the pick-up by a vehicle of some kind
- the preparation of the medications for discharge
- the gathering of prescriptions
- the scheduling of the follow-up appointments with the healthcare providers

The nursing assistant may have some input on this process since he is on the front lines of care. If the family communicates any important information to you, report it to the nurse. You may hear or be told directly about information regarding the time of pick-up, type of vehicle coming for the pick-up, and any special requests.

9 Describe the nursing assistant's role in discharge of a resident.

The discharge process is official after the physician formally writes an order to discharge the resident home or to another facility. The nurse will then complete a set of instructions for the resident to follow after discharge. Before the resident leaves the room, the nurse should come to the room, bring the medications and prescriptions, and review the instructions. Figure 14-25 shows an example of discharge instructions.

This is a stressful time for the resident, and it is best for family and friends to be able to hear the instructions. There may be a tendency for caregivers to want to continue relationships with discharged residents. For your safety, it is not a good idea to share your home address or telephone number with residents or their families. After the nurse leaves the room, if anyone has any additional questions, you must get the nurse to return to answer the questions. Do not try to answer any questions yourself.

After the formal discharge has been written, you should gather all of the belongings and carefully pack them for the move. You may be responsible for checking off each item on the original belongings list as it is packed so that everything is included. Your supervisor may arrange for a second staff member to be present as a witness.

The valuables packet or envelope is normally checked off by the nurses. When the moment arrives for the actual move to the vehicle, you are responsible for the resident successfully reaching the vehicle without incident. This means you must stay with the resident until you carefully assist the person and all belongings into the vehicle and *cautiously* close the door. Your responsibility does not end until the vehicle doors are all closed securely.

Discharge Instructions

Patient's Name: Caroyl Crawford

Treatments: Check blood sugar following your doctor's order. Call if blood sugar below 70 or over 110.

Medications: Follow doctor's order for insulin.

Diet: 1500 calorie ADA diet; See your dietician for questions.

Activity: Carefully follow doctor's orders for exercise and activity.

Appointments: Feb. 8, 2002 Dr. Steve Singer 11 Linden St. Telephone 555-1274.

Other: Call if you feel weak, dizzy, or notice any other unusual symptoms.

If you have any questions about these discharge instructions, please call.

Name: Sarah Harris RN, Dr. Maury's office

Telephone Number: 555-3885 extension 3303

Disharge instructions given by Diana Dugan, RN

Discharge instructions given to patient X or family member

Patient or Family Member Signature: David Crawford

Date: Jan 10, 2001

Figure 14-25.

Discharging a Resident

Follow all standard and/or transmission-based precautions. Follow all rules for body mechanics.

Collect equipment:
- **cart for belongings • wheelchair or stretcher**
- **gloves for equipment/unit cleaning**

PREPARE:

1. **Double-check with the nurse that the discharge instructions, including medications, prescriptions, and doctor's appointment along with the valuables envelope, have been given to the resident and that the people have arrived to pick up the resident.**
2. **Perform the "5 Stars."**

3. **Assist the resident in getting dressed, if appropriate to the situation. Double-check that all IV tubing has been removed by the nurse, if appropriate.**
4. **Carefully pack up all of the resident's belongings on the cart. Get another staff member to help move the belongings on the cart.**
5. **Allow the resident to say goodbye to a roommate and the unit staff.**

PERFORM:

6. **Lock the wheelchair or stretcher. Transfer the resident to the wheelchair or stretcher. (See Chapter 17) Bring the resident to the vehicle.**
7. **Lock the wheelchair or stretcher and carefully transfer the resident to the vehicle with assistance, if needed. (See Chapter 17)**
8. **Transfer all belongings to the vehicle. If medical records are being transferred, give these to the driver of the vehicle.**
9. **Say goodbye to the resident. Your responsibility ends when the resident has been placed inside the vehicle and the door is securely closed.**

FINISHING TOUCHES:

10. **Report to the nurse that the discharge is completed.**
11. **Arrange for or perform unit cleaning (Chapter 15) and equipment cleaning (Chapter 11) per facility policy.**

10 Explain the proper response if a resident wants to leave the facility against medical advice (AMA).

Sometimes a resident decides to leave a center or facility without the approval of the doctor. This is called leaving **AMA** or "against medical advice." When this occurs, a careful process must be followed in order to protect the facility along with all of the staff. If you see any signs that a resident is considering leaving the facility, immediately notify the nurse in charge of that resident.

★ *"Don't Delay. Report Right Away!"*

For example, some of the things you might notice are: if a resident is anxious and mentions a desire to leave, and/or if a resident gathers her belongings.

The nurse may then present the resident with a document called an AMA form that the resident is asked to sign before leaving the facility. It is very important that the resident sign this form before leaving the facility. Should the resident become injured, for example, after walking out of the facility, a signed AMA form may provide some protection from liability for the facility and the staff.

Stop abuse during admission, transfer, discharge, and physical exams!

The following situations are examples of abuse during the process of admission, transfer, discharge, and physical exams:

1. A resident is brought to a new room and left there alone in a wheelchair by a transport person. The transport person does not inform any staff member of the resident's arrival. The resident has no access to a signal light and falls while trying to get out of the chair.

2. A resident is transferred to another unit with all belongings by a nursing assistant. The nursing assistant leaves the resident in the new room alone and never reports to any staff member on the new unit that the resident has arrived. The resident has diabetes, an endocrine disorder, has a severe drop in blood sugar, and passes out in the room.

3. A resident is brought to a vehicle to be discharged and the nursing assistant stands behind the wheelchair and lets the family member transfer the resident to the car. The family member cannot handle the weight of the resident alone, the resident falls and breaks a hip, requiring admission to a hospital.

4. During a physical exam, a nursing assistant leaves a resident on an examining table, knowing the resident is confused and steps out to make a personal phone call. The resident falls off the examining table and gets a concussion (head injury causing a bruise to the brain due to a severe blow to the head).

These examples are all easily avoided. When cautious, considerate care is given to residents, the chance of accidents or injuries occurring is greatly reduced.

Summary

Residents who need to be admitted to a facility face many challenges in adjusting to their new home. You can provide a great deal of assistance with this transition. An in-house transfer (within a facility) means having to be separated from caring staff members and roommates. It is important for you to be aware of the emotional challenges of a transfer.

A resident's discharge home can be an exciting and happy time for a family. Staff members can make this move run smoothly by carefully following the discharge policies. The discharge to another facility should also be handled professionally. Residents may be upset when they are moving out of their home.

Physical exams sometimes cause anxiety for residents. The healthcare team can reduce this anxiety by being there for the resident and assisting the examiner so that the process runs smoothly.

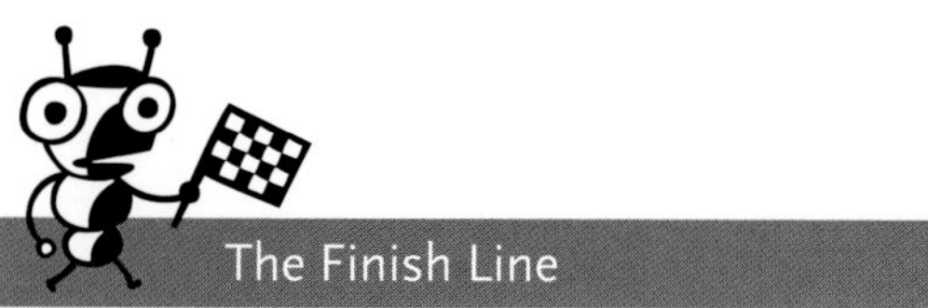

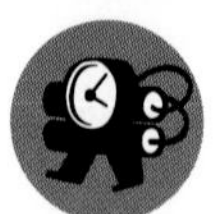

What's Wrong With This Picture?

These positions are mislabeled. Fix each of the mistakes.

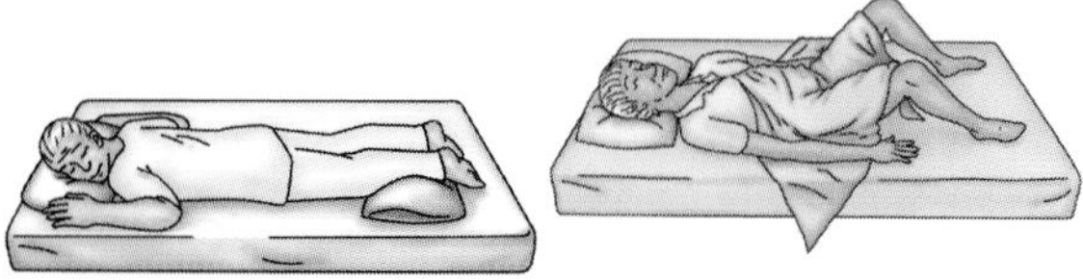

1. Fowler's position 2. supine position

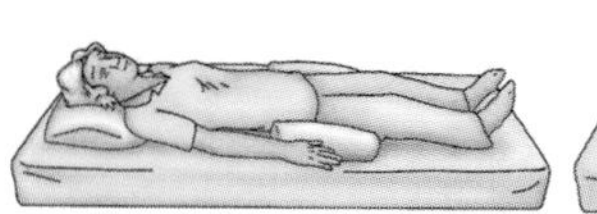

3. lithotomy position

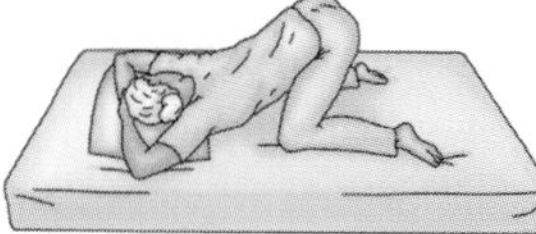

4. lateral position

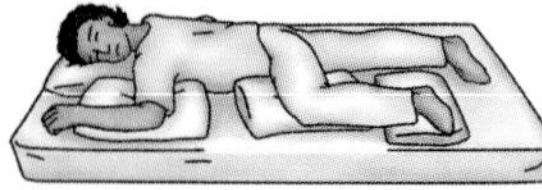

5. dorsal recumbent position

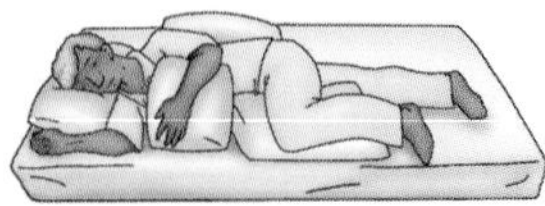

6. knee-chest position

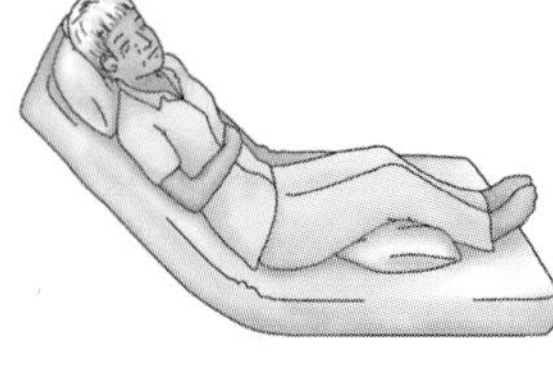

7. prone position

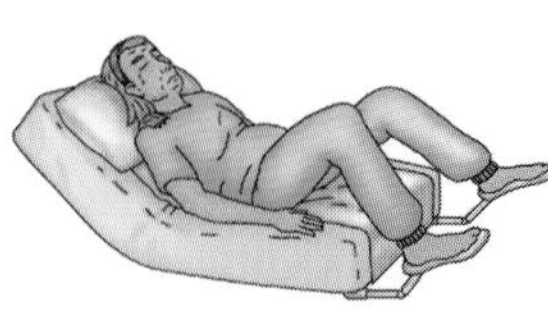

8. Sims' position

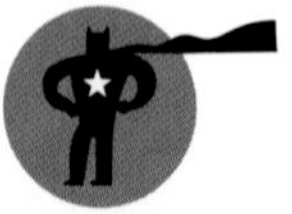

Star Student Central

1. Do you have any ideas about how to make the lives of residents in facilities more involved, active, and enjoyable? Write down at least three interesting ideas that might improve the lives of residents everywhere. Make each idea simple and inexpensive, with the goal being to show that you care about the residents.

2. Consider the experiences you have had either having a physical exam or going with someone to the doctor or other healthcare provider. Do you have pleasant or unpleasant memories of any of these experiences? Make two columns on a notepad and begin thinking about things you liked and disliked about your visits to these places. List at least three to five good things the office staff did to help make you or someone else feel more comfortable. Then make a list of three to five things that you did not like about the appointment. Examine the practices of other places and look at the good and bad things you have seen. You can learn from these experiences.

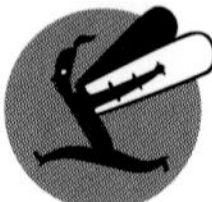

You Can Do It Corner!

1. Name seven questions families might ask when choosing a facility. (LO 2)
2. Name five ways you can assist your residents with their emotional adjustment to a new facility. (LO 3)
3. Identify the type of bed to have ready if a resident is to arrive on a stretcher. (LO 4)
4. How should you refer to the resident and her family members at the first meeting? (LO 4)
5. During orientation of the resident, name at least four things you need to orient the new person to the new home. (LO 4)
6. Identify four possible problems to consider when trying to ensure the safety of a new resident. (LO 4)
7. What are some changes residents may have made before moving into a long-term care facility? (LO 3)
8. Name at least six responsibilities of a nursing assistant during a physical exam. (LO 5)
9. During the transfer of a resident, list three important things to remember to do when you arrive at the new unit. (LO 7)
10. During the transfer of a resident outside of the facility or the discharge of a resident, you have been asked to bring the resident to the family's vehicle. Identify your responsibilities once you

reach the vehicle. When does your responsibility for this resident officially end? (LO 9)

11. What are two positions that can never be used without a doctor's order? (LO 6)
12. List two signs that a resident may leave a facility AMA. (LO 10)
13. What should you do if a family member tells you any important information during a discharge? (LO 9)

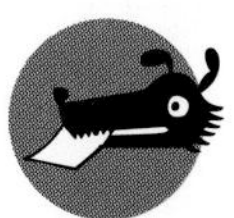

Star Student's Chapter Checklist

1. I have read my textbook chapter.
2. I have reviewed my own "Pocketful of Terms."
3. I have listened to my tutor tape.
4. I have reviewed and highlighted my class notes.
5. I have read and completed any handouts from this chapter.
6. I have completed "The Finish Line."
7. Star Time! Choose your reward!

15

Creating a Comfortable Room: Bedmaking and Unit Care Skills

Look Like a Star!

Look at the **Learning Objectives** and **The Finish Line** before you begin reading this chapter.

Look at your pocket calendar.
With your pencil, put a bracket (   ) around a study period every single day.

Look at your homework for this chapter.
Plug each piece of homework into a certain time slot.

Look at the **Star Student's Chapter Checklist** at the end of this chapter. Check off each item as it is completed.

"Egyptian Proverb:
The worst things:
To be in bed and sleep not
To want for one who comes not
To try to please and please not."

F. Scott Fitzgerald, 1896-1940

"Oh it's nice to get up in the mornin'/But it's nicer to lie in bed."

Sir Harry Lauder, 1870-1950

Learning Objectives

1. **Spell and define all STAR words.**
2. **Discuss the importance of rest.**
3. **Define "insomnia" and describe five types of sleep disorders.**
4. **Identify six factors that can affect your resident's ability to sleep.**
5. **List standard unit equipment and discuss "The Five Steps to Quality Unit Care."**
6. **Explain the four kinds of facility beds and discuss "The Art of Bedmaking I and II."**
7. **Summarize twelve steps in unit cleaning.**

Successfully perform these Practical Procedures

Making the Closed Bed

Making the Open Bed

Turning a Resident to One Side

Making the Occupied Bed

Making the Surgical/Stretcher Bed

Alcmaeon: One Theory About the Nature of Sleep

In the 6th century, medicine was taught in places where teachers, students, and philosophers gathered together. Crotona was one of these places, or "medical schools." Crotona was in Sicily, south of Italy. Alcmaeon was one of the teachers at the Crotona school. He believed that harmony inside the body would maintain health. He thought that the cause of disease was a change in the harmony of the body.

He also had interesting ideas about when sleep occurs. He thought that sleep was something that occurred when the blood vessels of the brain were filled. When the blood drained out of the brain, the person would awaken.

1 Spell and define all STAR words.

biorhythms: natural rhythms or cycles in bodily functions.

Chux: a name brand for small, absorbent pads placed beneath residents to protect furniture or linen.

circadian rhythm: the 24-hour day-night cycle.

closed bed: bed completely made with the bedspread in place.

cotton draw sheet: half-sheet used to protect the bottom sheet and the mattress, and for lifting and moving residents.

incontinent: lack of voluntary control of urine or bowel movements.

insomnia: persistent inability to sleep.

mitered corner: military-style corner used to corner sheets on beds in healthcare facilities.

occupied bed: a bed made while the resident is in the bed; resident is turned from side to side in order to change the linen.

open bed: bed made with linen folded down to the foot of the bed.

parasomnias: sleep disorders.

rest: period of inactivity during which one's energy may be restored.

suction containers: containers, usually plastic, used to collect drainage from a body cavity.

surgical bed: bed made so that a person can easily move onto it from a stretcher.

unit cleaning: special cleaning methods used to clean a unit after a resident leaves the room due to discharge, transfer, or death.

unoccupied bed: a bed made while no resident is in the bed.

"The Mints and the Rose"

Upon checking into a nice motel, the couple walks slowly to their room carrying an enormous amount of luggage along with three little children who have been riding in a hot car all day saying: "Are we there yet?" every five minutes. They open the door to the room and walk over to the bed and immediately see a pink rose along with a mint on each pillow. This brings a sudden smile to each face; the children grab the mints, the Mom picks up the lovely rose, and the Dad sits down and smiles. So the end of a long, tiring day turns into a happy moment due to a tiny extra comfort, the mints and the rose.

You can positively affect your resident's ability to rest and sleep. You can do these kinds of thoughtful little things for your residents and your family members, too. One extra little kindness may make the difference between having a difficult time going to sleep, or falling asleep feeling comforted and safe.

2 Discuss the importance of rest.

Rest is a period of inactivity during which one's energy may be restored. Sleep and rest are two of our basic needs, as described in Chapter 8. We cannot survive long without sleep. Our bodies must have it to replace old cells with new ones and provide new energy to our organs. It is also believed that the brain gathers all things learned throughout the prior day in order to properly rest and store the information.

The study of the rhythms of the body is called biorhythmology. Our **biorhythms**, or our natural rhythms or cycles related to our bodily functions, are being studied by researchers to learn more about why people seem to have different sleep cycles.

Sleep in your genes?

Have you ever wondered why two children in the same family have totally different sleep cycles? During non-school times, one child wakes up early in the morning and falls asleep at 10:00 p.m. while the other wakes up sometime after 12:00 noon and stays up well past midnight. Some people believe this is not just by chance; our sleep cycles might just be in our genes!

The most famous biorhythm is the **circadian rhythm**. This is our 24-hour day-night cycle and usually appears in infants when they are about three weeks old. Infants who are about six months in age should have established a fairly regular sleep-wake cycle, if the parents are lucky.

3 Define insomnia and describe five types of sleep disorders.

The inability to sleep adequately is called **insomnia**. A person may have a persistent inability to fall asleep, might not stay asleep through the night, or may wake up too early in the morning. There are many different causes of insomnia. Ways to help your residents sleep better will be described later in this chapter. Some of the many reasons for the elderly developing sleep disorders, called **parasomnias**, are anxiety, fear, breathing difficulty, noise, or hunger or thirst. Some common sleep disorders are described below:

Parasomnias

Somnambulism: sleepwalking; resident needs protection; may not be aware of dangers

Sleeptalking: talking during sleep; usually a problem only when it upsets other people

Nocturnal enuresis (bed wetting): urination during sleep; affects more males than females, usually over age three

Nocturnal erections (penile engorgement): usually start with adolescence; does not affect sleep

Bruxism: teeth-grinding and clenching the teeth; may eventually cause headaches, jaw discomfort, neck aches, and tooth loosening

4 Identify six factors that can affect your resident's ability to sleep.

Many factors exist within a facility that may affect the quality of your resident's sleep. The more you pay attention to these factors and try to improve the situation, the better your residents will sleep.

Factors Affecting a Resident's Quality of Sleep

1. **Environment**: Your resident may have been used to sleeping with a mate or perhaps all alone while at home. It is a major change to adjust to a roommate. Even if your married residents sleep in the same room at the facility, their ability to sleep may decrease because they are no longer in their own home.

   Make sure the mattress fits your resident. Some tall people may require an extra-long mattress. An obese person may need an extra-wide bed. If it is possible to get a different style of mattress or pillow that better suits your resident, ask the nurse.

   Noise level and/or lighting can also affect a resident's ability to sleep. Noise should be kept to a minimum. The simple closing of a door at night might help the resident sleep better. Darkness is very important to some residents. Blinds or shades help darken a room for sleep. Other residents prefer to sleep with a light on.

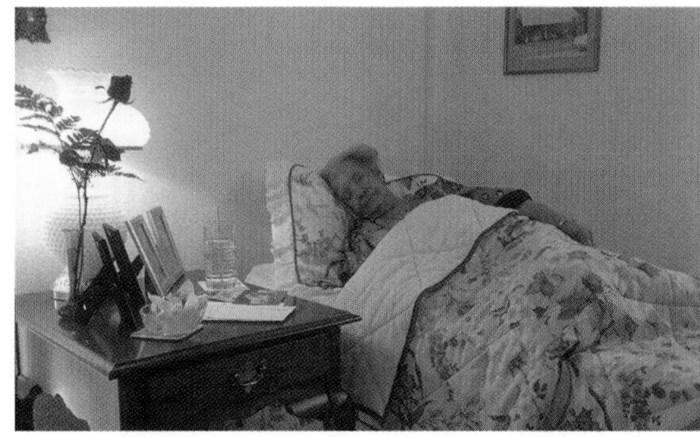

Figure 15-1. Some residents may prefer leaving a light on while sleeping or resting.

   Problems with odors and inadequate ventilation should also be taken into account. Older people may be **incontinent** (unable to control urine or bowels) or have problems with their GI systems that cause smells to linger temporarily. Diseases sometimes cause strong odors as well.

   When odors occur, staff should work together to try to locate the cause. Opening a window may work. Incontinent brief changes should be done as soon as possible.

   Temperature problems can affect sleep. Some people will want to be colder than others during the night. Help your residents by finding a comfortable temperature for everyone.

2. **Anxiety:** The resident may have a very real fear or anxiety about being alone if in a private room. It is possible your resident feels alone even in a semi-private room, when separated from a mate due to death or illness. The following things may help reduce anxiety:
   - making sure the resident is comfortable and has enough pillows and blankets
   - sitting with the resident for a short time, using touch and soothing words
   - offering back massages
   - making sure the resident is clean, has been to the bathroom, and has been given mouth care

3. **Illness:** A resident in pain or discomfort may be unable to get a good night's sleep until the source of the discomfort or pain is found. Because you are on the front line of care, you may see things the nurses do not. Be alert for any signs of pain or discomfort and pass this information to the nurses promptly.

4. **Aging changes:** Certain body changes that occur naturally with aging can prevent residents from getting a restful sleep. Many elderly people sleep

fewer hours (as few as six hours a night) and take longer to fall asleep. Hormonal changes also cause difficulty sleeping. Elderly people often have to get up in the night to urinate and then find it difficult to fall back to sleep. They may take frequent naps during the day, which also affects sleep at night. A lack of regular, moderate exercise affects sleep as well.

Nurses should always be made aware of any changes in the resident's sleep cycle. The nurse can then discuss with the doctor whether tests should be ordered to check on thyroid hormone levels, for example. If the resident frequently gets up in the night to go to the bathroom, nursing assistants can try taking the resident to the bathroom right before going to bed. A fluid restriction may be ordered after a certain time in the evening. Encourage residents to exercise moderately, following their care plan. Exercise often helps people sleep longer and more soundly.

5. **Dietary habits:** Some diets increase or decrease overall ability to sleep. Drinking or eating products with caffeine, such as soda or chocolate, may prevent sleep. Residents can limit themselves to caffeine-free drinks only. However, it is important to note that dehydration is a major problem in long-term care, and fluids should be encouraged. A resident's love of chocolate might be satisfied by offering a chocolate dessert only at lunchtime. Residents who have trouble falling asleep and can drink a glass of warm or cold milk, if they are not allergic. The special substance in milk, L-tryptophan, aids in falling asleep.

6. **Medications, alcohol, and drugs:** The nurse and doctor will need to assess the medications the resident is taking if a change in sleep cycle occurs. The nurse may alert you when a new medication has been started to watch for any changes and report them. You should be on the lookout for any evidence of unusual sleepiness or sudden inability to fall asleep. Should the resident suddenly fall asleep at breakfast, for example, the nurse would evaluate whether a new medication might have caused this problem.

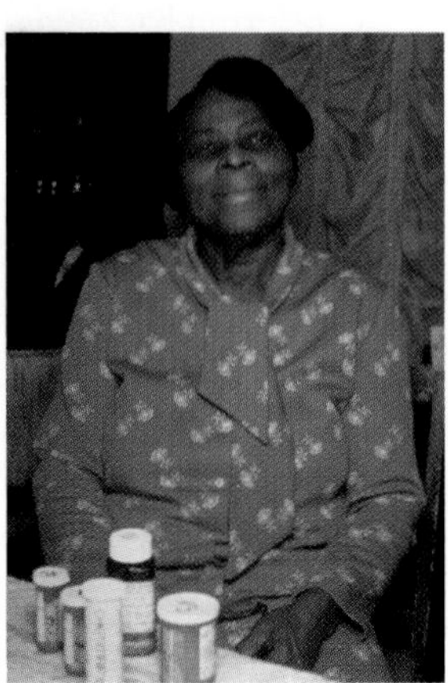
Figure 15-2. Medications can interfere with a resident's ability to sleep.

Some facilities allow residents to drink alcoholic beverages at mealtimes or smoke in certain locations outside the facility. Alcoholic drinks, like beer or wine, or smoking may cause the resident to have difficulty sleeping. Nicotine stimulates the body and may interfere with restful sleep.

Should your resident develop a problem sleeping, a care conference might be planned to try to solve this situation. Sometimes family members are asked to participate. Nursing assistants should always be asked to offer their valuable advice since they provide the majority of resident care.

5 List standard unit equipment and discuss "The Five Steps to Quality Unit Care."

The residents' units are their living spaces and their bedrooms all in one. It is extremely important that you always keep the units safe, clean, and neat, while keeping their freedom of choice intact. An example of the standard resident unit was first described in Chapter 10. Each unit may have slightly different equipment, because residents may bring furniture or other belongings from their homes. Personal items that bring the resident happiness should be encouraged. Box 15-1 repeats the standard unit equipment listed in Chapter 10.

Standard Unit Equipment Box 15-1

1. Bed
2. Bedside stand and possibly a dresser
3. Overbed table
4. One or two chairs
5. Washbasin for bathing
6. Emesis or kidney basin
7. Bedpan for both men and women and a urinal for men
8. Water pitcher and cup
9. Privacy screen or privacy curtain
10. Call system or call light

Once personal items are in place within a resident room or unit, you must NEVER move them without the resident's permission. Remember, this is the resident's home and you have no right to move these items unless there is a safety hazard. If a safety hazard exists, inform the nurse, and let the nurse handle the situation.

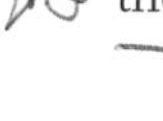

Making fun is not funny!

Making fun of any resident's personal items is inappropriate and cruel. This could be anything that might make the resident, a friend, or family member feel badly or be insulted. For example, you must never make fun of people shown in photographs or of a resident's special religious clothing or accessories. Any time a nursing assistant or any other staff member makes fun of residents or their belongings, it is verbal abuse.

The bedside stand is used for storing equipment like bath basins, urinals, and bedpans. Toothbrushes, toothpaste, combs and brushes, and other items may also be placed in the bedside stand but have to be kept separate from basins, urinals, and bedpans. Personal articles are usually in the top drawer; basins are generally placed in the top shelf in the section underneath and bedpans and urinals are in the lower shelf in the section underneath. A telephone and/or a radio, along with other personal items like greeting cards, may be placed on the top of the stand.

The overbed table is usually used for residents' meals whenever they do not eat in a dining room. It must be kept clean and free of clutter. Do not put bedpans or urinals on overbed tables because these tables are used for food. Right before mealtime, all overbed tables must be cleared of extra things so that the meal tray may slide smoothly onto it. A water pitcher and cup are routinely kept on the overbed table.

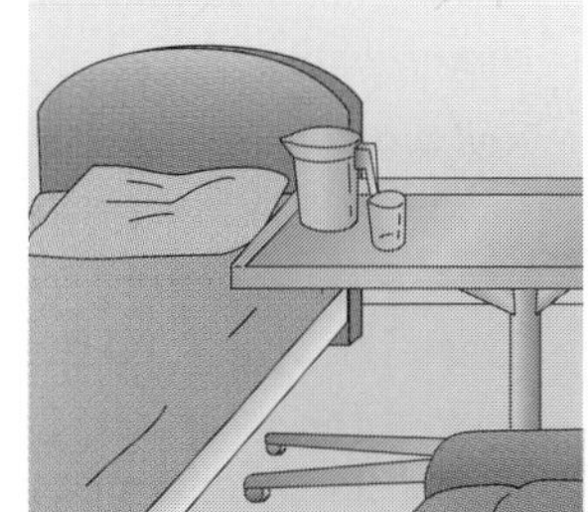

Figure 15-3. **Keep overbed tables clean and free of clutter.**

Watch those fingers and toes!

Have you ever been in a facility and had your toes jammed by a staff member moving the overbed table? Serious injury may be caused by carelessness with equipment. For example, if a resident with diabetes (a chronic illness that can cause poor circulation) is hit in the foot, the resulting injury may require an amputation (surgical removal of a body part) of the toes or foot. These things can happen, so it is best to take great care when moving any kind of equipment.

General care of the unit must be done whenever needed throughout the resident's day. You should clean up spills promptly. Bedpans and urinals must be cleaned and emptied after securing the residents. Crumbs should be removed from the bed right after meals. Some of these responsibilities listed below may not be a part of the nursing assistants' tasks.

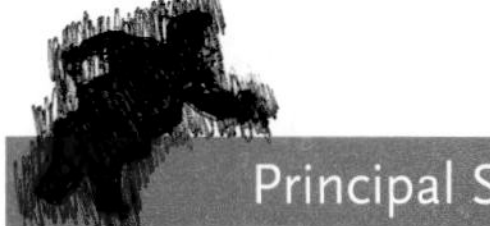

Principal Steps

The Five Steps in Quality Unit Care

Before leaving a resident's room and at least once a shift:

1. *Re-stock all resident supplies, including facial tissues, bathroom tissue, paper towels, soap, or anything else needed. If not your responsibility, write out a supply order for the appropriate department to fill.*
2. *Repair orders must be filled out for all resident equipment whenever needed. Check equipment daily to make sure it is working properly and not damaged in any way. Cords may be frayed or cracked; other equipment may not work, such as TVs or radios. Toilet or sinks may not work properly.*

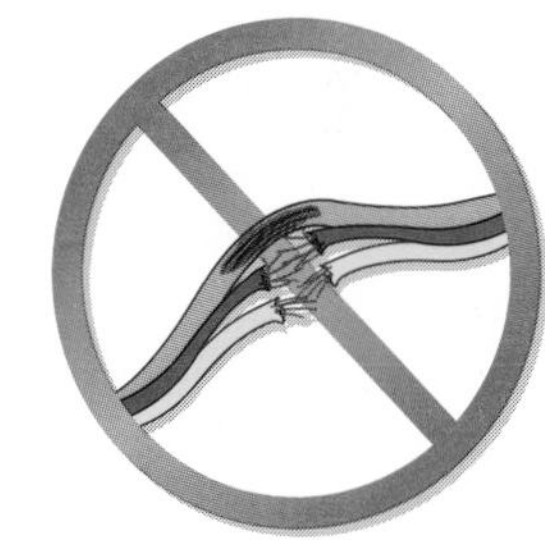

Figure 15-4.

3. *Refill water pitchers p.r.n. (when necessary) or on a regular schedule unless resident is N.P.O. (nothing by mouth) or has a fluid restriction. Promptly report to a nurse if a resident is not drinking his fluids.*
4. *Refresh the room. Using a paper towel wet with water (or other facility-approved cleaning fluid), wipe off any tops to the bedside stand or overbed table whenever they need light cleaning. When cleaning these items, move the damp paper towel away from you so as to not wipe dirt or dust onto your uniform.*
5. *Remove anything that might cause odors or safety hazards, like trash, clutter or spills. Dispose of any disposable supplies and trash. Dispose of and replace any equipment that is stained or has an odor. Label new item with name and room number according to facility policy. Replace call light within resident's reach.*

6 Explain the four kinds of facility beds and discuss "The Art of Bedmaking I and II."

The resident's bed is a place in which he or she will

spend a great deal of time. It is important for nursing assistants to understand that a neat, well-made bed can help the resident sleep better each night. In addition, possible complications can be prevented. A clean, neat, dry bed helps prevent skin breakdown and odors and increases overall comfort. Skin breakdown is an enormous problem in long-term care facilities and is covered in detail in Chapter 24.

There are four basic types of beds: closed, open, occupied, and surgical (also called postoperative, post-op, recovery, gurney, or stretcher bed). A **closed bed** is usually made for a resident who will be out of bed all day. It may also be made for a new resident who will be admitted to the facility. Closed beds are in empty rooms as well. A closed bed is turned into an **open bed** by folding the linen down to the end or foot of the bed. This makes it easier for a resident to get into the bed in the afternoon for a nap or at bedtime. You will also open a bed when a new resident has been assigned to that room.

An **occupied bed** is made for residents who have a doctor's order to stay in bed at all times. These orders may be called "absolute bedrest (ABR)," "strict bedrest," or "complete bedrest (CBR)." The resident must stay in the bed while you are making it. This type of bed may be completed more safely working with a co-worker. Follow the 5 Stars and 3 Rs when making an occupied bed. Remember to lock the bed wheels, and, even if you are working with a co-worker, only one side rail should be lowered at a time.

An **unoccupied bed** is just that. No one is in the bed while you are making it.

A **surgical bed** is made so that it can easily accept a resident who must return to bed on a stretcher. Residents on a stretcher are usually returning from some kind of treatment or possibly a visit to a clinic or hospital. Nursing assistants must use caution when transferring residents from a stretcher to a bed. The bed and stretcher wheels must be locked and the bed and stretcher must be close together during the transfer. (See Chapter 10.)

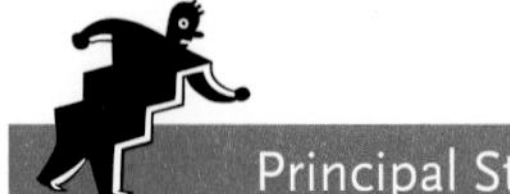

Principal Steps

The Art of Bedmaking I

Linen Handling

1. *Before getting clean linen, you must wash your hands. Gather linen in order of placement on the bed. This means first pick up mattress pad, then all sheets, blankets, bedspreads, and pillow cases. Note: If there is no clean linen available, see your supervisor immediately. Do not allow your resident to remain in or on soiled linen for any length of time.*
2. *Re-cover the linen cart if facility policy.*
3. *Carry clean linen AWAY from your uniform.*
4. *Bring linen into one resident's room at a time. Put it down after flipping the stack of linens so that the first item on the bed (mattress pad) is now on the top of the stack.*

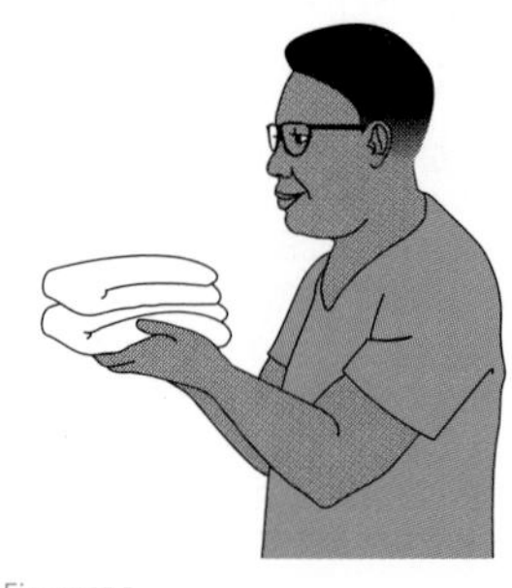

Figure 15-5.

5. *Never pick up linen from one resident's room and transfer it to another resident's room for any reason. You could spread dangerous microorganisms.*
6. *You may place clean linen on a facility-approved spot in a resident room. This may be the large chair in the room or the overbed table or bedside stand. Never place clean linen on the floor or on a contaminated area.*
7. *Make the appropriate bed using proper infection control principles and body mechanics techniques. Wash hands when required and bend knees and raise height of bed for back safety.*
8. *Never shake bed linen. This may spread airborne contaminants.*
9. *Roll dirty linen away from you as you remove it from the bed. Make sure you wear gloves if removing linen soiled with blood or body wastes, such as urine or feces.*
10. *Look at the sheets and bed linens carefully for any personal belongings like dentures, hearing aids, rings, watches, money, or other items. Remove crumbs from mattress.*
11. *Place used linen into a pillowcase or laundry bag, if facility policy, or into a linen hamper, if available. Linen hampers may be kept within the room or in a hallway or other area and should also be covered after use. Some facilities have rules regarding the placement of clean and dirty containers. Follow your facility policy regarding the placement of these containers. Never place used linen on the floor or on ANY piece of furniture within the room. Some facilities have rules for placing linen with blood or body fluids or linen that is heavily soiled in special bags. Wash your hands after working with soiled linens.*

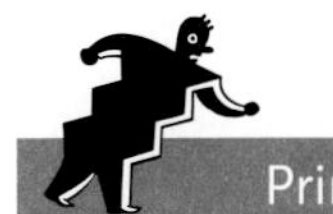

Principal Steps

The Art of Bedmaking II

The Safety and Comfort of You and Your Residents

1. *Remember, the "5 Stars and 3 Rs" apply to bedmaking, too. Make all beds using proper infection control and body mechanics techniques. Wash hands, and put on gloves when required. Bend knees and raise height of bed for back safety. Get help when necessary from one or more co-workers.*
2. *Change bed linen when wet, soiled, or when it is too wrinkled for comfort. This means change linen every time the linen requires it. Never take shortcuts with changing linen. Residents can develop pressure sores if left in wet, soiled, or wrinkled linen.*
3. *To save your energy, make one side of the bed completely and then go to the other side of the bed to complete your bedmaking. This prevents you from going side-to-side many times. You will have to make many beds in a day; it is worth it to save your energy.*
4. *Keep beds wrinkle- and crumb-free.*
5. *Remove lumps of any kind in the bed. Order or ask the nurse for a new mattress if a lumpy mattress cannot be smoothed. Lumps, crumbs, and wrinkles irritate skin and cause pressure sores.*
6. *Remove and change disposable pads, sometimes called* **Chux**, *whenever they become soiled or wet. Dispose of them according to facility policy.*
7. *A* **cotton draw sheet**, *sometimes called a "crib sheet" or a "half-sheet," is used to provide an extra layer of linen over the area of the bed that may get wet or soiled. See Figure 15-7. It is best not to use plastic or rubber draw sheets on residents' beds. Even when we are careful, these sheets or pads can rub against the resident's skin and cause sores.*
8. *With a manual bed (See Chapter 10), the handles that control the bed height, etc. must not be left out or up. Anyone could trip and fall over them.*
9. *Remember to follow the Five Steps in Quality Unit Care from Learning Objective 5.*

Figure 15-6. **Absorbent pads.**

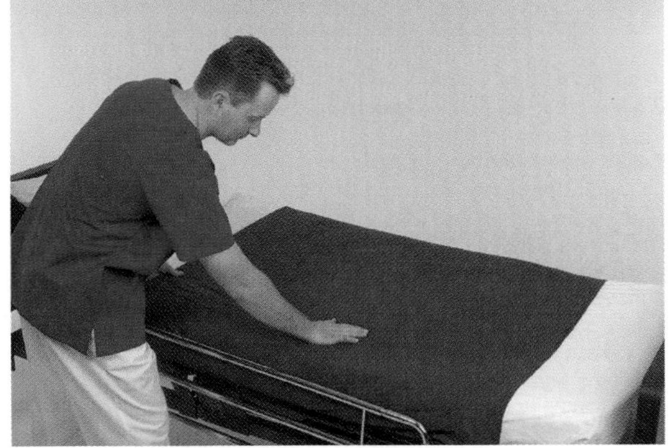

Figure 15-7. **A draw sheet.**

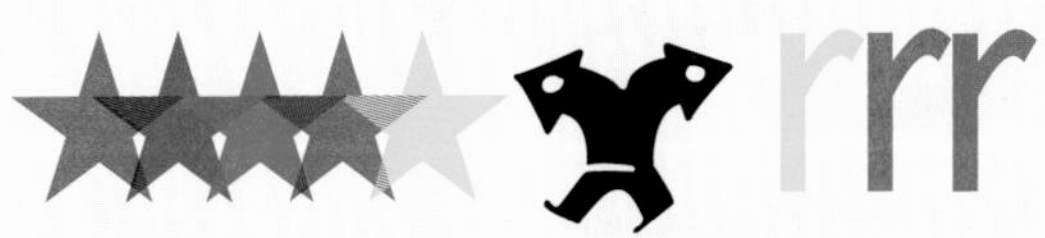

Beginning Steps

★ RESPECT
Knock first, ask and receive permission to enter a resident's room.

★ INFECTION CONTROL
Wash hands.

★ COMMUNICATION
Greet and identify the resident. Identify yourself. Explain the procedure, encouraging the resident to be as independent as possible throughout.

★ BED SAFETY
Lock bed wheels. Raise bed to safe working height. Lower one side rail if required.

★ PRIVACY
Provide for privacy by closing the door and covering the resident appropriately.

Ending Steps

★ RESIDENT SAFETY AND COMFORT
Secure the resident, lowering the bed, and raising the side rails if ordered. Check that the resident is comfortable and properly aligned.

★ PRIVACY
Remove any added privacy measures, such as a drape or a privacy screen.

★ ESSENTIALS
Place the call light, fresh beverage, and other items within reach.

★ COURTESY
Ask the resident if he or she needs anything else. Say thank you and goodbye.

★ INFECTION CONTROL
Wash hands.

r **Report** your care and any important observations to the nurse.

r **Record** your care and any important information/observations such as vital signs in the appropriate place.

r **Recheck** your resident for any changes as directed by the nurse!

Making the Closed Bed

Follow all standard and/or transmission-based precautions. Follow all rules for body mechanics.

Collect equipment:

- mattress pad, if needed • 1 draw sheet (or half-sheet)
- 2 large sheets or 1 large sheet and fitted sheet
- disposable pads (Chux) or "crib" sheet
- blankets and bedspread, if new ones needed
- correct number of pillow cases • pillow, if needed

1. Unit cleaning might have been completed before making the bed. If not, the bed linens must be removed and placed in the hamper or laundry bag before you make a new bed. Make sure that your supervisor or the housekeeping staff have verified that the bed should be made.

PREPARE:

2. Perform the "5 Stars."

3. Using handles, if available, slide mattress toward the head of the bed (HOB).

PERFORM:

4. Place the mattress pad on the bed using elastic at corners, if available.
5. Place bottom sheet on bed without shaking the linen. If using creased sheets, the sheet must be placed with the pressed crease EXACTLY in the center of the mattress. (Figure 15-8) The seams on both ends must be placed DOWN. (If using a fitted bottom sheet, place right-side up and tightly pull the ends over all four corners of the bed.)

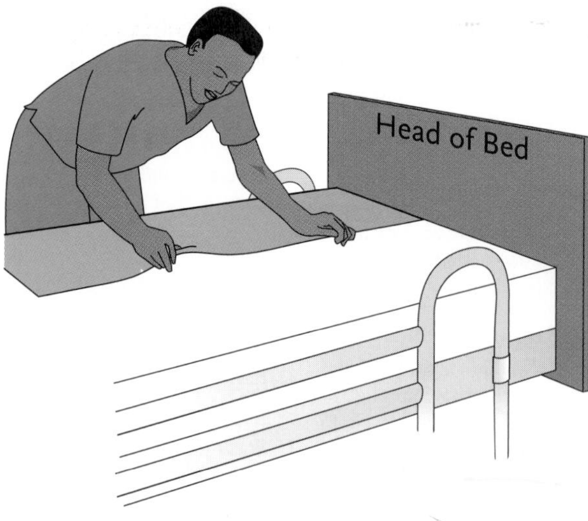

Figure 15-8.

6. Tuck the bottom sheet at the HOB.
7. Make a **mitered corner** at the HOB. This is a special corner used in facilities and in the military.
   a. Take your hand and, moving down about one foot (12 inches) from the HOB, pick up the sheet and place it on the bed. It should form a triangle (Figure 15-9).

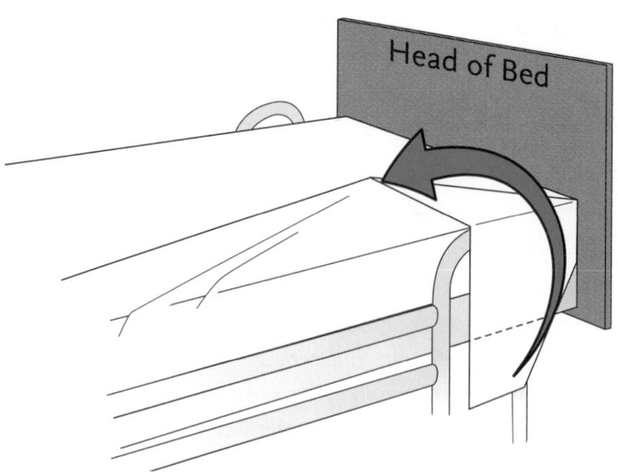

Figure 15-9.

   b. Tuck in the part of the sheet hanging off the side of the bed. (Figure 15-10)

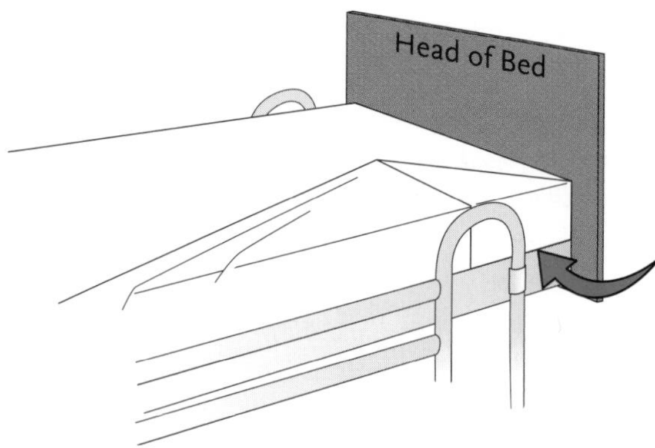

Figure 15-10.

   c. Holding the tuck tightly with one finger, fold down the triangle and tuck it in at the side of the bed (Figure 15-11). (Stop here if using Chux or draw sheet.)

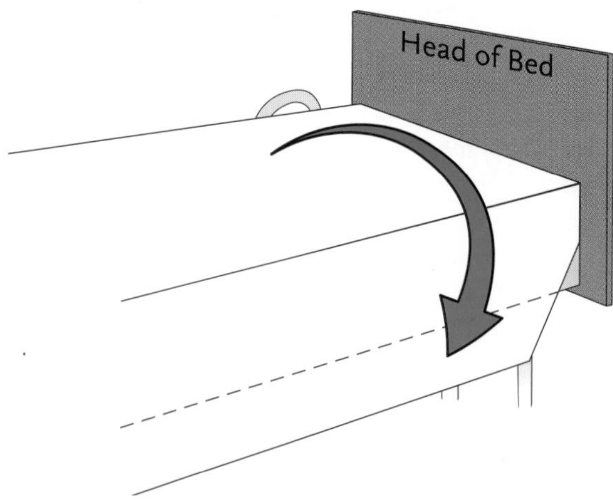

Figure 15-11.

8 If using Chux, place them in the center of the bed in the center of the bottom sheet. If using a cotton draw sheet, place the draw sheet on the bed over or under the Chux

with the draw sheet top about even with the resident's shoulders and the draw sheet bottom about even with the hips or knees. The pressed crease must be EXACTLY in the center of the bed (Figure 15-12).

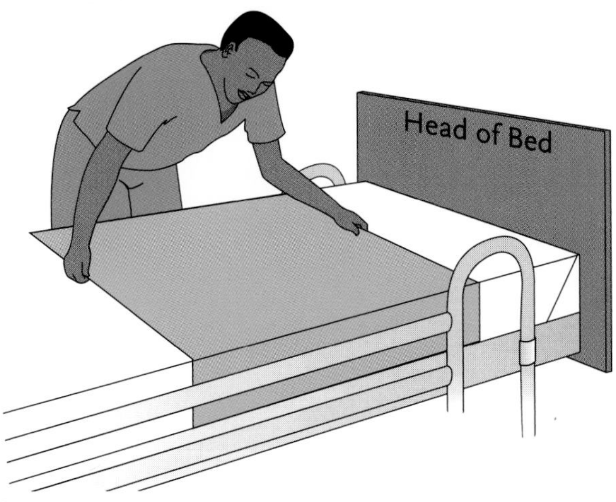

Figure 15-12.

TIGHTLY tuck the bottom sheet and the draw sheet TOGETHER along the side of the bed, moving from the HOB to the foot of the bed (FOB).

9. Place the top sheet on the bed with the pressed crease EXACTLY in the center of the bed. The seam must be UP. (STOP here if using a blanket and/or bedspread.)
10. Place the blanket on the bed RIGHT SIDE UP, making sure you have enough to tuck on both sides.
11. Place the bedspread on the bed RIGHT SIDE UP, making sure you have enough to tuck on both sides.
12. Now, tuck in all three: the top sheet, blanket, AND bedspread at the FOB. Leave enough toe room for comfort.
13. Still at the FOB, go to the side of the bed, make a mitered corner with ALL three items, the top sheet, blanket, AND the bedspread. (Figure 15-13) Tuck in the loose linen hanging over the side. Another tuck is NOT NEEDED. These hang down at the side.

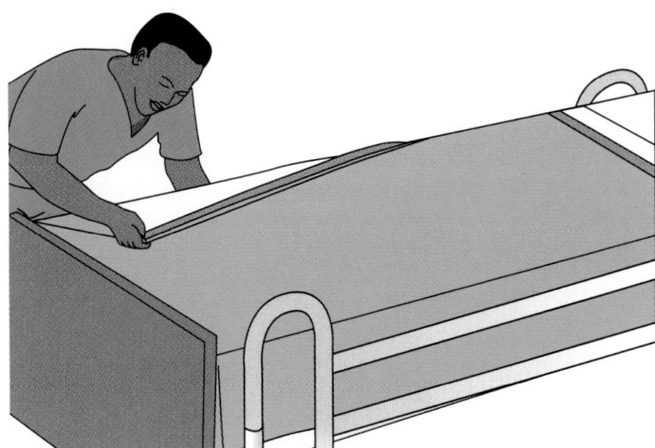

Figure 15-13.

14. Go over to the other side of the bed and fold the top linen to one side so that you may now tuck the leftover bottom linen.
    a. Make another mitered corner at the HOB, and tuck both the bottom sheet and the draw sheet all the way down the side of the bed (Figure 15-14).

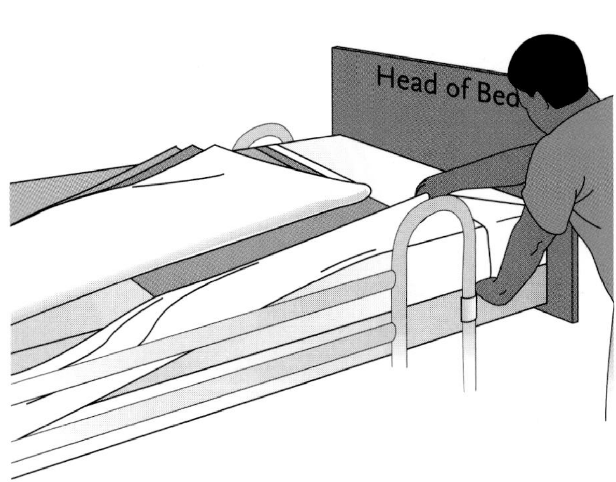

Figure 15-14.

    b. Going to the FOB on the same side, make a mitered corner with the top sheet, blanket, and bedspread.
    c. Make a 5-inch cuff at the HOB with the top sheet folding it over the blanket and bedspread.
15. Put the pillow cases on the pillows with the zipper or tag of the pillow on the inside. Do not touch pillowcase to your uniform.
16. Place pillows with opening AWAY from the door. Using both hands, make a neat fold in the open end of the cases (Figure 15-15).

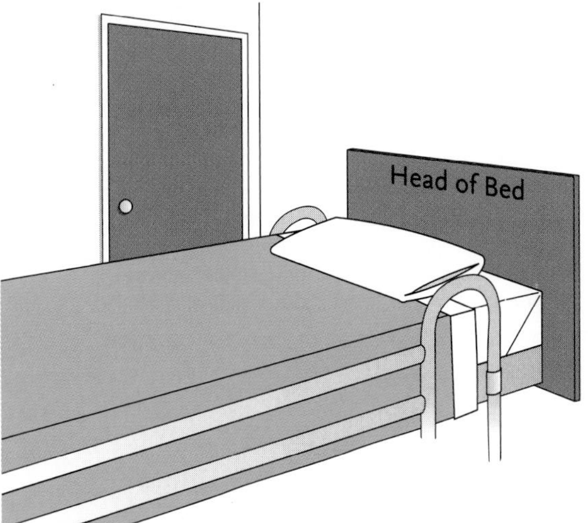

Figure 15-15.

17. The final bed will look like this (Figure 15-16).

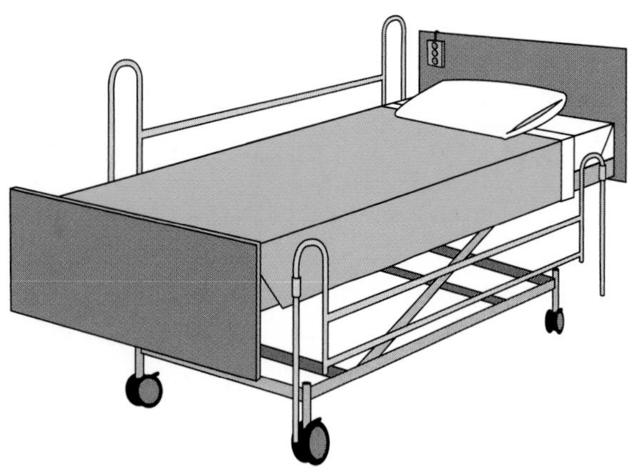

Figure 15-16.

FINISHING TOUCHES:

18. Before leaving room, make sure bed is wrinkle-free.
19. Perform the "5 Stars and 3 Rs."

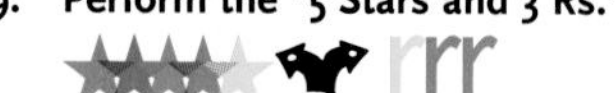

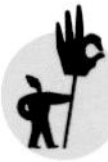

Seams and the Skin

Residents' skin may be very fragile. Even a tiny seam rubbing against the resident's skin can cause the skin to tear or crack. It is important to follow rules for seams on linens for residents.

When trying to remember the seam placement on the bottom and top sheets, you may find this helpful:

BOTTOM SHEET: *Seam DOWN = Bottom-DOWN*

TOP SHEET: *Seam UP = Top-UP*

And, a resident's cheek should not rest against a seam on a pillow.

Making the Open Bed

Follow all standard and/or transmission-based precautions. Follow all rules for body mechanics.

Collect equipment:

- mattress pad, if needed • 1 draw sheet (or half-sheet)
- 2 large sheets or 1 large sheet and fitted sheet
- disposable pads (Chux) or "crib" sheet
- blankets and bedspreads, if new ones needed
- correct number of pillow cases • pillow, if needed

PREPARE:

1. Perform the "5 Stars."

2. Make a closed bed, shown above.

PERFORM:

3. Stand at the HOB. Grasp the top sheet, blanket, and bedspread and fanfold them down to the FOB (Figure 15-17).

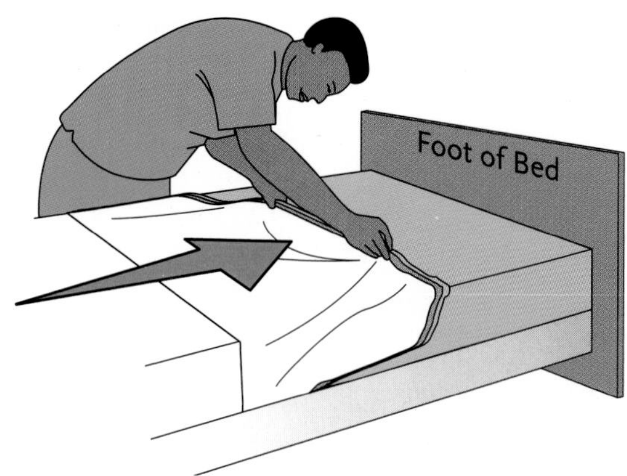

Figure 15-17.

4. Fold them back up toward the HOB (Figure 15-18).

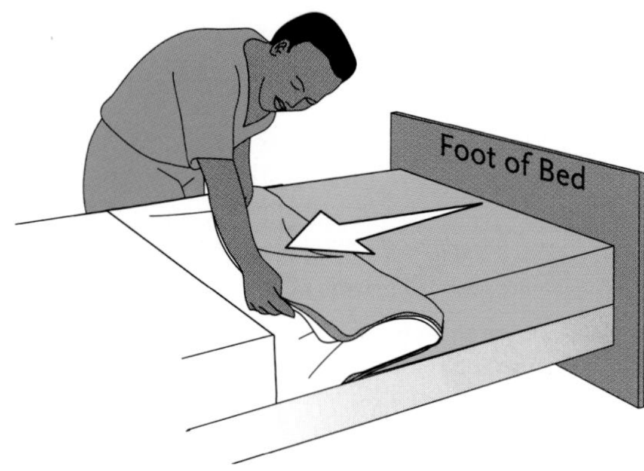

Figure 15-18.

5. Bring the cuff on the top linens to a point where it is one hand-width above the linen underneath. This is so that the resident will not grasp the linens and pull out the linen tucked in at the FOB.

FINISHING TOUCHES:

6. Make sure all linen is wrinkle-free.
7. Perform the "5 Stars and 3 Rs."

Turning a Resident to One Side

When making an occupied bed, the resident must be turned to one side at least twice during the procedure. This is a brief set of instructions on this procedure. This procedure is covered in much more detail in Chapter 17.

1. Perform the "5 Stars."

2. Remove and neatly fold the bedspread and blanket and place over the back of a chair.
3. Cover resident with used top sheet OR bath blanket.
4. When ready to turn resident to one side, first cross the resident's arms in the direction of the turn.

5. Cross resident's legs in the direction of the turn.
6. Carefully turn the resident toward you, protecting fragile arms and legs at all times.
7. Position the resident comfortably to one side with a pillow placed under the head. Take care not to catch arms or legs under the body or in the side rail. Raise side rail.
8. Cover resident with bath blanket or used top sheet.
9. When resident is comfortable, continue with step 5 in procedure on making the occupied bed.

Making the Occupied Bed

Note: Follow facility policy regarding the folding of linens under residents during this procedure. Lumpy rolls of linen may not be comfortable for residents for any length of time.

Follow all standard and/or transmission-based precautions. Follow all rules for body mechanics.

Collect equipment:

- mattress pad, if needed • 1 draw sheet (or half-sheet)
- 2 large sheets or 1 large sheet and fitted sheet
- pillow, if needed • correct number of pillow cases
- disposable pads (Chux) or "crib" sheet
- blankets and bedspread, if new ones needed

PREPARE:

1. Perform the "5 Stars."

2. Remove and neatly fold the bedspread and blanket and place over the back of a chair.

PERFORM:

3. Cover resident with used top sheet OR bath blanket.
4. Turn resident to one side away from you. Keep resident covered at all times with the top sheet or bath blanket (Figure 15-19).

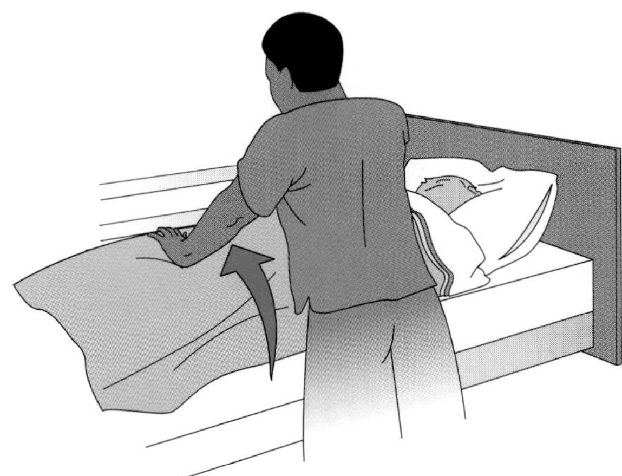

Figure 15-19.

5. Fanfold each piece of linen, one at a time, away from you and toward the resident. Check covers carefully for belongings like jewelry (Figure 15-20).

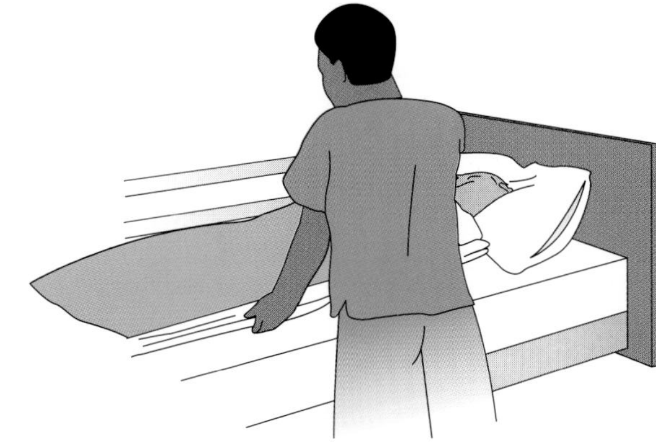

Figure 15-20.

6. Place the mattress pad on the bed using elastic at corners, if available. If not available, place the mattress pad with end at the edge of the foot of the bed (FOB).
7. Place bottom sheet on bed without shaking linen. This sheet must be placed with the pressed crease exactly in the center of the mattress. The seams on both ends must be placed down. (If using a fitted bottom sheet, place right-side up and tightly pull over all four corners of the bed.) Make a fanfold in the bottom sheet so that the linen forms a roll in the center of the bed against the resident.
8. Go to the HOB and tuck the bottom sheet at the head of the bed (HOB).
9. Make a mitered corner.
    a. Take your hand and, moving down about one foot (12 inches) from the HOB, pick up the sheet and place it on the bed. It should form a triangle.
    b. Tuck the part of the sheet hanging off side of the bed.
    c. Holding the tuck tightly with one finger, fold down the triangle and tuck it in at the side of the bed. (Stop here if using Chux or a draw sheet.)
10. If using Chux, place them in the center of the bed on top of the bottom sheet. If using a cotton draw sheet, place the draw sheet on the bed over or under the Chux. The draw sheet top should be about even with the resident's shoulders and the draw sheet bottom should be about even with the hips or knees. The pressed crease must be EXACTLY in the center of the bed. Form another roll with this linen under the resident. TIGHTLY tuck the bottom sheet AND the draw sheet together along the side of the bed, moving from the HOB to the foot of the bed (FOB).
11. Bring the side rail up and go to the other side of the bed. (Figure 15-21)

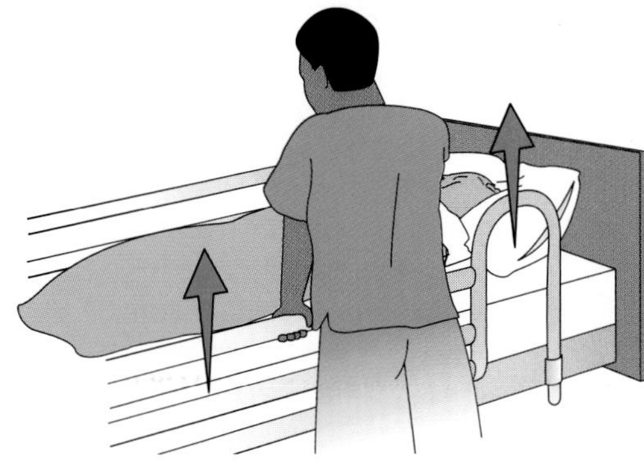

Figure 15-21.

12. Explain again to resident what next step will be. Lower side rail on the other side of bed. Turn resident carefully over fanfolded linen to other side of the bed (Figure 15-22).

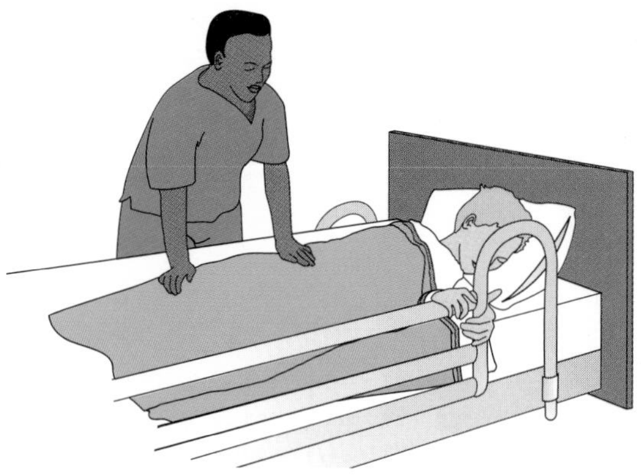

Figure 15-22.

13. Pull out the dirty linen and place in hamper or laundry bag. You must have the bag right next to you and the bed or you must raise the side rail while you place it in the hamper or bag. If using a hamper, wash your hands before you return and continue.
14. Pull the clean linen through as quickly as possible. Start with the mattress pad and wrap around corners.
15. Pull the bottom sheet and then the draw sheet and Chux through. Tuck and miter the bottom sheet at the HOB. Tuck the bottom sheet and the draw sheet together all the way down the side of the bed (Figure 15-23).

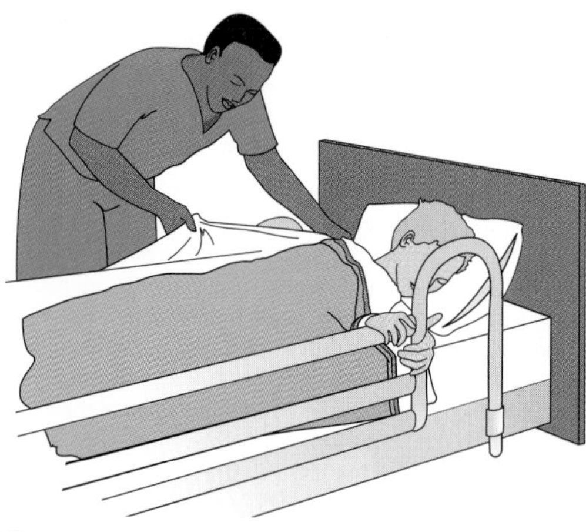

Figure 15-23.

16. Turn the resident so that she is on her back. Replace the top sheet OR the bath blanket with a new top sheet, making sure you do not expose the resident. Place the top sheet on the bed with the pressed crease EXACTLY in the center of the bed. The seam must be up. Allow enough room for toe comfort.
17. Place the blanket on the bed RIGHT SIDE UP, making sure you have enough to tuck on both sides.
18. Place the bedspread on the bed RIGHT SIDE UP, making sure you have enough to tuck on both sides.
19. Now tuck in all three, the top sheet, blanket and bedspread at the FOB.
20. Going first to one side of the bed, then the other, make another mitered corner with ALL three items, the top sheet, blanket AND the bedspread. Tuck in the loose linen hanging over the side and STOP THERE! Another tuck IS NOT NEEDED! These hang down at the side.
21. Make a 5-inch cuff at the HOB with the top sheet, folding it over the blanket and bedspread.
22. Change pillow cases with the zipper or tag of the pillow on the inside and making a neat fold in the open end of the cases. Carefully replace under the head of resident with the open end of the pillow case away from the door.

FINISHING TOUCHES:

23. Before leaving room, make sure bed is wrinkle-free. Check for comfort by straightening all linen, blankets, bedspreads, and pillowcases.
24. Perform the "5 Stars and 3 Rs."

 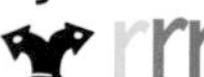

Making an occupied bed is a great opportunity to observe a resident's skin for signs of breakdown. Bed-bound residents are at great risk. You will learn more about skin breakdown in Chapter 24.

Making the Surgical/Stretcher Bed

Follow all standard and/or transmission-based precautions. Follow all rules for body mechanics.

Discuss the preparation for the arrival of a resident on a stretcher with the nurse. When preparing a room for a person returning on a stretcher, you may need to set up certain equipment in the room. Check with the nurse for instructions on gathering any extra equipment/supplies.

PREPARE:

1. Perform the "5 Stars."

2. Follow facility policy for making this type of a bed. The following is just one method for making a stretcher bed.
3. Make a bed just like the closed bed except DO NOT TUCK THE TOP SHEET, BLANKET, AND BEDSPREAD IN AT THE FOB.

PERFORM:

4. Fold the top sheet, blanket and bedspread down from the HOB and up from the FOB. (Figure 15-24)

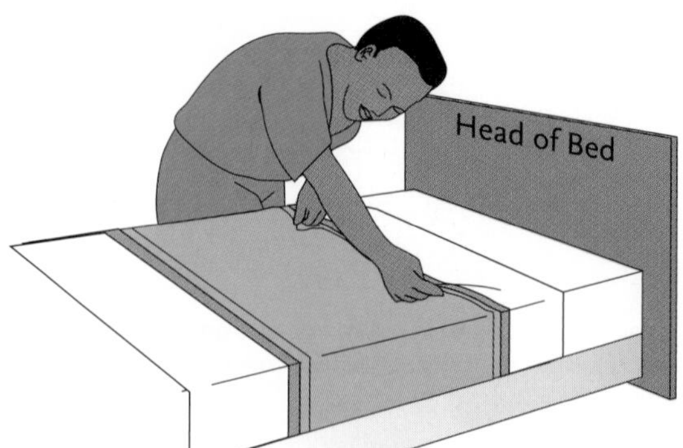

Figure 15-24.

5. **Go to the side of the bed. Grasp the top linens and fold over on both sides to form a perfect triangle. (Figure 15-25)**

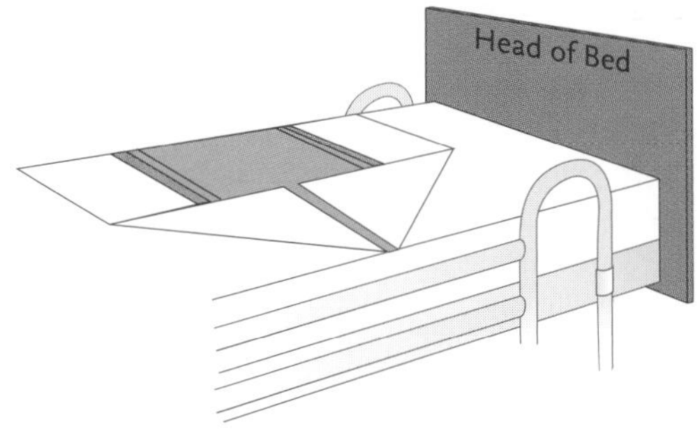

Figure 15-25.

6. **Fanfold the linen triangle into layers over to the opposite side of the bed. Leave the tiny tip of the triangle hanging over the linen so that it can be grasped quickly and pulled over the resident upon returning to the bed. This provides needed warmth quickly to the resident (Figure 15-26).**

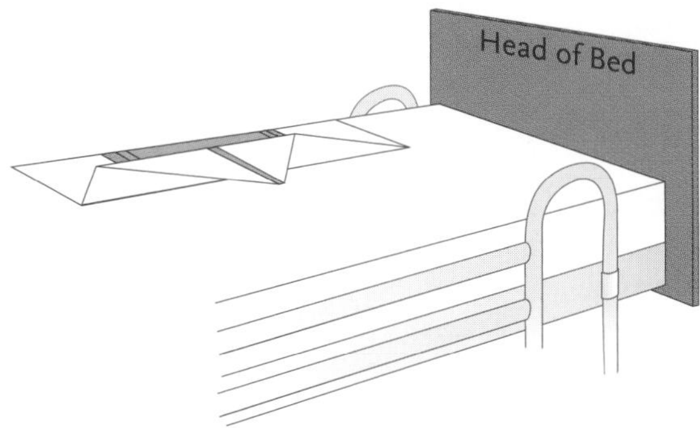

Figure 15-26.

7. **Put on clean pillowcase and place the pillow upright against the HOB. Some facilities ask that you place the clean pillow somewhere off the bed, such as on the overbed table or a clean chair.**

FINISHING TOUCHES:

8. **Move all furniture to make room for the stretcher.**
9. **Perform the "5 Stars and 3 Rs."**

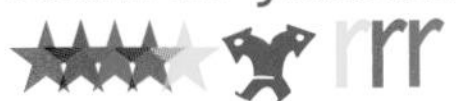

PLEASE NOTE THE FOLLOWING:

a. PLACE CALL LIGHT WITHIN REACH AFTER RESIDENT RETURNS TO BED.

b. LEAVE BED AT STRETCHER HEIGHT.

c. LEAVE BOTH SIDE RAILS DOWN!

Give prompt, compassionate care!

Some residents will unintentionally soil or wet the bed or a chair. Empathize with a resident in this situation. The odor from a soiled or wet bed is usually strong and there can be a serious danger to the resident's fragile skin. When you find that a resident has wet or soiled his or her bed, you must act immediately and change the sheets, along with all clothing and pads. Do so in a compassionate and respectful manner. Act professionally; never draw attention to the resident or tell other residents what happened. It is also very important that you clean the resident and make him feel comfortable again. When a resident is left in a wet bed for any length of time, it may be considered physical and emotional abuse, as well as neglect.

7 Summarize twelve steps in unit cleaning.

Nursing assistants may be responsible for **unit cleaning** and preparation for a new resident. Facilities will follow certain steps when cleaning units. For example, they may have a six-step process that must always be followed by staff. Whatever the policy at your facility, follow it carefully to protect you, other staff members, and future residents and visitors.

Remember that residents' belongings are very important to them. Consider for a moment the steps you take upon checking out of a motel or leaving a family member or friend's home at the end of a visit. It is important to be very thorough in order not to forget anything. It is best to keep this in mind every time you transfer or discharge a resident and have to do unit cleaning. Treat all residents' personal items with the utmost respect. Carefully follow facility policy regarding any forgotten belongings. Report the situation to your supervisor so that family can be notified.

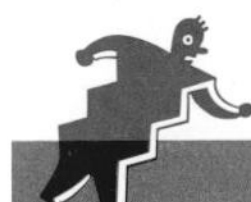

Principal Steps

Unit Cleaning

1. *Transfer or discharge the resident following facility policy, then wash your hands. (See Chapter 14.) It is important that you always carefully check the room for belongings before a resident leaves. If you find any belongings, notify the nurse so that they can be returned to the resident. Do not forget to double-check the closet, under the bed, all drawers including the small sliding drawer in the overbed table, the window sills, the bathroom, medicine cabinet, and behind the bathroom door!*
2. *Put on gloves, either regular or heavy-duty cleaning gloves, along with other PPE like a gown, following facility policy.*
3. *Remove all disposable and non-disposable equipment and supplies carefully, following your facility policy. These may include things like oxygen tubing,* ***suction containers*** *called canisters, facial tissue boxes, plastic*

water pitchers, and cups. Also remove towels, washcloths, and equipment that will be sent for cleaning.

4. *Raise the bed to a suitable height and lower both side rails to protect your back.*
5. *Remove pillow cases if pillows are still on bed. Some facilities use disposable pillows. The pillows are offered to the residents, who may accept or decline. If this is your facility's policy, dispose of leftover pillows in appropriate spot.*
6. *Carefully roll all bed linens away from you one piece at a time, watching for personal items. Remove linens and place in laundry bag or hamper.*
7. *Follow facility policy for cleaning the mattress and the bed itself. Make sure the area is well-ventilated when using strong cleaning solutions.*
8. *Clean all other unit items and equipment following facility policy. This may include items like the telephone, bed control and TV control, bedside stand, overbed table, chairs, bathrooms, windows and window sills, and ALL door handles. Write repair orders for any damaged or broken furniture.*

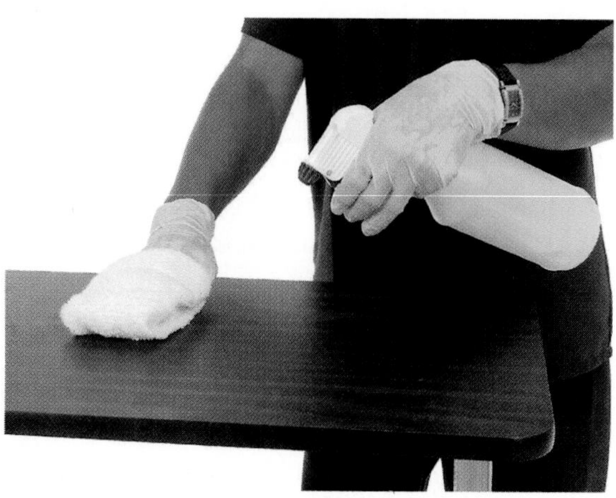

Figure 15-27.

9. *Remove all PPE and wash hands.*
10. *Prepare to make the new bed. Put on a second set of clean gloves when making a bed for a new resident. Make a neat, wrinkle-free bed. (See the Practical Procedure on Making a Closed Bed.)*
11. *Follow facility policy for placing equipment and supplies in the room for a new resident.*
12. *Wash hands.*

Summary

When nursing assistants work hard to ensure the comfort of their residents, residents may sleep better and wake up with more energy. This makes your overall job easier and more pleasant. Sometimes a few small comfort techniques can make the facility seem sunnier and a nicer place to live and work each day.

Proper bedmaking protects a resident's skin from preventable skin breakdown. Keeping residents' rooms clean and neat protects their health and allows for safe care.

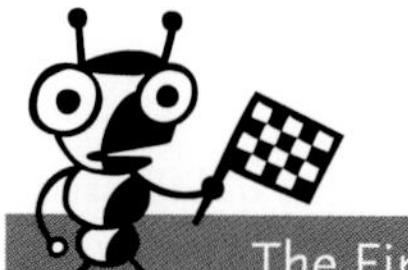

The Finish Line

What's Wrong With This Picture?

Look at the portion of the Principal Steps shown below. There are three errors included. Correct the three errors.

Linen Handling

1. *Get your clean linen and wash your hands. Gather linen in order of placement on the bed. This means first pick pillow cases, then blankets, bedspreads, sheets, and mattress pad. Note: If there is no clean linen available, see your supervisor immediately. You can only allow your resident to remain in or on soiled linen for an hour at a time.*

The definitions of the following sleep disorders are incorrectly listed. Write the correct definition for each sleep disorder.

Somnambulism: bed wetting

Sleeptalking: grinding and clenching teeth

Nocturnal enuresis: penile engorgement

Nocturnal erections: sleepwalking

Bruxism: talking during sleep

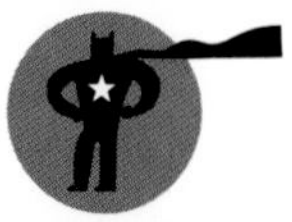

Star Student Central

1. Contact the hospitality director of a major hotel

in your area. Ask them what their beliefs are regarding the comfort of their guests. Write down any good ideas and tips and bring them in to share with your class.

2. Contact a local sleep center or sleep clinic. Arrange for a visit to the center and collect pamphlets about sleep that might be helpful to your class.

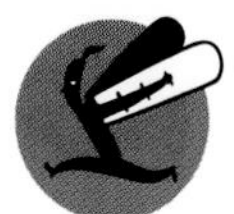

You Can Do It Corner!

1. List the five steps to quality unit care. (LO 5)
2. Name and explain at least eight of the "rights" to a good night's sleep. (LO 4)
3. Why is it important that linen always be changed when it is wet, damp, or soiled? (LO 6)
4. What are some reasons our bodies must have sleep? (LO 2)
5. List six factors that may improve your resident's ability to sleep. (LO 4)
6. What is insomnia? (LO 3)
7. What two things does a clean, neat, dry bed help prevent? (LO 6)
8. List six tips to improve a resident's ability to sleep. (LO 4)
9. Clean linen is never transferred from one resident room to another resident room, even when you are short of linen. Why not? (LO 6)
10. List twelve steps in unit cleaning. (LO 7)

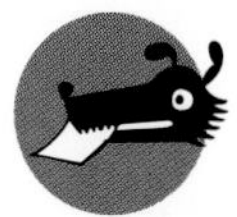

Star Student's Chapter Checklist

1. I have read my textbook chapter.
2. I have reviewed my own "Pocketful of Terms."
3. I have listened to my tutor tape.
4. I have reviewed and highlighted my class notes.
5. I have read and completed any handouts from this chapter.
6. I have completed "The Finish Line."
7. Star Time! Choose your reward!

16

Your Role:
The Vital Signs

Look Like a Star!

Look at the Learning Objectives and The Finish Line before you begin reading this chapter.

Look at your pocket calendar.
With your pencil, put a bracket ( ) around a study period every single day.

Look at your homework for this chapter.
Plug each piece of homework into a certain time slot.

Look at the Star Student's Chapter Checklist at the end of this chapter. Check off each item as it is completed.

"The same heart beats in every human breast."

Matthew Arnold, 1822-1888

"Once Antigones was told his son was ill, and went to see him. At the door he met some young beauty. Going in, he sat down by the bed and took his pulse. 'The fever,' said Demetrius, 'has just left me.' 'Oh, Yes,' replied the father, 'I met it going out at the door.' "

Plutarch, A.D. 46-120

Learning Objectives

1. Spell and define all STAR words.
2. Discuss the relationship of vital signs to health and well-being.
3. Name six factors that affect body temperature.
4. Identify five symptoms of a fever.
5. Compare the two temperature scales.
6. Identify the four sites on the body that are used for measuring temperature.
7. Identify the four main types of thermometers.
8. Describe three types of glass thermometers and explain the care of a glass thermometer.
9. List reasons an oral temperature should not be taken and perform taking a temperature at each of the four sites.
10. Identify the seven primary pulse sites and the most commonly used site.
11. List eight factors affecting pulse rate and three things to observe when taking a pulse.
12. Explain the apical pulse and the pulse deficit.
13. Identify three observations to record when taking respirations.
14. Identify nine factors that will affect blood pressure and two things to observe when taking blood pressure.
15. Identify the device used to take a blood pressure reading.
16. Describe how to recognize pain and list seven measures used to manage pain.
17. Explain the primary reasons to check a resident's neurological signs.

Successfully perform these Practical Procedures

Cleaning a Glass Thermometer

Taking an Oral Temperature using a Glass, Electronic, or Digital Thermometer

Taking a Tympanic Temperature

Taking an Axillary Temperature using a Glass, Electronic, or Digital Thermometer

Taking a Rectal Temperature using a Glass or Electronic Thermometer

Taking the Radial Pulse

Taking the Apical Pulse

Taking the Pedal Pulse

Taking the Apical-Radial or Apical-Pedal Pulse

Counting Respirations

Taking Blood Pressure

Observing Neurological Signs

René Théophile Hyacinthe Laënnec: The Invention of the Stethoscope

In 1816, René Théophile Hyacinthe Laënnec had difficulty hearing the heartbeat of a woman of great size. He solved the problem creatively. Using a rolled piece of paper, he placed his ear to one end of the paper and placed the other end of the paper over the heart. He realized he could actually hear the heartbeat! This ability to hear the beat of the heart so clearly was the beginning of what we now call the stethoscope.

1 Spell and define all **STAR** words.

apical pulse: the number of heartbeats heard when using a stethoscope on the left side of the chest under the nipple.

apnea: the absence of breathing; may be temporary and is due to a physical problem.

axilla: the armpit (axillae: plural form, meaning the armpits).

axillary: pertaining to the axilla or the armpit.

blood pressure: a measurement of the pressure of the blood on the walls of the arteries in the body.

BPM: beats per minute.

brachial pulse: the pulse in the upper arm; used to take the blood pressure in the arm.

bradycardia: a slow heart rate; under 60 beats per minute (BPM).

Celsius: official scientific name for the centigrade temperature scale; on this scale the boiling point of water is 100 degrees and the freezing point of water is 0 (zero) degrees.

centigrade: thermometer divided into 100 degrees.

Cheyne-Stokes respiration: a type of respiration where a person will have periods of apnea lasting at least 10 seconds along with alternating periods of rapid, deep breathing and slow, shallow breathing.

diastolic blood pressure: the pressure of the blood on the walls of the arteries when the heart is not contracting or when the heart is relaxed or at rest; this occurs between heartbeats.

dyspnea: difficulty breathing.

eupnea: normal respirations.

expiration: when air is removed from the lungs during breathing.

Fahrenheit: a temperature scale where the boiling point of water is 212 degrees and freezing point of water is 32 degrees.

inspiration: when air is brought into the lungs during breathing.

insulation: a material that prevents heat from being allowed into or out of a structure.

irregular: not steady; not following an even pattern.

legal jeopardy: the state of possibly being liable, or possibly being held legally responsible for some act.

orthopnea: when a person can only breathe while sitting up or in a standing position.

pedal pulse (also called dorsalis pedis pulse): the pulse used to assess blood circulation in the lower extremities; located on the top of the foot.

pinna: the auricle of the ear, the part of the ear on the outside of the body.

probe cover: a hard plastic sheath used to cover the probe on an electronic thermometer.

radial pulse: the pulse used most often to count the heartbeat; found on a spot over the radial artery in the arm at the wrist; located on the thumb-side of the body.

rectal: pertaining to the rectum.

regular: steady; following an even pattern.

sheath: a protective cover fitting over something.

sphygmomanometer: a device used to measure the blood pressure.

stethoscope: an instrument used by people in the healthcare field to hear sounds produced inside the human body, like the heartbeat or pulse, breathing sounds, or bowel sounds.

systolic blood pressure: the pressure of the blood on the walls of the arteries when the heart is contracting, or working to pump the blood out from the left ventricle into the body through the aorta.

tachycardia: fast heartbeat; over 100 beats per minute.

tachypnea: rapid respirations.

thermometer: a device used for measuring the amount of heat or cold.

thermostat: an automatic device for regulating temperature.

tympanic: pertaining to the tympanum or the middle ear.

2 Discuss the relationship of vital signs to health and well-being.

The vital signs are temperature, pulse, respiration, and **blood pressure**. Vital signs are very important readings that can tell healthcare providers whether the body is in a state of health and well-being or illness. When people are asked whether they go to the doctor each year for an annual check-up, some people may respond: "Why? My body will tell me if there is a problem and THEN I will go to the doctor." Unfortunately, it may be too late by the time your body "announces" there might be a problem. Problems such as high blood pressure, also known as the "silent killer," and certain kinds of heart problems, are sometimes only found during a visit to the doctor's office. You cannot look at another person and be able to tell if he has high blood pressure or an irregular pulse. Sometimes even a fever can hide itself. The first sign of a fever may be when a caregiver is washing a resident's face and notes that the resident's forehead is quite warm.

Think for a moment about the vehicles we drive. Cars and trucks require periodic safety checks in order to keep them running smoothly. If we don't take care of our vehicles, we may not be able to rely on them for regular transportation. Our bodies are a little like these cars. We need to rely on our bodies to be healthy! Good health allows us to move from day to day and week to week being able to fulfill all of our responsibilities.

Nurses and doctors are always on the lookout for signs of a problem or an illness. Sometimes the first sign that a person is ill is a change in the vital signs. When one or more vital signs is too high or too low, it signals a potential health problem.

Measuring weight was covered in Chapter 14. Weight is often measured along with vital signs, not just at admission. Unintended weight loss is a big concern and is often a sign of a health problem. Monitoring and promptly reporting any weight loss, no matter how slight, is a very important part of the regular care of all residents.

Residents usually have vital signs checked periodically throughout the day. This is important because it helps in recognizing changes, even small ones. When recording your residents' vital signs, know your facility's policy on how to document them in the chart.

3 Name six factors that affect body temperature.

Body temperature is controlled by the hypothalamus in the brain. The hypothalamus regulates our body temperature by carefully balancing the amount of heat the body makes with the amount of heat the body loses. The hypothalamus is considered to be our body's **thermostat**, keeping our temperature set at a certain point. A normal temperature is a sign of well-being. A low or high temperature may mean a resident has a problem or an illness. There are many factors affecting body temperature. Some of these factors include the following:

1. **The age of the person:** Our fat layer usually acts as **insulation**, protecting our bodies from heat and cold, like the insulation in the walls of a home or apartment. Elderly people normally have less of a fat layer in their bodies, so they may not be able to prevent heat loss. Poor circulation may also be a factor. Since blood circulation plays an important part in body temperature regulation, poor circulation may cause changes in body temperature. A common sign of poor circulation in older people may be cold feet.

2. **Amount of exercise:** The contraction of muscles stimulates the production of heat. Exercise, then, may actually increase body temperature. With permission from a doctor, exercise can be very important for overall health and well-being. However, elderly people should never exercise to a point where they are overtired or exhausted.

3. **Our circadian rhythms:** The circadian rhythm can affect body temperature, as discussed in Chapter 15. Average temperature readings change throughout a normal 24-hour day. People may have lower average temperatures in the morning and higher temperatures at night.

4. **Our emotions:** We show many emotions each day. Our emotions may cause our vital signs to change. Temperature may be heavily affected by anxiety because, during stress, our fight-or-flight response kicks into gear, causing certain hormones to be released into our systems. This hormonal shift may increase our body temperature.

5. **Illnesses:** Illnesses, such as infections, may cause an increase in body temperature. Some infections also cause dehydration, which occurs when the body loses too much fluid. When our body's "fluid levels" are too low, our body temperature may increase in response. Certain other illnesses, like diabetes, cause poor circulation and can also affect body temperature.

6. **A person's surroundings:** Sometimes the resident's room may be too hot or too cold, and may

influence body temperature. Healthcare team members may have the temperature of the resident's room adjusted if they believe a resident is uncomfortable. Residents should only be out in extremely cold or hot weather for very short periods of time. Residents may become chilled or overheated very easily. Drafts in a room may also increase the risk of chills. Residents may require extra blankets to help them stay warm in bed or in a chair.

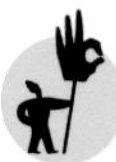

Am I hot or do I have a fever?

If a temperature is taken in the morning while the person is still in bed, the temperature may temporarily read slightly higher than normal. Extra heat may be kept inside the body, especially when we are dressed in very heavy pajamas or nightgowns and covered with a lot of blankets. When suspecting a fever in an adult or a child in the morning, it is a good idea to wait a few minutes and allow the person to get up, if possible, before taking the temperature. This will give you a more accurate temperature reading. If an important decision rests on a temperature reading, you want it to be accurate. You would not want a resident to go to an activity outside of the facility with a fever.

4 Identify five symptoms of a fever.

Residents who develop a fever may show many symptoms in addition to the temperature reading. Those symptoms include headaches, fatigue, muscle aches, and chills. The skin might feel hot to the touch and look flushed.

Residents with darker skin tones might show very subtle skin color changes with a fever. In this case, you may have to feel the forehead for warmth when suspecting a fever.

If you suspect a fever, always take a temperature. Fevers develop quickly. It is possible to catch an infection early and prevent complications from occurring.

5 Compare the two temperature scales.

Thermometers may measure in either degrees **Fahrenheit** (F) or **Celsius** (C). Fahrenheit and Celsius are two different scales that are used to measure temperature. Fahrenheit is a temperature scale in which the boiling point of water is 212 degrees and the freezing point of water is 32 degrees. The Celsius thermometer is divided into 100 degrees. Celsius is the official scientific name for the **centigrade** temperature scale. On the Celsius scale, the boiling point of water is 100 degrees and the freezing point of water is 0 degrees.

In degrees Fahrenheit (F), each long line represents one degree and each short line represents two-tenths of a degree. In degrees Celsius (C), the long lines represent one degree and the short lines represent one-tenth of a degree. In the United States, you might see the Fahrenheit scale used more often. In almost all other countries, the Celsius scale tends to be used along with the metric system of measurement.

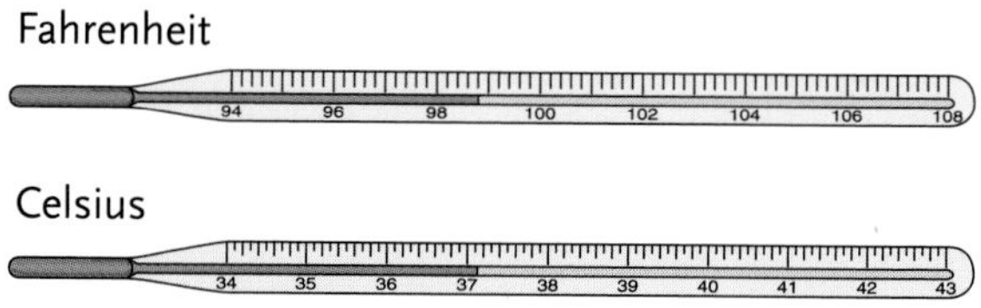

Figure 16-1. **Fahrenheit and Celsius thermometers.**

6 Identify the four sites on the body that are used for measuring temperature.

There are four main sites on the body for measuring a temperature: oral, **tympanic**, **axillary**, and **rectal**. The oral temperature is the most common site. The rectal site is considered by some to be the most accurate, while the axillary is considered to be the least accurate site. Box 16-1 identifies the various sites and normal ranges.

Body Sites for Measuring Temperature Box 16-1

1. mouth (oral)	NORMAL READING: 98.6 F/37 C
2. ear (tympanic or aural)	NORMAL READING: 98.6 F/37 C
3. underarm (axillary)	NORMAL READING: 97.6 F/36.5 C
4. rectum (within the rectum)	NORMAL READING: 99.6 F/37.5 C

7 Identify the four main types of thermometers.

There are four main types of thermometers: mercury glass, tympanic, electronic, and digital. The mercury glass, the electronic, and the digital thermometer may all be used to take an oral (in the mouth), a rectal (in the rectum), or an axillary (in the underarm or **axilla**) temperature. A tympanic thermometer is used to take a temperature in the ear. Disposable thermometers are used in some facilities; however, some doctors and nurses feel these are not as accurate as the other methods.

1. The mercury glass thermometer

A mercury glass thermometer may measure in Fahrenheit or Celsius. The mercury is inside a glass tube. When placed inside one of the temperature sites, body heat causes the mercury to heat up and expand within the glass tube. The mercury moves up the tube until it stops at the correct temperature.

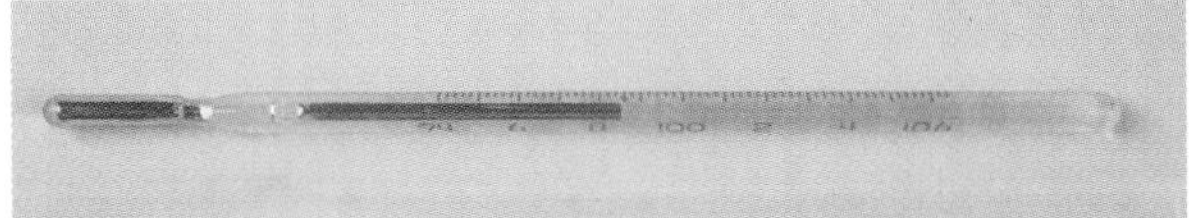

Figure 16-2. **A mercury glass thermometer.**

2. The tympanic thermometer

The tympanic or aural thermometer is used to measure the temperature reading in a person's ear. It works using a special sensor that detects heat from the tympanic membrane (eardrum) and is able to register the amount of heat on a tiny screen in a matter of seconds. Facilities generally like this style of thermometer because it measures the reading fairly quickly. However, some facilities ask that a reading be taken in both ears to reduce the risk of an inaccurate reading. It is also very important to follow the instructions for taking this type of temperature to try to be as accurate as possible. Ear injury is possible with this thermometer. Hearing aids may need to be carefully removed during this procedure. Ear wax may also cause an inaccurate reading.

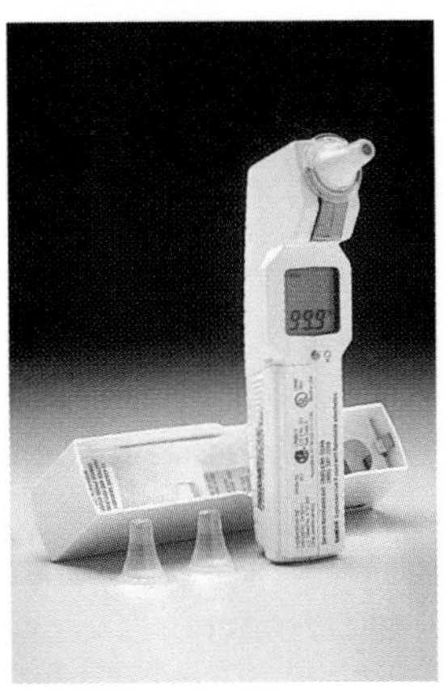

Figure 16-3. **A tympanic thermometer.**

3. The electronic thermometer

The electronic thermometer is a battery-operated device that is stored in a wall unit for recharging when not in use. There are many different styles of electronic thermometers, but most of them record the temperature reading in two to 60 seconds. A coiled probe that is color-coded blue or red plugs into the base unit. The red probe is used when taking a rectal temperature, and the blue probe is used for an oral or axillary temperature. The probe must first be covered with a disposable **probe cover** before use. The probe cover is used for a single resident and then carefully disposed of into a facility-approved container. Nursing assistants must NEVER use the probe cover on more than one resident.

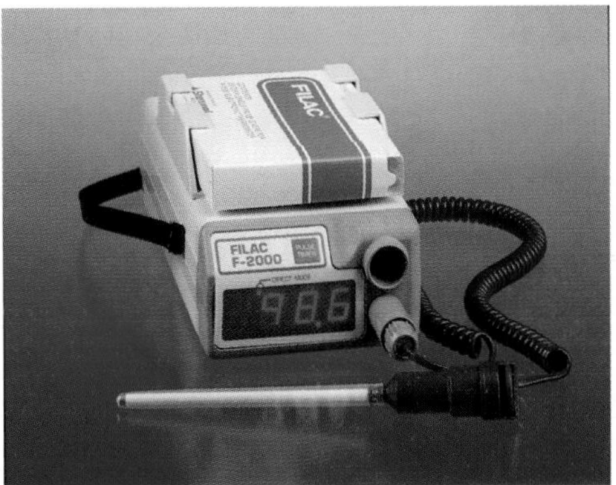

Figure 16-4. **An electronic thermometer.**

4. The digital thermometer

A digital thermometer is often the style used in the home. This style is easy-to-use and helps prevent the transfer of infection due to a disposable plastic **sheath** used to cover the probe. The sheath is used once and then disposed of in a facility-approved container. The temperature appears on a tiny screen after a period of about 60 seconds. Some units beep while others blink, and some register the reading without a light or a sound. These models are battery-operated and require that the battery be replaced periodically. Some may also have a small re-charging unit within the facility.

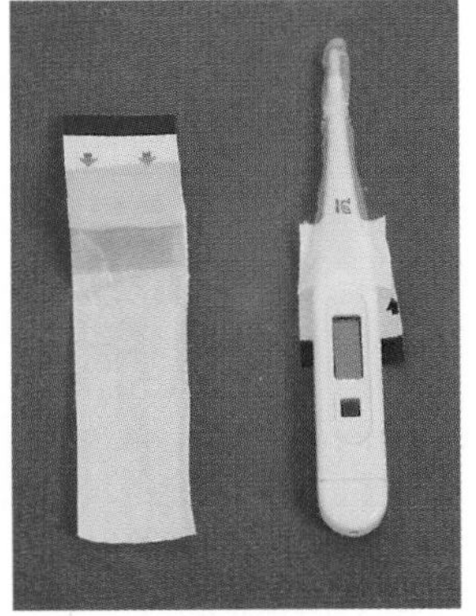

Figure 16-5. **A digital thermometer.**

8 Describe three types of glass thermometers and explain the care of a glass thermometer.

There are three types of glass thermometers. The oral thermometer, sometimes color-coded blue at one end, is used to take temperatures in the mouth or under the arm. The security thermometer usually has a stubby bulb shaped like a pear. The end of a security thermometer may be blue or green if used for oral temperatures, or red when used for rectal temperatures. The clear glass thermometer does not have any color coding. This type of glass thermometer may be used for infants or the elderly. Figure 16-6 shows the three types of glass thermometers. If you're dealing with a confused or agitated resident, never use a glass thermometer for an oral or rectal temperature. If in doubt, check with your supervisor.

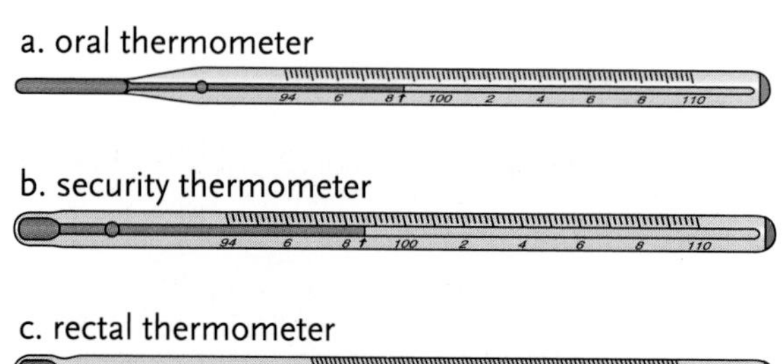

Figure 16-6. **a. Oral thermometer, color-coded blue. b. Security thermometer. c. Rectal thermometer.**

Glass thermometers need to be handled very carefully. Gloves should be used with disposable plastic sheaths for oral thermometers, because when you remove the sheath, your hands can come into contact with the body fluids from the mouth. Glass thermometers may also be very slippery and could drop and break. When mercury thermometers are broken, the mercury is dangerous and might have to be cleaned up by a toxic-clean-up crew. If a glass mercury thermometer breaks, you need to immediately notify your supervisor.

Glass thermometers should be cleaned after each use. You must follow your facility policy when cleaning mercury thermometers. Some facilities require a special disinfecting solution when cleaning glass thermometers. If soap and water are used to clean glass thermometers, the water used to wash and rinse the thermometers must never be hot. Use cool water to clean glass thermometers because hot water might heat the mercury and cause the glass to break.

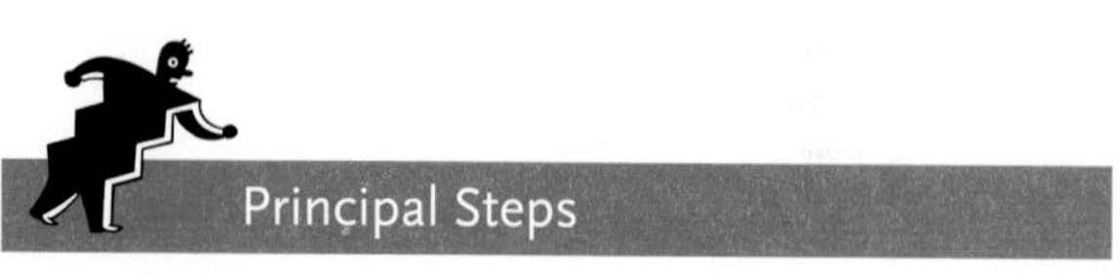

Safe Use of a Glass Thermometer

1. *Look at the thermometer before picking it up; it may be chipped or cracked.*
2. *When using a plastic sheath, body fluids from the mouth may get onto the nursing assistant's hands. Always put gloves on before picking up a glass thermometer.*
3. *Before using on a resident, carefully inspect again for chips or cracks.*

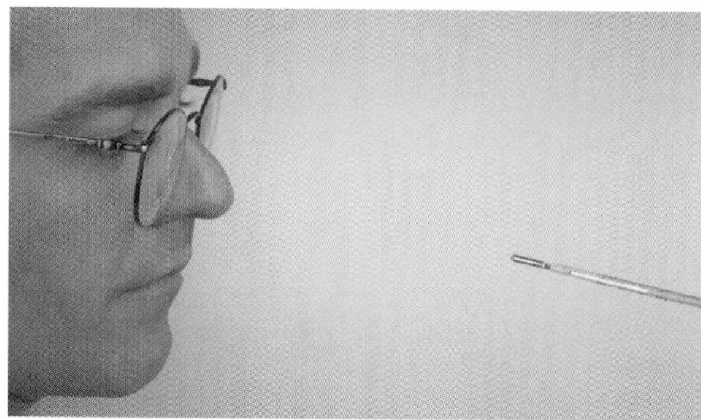

Figure 16-7. **Inspect the thermometer for chips or cracks.**

4. *Use only an oral thermometer (blue-tip or clear-tip) for oral or axillary temperatures. Use only a rectal (red-tip) thermometer for rectal temperatures.*
5. *Shake down the thermometer before applying a sheath (plastic cover). Hold it tightly while shaking to avoid dropping and breaking the thermometer. (See Principal Steps: How to Shake Down a Glass Thermometer.)*
6. *For oral temperatures, insert into the mouth bulb-end first, without hurting any part of the resident's mouth, teeth, or tongue.*
7. *For rectal temperatures, always lubricate the bulb tip of the thermometer before placing it into the rectum.*
8. *For rectal temperatures, insert the bulb tip only one-half inch for children and one inch for adults.*
9. *Hold the thermometer in place the entire time when taking oral, rectal, or axillary temperatures. Never allow the resident to fall back on a rectal thermometer.*
10. *Remove the sheath, discard in wastebasket, and wipe the thermometer using a tissue or alcohol wipe before reading the temperature.*
11. *Clean thermometer. (See following procedure.) Always shake down the thermometer when finished cleaning.*

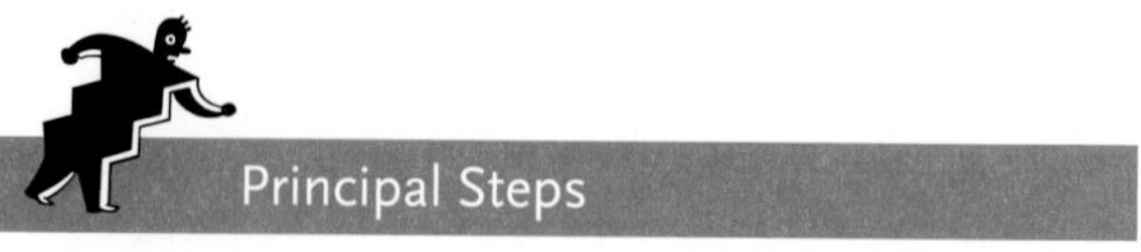

How to Shake Down a Glass Thermometer

1. *Before using and after cleaning, you must always shake down a glass thermometer. This prevents possi-*

ble errors when the next temperature is taken.

2. *Before or after a temperature reading, with gloves on, prepare to shake down.*
3. *Stand clear of people and objects when shaking down. Be careful not to poke yourself in the face or eye with the thermometer.*
4. *Hold thermometer firmly at the stem end with thumb and first two fingers and shake down using a "snapping" motion with your wrist.*
5. *Shake down until the mercury is below the first number on the thermometer.*

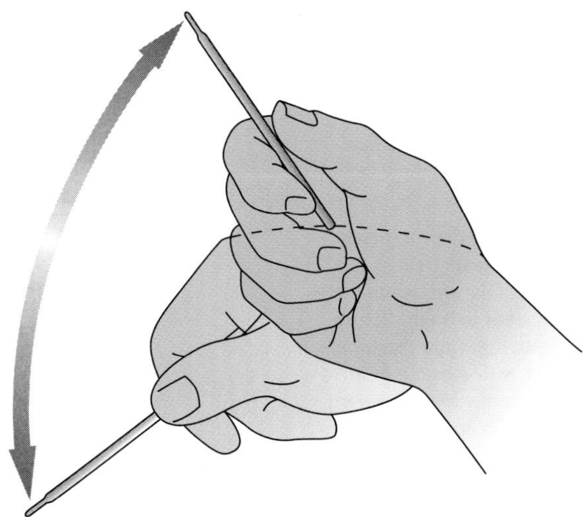

Figure 16-8.

Principal Steps

How to Read a Glass Thermometer

1. *Complete the procedure for Taking an Oral Temperature Using a Glass Thermometer.*
2. *Remove the sheath, discard in wastebasket, and wipe the thermometer from stem to bulb using a tissue or alcohol wipe before reading the temperature.*
3. *Hold the thermometer by the stem up to the light at eye level. Read the temperature at the number where the mercury stops. If you cannot see where the mercury stops, rotate the thermometer between thumb and index finger to find the mercury.*
4. *Always read a glass thermometer to the closest two-tenths of a degree. Each short line is two-tenths or .2, .4, .6, .8. A glass temperature reading is usually written in Fahrenheit (F) using even numbers.*
5. *If unable to read the temperature, ask another staff member for assistance. Never guess the reading!*

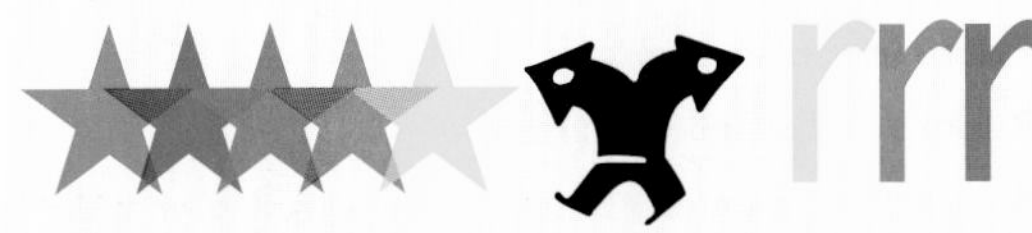

Beginning Steps

★ RESPECT
Knock first, ask and receive permission to enter a resident's room.

★ INFECTION CONTROL
Wash hands.

★ COMMUNICATION
Greet and identify the resident. Identify yourself. Explain the procedure, encouraging the resident to be as independent as possible throughout.

★ BED SAFETY
Lock bed wheels. Raise bed to safe working height. Lower one side rail if required.

★ PRIVACY
Provide for privacy by closing the door and covering the resident appropriately.

Ending Steps

★ RESIDENT SAFETY AND COMFORT
Secure the resident, lowering the bed, and raising the side rails if ordered. Check that the resident is comfortable and properly aligned.

★ PRIVACY
Remove any added privacy measures, such as a drape or a privacy screen.

★ ESSENTIALS
Place the call light, fresh beverage, and other items within reach.

★ COURTESY
Ask the resident if he or she needs anything else. Say thank you and goodbye.

★ INFECTION CONTROL
Wash hands.

Report your care and any important observations to the nurse.

Record your care and any important information/observations such as vital signs in the appropriate place.

Recheck your resident for any changes as directed by the nurse!

Cleaning a Glass Thermometer

Follow all standard and/or transmission-based precautions. Follow all rules for body mechanics.

Collect equipment: • soap, water and paper towels

1. Apply gloves.
2. Carefully check thermometer for cracks or chips.
3. Wet and clean in cool soapy water.
4. Rinse completely with cool water and dry with a paper towel.
5. Disinfect with facility-approved disinfectant.
6. Rinse completely with cool water and dry.

7. Shake thermometer down.
8. Return to storage site.
9. Remove gloves and wash hands.

If a glass thermometer breaks during cleaning or at any other time, secure the resident and anyone else nearby. Do not touch or let anyone else touch the mercury or the glass. Call your supervisor immediately. You must NEVER clean up the mercury by yourself!

9 List reasons an oral temperature should not be taken and perform taking a temperature at each of the four sites.

Do not take an oral temperature on a person:

- who is under the age of 6
- who is having hot or cold applications to the neck
- who cannot handle a thermometer in the mouth and keep the mouth closed
- who cannot breathe through the nose
- who sneezes or coughs a lot, such as someone who has severe allergies
- who has sores, redness, swelling, or pain in her mouth
- who is confused, disoriented, or restless
- who is unconscious
- who is on oxygen therapy by mouth or nose
- who has a nasogastric tube
- who has just had face or neck surgery
- who has paralysis from a CVA or from some other reason
- who is likely to have a seizure
- who has an injury to the face or neck

Taking an Oral Temperature Using a Glass, Electronic, or Digital Thermometer

Follow all standard and/or transmission-based precautions. Follow all rules for body mechanics.

Collect equipment:

- **two sets of gloves • glass, electronic, or digital thermometer • two sheaths (if using glass or digital thermometer)**
- **pen and pad • plastic probe covers (if using an electronic thermometer) • trash container next to bed**

PREPARE:

1. **Perform the "5 Stars."**

2. **Apply gloves.**
3. **Check to see if resident has had food or fluids, smoked, or chewed gum in the last 15 minutes. These activities may increase the heat inside the mouth and cause a higher temperature. If so, WAIT 15 to 30 minutes or follow facility policy.**

PERFORM:

For a glass thermometer:

4. **Clean and carefully shake down thermometer. Cover thermometer with disposable sheath.**
5. **Ask resident to open mouth. Insert thermometer slowly and carefully to one side of mouth under the tongue.**
6. **Ask resident to gently close mouth around thermometer but NOT to bite down. Hold in place if necessary. Ask resident to breathe through nose.**
7. **Leave thermometer in place for three to five minutes or follow facility policy.**
8. **Remove thermometer and sheath using a tissue. Discard tissue and sheath in trash. Before reading, wipe thermometer with a tissue or an alcohol wipe from stem to bulb end.**
9. **Read thermometer at eye level holding the stem towards the light.**
10. **Place thermometer on paper towel. (Skip to step 11.)**

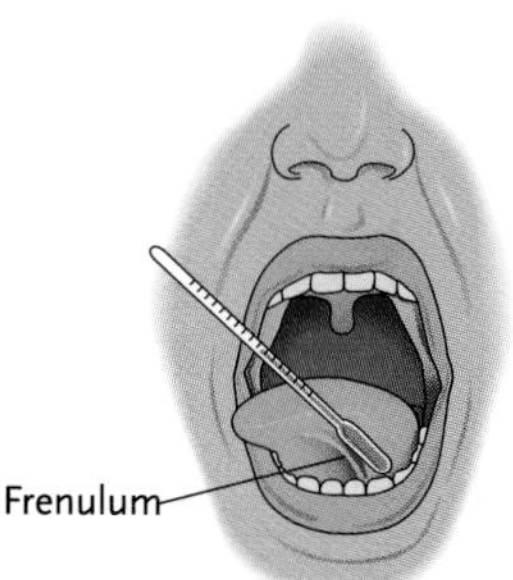

Figure 16-9.

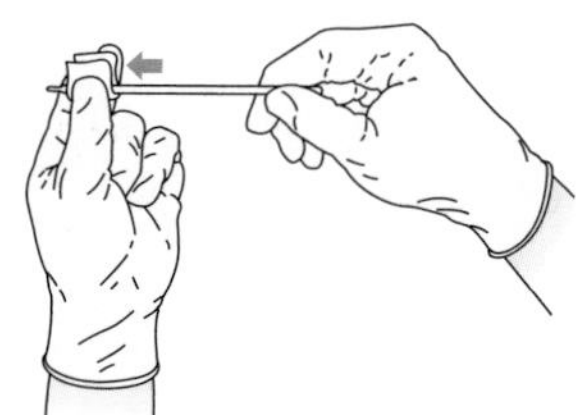
Figure 16-10.

For an electronic thermometer:

4. **Remove probe from base unit and insert in probe cover. Make sure cover clicks into place.**
5. **Ask resident to open mouth. Insert thermometer slowly and carefully to one side of mouth under the tongue.**
6. **Leave in place until thermometer blinks or beeps.**
7. **Ask resident to relax mouth and remove probe slowly.**
8. **Read temperature on display screen.**
9. **Press button to remove probe cover and direct cover into a facility-approved waste container.**
10. **Replace probe in thermometer base unit. (Skip to step 11.)**

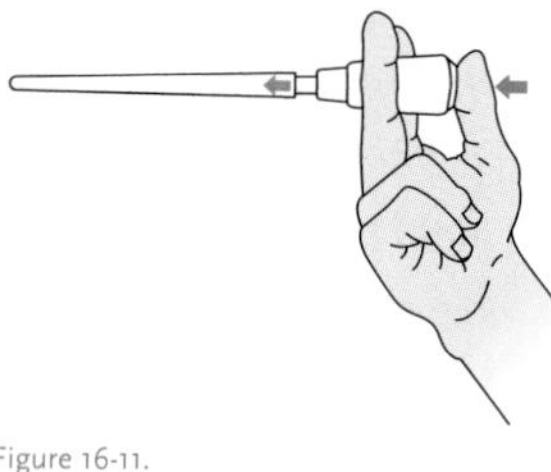
Figure 16-11.

For a digital thermometer:

4. **Insert thermometer into sheath. Turn on thermometer and wait until "ready" sign appears on the display screen.**
5. **Ask resident to open mouth. Insert thermometer slowly and carefully to one side of mouth under the tongue.**

6. Leave in place until thermometer blinks or beeps.
7. Ask resident to relax mouth and remove thermometer slowly.
8. Read temperature on tiny display screen.
9. Using tissue, remove and dispose of sheath in facility-approved waste container.
10. Replace thermometer into case.

FINISHING TOUCHES:

11. Remove gloves and dispose of them in trash. SECURE THE RESIDENT.
12. Wash hands and return to bedside. Write temperature reading on your pad, including method used (oral),next to resident name.
13. Perform the "5 Stars and 3 Rs."

For a glass thermometer:

14. Using paper towel, pick up thermometer. Clean it according to facility policy, and return to storage area. Wash hands again.

For an electronic thermometer:

14. Return electronic thermometer to charger.

Taking a Tympanic Temperature

Follow all standard and/or transmission-based precautions. Follow all rules for body mechanics.

Collect equipment:
- tympanic thermometer • pen and pad
- two sheaths (in case one sheath cracks)
- trash container next to bed

PREPARE:

1. Perform the "5 Stars."

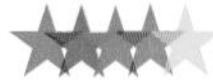

PERFORM:

2. Pick up tympanic thermometer and insert in plastic cover. Make sure cover locks into place.
3. Stand to the front of the person's head. Make sure hearing aid is carefully removed and that wax does not block ear canal.
4. Turn on thermometer. Wait until "ready" sign appears.
5. Pull on ear following guidelines below:

   Adults: pull up/back on pinna or outer edge of ear.

   Infants and Children: pull ear straight back.

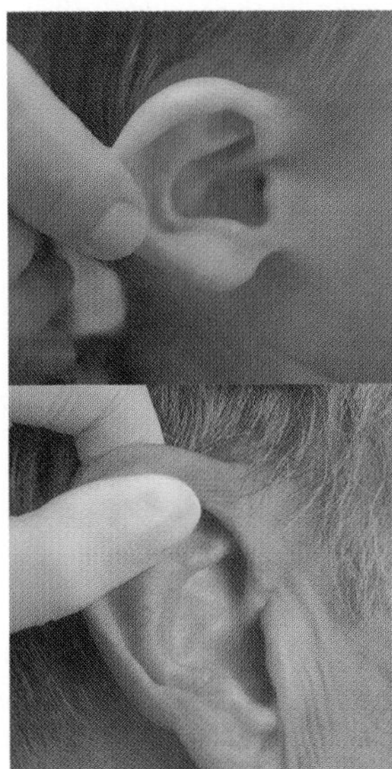

Figure 16-12.

6. Gently insert covered thermometer tip into ear. Make sure you have a good seal.
7. To take the temperature, press the button and hold for one full second. (To make sure you wait one second, say the words "one one-thousand.")
8. Remove from ear and read temperature on display screen.
9. Remove plastic cover by pressing button and directing it into the trash OR using your gloved hand if no button.
10. If facility policy is to take reading in both ears, repeat procedure using CLEAN PLASTIC COVER for the other ear.
11. Turn thermometer off. (Some of these have an auto-off.)
12. Replace tympanic thermometer into holder, if available.

FINISHING TOUCHES:

13. SECURE THE RESIDENT.
14. Wash hands and return to bedside. Write down the temperature on your pad, including method used, next to resident name.
15. Perform the "5 Stars and 3 Rs."

16. Return tympanic thermometer to storage area.

The axillary area needs to be clean and dry for an accurate temperature reading. A resident should be lying flat in bed when an axillary temperature is taken. A glass thermometer must be held in place under the arm for 10 full minutes for an accurate reading. The arm should be placed over the chest to hold the thermometer in place. The thermometer should not be jabbed under the arm.

Taking an Axillary Temperature Using a Glass, Electronic, or Digital Thermometer

Follow all standard and/or transmission-based precautions. Follow all rules for body mechanics.

Collect equipment:
- glass, electronic, or digital thermometer
- two sheaths (if using a glass or digital thermometer)
- pen and pad • plastic probe covers (if using an electronic thermometer) • trash container next to bed

PREPARE:

1. Perform the "5 Stars."

PERFORM:

For a glass thermometer:

2. Clean and carefully shake down thermometer. Cover thermometer with disposable sheath.
3. Pull down bed linens and open gown or pajamas to

expose underarm (axilla) area.

4. Place mercury (bulb) end of the thermometer into the center of the underarm area.
5. Make sure arm is close against the side or arm is resting on chest.
6. Hold thermometer in place for 10 minutes or according to facility policy.

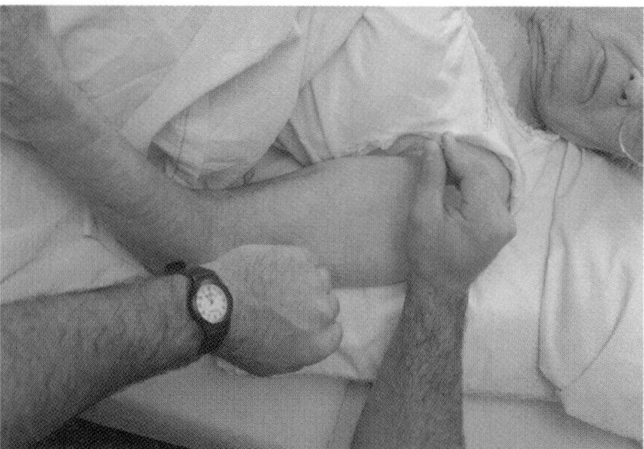

Figure 16-13.

7. Remove thermometer and remove sheath using a tissue. Discard tissue and sheath in trash.
8. Read thermometer at eye level, holding towards the light.
9. Place thermometer on clean paper towel. (Skip to step 10.)

For an electronic thermometer:

2. Remove probe from base unit and insert probe in probe cover. Make sure cover clicks into place.
3. Pull down bed linens and open gown or pajamas to expose underarm (axilla) area.
4. Place covered probe into the center of the underarm area.
5. Pull arm over chest area to secure.
6. Leave in place until thermometer blinks or beeps.
7. Read thermometer on display screen.
8. Remove covered probe and press button, directing probe cover into trash.
9. Replace probe in thermometer base unit. (Skip to step 10.)

For a digital thermometer:

2. Insert thermometer into sheath. Turn on thermometer and wait until "ready" sign appears on the display screen.
3. Pull down bed linens and open gown or pajamas to expose underarm (axilla) area.
4. Place covered thermometer into the center of the underarm area.
5. Pull arm over chest area to secure.
6. Leave in place until thermometer blinks or beeps.
7. Remove covered thermometer and using tissue, remove sheath and discard in facility-approved container.
8. Read temperature on tiny display screen. Turn off thermometer and place it on clean paper towel.
9. Replace thermometer into case.

FINISHING TOUCHES:

10. SECURE THE RESIDENT.
11. Wash hands and return to bedside. Write down temperature on your pad, including method used, next to resident name.
12. Perform the "5 Stars and 3 Rs."

For a glass or digital thermometer:

13. Using paper towel, pick up thermometer. Clean it according to facility policy, and return to storage area. Wash hands again.

For an electronic thermometer:

13. Return electronic thermometer to charger.

Rectal thermometers should be lubricated and inserted carefully not more than one-half inch for children and one inch for adults. Some people believe this method is one of the most accurate methods. However, it also can be a risky method. When you place a rectal thermometer into the rectum, you must stay with the resident for the entire time the thermometer is in place. You must also hold the thermometer the entire time it is in the rectum. Stimulation of the rectal area by the thermometer may temporarily increase the heartbeat and blood pressure. This could cause problems for a person with heart disease.

Taking a Rectal Temperature using a Glass or Electronic Thermometer

Follow all standard and/or transmission-based precautions. Follow all rules for body mechanics.

Double-check with the nurse:
"Is a rectal temperature appropriate for this resident?"

Collect equipment:
- two sets of gloves • two clean paper towels
- two clean tissues • glass or electronic thermometer
- two sheaths (*rectal* probe if using an electronic thermometer) • plastic probe covers • lubricant jelly
- pen and pad • trash container next to bed

PREPARE:

1. Perform the "5 Stars."

2. Apply gloves.
3. Place thermometer on clean paper towel on overbed table. Open lubricant. Squeeze a small amount onto the paper towel.

4. *For a glass thermometer:* Clean and carefully shake down thermometer.

   For an electronic thermometer: Make sure thermometer is working.

5. Make sure the bed is flat and turn resident to one side. Position comfortably.

PERFORM:

6. Pull back bed linens and gown or pajamas to expose buttocks.

7. *For a glass thermometer:* Dip the sheathed mercury bulb end of the thermometer into lubricant on the paper towel.

   For an electronic thermometer: Apply plastic probe cover. Apply lubricant to the plastic probe cover.

8. Pull back top of buttocks to expose the anus, and gently and carefully insert the lubricated end of the thermometer into the rectum following the guidelines below:

   a. Adults: Insert NOT MORE than one inch.

   b. Infants and children: Insert NOT MORE than one-half inch.

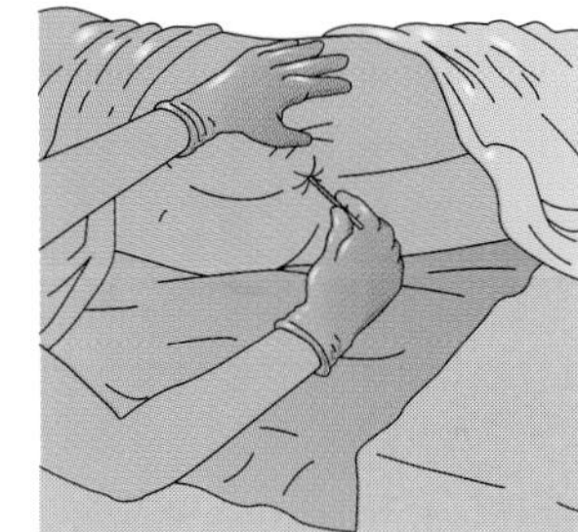

Figure 16-14.

   Never force or push thermometer into the rectum. If you are unable to insert, STOP and call for the nurse.

9. Hold the thermometer in place for the entire time. Do not allow resident to fall back on the thermometer. Serious internal damage could occur.

10. *For a glass thermometer:* Hold thermometer in place for three to five minutes or according to facility policy.

    For an electronic thermometer: Hold thermometer in place until it blinks or beeps.

11. *For a glass thermometer:* Carefully remove thermometer, remove sheath using tissue and discard sheath in trash. Wipe thermometer from stem to bulb end using a tissue or an alcohol wipe.

    For an electronic thermometer: Carefully remove thermometer. Remove probe cover using button, and direct probe cover into trash container.

12. *For a glass thermometer:* Read temperature at eye level, holding it towards the light. Place thermometer and tissue on clean paper towel.

    For an electronic thermometer: Read temperature BEFORE you insert probe back into thermometer base unit. If you read after you insert the probe, the numbers will have disappeared from the display screen.

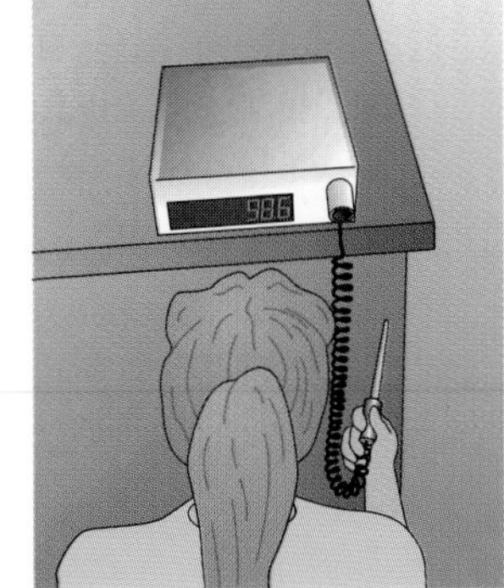

Figure 16-15.

FINISHING TOUCHES:

13. Using a tissue, wipe the anal area and dispose of tissue in trash.

14. Remove gloves and dispose of them in trash. Cover resident. SECURE THE RESIDENT.

15. Wash hands and return to bedside. Write down temperature reading on pad, including method used (rectal), next to resident name.

16. Perform the "5 Stars and 3 Rs."

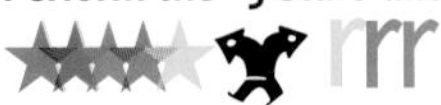

17. *For a glass thermometer:* Put on second set of gloves. Pick up thermometer and dispose of paper towels in trash. Clean thermometer according to facility policy, and return it to storage area. Remove gloves and wash hands again.

    For an electronic thermometer: Return electronic thermometer to charger.

---

10 Identify the seven primary pulse sites and the most commonly used site.

When the left ventricle of the heart contracts, it causes a wave of blood to move through an artery. This "pulse" is what you feel at the wrist or at another pulse site. The pulse count is the number of times

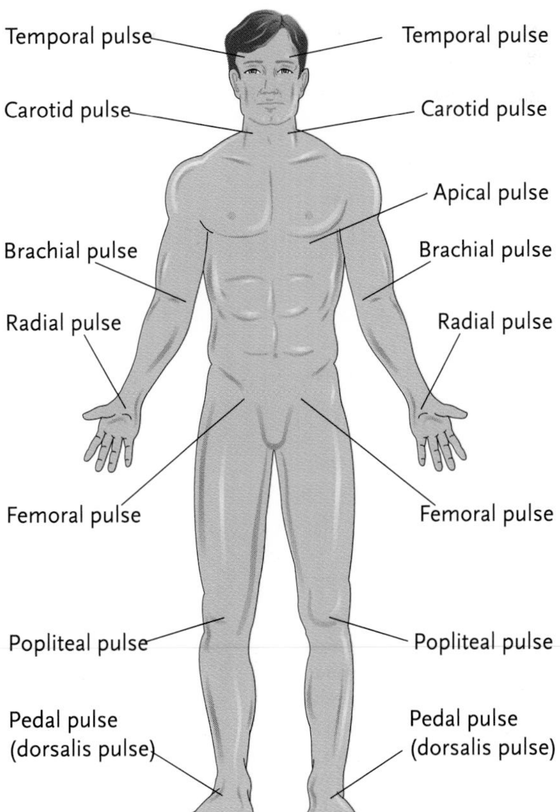

Figure 16-16.

the heart beats in 60 seconds, or one minute. Sometimes the abbreviation **BPM** (beats per minute) may be used after a pulse count. The heartbeat or pulse is measured by the fingers or by certain types of electronic devices that automatically measure the pulse. There are many areas on the body where a pulse can be felt. These pulse sites are shown in Figure 16-16.

The **radial pulse** is the most common site for counting pulse beats. This pulse is found in the lower arm at the wrist on the thumb-side of the body. The word "radial" comes from the radial artery in the arm and is similar to the word "radius," one of the bones in the lower arm. A pulse may be identified as **regular**, having the same amount of time between the beats, or **irregular**, having different amounts of time between the beats.

Taking the Radial Pulse

Follow all standard and/or transmission-based precautions. Follow all rules for body mechanics.

Collect equipment:

- **pen and pad • watch with a second hand or second counter • trash container next to bed**

PREPARE:

1. **Perform the "5 Stars."**
2. **Place resident in comfortable position sitting or lying down.**

PERFORM:

3. **Rest resident's arm on overbed table or on bed linens.**
4. **Lift wrist and locate radial pulse using the first two or three fingers of your hand. Do not press too hard or you may close the artery.**
5. **Look at your watch and wait until the second hand gets to the "12"or the "6."**
6. **Begin counting the pulse.**
7. **Some facilities require nursing assistants to count the pulse for one full minute (60 seconds). Others allow the pulse to be counted for 30 seconds. If irregular, always count a pulse for one full minute (60 seconds).**

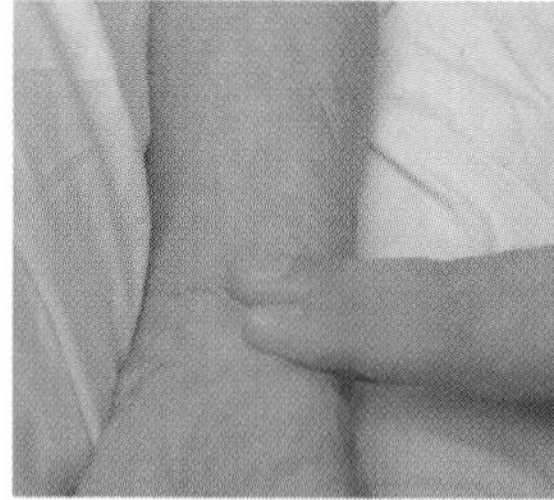

Figure 16-17.

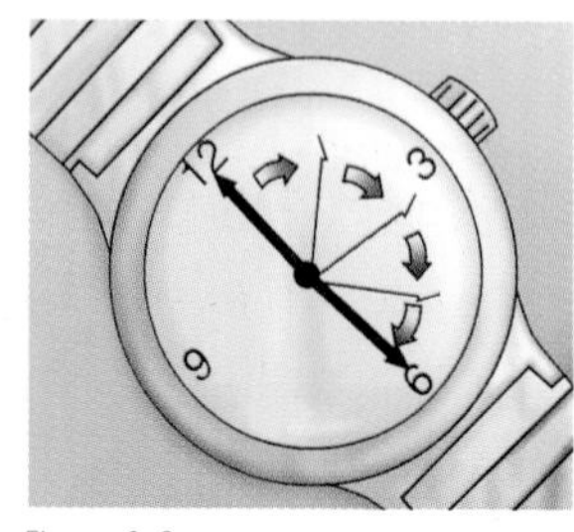

Figure 16-18.

Record the resident's pulse.

a. **If counted for 30 seconds, double your count so the number reflects the beats in one full minute. Follow steps below:**

   Pulse in 30 sec. = 40 beats

   40 beats x 2 = 80 beats

   Write it as 80.

b. **If counted for one full minute (60 sec.):**

   Pulse in one min. = 68 beats
   Write it as 68.

FINISHING TOUCHES:

8. **SECURE THE RESIDENT.**
9. **Wash hands and return to bedside. Write down the pulse on your pad next to resident name.**
10. **Perform the "5 Stars and 3 Rs."**

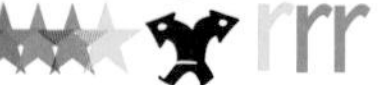

11 List eight factors affecting pulse rate and three things to observe when taking a pulse.

The pulse is affected by many different factors. Nurses and doctors have to evaluate all of the possible causes for an increase or decrease in a resident's pulse rate. Normal pulse rate is 60 to 100 beats per minute. When a pulse is too high, a person has **tachycardia**. If it is too low, a person has **bradycardia**.

Factors Affecting Pulse Rate

1. **Age:** The pulse tends to increase with age.
2. **Sex:** A male may have a slightly lower pulse rate than a female.
3. **Exercise:** When we exercise, our pulse rate will normally increase. However, someone who has exercised regularly for years may have a lower pulse, which can be normal for that person.
4. **Position Changes:** When we change position and sit down, our pulse may increase slightly as the heart tries to circulate the blood with the knees bent.
5. **Stress:** The sympathetic nervous system may be stimulated by fear, anxiety, and also pain. These factors may cause the pulse to increase.
6. **Hemorrhage:** When we begin to lose blood, our

pulse rate will usually increase at first. The heart tries to work harder to circulate the blood.

7. **Medications:** Medications can increase or decrease the heart rate.
8. **Fever and illness:** When we are ill and have a fever, our blood vessels may dilate or open up wider due to the rise in temperature. A decrease in blood pressure may then occur due to the dilated blood vessels. The heart may then respond by working harder and increasing the pulse rate.

When checking a resident's pulse, observe for the following:

- The pulse rate: The number of pulses in one minute (The normal range is 60 to 100 beats per minute).
- The overall pattern of the pulse: Is the pulse regular or irregular?
- The quality or type of pulse: Is the pulse strong or weak?

12 Explain the apical pulse and the pulse deficit.

The **apical pulse** is heard by listening directly over the heart with a **stethoscope**. This type of pulse is checked on residents who have a weak radial pulse or an irregular pulse. It may also be taken on infants and people with known heart disease.

Another reason for taking an apical pulse is to compare the apical pulse to a pulse somewhere else in the body, such as the arm or the foot. In some cases, the apical and radial or **pedal pulses** differ. This is significant when evaluating the circulation or a heart problem. The doctor or nurse may ask you to take an apical-radial pulse or an apical-pedal pulse. This allows the healthcare provider to evaluate the circulation to the arms or the feet.

An apical pulse is normally the same as a radial or a pedal pulse. When the radial or pedal pulse is less than the apical pulse, the resident may have poor circulation to that extremity. The apical pulse will always be the same or higher than any other pulse on the body. It will never be lower than another pulse on the body.

The pulse deficit is the difference between an apical pulse and a radial or pedal pulse. An explanation of pulse deficit is shown below.

Figuring a Pulse Deficit

Apical Pulse	Radial or Pedal Pulse
Pulse in 60 sec.= 80 beats	Pulse in 60 sec. = 68 beats

Pulse Deficit: 80 minus 68 = 12 (80–68=12)
The pulse deficit is 12.

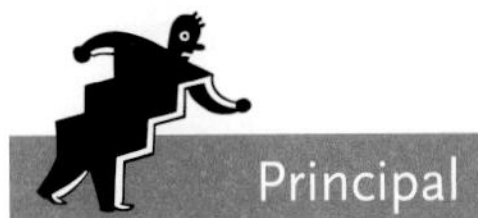

Principal Steps

Using a Dual-Sided Stethoscope

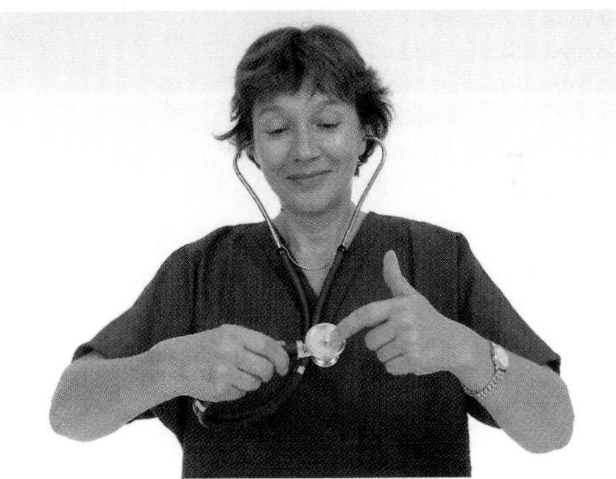

Figure 16-19.

1. *Clean earpieces and diaphragm of stethoscope with alcohol wipes.*
2. *Place earpieces in ears.*
3. *Tapping lightly on the diaphragm (larger round side of the stethoscope), note whether or not you can hear the light tapping. If you can hear the tapping, the diaphragm side of the stethoscope is ready to be used.*
4. *If you cannot hear the tapping, this means that the pediatric bell side (smaller round end of the stethoscope) is ready to be used.*
5. *Normally, use the diaphragm side of the stethoscope.*
6. *Use the pediatric bell side when you have trouble hearing a pulse or a blood pressure with the diaphragm side of the stethoscope.*

Taking the Apical Pulse

Follow all standard and/or transmission-based precautions.
Follow all rules for body mechanics.

Collect equipment:

- **two alcohol wipes • pen and pad • dual-sided stethoscope**
- **watch with a second hand or second counter**
- **trash container next to bed**

PREPARE:

1. Perform the "5 Stars."

2. Place resident in comfortable position lying down.
3. Clean both earpieces along with the diaphragm and bell sides of stethoscope.

PERFORM:

4. With permission of resident, place diaphragm of stethoscope under clothing on apical pulse site (on the left side of resident's chest, just below the nipple). See Figure 16-20. You may have to move stethoscope to locate loudest pulse sound. You may also "flip" the stethoscope head to the bell side to hear a louder pulse sound.

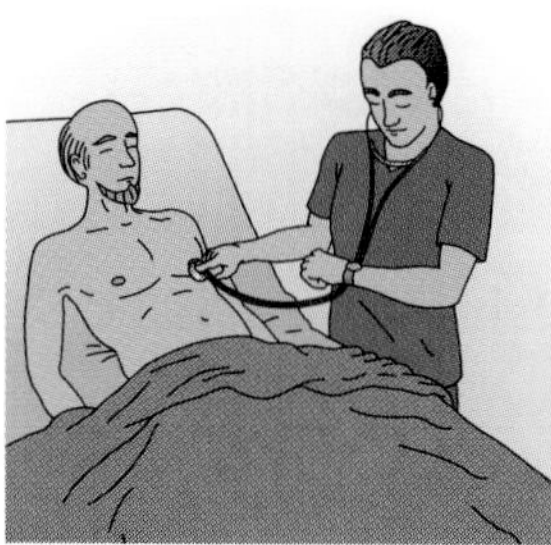

Figure 16-20.

5. Hold diaphragm or bell with two fingers firmly on chest.
6. Look at your watch and wait until the second hand gets to the "12" or the "6."
7. Count pulse for one full minute (60 seconds).
8. Replace clothing and move resident to comfortable position.

FINISHING TOUCHES:

9. SECURE THE RESIDENT.
10. Wash hands and return to bedside. Write down the pulse on your pad, including method used (apical), next to resident name.

    Pulse in 60 sec. = 80 beats
    Write it as 80.

12. Perform the "5 Stars and 3 Rs."

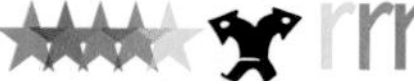

Taking the Pedal Pulse

Follow all standard and/or transmission-based precautions. Follow all rules for body mechanics.

Collect equipment:
- pen and pad • watch with a second hand or second counter • trash container next to bed

PREPARE:

1. Perform the "5 Stars."

2. Place resident in comfortable position lying down.

PERFORM:

3. Standing to side of bed or at FOB, pull back the bed linens, exposing one foot.

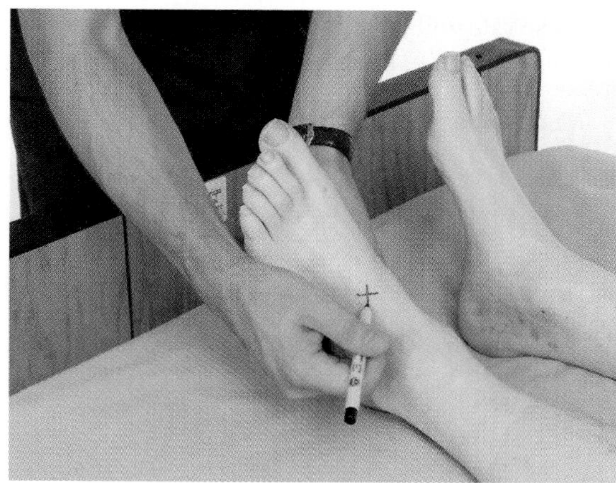

Figure 16-21. Approximate location of the pedal pulse.

4. Locate the pedal pulse in the foot using two fingers of your hand. Do not press too hard or you may close the artery.
5. Look at your watch and wait until the second hand gets to the "12" or the "6."
6. Begin counting the pulse.
7. Count for not more than 15 seconds. (The pedal pulse may be faint and difficult to count for more than 15 seconds. Ask for assistance if you have difficulty finding or counting pedal pulse.) Multiply your count by four for a 60-second reading.

FINISHING TOUCHES:

8. SECURE THE RESIDENT.
9. Wash hands and return to bedside. Write down the pulse on your pad, including method used (pedal), next to resident name.

    Number of beats in 15 seconds multiplied by 4 equals beats per minute.

    Pulse in 15 sec. = 20 beats
    20 beats x 4 = 80 beats
    Write it as 80.

10. Perform the "5 Stars and 3 Rs."

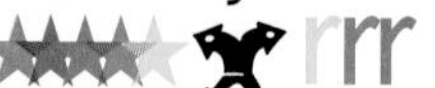

Taking the Apical-Radial or Apical-Pedal Pulse

Ask a co-worker to assist you!

Follow all standard and/or transmission-based precautions. Follow all rules for body mechanics.

Collect equipment:
- two alcohol wipes • pen and pad• dual-sided stethoscope
- watch with a second hand or second counter
- trash container next to bed

PREPARE:

1. Perform the "5 Stars."

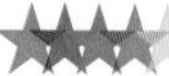

2. Place resident in comfortable position lying down.

3. **Clean both earpieces along with the diaphragm and bell sides of stethoscope.**

PERFORM:

4. **With permission of resident, one person places the diaphragm of stethoscope under clothing on apical pulse site (on the left side of resident's chest, just below the nipple). You may have to move stethoscope to locate loudest pulse sound. You may also "flip" the stethoscope head to the bell side to hear a louder pulse sound.**

   Hold diaphragm or bell with two fingers firmly on chest.

5. **The second person lifts the wrist or places two fingers on the foot and locates the radial or pedal pulse.**

6. **Wait until the second hand on a watch gets to the "12" or the "6." When it does, say "start," and both people will count a pulse for one full minute (60 seconds). Say "stop" after one minute.**

7. **Replace clothing and move resident to comfortable position.**

FINISHING TOUCHES:

8. **SECURE THE RESIDENT.**

9. **Wash hands and return to bedside. Write down both pulses on your pad, including method used (apical-radial or apical-pedal) next to resident name.**

APICAL PULSE:	RADIAL or PEDAL PULSE:
Pulse in 60 sec. = 80 beats	Pulse in 60 sec. = 68 beats
20 beats x 4 = 80 beats	17 beats x 4 = 68 beats

   PULSE DEFICIT:

   80 minus 68 = 12

   The pulse deficit is 12.

10. **Perform the "5 Stars and 3 Rs."**

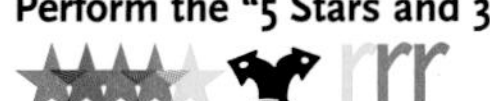

13 Identify three observations to record when taking respirations.

Respiration is the act of **inspiration** (breathing in) and **expiration** (breathing out). Each respiration consists of an inspiration and an expiration. The normal respiration rate for adults ranges from 12 to 20 breaths per minute.

When counting respirations, nursing assistants must look at the number of respirations per minute and whether they are regular or irregular. In addition, nursing assistants observe and report difficulty breathing. Difficulty breathing is called dyspnea, and may be identified when a resident has shortness of breath (SOB) or complains of painful breathing. Box 16-2 identifies the things to look for when watching a person breathe.

Observing Respirations — Box 16-2

Observe the resident for the following:

1. The respiratory rate: How many times does the resident breathe in one minute (12-20)?
2. The overall pattern of respirations: Is breathing regular or irregular?
3. The quality or type of breathing: Is SOB or dyspnea noted? Does the resident have noisy breathing? Normal breathing is quiet. Is the breathing deep or shallow?

Some of the different types of respiration you will see are outlined below.

Different Types of Respirations

apnea: the absence of breathing; may be temporary.

dyspnea: difficulty breathing.

eupnea: normal respirations.

orthopnea: the ability to only breathe sitting up or in a standing position.

tachypnea: rapid respirations.

Cheyne-Stokes respiration: type of respiration with periods of apnea lasting at least 10 seconds along with alternating periods of rapid, deep breathing and slow, shallow breathing.

Counting Respirations

Follow all standard and/or transmission-based precautions. Follow all rules for body mechanics.

NOTE: Because people may breathe more quickly if they know they are being observed, count respirations immediately after taking the pulse. Do not make it obvious that you are observing the resident's breathing.

Collect equipment:
• pen and pad • watch with a second hand or second counter • trash container next to bed

PREPARE:

1. **Perform the "5 Stars."**

2. **While continuing to hold the wrist after taking the resident's pulse, look at the resident's chest and count the number of times the resident breathes.**

PERFORM:

3. Follow these steps:
   a. Look at the rise and fall of the chest or abdomen. If unable to see the chest or abdomen rise and fall, you may place your hand on the chest with the resident's permission and count the respirations in this way.
   b. One chest (or abdomen) rise and fall equals one respiration.
4. Look at your watch and wait until the second hand gets to the "12" or the "6."
5. Begin counting the respirations.
6. Count for one minute (60 seconds). Some facilities allow the respirations to be counted for 30 seconds.

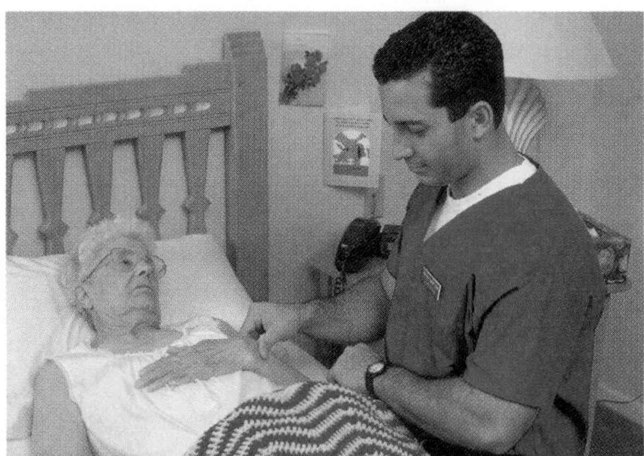

Figure 16-22.

7. If irregular, count respirations for one full minute (60 seconds).

FINISHING TOUCHES:

8. SECURE THE RESIDENT.
9. Wash hands and return to bedside. Write down the respiration on your pad next to resident name.

   If counted for 30 seconds, follow the examples below:

   Respirations in 30 sec. = 10

   10 x 2 = 20

   Write it as 20.

   Respirations in 30 sec. = 8

   8 x 2 = 16

   Write it as 16.

   If counted for one full minute:

   Respirations in one min. = 20

   Write it as 20.

10. Perform the "5 Stars and 3 Rs."

14 Identify nine factors that will affect blood pressure and two things to observe when taking blood pressure.

Blood pressure is the measurement of the force of the blood against the walls of blood vessels called arteries. Arteries carry blood away from the heart. The left ventricle of the heart causes the blood to surge out of the heart and travel to all corners of our body. The force of this movement of blood is the blood pressure. A blood pressure reading is written with two numbers, for example, 120/80.

The top number in a blood pressure reading is called the **systolic blood pressure**. This is the pressure of the blood on the walls of the arteries when the heart is contracting, or working to pump the blood out from the left ventricle into the body. The blood is pumped out through the aorta, the largest artery in the body. This number is the higher of the two numbers because there is more force when the blood is being pumped out into the body. Normal systolic blood pressure for an adult is between 100 and 140.

The bottom number is the **diastolic blood pressure**. One way to remember the word diastolic is to think diastolic-down, or the lower reading of the blood pressure. The lower reading is the pressure of the blood when the heart is relaxed. This relaxation occurs when the heart is not contracting and occurs between the heartbeats. Normal diastolic blood pressure for an adult is between 60 to 90.

The number is written in this way: systolic/diastolic, for example, 120/80. Again, the normal range of blood pressure for an adult is 100/60 to 140/90. When blood pressure is too high it is called hypertension. When it is too low, it is called hypotension.

Factors Affecting Blood Pressure

1. **Age:** Elderly residents with circulatory disorders may have an increased systolic reading.
2. **Exercise:** Physical activity generally increases the blood pressure.
3. **Stress:** The sympathetic nervous system may increase blood pressure during times of stress.
4. **Race:** Certain races may tend to have a higher blood pressure. For example, some African Americans have a tendency toward high blood pressure.
5. **Obesity:** Blood pressure may increase in persons who are overweight.

6. **Gender:** Hormones may cause differences in blood pressure between men and women.
7. **Medications:** Medications can increase or decrease the blood pressure.
8. **Time of Day:** Blood pressure may be lower in the morning and may increase later in the day.
9. **Illness:** Certain diseases may have an effect on blood pressure. Dehydration may increase the blood pressure.

Observing Blood Pressure

Observe the resident for the following:

1. The blood pressure reading: The normal reading should be from 100/60 to 140/90.
2. The quality or type of sounds: Are the sounds you hear when listening with your stethoscope strong or weak?

15 Identify the device used to take a blood pressure reading.

Blood pressure is measured with a device called a **sphygmomanometer**. You will need to gather alcohol wipes, a stethoscope, a blood pressure cuff, and a sphygmomanometer when preparing to take a blood pressure. Some facilities do not allow nursing assistants to take blood pressure readings.

You must carefully choose the correct size cuff to take a blood pressure reading. You can choose from a standard size, a pediatric size, or a large-sized cuff. Check with the nurse if you have questions about the size of the blood pressure cuff. If you use the wrong size blood pressure cuff, you may not get an accurate blood pressure reading. If the cuff is too tight, you may get a reading that is too high. If the cuff is too loose, you may get a reading that is too low.

The pulse used to take a blood pressure reading is normally the **brachial pulse**. This is the pulse located on the inside of the arm (opposite of the elbow) about one inch above the crease in the arm.

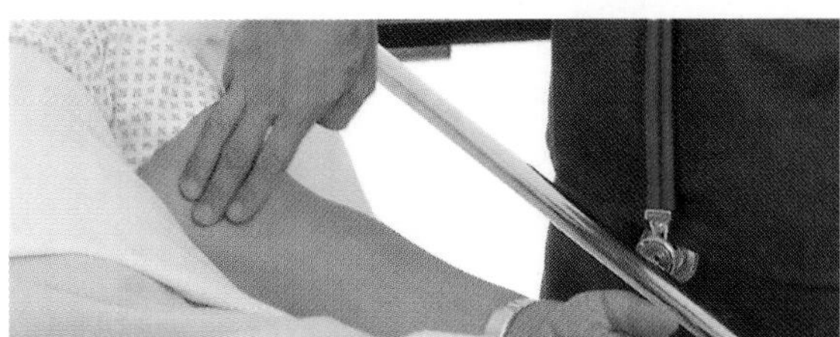

Figure 16-23. You locate the brachial pulse using the first three fingers of your hand.

Types of Sphygmomanometers

1. Aneroid sphygmomanometer. This device has a round gauge that may be attached to the wall in the room or may be portable. It may also hook onto clothing.

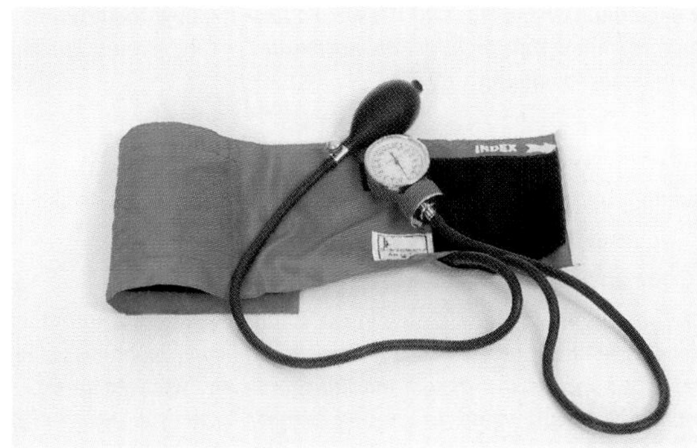

Figure 16-24. An aneroid sphygmomanometer.

2. Electronic sphygmomanometer. This device works automatically to measure the blood pressure for the staff. Nursing assistants will not have to listen for the sounds with their stethoscopes when using this type of machine. Because these devices may be extremely sensitive, it is important for the nursing assistant to ask the resident to keep his or her hand still when using this device. If the hand moves even slightly, the reading may not be accurate.

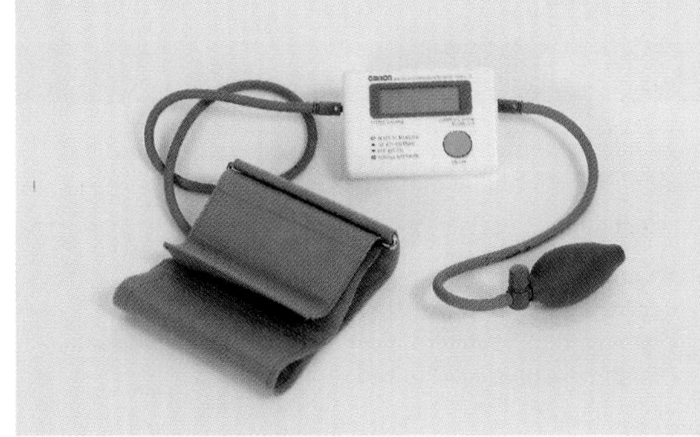

Figure 16-25. An electronic sphygmomanometer.

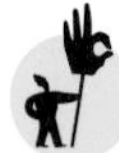

LSS Blood Pressures

There are times when special blood pressure readings may be ordered for a resident. The order may be written as LSS blood pressures. This means that you will have to take the resident's blood pressure reading three separate times. You will take the blood pressure reading while the resident is lying down, then sitting, and then standing. You will report and record all three readings. An example is L=100/80, S=120/82, and S=120/86.

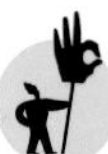

What if you can't hear it the first time?

When you are unable to hear the blood pressure the first time you pump up the blood pressure cuff, you must deflate the cuff completely (allow all of the air out of the cuff) and WAIT 30 to 60 seconds before you begin pumping up the cuff the second time to allow the artery to relax completely. You might get an inaccurate reading if you pump the cuff up again too quickly.

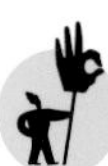

Higher Blood Pressures

When you begin to release the air in the cuff and you hear a sound immediately, this may mean the resident has a higher blood pressure. When this happens, first deflate the cuff completely. Wait the 30-60 seconds and then re-inflate to a higher number. When you deflate the second time, you should not hear the sound immediately.

Never guess!

When taking vital signs, readings may be difficult to get on some residents. If you are unable to get a vital sign reading on a resident, NEVER record a guess of the reading. By guessing the reading, you may put the life of the resident in danger. If you make up a reading, nurses and doctors may not find out the person has a fever or that the pulse, respiration, or blood pressure is too high or too low. The person could die if you falsify information and make up a vital signs reading. When you falsify a resident's information, it is physical abuse and you may put yourself in ***legal jeopardy****. You may be held liable, or legally responsible.*

Taking Blood Pressure

Follow all standard and/or transmission-based precautions. Follow all rules for body mechanics.

Collect equipment:

- **correct size blood pressure cuff • pen and pad**
- **sphygmomanometer • alcohol wipes • stethoscope**
- **trash container next to bed**

PREPARE:

1. **Perform the "5 Stars."**

2. **Place resident in comfortable position sitting or lying down. Make sure resident has rested after exercise for 15 to 30 minutes before taking a blood pressure.**
3. **Decide on the left or the right arm. The arm must be at the same level as the heart with the palm up and completely relaxed. No blood pressures may be taken on an arm:**
   - **with an intravenous line**
   - **on the side of a mastectomy (or any breast surgery)**
   - **being used for dialysis**
   - **with a cast**
   - **with any injury, burn, surgery**
   - **paralyzed due to a stroke**

PERFORM:

4. **Prepare to take the blood pressure. Make sure blood pressure cuff is deflated (without air) by flattening or squeezing the cuff to let air out. Clean diaphragm of stethoscope with an alcohol wipe.**
5. **Do not take a blood pressure over clothing. Either move the sleeve up or ask the resident to move the sleeve up the arm. Do not wrap the cuff too tightly.**
6. **Locate brachial pulse using the first three fingers of your hand. Feel the pulse for a few seconds.**
7. **Wrap blood pressure cuff around arm in this manner:**
   a. **If the cuff has arrows showing the spot to place over the brachial pulse, place either left or right arrow exactly over the brachial pulse on that arm. (Figure 16-26)**
   b. **If there is no arrow on the cuff, place the center of the bladder of the cuff exactly over the brachial artery.**
   c. **Wrap cuff snugly around the upper arm, about one inch above the crease in the elbow.**

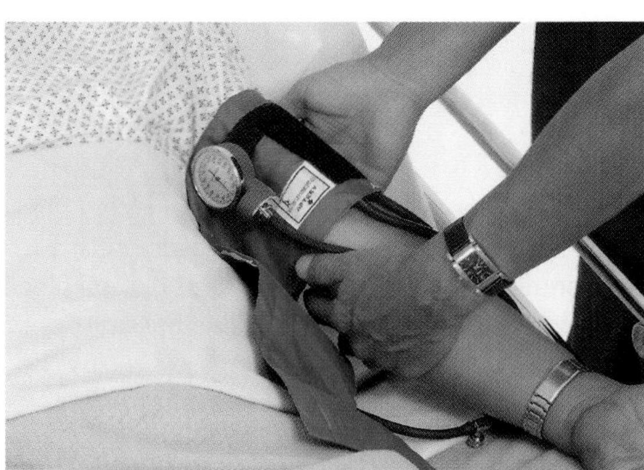

Figure 16-26.

8. **Close the knob (valve) on the end of the tubing by turning it clockwise. Do not over-tighten valve or it will be harder to reopen. (Figure 16-27)**

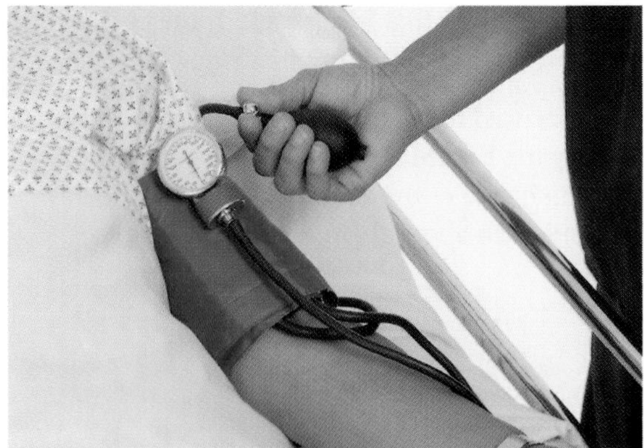

Figure 16-27.

9. **Position blood pressure gauge (with numbers) so that you can see it clearly.**

10. **Place the earpieces of the stethoscope in your ears.**
11. **Place the diaphragm of the stethoscope directly over the brachial pulse and hold firmly in place with the first two fingers of one hand.**
12. **a. Pump up the cuff according to facility policy. Some facilities have nursing assistants pump up to 160 to 180 mm Hg. (mercury).**

    b. Other facilities ask that the blood pressure be pumped up about 30 mm Hg higher than the most recent systolic blood pressure reading. (For example, if the most recent reading was 130 over 80, then the cuff would be pumped up to 160.)
13. **SLIGHTLY turn and open the knob (valve) and deflate the cuff slowly.**

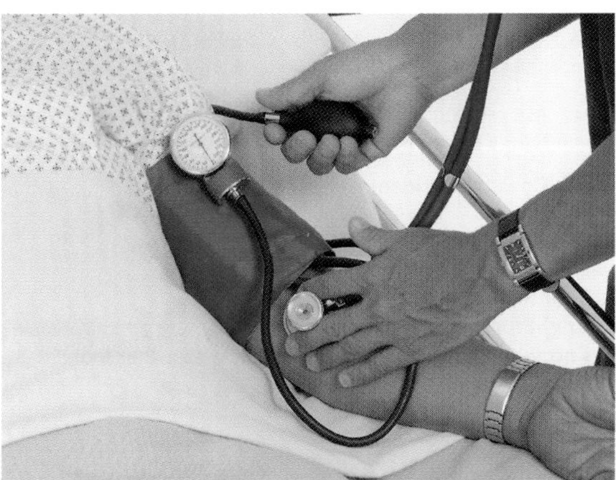

Figure 16-28.

14. **Listen for the first sound of the pulse. This is the higher, or systolic, reading.**
15. **Listen for the point when the sound of the pulse disappears. This is the lower, or diastolic, reading.**
16. **Immediately let the rest of the air out of the cuff (deflate). Remove the cuff carefully from the resident's arm.**
17. **Write down the blood pressure reading on your pad next to resident name.**

FINISHING TOUCHES:

18. **Perform the "5 Stars and 3 Rs."**

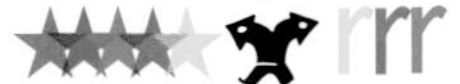

19. **Clean stethoscope with alcohol wipes. Clean the blood pressure cuff according to facility policy and return to storage area. Wash hands again.**

16 Describe how to recognize pain and list seven measures used to manage pain.

Pain is an important condition to observe and report with your residents. Some even call pain the fifth vital sign, because it is as important to monitor pain as it is to monitor the other vital signs.

Pain is a very difficult thing to cope with. It can affect your residents' daily lives to the point that their ability to perform ADLs is restricted. Pain can swiftly drain energy and hope.

All caregivers are responsible for recognizing pain and taking appropriate action to provide pain management. As the person who will be with your residents more often than others, you play a significant role in noticing and managing pain. Follow the guidelines below to recognize and reduce pain.

Pain Recognition

- Notice individual signs of pain specific to each resident. Work with family and friends who can assist with recognition of unrelieved pain.
- Monitor the resident's response to pain medication.

Measures to Reduce Pain

- Report complaints of pain or unrelieved pain promptly to the nurse.
- Constantly check on the resident.
- Offer back rubs often.
- Assist in frequent changes of position. Use extreme care when moving, lifting, or transferring a resident in pain.
- Offer warm baths or showers.
- Encourage slow, deep breaths when the resident has difficulty breathing or is in pain.
- Always be patient, caring, gentle, and sympathetic.

17 Explain the primary reasons to check a resident's neurological signs.

Neurological signs are taken on some residents to look for a change in the nervous system. A change in the neurological signs may indicate the resident is developing a problem with his or her nervous system or circulatory system. The reaction of the pupil, for example, can show the blood flow within the brain. When a pupil is dilated (large), the blood flow inside the brain may be decreased.

When the movement of the extremities, or the arms and the legs, is affected, it can be a sign of a change in the nervous system. Whenever you notice a change in a resident's ability to move arms and/or legs, pupil response to light, or orientation, you must immediately notify the nurse. Also report if hand grasp is weaker on one side or if pupil size has changed.

Observing Neurological Signs

Follow all standard and/or transmission-based precautions. Follow all rules for body mechanics.

Collect equipment:
- penlight or regular flashlight • pen and pad
- watch with a second hand or second counter
- trash container next to bed

PREPARE:

1. Perform the "5 Stars."

2. Place resident in comfortable position lying down.

PERFORM:

3. Orientation:

- Is the resident oriented (x 3) to person, place, and time?
- Is the resident oriented x 2 or x 1?
- Is the resident disoriented, or oriented x 0?
- Is the resident able to make sense when she talks?

4. Eye Opening:

- Does the resident open his eyes right away when you speak to him?
- Does the resident open his eyes only when asked using a loud voice?
- Does the resident not open his eyes?

5. Checking pupil size:
   a. Stand directly in front of resident. Turn on flashlight.
   b. Move flashlight from the side of the head directly over one eye and watch for any change at all in pupil size. (Figure 16-29)

   Does the pupil get smaller? get bigger? stay the same size?

   Facilities will usually have a chart with tiny dots that show possible pupil sizes. Nursing assistants should ask a nurse for guidance when using this chart for the first time.

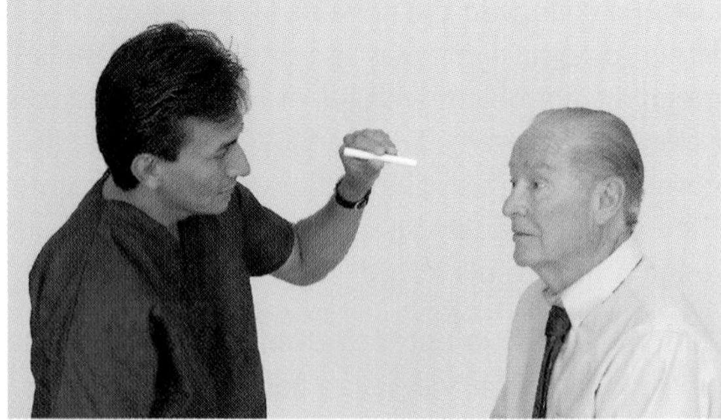

Figure 16-29.

   c. Check other pupil. Both pupils should react the same to the light.
   d. Look at the neurological signs form or guide card and find the dot size that most closely matches the size of the pupil AFTER the light shines on it.

6. Measuring hand grasp:
   a. Stand in front of the resident. The resident may sit or stand.
   b. Take both resident's hands in your hands.
   c. Ask the resident to squeeze your hands on your count of "three." Does the resident have:

- equal hand strength, strong?
- equal hand strength, weak?
- left hand stronger?
- right hand stronger?
- no hand grasp in one hand?
- no hand grasp in both hands?

7. Foot Strength:
   a. The resident must lie in bed for this procedure.
   b. Stand at the foot of the bed. Pull aside the lower bed linens.
   c. Ask resident to push on your hands as you hold your hands against the bottom of both feet. (Figure 16-30)
   d. Does the resident have:

- equal foot strength, strong?
- equal foot strength, weak?
- left foot stronger?
- right foot stronger?
- no foot strength or ability to push with either foot?
- no foot strength in both feet?

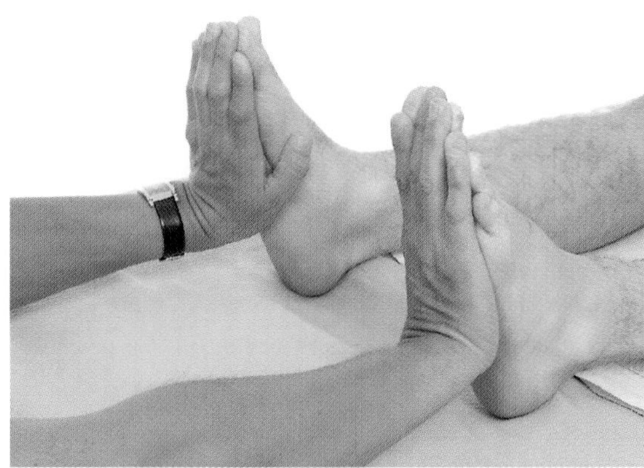

Figure 16-30.

8. Leg Strength:
   a. The resident must lie in bed for this procedure.
   b. Stand at the foot of the bed. Pull aside the lower bed linens, taking care to protect the resident's privacy.
   c. Ask resident to lift one leg as high as he can and slowly lower it back down.
   d. Ask the resident to lift the other leg as high as he can and slowly lower it back down.
   e. Answer these questions regarding the resident's legs. Can the resident:

- raise both legs equally?
- lift the left foot higher?
- lift the right foot higher?
- not lift either leg?

FINISHING TOUCHES:

9. **SECURE THE RESIDENT.**
10. **Wash hands and return to bedside. Write down the neurological signs results on your pad next to resident name.**
11. **Perform the "5 Stars and 3 Rs."**

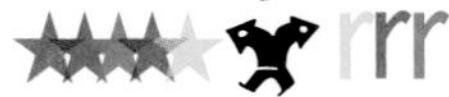

When recording, follow facility policy regarding neurological signs.

Summary

The vital or cardinal signs are one important method of determining the overall health of your residents. In this book, you will see that noticing and reporting change, any change, in a resident is perhaps the most important part of being a nursing assistant. These vital signs may show subtle or distinct changes that can alert the staff to important changes in a resident's condition. When these changes are detected early, doctors and nurses may help the resident return to good health. Thus, when a vital sign is abnormal, it is extremely important that you notify the nurse immediately.

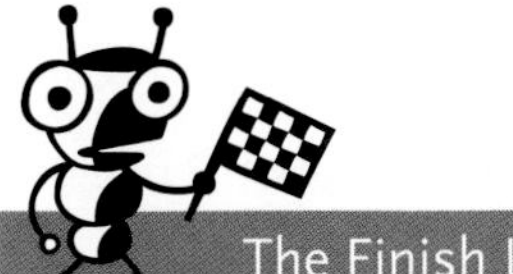

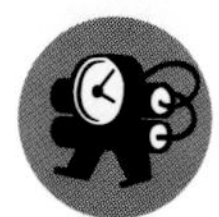

What's Wrong With This Picture?

These sentences all have errors in them. Find each of the mistakes and rewrite the sentences to make true statements.

1. Dehydration may decrease blood pressure.
2. Exercise may cause our body temperature to decrease.
3. Normal axillary temperature is 99.6 degrees Fahrenheit.
4. Normal oral temperature is 97.6 degrees Fahrenheit.
5. Normal rectal temperature is 98.6 degrees Fahrenheit.
6. You should wait five minutes before taking an oral temperature after a person has eaten, drunk, smoked, or chewed gum.
7. Glass thermometers should be rinsed in hot water during the cleaning process.
8. Normal adult pulse is 80 to 100 beats per half-minute.
9. Bradycardia is when the pulse or heartbeat is too fast.
10. Normal respirations are 14 to 22 per minute.
11. An apical pulse is always lower than a radial pulse or a pedal pulse.
12. To get a pulse deficit, you must subtract the apical pulse from the radial or the pedal pulse.
13. A normal adult systolic blood pressure should be between 90 and 140.
14. A normal adult diastolic blood pressure should be between 80 and 100.
15. In between blood pressure readings, it is best to wait at least 15 to 20 seconds before taking the second reading.
16. The radial pulse is the pulse used for taking a blood pressure in the arm.
17. The brachial pulse is the pulse used to take a blood pressure in the leg.
18. You should leave a glass thermometer in place in the mouth for five to 10 minutes.
19. Electronic or digital thermometers should be left in place for two to three minutes.

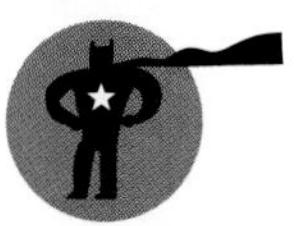

Star Student Central

1. Find a few people and ask permission to take their radial pulse. Use correct procedure (wash hands, ID, explain procedure). Document the pulse for each person in your notes.
2. Next, ask permission to take their respiration. Use correct procedure (wash hands, ID, explain procedure). Document the respiration for each person in your notes.
3. After you feel fairly comfortable taking pulse and respirations, practice this procedure:

a. Take the pulse of an adult friend or family member. Remember the number.

b. While still holding the arm of the person, look at the chest and begin taking the respirations. (When we tell people we are taking their respirations, sometimes they breathe differently.)

c. When finished, write down both numbers in your notes.

4. Arrange for an adult friend or family member to help you. You will need a tiny flashlight and a semi-dark room. Stand in front of the person and bring the light from the side of the person's head over the front of one eye for just a second, then quickly pull the light back to the side of the head. What happens to the pupil when light hits it? (Always shine the light only once on each pupil.)

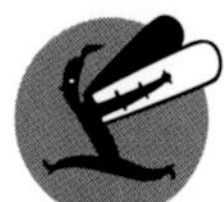

You Can Do It Corner!

1. You take an oral temperature on your resident and get a reading of 98.6 F. You know that if you took a rectal temperature, it would be approximately ____________ F. (LO 6)
2. The six factors that affect body temperature are age of the person, circadian rhythm, emotion, illness, exercise, and ____________. (LO 3)
3. The oral, security, and rectal are all types of ____________ thermometers. (LO 8)
4. Blood pressure is measured with a device called a ____________. (LO 15)
5. Vital signs include temperature, respiration, blood pressure, and ____________. (LO 2)
6. A resident who cannot breathe through his nose should not have an ____________ temperature taken. (LO 9)
7. Symptoms of a fever include skin feeling hot and looking flushed, headaches, muscle aches, chills, and ____________. (LO 4)
8. A temperature may be taken with a mercury glass, tympanic, digital, or ____________ thermometer. (LO 7)
9. If the apical pulse is 85 and the radial pulse is 69, the pulse deficit is ____________. (LO 12)
10. Why should you count respirations directly after taking the pulse? ____________. (LO 13)
11. The pulse count is the number of times the ____________ beats in one minute. (LO 10)
12. In degrees Fahrenheit (F), each long line represents one degree and each short line represents ____________ of a degree. (LO 5)
13. Whenever you notice a change in a resident's ability to move arms and/or legs, orientation, or ____________ you must immediately notify the nurse. (LO 17)
14. You must observe two things when taking a blood pressure: the blood pressure reading and ____________. (LO 14)
15. Normal pulse rate is ____________ beats per minute. (LO 11)

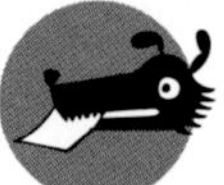

Star Student's Chapter Checklist

1. I have read my textbook chapter.
2. I have reviewed my own "Pocketful of Terms."
3. I have listened to my tutor tape.
4. I have reviewed and highlighted my class notes.
5. I have read and completed any handouts from this chapter.
6. I have completed "The Finish Line."
7. Star Time! Choose your reward!

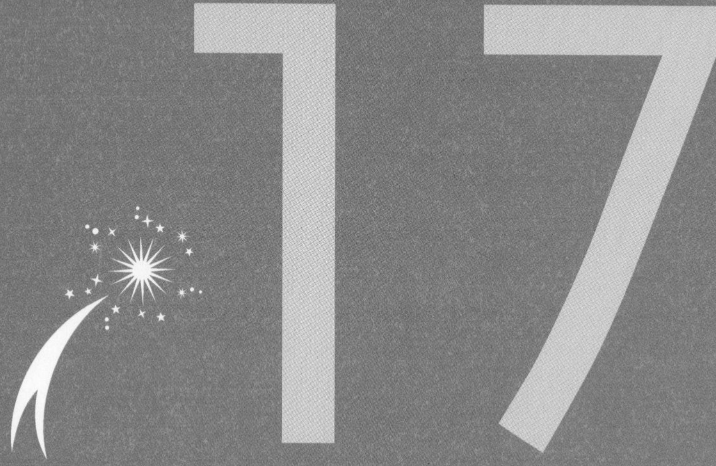

Your Guide: Moving, Lifting and Positioning

Look Like a Star!

Look at the Learning Objectives and The Finish Line before you begin reading this chapter.

Look at your pocket calendar.
With your pencil, put a bracket ( ) around a study period every single day.

Look at your homework for this chapter.
Plug each piece of homework into a certain time slot.

Look at the Star Student's Chapter Checklist at the end of this chapter. Check off each item as it is completed.

"Take her up tenderly/Lift her with care..."

Thomas Hood, 1798-1845

"The superior man is the providence of the inferior. He is eyes for the blind, strength for the weak, and a shield for the defenseless. He stands erect by bending above the fallen. He rises by lifting others."

Robert Green Ingersoll, 1833-1899

Learning Objectives

1. **Spell and define all STAR words.**
2. **Explain why it is necessary to maintain good body alignment and list the ten rules of proper body mechanics.**
3. **Explain why regularly-scheduled positioning changes are a vital part of quality care for residents who are confined to bed.**
4. **Explain why transfers lead with the strong side of the body and demonstrate the use of a gait/transfer belt and a sliding board.**

Successfully perform these Practical Procedures

Locking Arms with a Resident and Raising Head and Shoulders

Moving a Resident up in Bed with a Lift/Draw Sheet: Two Co-Workers

Moving a Resident to the Side of the Bed with a Lift/Draw Sheet: Two Co-Workers

Moving a Resident to the Side of the Bed: One Worker

Turning Your Resident Toward You

Turning Your Resident Away from You

Logrolling Using a Lift/Draw Sheet: Two Co-Workers

Assisting a Resident to the Side of the Bed: Dangling

Using a Sliding or Transfer Board

Transfer from Bed to Chair/Wheelchair with a Gait/Transfer Belt

Transfer from Bed to Chair/Wheelchair without a Gait/Transfer Belt

Transfer from Bed to Chair/Wheelchair with Walker Assist

Transfer to and from Toilet from a Wheelchair

Transfer to and from a Shower Chair from a Wheelchair

Transfer to a Car from a Wheelchair

Using a Mechanical Lift to Transfer to Wheelchair or Chair: Two or Three Co-Workers

Transfer from Stretcher to Bed Using a Transfer Sheet: Four Co-Workers

Transfer from Bed to Stretcher Using a Transfer Sheet: Four Co-Workers

A View from the Past: "Falling into Life"

"Having lost the use of my legs during the polio epidemic that swept across the eastern United States during the summer of 1944, I was soon immersed in a process of rehabilitation that was. . .as much spiritual as physical. That was a full decade before the discovery of the Salk vaccine ended polio's reign as the disease most dreaded by America's parents and their children. Treatment of the disease had been standardized by 1944: following the initial onslaught of the virus, patients were kept in isolation for a period of ten days to two weeks. Following that, orthodox medical opinion was content to subject patients to as much heat as they could stand. Stiff paralyzed limbs were swathed in heated, coarse woolen towels known as 'hot packs.' As soon as the hot packs had baked enough pain and stiffness out of a patient's body so that he could be moved on and off a stretcher, the treatment was ended, and the patient faced a series of daily immersions in a heated pool. I would ultimately spend two full years at the appropriately named New York State Reconstruction Home. . .We would learn during our days in the New York State Reconstruction Home to confront the world that was. . .My future had arrived."

Leonard Kriegel

1 Spell and define all STAR words.

body alignment: body positioning that promotes proper body functioning; posture.

body mechanics: the way the parts of the body work together whenever a person moves.

bony prominences: areas of the body where the bone lies close to the skin, including elbows, shoulder blades, tailbone, hip bones, ankles, heels, the back of the neck, and the back of the head.

dangling: position with the resident sitting to the side of the bed with legs over the side.

gait belt: transfer belt used to assist with walking.

lift sheet: small sheet placed under the resident from the shoulder to the hips; also called a draw sheet.

logrolling: turning a resident all at once while keeping the spine straight.

mechanical lift: special piece of equipment used to lift and transfer a resident from one area to another or to lift and weigh a resident.

transfer belt: gait belt.

transfer: moving a resident, e.g. from a bed to a chair.

turn sheet: lift sheet.

2 Explain why it is necessary to maintain good body alignment and list the ten rules of proper body mechanics.

The positioning of the body plays an important part in the proper functioning of the body. **Body alignment** is also known as good posture. Good body alignment assists the body in achieving balance without causing any muscle or joint strain. In addition, good body alignment allows the body to function at its highest level. The lungs are able to expand and contract, the blood circulation moves more smoothly through the body, the food digests effortlessly, and the kidneys are able to better cleanse the body of wastes. Also, good body alignment helps prevent the complications of immobility, such as contractures and muscle atrophy.

You first learned about **body mechanics** in Chapter 12. When you do not transfer and lift using good body mechanics, you and your residents can be injured. The following ten rules will help you remember to use proper body mechanics:

1. **Assess the load.** Before attempting a lift, assess the weight of the load to determine if you can safely move the object without help. Know the lift policies at your facility. Never attempt a lift you do not feel comfortable doing. Consider using assistive devices as necessary. When you are satisfied that you can perform the lift alone or you have enough help to perform the lift, prepare the environment.
2. **Think ahead, plan, and communicate the move.** Scan the environment for any objects in your path or any potential risks, such as a wet floor. Ensure the pathway is clear. Account for hazards, like high-traffic areas, combative residents, residents losing balance, or a loose toilet seat. Decide exactly what you are going to do together and agree on the verbal cues you will use before attempting to **transfer**.
3. **Check your base of support and be sure you have firm footing.** Use a wide but balanced stance to increase your base of support, and keep this stance when walking. Do you have enough room to maintain a wide base of support? Are you and your resident wearing slip-resistant shoes?
4. **Face what you are lifting.** Your feet should always face the direction you are moving. This enables you to move your body as one unit and keeps your back straight. Twisting at the waist increases the likelihood of injury.
5. **Keep your back straight.** Keeping your head up and shoulders back will keep the back in the proper position. Take a deep breath to help you regain correct posture.
6. **Begin in a squatting position and lift with your legs.** Bend at the hips and knees and use the strength of your leg muscles to stand and lift the object. You will need to push your buttocks out to accomplish this. Before you stand erect with the object you are lifting, remember it is your legs, not your back, that will enable you to lift. You should be able to feel your leg muscles as they work. Lifting with the large leg muscles decreases stress on the back.
7. **Contract (tighten) your stomach muscles when beginning the lift.** This will help to take weight off the spine and maintain alignment.

8. **Keep the object close to your body**. This decreases the length of the lever arm (distance from your center of gravity to the object being carried) and the stress to your back. Lift objects to your waist. Carrying them any higher can compromise your balance.
9. **Do not twist**. Turn and face the area you are moving the object to and then set the object down. Twisting increases the stress on your back and should always be avoided. The muscles that you use to twist are not that strong; therefore twisting is not as stable as turning your whole body as one unit.
10. **Push or pull when possible rather than lifting**. When you lift an object, you must overcome gravity and be able to balance the load. When you push or pull an object, you only need to overcome the friction between the surface and the object. Your can use your body weight to move the object, rather than your lifting muscles. Push rather than pull whenever possible, and stay close to the object to decrease the length of the lever arm. Use both arms and tighten the stomach muscles.

Safety, not speed!

Repositioning your residents can be a challenging procedure. The simple act of turning a resident may sometimes break a bone, tear fragile skin, or tug too hard on tubing such as catheters or IVs. It is extremely important for nursing assistants to take great care when moving and positioning residents. Moving too quickly during these procedures can cause serious injury and the potential for many complications. Moving residents in a hasty or rough manner may be considered abuse.

3 Explain why regularly-scheduled positioning changes are a vital part of quality care for residents who are confined to bed.

Many facilities have regularly-scheduled positioning changes posted in residents' rooms. Residents need to be turned frequently so that pressure on skin surfaces of the body alternates from one side to the other. Too much pressure on one area for too long can cause a decrease in circulation. This increases the risk of pressure sores and other problems like muscle contractures. Constant pressure over **bony prominences** causes the greatest risk of pressure sores or bedsores, a major problem in long-term care (More information on pressure sore prevention and care is in Chapters 19 and 24). To try to prevent these types of sores from occurring, many facilities have established turning schedules.

Nursing assistants must organize their days to carefully follow the posted turn schedules as closely as possible. You may have several residents who require frequent turning. The more residents requiring frequent turning, the more organized you must be in order to make sure your residents change positions often. Special sheets called **lift sheets** or **turn sheets** are sometimes used to move residents in a safer manner.

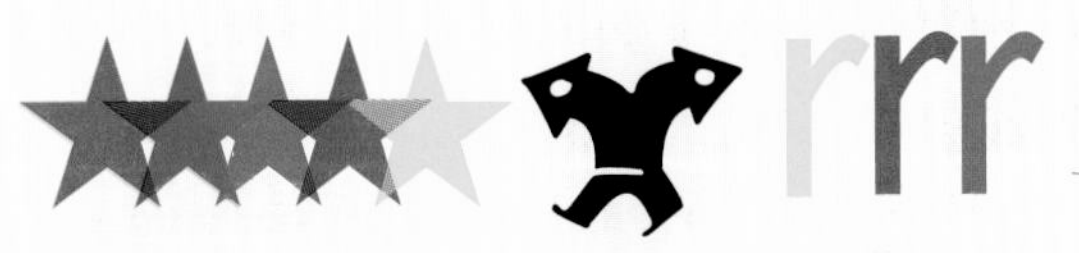

Beginning Steps

★ **RESPECT**
Knock first, ask and receive permission to enter a resident's room.

★ **INFECTION CONTROL**
Wash hands.

★ **COMMUNICATION**
Greet and identify the resident. Identify yourself. Explain the procedure, encouraging the resident to be as independent as possible throughout.

★ **BED SAFETY**
Lock bed wheels. Raise bed to safe working height. Lower one side rail if required.

★ **PRIVACY**
Provide for privacy by closing the door and covering the resident appropriately.

Ending Steps

★ **RESIDENT SAFETY AND COMFORT**
Secure the resident, lowering the bed, and raising the side rails if ordered. Check that the resident is comfortable and properly aligned.

★ **PRIVACY**
Remove any added privacy measures, such as a drape or a privacy screen.

★ **ESSENTIALS**
Place the call light, fresh beverage, and other items within reach.

★ **COURTESY**
Ask the resident if he or she needs anything else. Say thank you and goodbye.

★ **INFECTION CONTROL**
Wash hands.

r **Report** your care and any important observations to the nurse.

r **Record** your care and any important information/observations such as vital signs in the appropriate place.

r **Recheck** your resident for any changes as directed by the nurse!

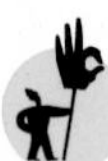

Communicate.

Any time you assist a resident, discuss with them what you would like to do. Promote their independence by allowing them to do what they can. The two of you must work together, especially during transfers!

Locking Arms with a Resident and Raising Head and Shoulders

Follow all standard and/or transmission-based precautions. Follow all rules for body mechanics.

1. **Perform the "5 Stars."**

PREPARE:

2. **Place pillow at the HOB up against the headboard.**
3. **Stand at the side of the bed and face the HOB.**
4. **Spread feet apart about 12 inches and slightly bend the knees to protect your back.**
5. **Gently slide one hand under the resident's near shoulder.**
6. **Gently slide the other hand under the resident's upper back.**

PERFORM:

7. **At the count of three, slowly and carefully raise the resident's head and shoulders and give care such as adjusting the ties on a gown.**

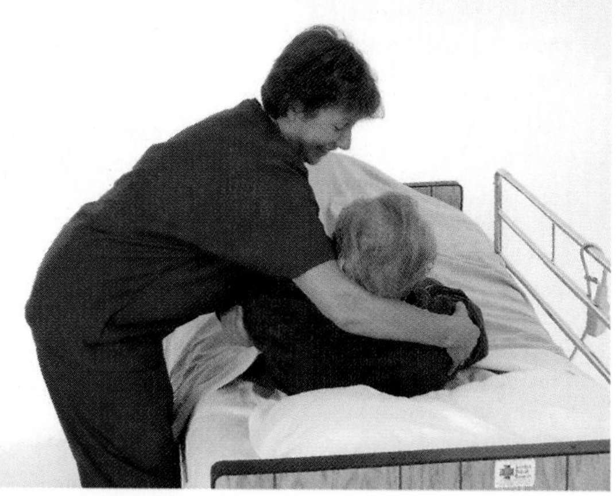

Figure 17-1.

FINISHING TOUCHES:

8. **Carefully reposition the pillow under the resident's head.**
9. **Straighten all of the bed linens. Secure and position the resident comfortably.**
10. **Perform the "5 Stars and 3 Rs."**

Moving a Resident up in Bed with a Lift/Draw Sheet: Two Co-Workers

Follow all standard and/or transmission-based precautions. Follow all rules for body mechanics.

Collect equipment: • lift sheet

1. **Perform the "5 Stars."**

PREPARE:

2. **Place pillow at the HOB up against the headboard.**
3. **Position lift sheet so that it is under the shoulders and hips of the resident (Figure 17-2).**
4. **Stand at the side of the bed and roll the lift sheet up toward the resident's body.**
5. **Spread feet apart about 12 inches and slightly bend the knees to protect your back.**

PERFORM:

6. **With hands and fingers facing upward, grasp the rolled edge of the lift sheet tightly at the shoulder AND the hips, and on the count of three, slowly and carefully move resident to the HOB. (Figure 17-3)**

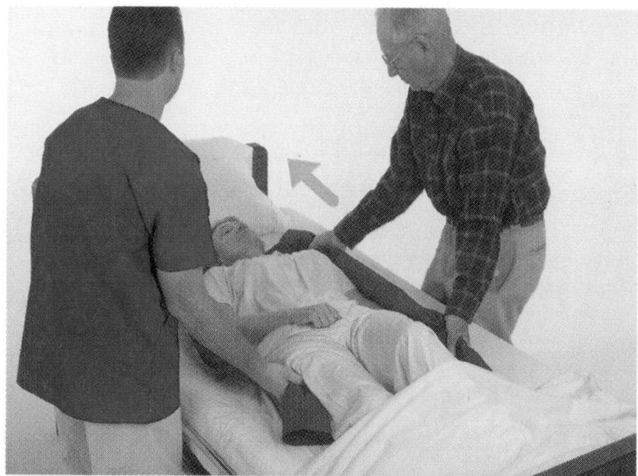

Figure 17-2.

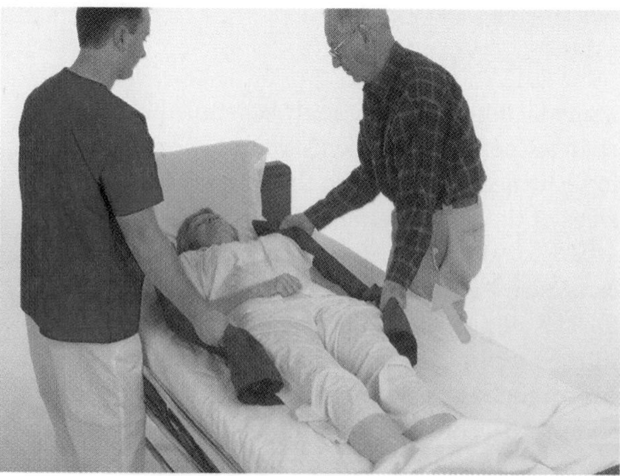

Figure 17-3.

FINISHING TOUCHES:

7. Carefully reposition the pillow under the resident's head.
8. Straighten all of the bed linens. Secure and position the resident comfortably.
9. Perform the "5 Stars and 3 Rs."

Moving a Resident to the Side of the Bed with a Lift/Draw Sheet: Two Co- Workers

Follow all standard and/or transmission-based precautions. Follow all rules for body mechanics.

Collect equipment:

- lift sheet

1. Perform the "5 Stars."

PREPARE:

2. Place pillow at the HOB up against the headboard.
3. Position lift sheet so that it is under the shoulders and hips of the resident.
4. Each co-worker stands on opposite sides of the bed and rolls up the lift sheet to better grasp it.
5. Spread feet apart about 12 inches and slightly bend the knees to protect your back.

PERFORM:

6. With hands and fingers facing upward, grasp the rolled edge of the lift sheet tightly at the shoulder AND the hips, and on the count of three, slowly and carefully move resident to the side of the bed.

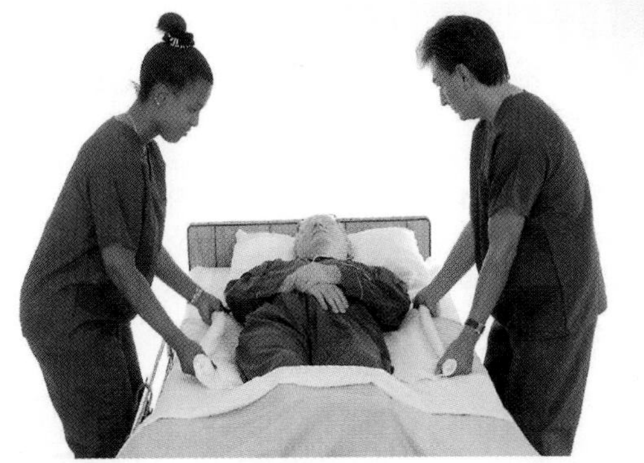

Figure 17-4.

FINISHING TOUCHES:

7. Carefully reposition the pillow under resident's head.
8. Straighten all of the bed linens. Secure and position the resident comfortably.
9. Perform the "5 Stars and 3 Rs."

Moving a Resident to the Side of the Bed: One Worker

Follow all standard and/or transmission-based precautions. Follow all rules for body mechanics.

1. Perform the "5 Stars."

PREPARE:

2. Place pillow at the HOB up against the headboard.
3. Stand at the side of the bed.
4. Spread feet apart about 12 inches and slightly bend the knees to protect your back.

PERFORM:

5. Gently slide hands under the head and shoulders of the resident and move the head and shoulders area toward you.
6. Gently slide hands under the mid-section of the resident and move the midsection area toward you.
7. Gently slide hands under the hips and legs area of the resident and move the midsection area toward you.

Figure 17-5.

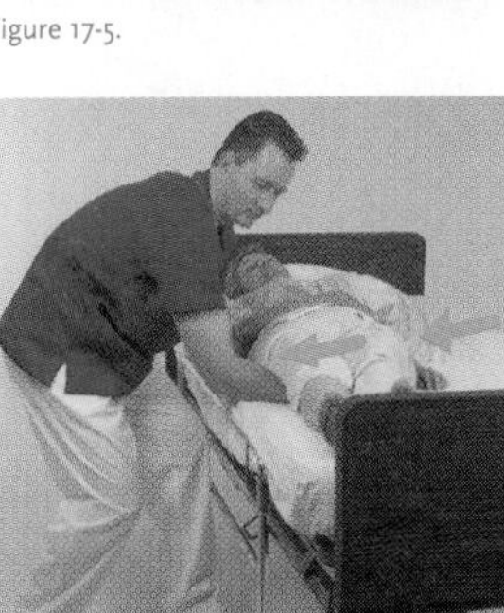

Figure 17-6.

FINISHING TOUCHES:

8. Carefully reposition the pillow under the head of the resident.
9. Straighten all of the bed linens. Secure and position resident comfortably.
10. Perform the "5 Stars and 3 Rs."

 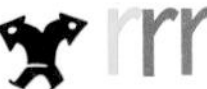

Turning Your Resident Toward You

Follow all standard and/or transmission-based precautions. Follow all rules for body mechanics.

1. Perform the "5 Stars."

PREPARE:

2. Stand at the side of the bed and spread feet apart about 12 inches and slightly bend the knees to protect your back.

PERFORM:

3. After carefully moving the resident to the side of the bed using the previous procedure, secure the resident, and move to the opposite side of the bed.

4. Cross the resident's arm furthest from you over the resident's chest.
5. Cross the resident's leg furthest from you over the resident's other leg.

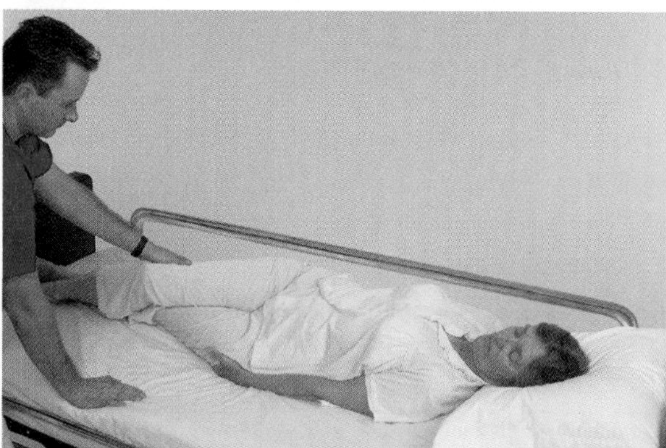

Figure 17-7.

6. Place one hand on the resident's shoulder and the other hand on the resident's hip.
7. Gently roll the resident toward your side of the bed.

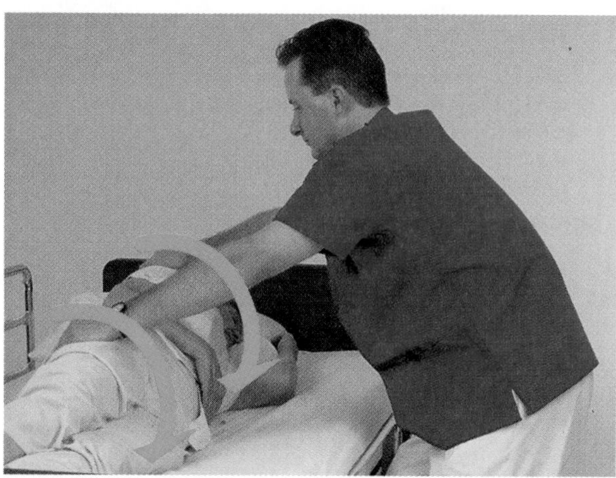

Figure 17-8.

FINISHING TOUCHES:

8. Carefully reposition the pillows under the head, back, and between the legs of the resident.
9. Straighten all of the bed linens. Secure and position the resident comfortably.
10. Perform the "5 Stars and 3 Rs."

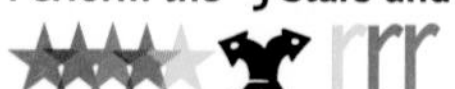

Turning Your Resident Away from You

Follow all standard and/or transmission-based precautions. Follow all rules for body mechanics.

1. Perform the "5 Stars."

If side rails are in use, side rail must be up on the opposite side of the bed and down on the side from which you will work.

PREPARE:

2. Stand at the side of the bed and spread feet apart about 12 inches and slightly bend the knees to protect your back.

PERFORM:

3. Carefully move the resident to the side of the bed following the prior procedure, and then stand on the side nearest the resident.
4. Cross the resident's arm nearest you over the resident's chest.
5. Cross the resident's leg nearest you over the resident's other leg.

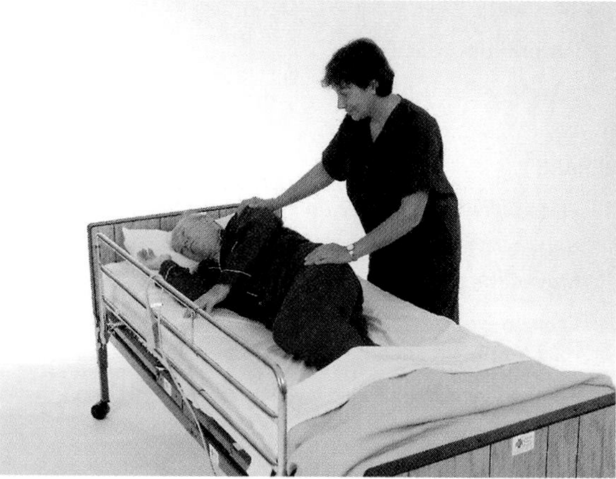

Figure 17-9.

6. Place one hand on the resident's shoulder closest to you and the other hand on the resident's hip closest to you.
7. Gently push the resident to the opposite side of the bed.

FINISHING TOUCHES:

8. Carefully reposition the pillow under the head, back, and between the legs of the resident.
9. Straighten all of the bed linens. Secure and position the resident comfortably.
10. Perform the "5 Stars and 3 Rs."

Logrolling Using a Lift/Draw Sheet: Two Co-Workers

Follow all standard and/or transmission-based precautions. Follow all rules for body mechanics.

Logrolling allows you to turn a resident all at once while keeping the spine straight.

Collect equipment:

- lift sheet

1. Perform the "5 Stars."

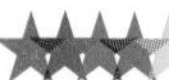

PREPARE:

2. Both co-workers stand on one side of the bed:
    a. One worker stands at the head and shoulders of the resident.
    b. One worker stands at the midsection of the resident.
3. Stand with feet spread apart about 12 inches and slightly bend the knees to protect your back.

PERFORM:

4. Place a pillow under the head to support the neck during the move.
5. Cross the resident's arm nearest you over the chest.
6. Roll up the edges of the draw sheet next to the body toward the resident, fingers pointed downward to better grasp it.
7. On the count of three, co-workers slowly roll the resident, using the draw sheet, all at once toward the side of the bed.

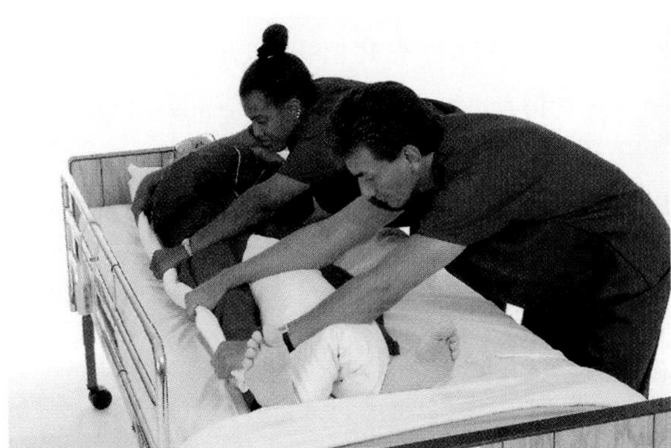

Figure 17-10.

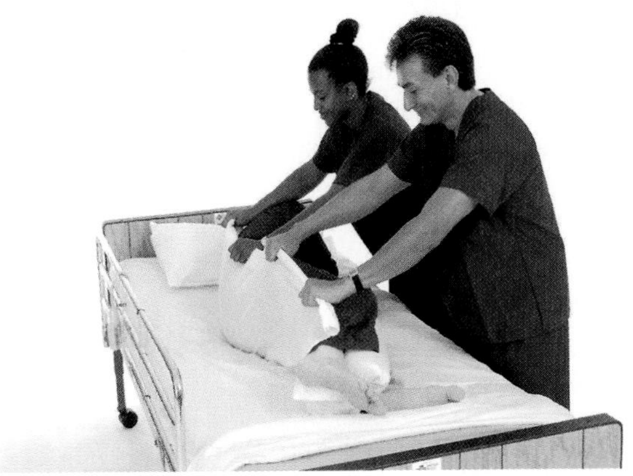

Figure 17-11.

FINISHING TOUCHES:

8. Carefully reposition the pillows under the head, back, and between the legs of the resident. Add pillows as needed.
9. Straighten all of the linens. Secure and position the resident comfortably.
10. Perform the "5 Stars and 3 Rs."

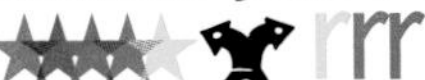

Assisting a Resident to the Side of the Bed: Dangling

Follow all standard and/or transmission-based precautions. Follow all rules for body mechanics.

Dangling moves the resident into a sitting position on the side of the bed with the legs hanging over the side.

1. Perform the "5 Stars."

PREPARE:

2. Raise the HOB to Fowler's position.
3. Stand at the side of the bed with the feet about 12 inches apart and bend the knees slightly to protect your back.

PERFORM:

4. Cross the resident's leg opposite you over the resident's other leg.
5. Gently slide one hand behind the resident's upper back closest to you and one hand under the knees and around the upper legs.

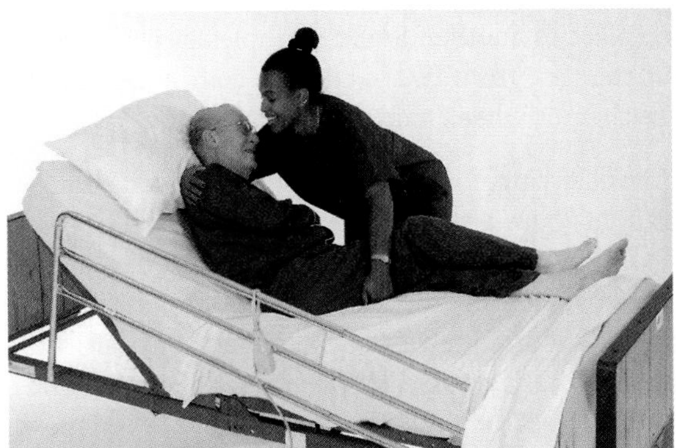

Figure 17-12.

6. Moving smoothly, slide the legs over the side of the bed and move the head and shoulders upward at the same time, so that the resident is now sitting to the side of the bed.

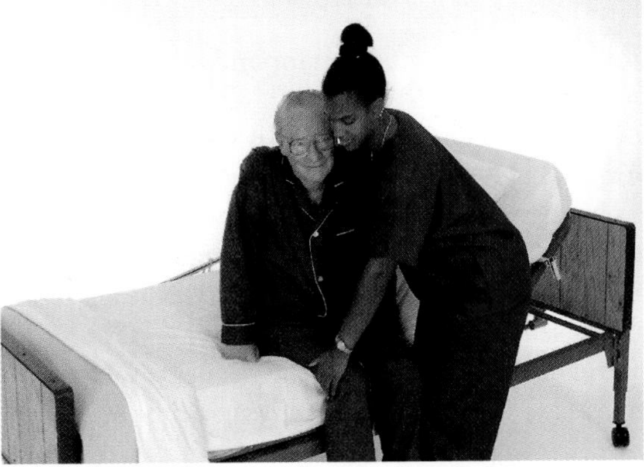

Figure 17-13.

7. **Ask the resident to immediately form a fist with both hands and push both fists into the bed for support.**
8. **If the resident feels faint, immediately allow his head and shoulders to move back down onto the pillow and call for the nurse.**
9. **Allow the resident to dangle for a period of time and then return the resident back to bed. Stay with the resident at all times.**
10. **Take vital signs if necessary.**

FINISHING TOUCHES:

11. **Carefully reposition the pillow under the resident's head.**
12. **Straighten all of the linens. Secure and position the resident comfortably.**
13. **Perform the "5 Stars and 3 Rs."**

4 Explain why transfers lead with the strong side of the body and demonstrate the use of a gait/transfer belt and a sliding board.

Transfers are done so that a resident can move from one place to another. Some examples of possible transfers are from bed to chair or commode, bed to stretcher, or wheelchair to toilet or vehicle.

In transferring, it is important to know that some residents have a strong side and a weak side. The weak side is called the "involved" or "affected" side. You must plan the move so that the strong side moves first and the weak side follows. It is difficult for a resident to move a weak arm and leg first and be able to bear enough weight to allow for the move.

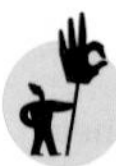

The strong arm transfers!

When transferring a resident with one weak side from one place to another, one method of remembering the correct position is the following: The "strong arm" transfers a resident.

While evaluating a resident for ambulation, staff members may determine that a resident would be safer if a gait belt is used. A **gait belt** or **transfer belt** is a heavy-duty belt with a strong buckle that is wrapped around a resident's waist and over clothes, and then secured. The buckle is usually positioned slightly off-center on the front of the body. A gait belt is not used to lift a resident; it is used to have greater control of the movement of the resident. When securing the belt, enough room should be left to insert two fingers into the belt. Care must be taken not to catch residents' breasts in the belt when tightening. The staff member who is using the belt should grasp it in the following manner:

Grasp belt in the center of the back of the belt with the dominant or strong hand, with fingers positioned up.

This allows maximum support of the resident during ambulation, and, should the resident begin falling, it may help you prevent injury.

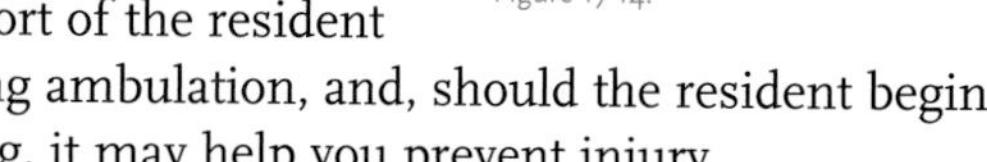

Figure 17-14.

Use a gentle rocking motion to take advantage of any momentum.

Sliding or transfer boards allow residents who use wheelchairs to transfer to vehicles, beds, shower chairs, and other areas without a lot of assistance from other people. Applying a small amount of cornstarch powder can make movement on a sliding board easier.

Mechanical lifts are tools to protect you and your resident. However, staff frequently avoid using available mechanical lifts. Learn to use the lifts available to you. Also learn to explain their use to your residents to ease their fears of them.

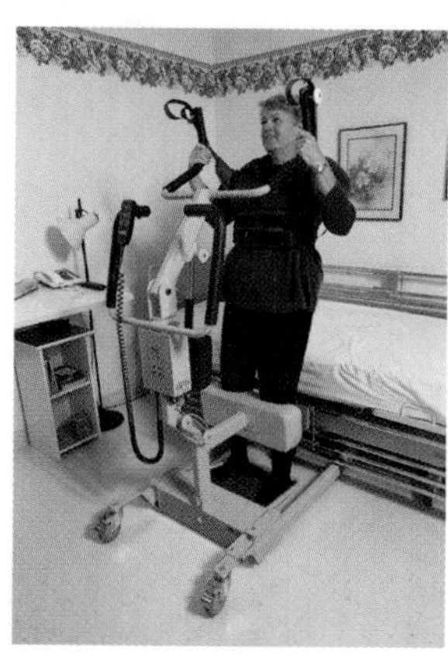

Figure 17-15. **(Photo of TotaLift-SPL courtesy of Wy'East Medical Corporation)**

Using a Sliding or Transfer Board

Follow all standard and/or transmission-based precautions. Follow all rules for body mechanics.

Collect equipment:
- **wheelchair • sliding board**
- **OPTIONAL: cornstarch powder**

1. **Perform the "5 Stars."**

PREPARE:

2. Position wheelchair at the side of the bed, sofa, or car at a slight angle on the resident's stronger side.
3. Lock wheelchair and remove arm- and footrests closest to resident.
4. Position the sliding/transfer board between the chair and the other surface (bed, chair, car).
5. Sprinkle with cornstarch powder if desired.

PERFORM:

6. Ask resident to slowly slide over the sliding board to the bed, chair, or car. Assist as necessary, watching your own body positioning.

FINISHING TOUCHES:

7. Carefully position resident, straighten all linens if in bed, and make sure resident is comfortable. Secure resident.

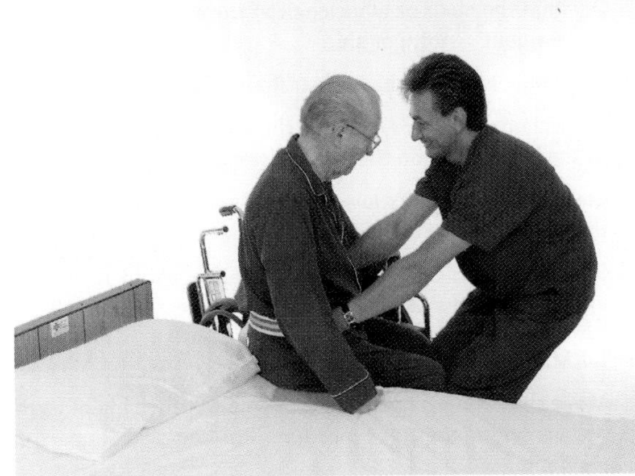

Figure 17-16.

8. Perform the "5 Stars and 3 Rs."

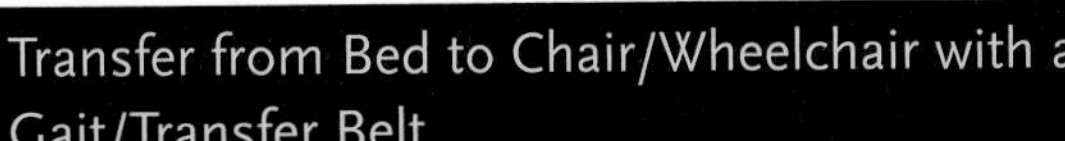

Transfer from Bed to Chair/Wheelchair with a Gait/Transfer Belt

Follow all standard and/or transmission-based precautions. Follow all rules for body mechanics.

Collect equipment:
- gait/transfer belt
- wheelchair or chair
- slippers or shoes • socks

1. Perform the "5 Stars."

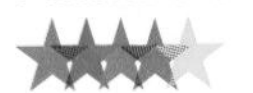

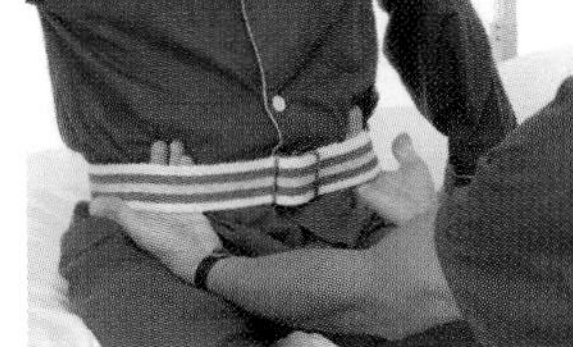

Figure 17-17.

PREPARE:

2. Position the chair or wheelchair at the side of the bed on the resident's stronger side.
3. Lock wheels of the wheelchair and remove the armrest and the footrest of the wheelchair closest to the bed.
4. Lower the HOB to its lowest flat position. The height of the bed has to be equal to or slightly higher than the chair.
5. Stand at the side of the bed with the feet about 12 inches apart and bend the knees slightly to protect your back.

PERFORM:

6. Move the resident to a sitting position at the side of the bed according to prior procedure. Put non-skid slippers on resident.
7. Wrap the transfer belt around the resident and secure.
8. Grasp the transfer belt at the sides with your fingers facing UP and place your feet and legs outside of the resident's feet and legs.
9. Ask resident to work with you, explaining again what you will do. On the count of three, using your legs to lift, bring the resident to a standing position.

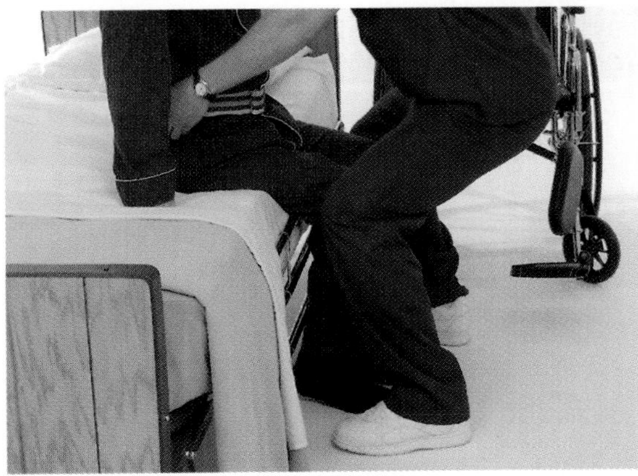

Figure 17-18.

10. Ask the resident to reach over and grasp the arm of the wheelchair with his strong arm.
11. Ask the resident to pivot his foot and move up against the front of the chair or wheelchair.
12. Bending your knees again, assist the resident to sit down and move to the back of the chair.

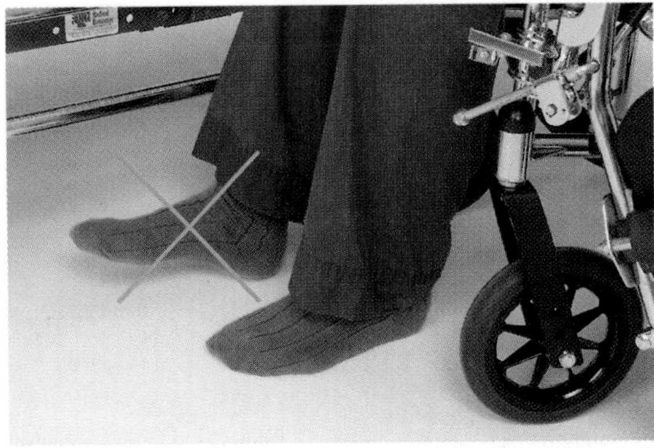

Figure 17-19. Residents should wear non-skid slippers during transfers.

FINISHING TOUCHES:

13. Remove the gait/transfer belt.
14. Replace the armrest on the wheelchair.
15. Carefully position the resident and make sure the resident is comfortable. Secure the resident.

16. Perform the "5 Stars and 3 Rs."

TO RETURN TO BED, REVERSE THE ABOVE PROCEDURE.

Transfer from Bed to Chair/Wheelchair without a Gait/Transfer Belt

Follow all standard and/or transmission-based precautions. Follow all rules for body mechanics.

Collect equipment:
- wheelchair or chair
- slippers or shoes • socks

1. Perform the "5 Stars."

PREPARE:

2. Position the chair or wheelchair at the side of the bed on the resident's stronger side.
3. Lock wheels of the wheelchair and remove the armrest and the footrest on the side closest to the bed.
4. Lower the HOB to its lowest flat position. The height of the bed has to be equal to or slightly higher than the chair.
5. Stand at the side of the bed with the feet about 12 inches apart and bend the knees slightly to protect your back.

PERFORM:

6. Move the resident to a sitting position at the side of the bed according to prior procedure. Put non-skid slippers on resident.
7. Place your hands well under the arms of the resident so that your fingers are not in the underarm or axilla.
8. Place your feet and legs outside of the resident's feet and legs.
9. Ask the resident to place his hands on your shoulders.
10. On the count of three, using the strong muscles of your legs to lift, bring the resident to a standing position.
11. Ask the resident to reach over and grasp the arm of the wheelchair with his strong arm.
12. Ask the resident to pivot his foot and move up against the front of the chair or wheelchair.

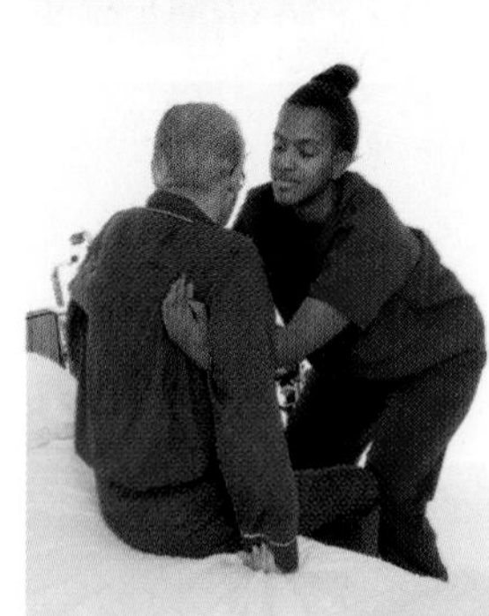

Figure 17-20.

13. Bending your knees again, assist the resident to sit down and move to the back of the chair.

FINISHING TOUCHES:

14. Carefully position the resident and make sure the resident is comfortable. Secure the resident.

15. Perform the "5 Stars and 3 Rs."

TO RETURN TO BED, REVERSE THE ABOVE PROCEDURE.

Transfer from Bed to Chair/Wheelchair with Walker Assist

Follow all standard and/or transmission-based precautions. Follow all rules for body mechanics.

Collect equipment:
- walker • wheelchair or chair • slippers or shoes • socks

1. Perform the "5 Stars."

PREPARE:

2. Position the chair or wheelchair at the side of the bed on the resident's stronger side.
3. Lock wheels of the chair. Clear floor of any obstacles.
4. After choosing a side, remove the armrest and the footrest of the wheelchair on the side closest to the bed.
5. Lower the HOB to its lowest flat position. The height of the bed has to be equal to slightly higher than the chair.
6. Stand at the side of the bed with the feet about 12 inches apart and bend the knees slightly to protect your back.

PERFORM:

7. Move the resident to a sitting position at the side of the bed according to prior procedure. Put non-skid slippers on resident.
8. Place your hands well under the arms of the resident so that your fingers are not in the underarm or axilla.
9. Place your feet and legs outside of the resident's feet and legs.
10. Ask the resident to place his hands on your shoulders.
11. On the count of three, using the strong muscles of your legs to lift, bring the resident to a standing position.
12. Place the walker in front of the resident and ask the resident to place his hands on the walker.
13. Ask the resident to slowly move the walker so that he is in front of the wheelchair or chair.
14. Ask the resident to take the strong hand off of the walker

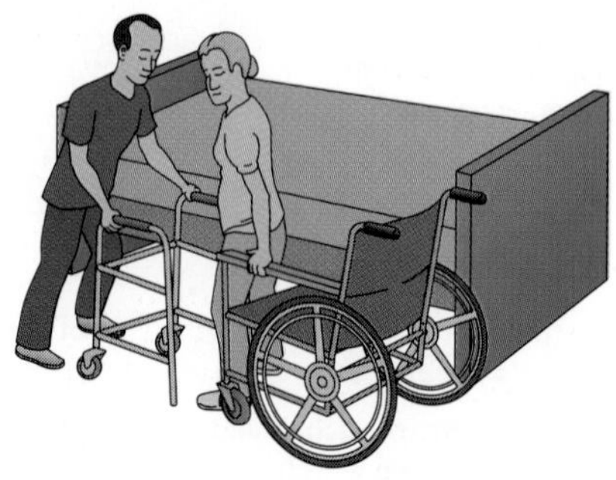

Figure 17-21.

and reach over and grasp the arm of the wheelchair.

15. Ask the resident to move up against the front of the chair or wheelchair.
16. Ask the resident to remove the second hand from the walker, sit down in the chair or wheelchair, and move to the back of the chair.

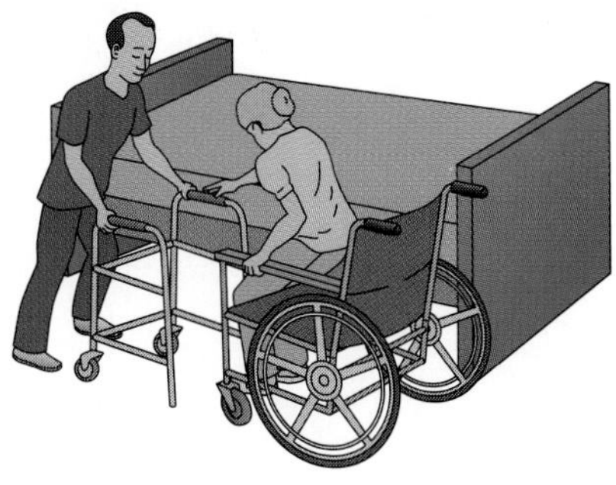

Figure 17-22.

FINISHING TOUCHES:

17. Carefully position the resident and make sure the resident is comfortable. Secure the resident.
18. Perform the "5 Stars and 3 Rs."

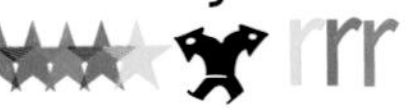

TO RETURN TO BED, REVERSE THE ABOVE PROCEDURE.

Transfer to and from Toilet from a Wheelchair

Follow all standard and/or transmission-based precautions. Follow all rules for body mechanics.

Collect equipment:
- two pair of disposable gloves • wheelchair
- slippers or shoes • socks

1. Perform the "5 Stars."

2. Apply gloves.

PREPARE:

3. Transfer resident to wheelchair using prior procedure.
4. Move resident into the bathroom. Close the door.
5. Place wheelchair close to the toilet at an angle on the side of the toilet with the most room. Lock wheelchair.

PERFORM:

6. Ask the resident to push against the armrests of the wheelchair and come to a standing position, immediately reaching for and grasping the hand bar.

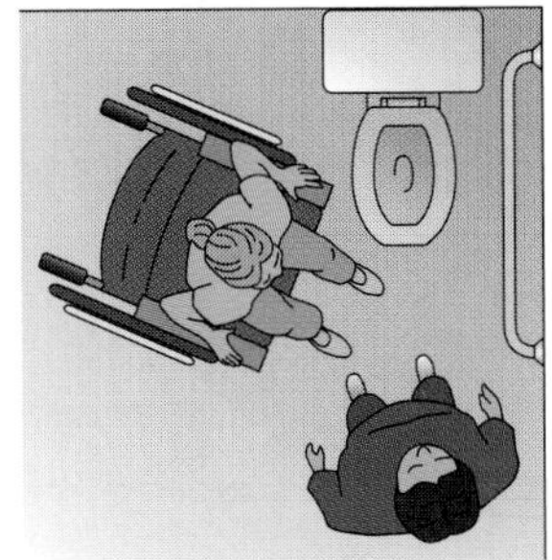

Figure 17-23.

7. Ask the resident to pivot his foot and back up so that he can feel the front of the toilet with the back of his legs.
8. Assist the resident to pull down clothing and slowly sit down onto the toilet.
9. When the resident is finished, assist the resident in cleaning his perineal area or buttocks and remove and dispose of your gloves.
10. Pull up clothing and transfer the resident back to the wheelchair. Assist resident to the sink to wash hands. Wash your hands.

FINISHING TOUCHES:

11. Return the resident to the bed or other area. Carefully position the resident and make sure the resident is comfortable. Secure the resident.
12. Perform the "5 Stars and 3 Rs."

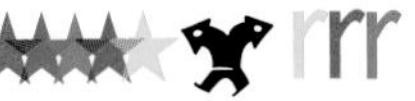

Transfer to and from a Shower Chair from a Wheelchair

Follow all standard and/or transmission-based precautions. Follow all rules for body mechanics.

Collect equipment:
- wheelchair • shower chair • two bath towels
- bath supplies • slippers or shoes • socks

1. Perform the "5 Stars."

PREPARE:

2. Transfer resident to wheelchair using prior procedure.
3. Move resident into the shower room.
4. Place wheelchair close to the shower chair at an angle on the side with the most room. Lock wheelchair and shower chair, if on wheels.

PERFORM:

5. Remove gown or clothes. Have the resident hold onto the grab bars and push against the arm rests of the wheelchair and come to a standing position.
6. Ask the resident to pivot his foot and back up so that he feels the front of the shower chair with the back of his legs.
7. The resident should then grasp the shower chair armrest (if available) and slowly sit down onto the shower chair.

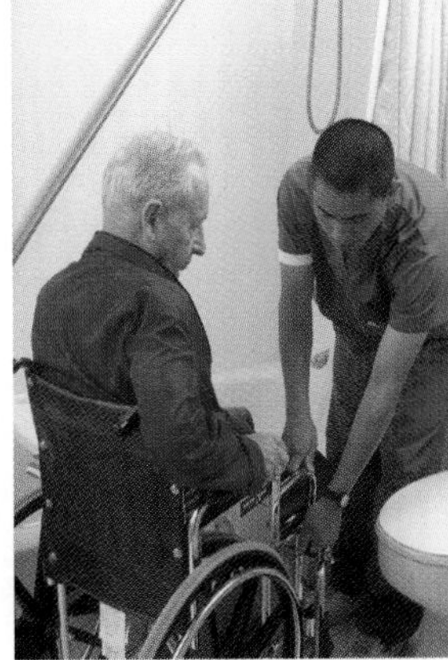

Figure 17-24.

8. When the resident is finished showering, wrap resident in towel. Assist the resident to sit in a chair and provide him

with another towel for drying. Offer assistance in drying hard-to-reach places. Assist resident in getting dressed.

9. Transfer resident back to the wheelchair. Make sure you lock both chairs before the transfer.

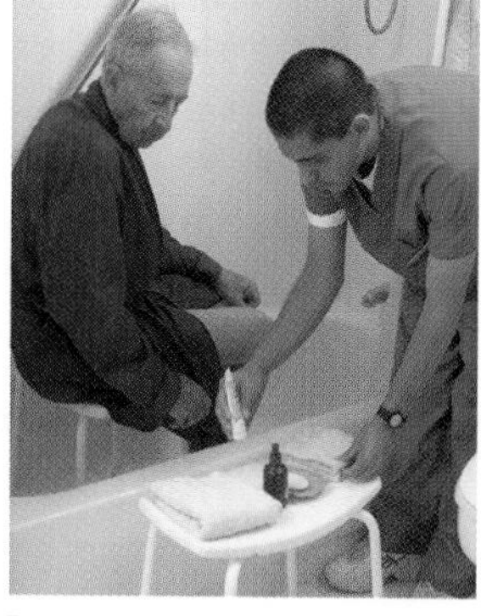

Figure 17-25.

FINISHING TOUCHES:

10. Return the resident to the bed or other area. Carefully position the resident and make sure the resident is comfortable. Secure the resident.

11. Perform the "5 Stars and 3 Rs."

Transfer to a Car from a Wheelchair

Follow all standard and/or transmission-based precautions. Follow all rules for body mechanics.

Collect equipment:
- wheelchair

1. Perform the "5 Stars."

PREPARE:

2. Transfer resident to wheelchair using prior procedure.
3. Move resident outside to the car.
4. Place wheelchair close to the car at an angle with the car's open door on the resident's stronger side
5. Lock wheelchair. Remove footrests.

PERFORM:

6. Ask the resident to push against the arm rests of the wheelchair and come to a standing position.
7. Ask the resident to stand, grasp the car, and pivot his foot.

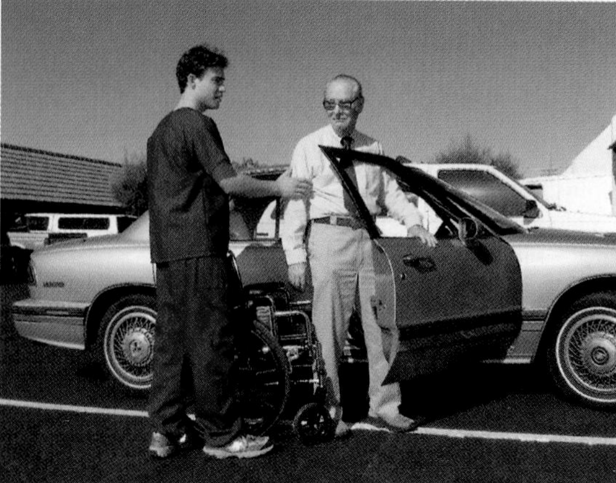

Figure 17-26.

8. The resident should then sit on the car seat and lift one leg, and then the other, into the vehicle.

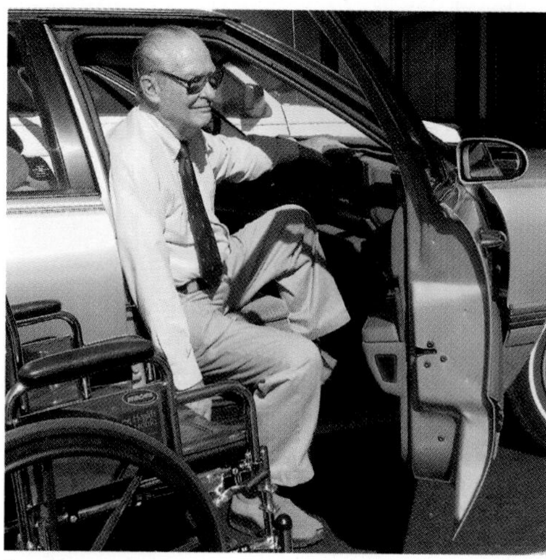

Figure 17-27.

FINISHING TOUCHES:

9. Carefully position the resident comfortably in the car. Assist in securing seat belt.
10. See that door can be safely shut and shut door.
11. Return the wheelchair to the appropriate site for cleaning and wash hands.

Using a Mechanical Lift to Transfer to Wheelchair or Chair: Two or Three Co-Workers

Follow all standard and/or transmission-based precautions. Follow all rules for body mechanics.

Collect equipment:
- **mechanical lift** or lift scale • washcloth or small towel

Before performing this procedure, you must check the weight limit of the lift, and make sure your resident is within the weight limit. Make certain you know how to use this lift.

1. Perform the "5 Stars."

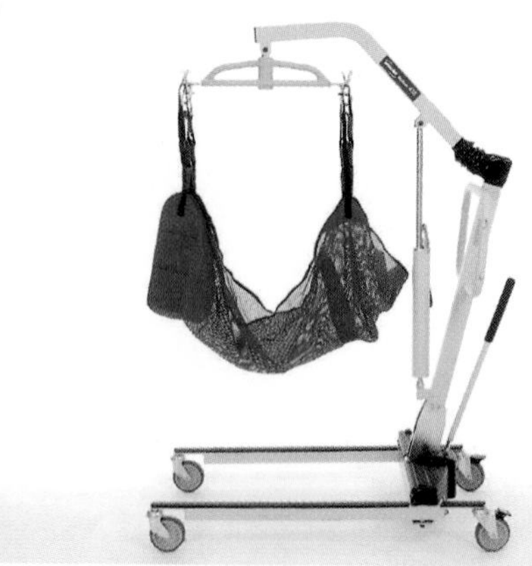

Figure 17-28.

PREPARE:

2. Depending upon the room set-up, place the wheelchair parallel to the bed facing the FOB. Pad the wheelchair with a bath blanket, blanket, or sheet.
3. Lock the wheelchair and remove the armrest and the footrest closest to the bed.
4. Select the correct size sling for resident size.
5. Correctly position the sling under the resident by turning the resident from side to side. Pad the sling, if necessary.
6. Position soft washcloth or small towel beneath the neck of the resident to prevent the sling from rubbing on the neck and shoulders of the resident.
7. Have resident cross arms over his chest.

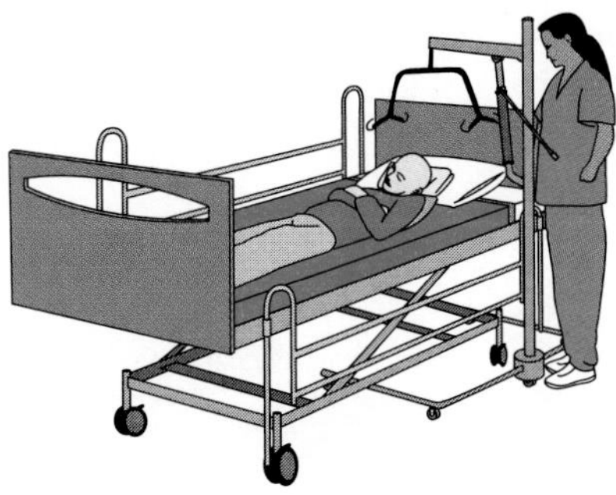

Figure 17-29.

PERFORM:

8. Move the lift over the resident and be careful that the bars do not hit anyone.
9. Attach the straps or clips securely to the sling. The hooks or clip openings should face away from the resident to avoid injury. Double-check connections before moving.
10. The resident should then be slowly raised in the lift until the bottom of the resident clears the bed. One worker pumps and another guides the resident, protecting the resident's legs and feet.
11. Move the lift to the wheelchair or chair and position directly over the chair.
12. One helper slowly lowers the resident into the chair while the second helper protects the legs and feet and guides the resident into the chair.
13. Make sure the resident is all the way at the back of the chair.

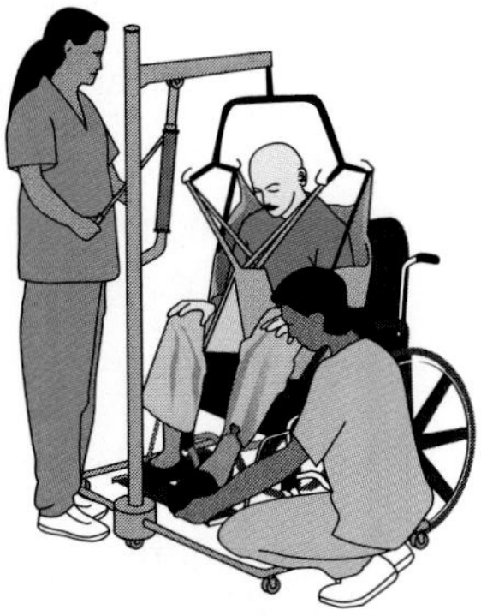

Figure 17-30.

FINISHING TOUCHES:

14. Detach the sling straps or hooks and chains, leaving sling in place.
15. Remove the lift from the wheelchair area.
16. Position the resident comfortably in the chair, and SECURE THE RESIDENT.
17. Place a wheelchair cushion, or other type of active or passive restraint, in place ONLY if ordered.
18. Place call light in reach of resident if the resident is to stay in room.
19. Wash hands.
20. Perform the "5 Stars and 3 Rs."

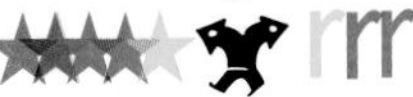

RETURN TO BED, REVERSE THE ABOVE PROCEDURE.

Transfer from Stretcher to Bed Using a Transfer Sheet: Four Co-Workers

Follow all standard and/or transmission-based precautions. Follow all rules for body mechanics.

Collect equipment:
- transfer sheet

1. Perform the "5 Stars."

PREPARE:

2. Place stretcher solidly against the bed, lock stretcher, and bring bed height up almost to the height of the stretcher. Remove stretcher safety belts.
3. Two helpers should be on each side of the resident.
4. Each helper rolls the sides of the transfer sheet and prepares to move the resident. It may be your facility policy to allow some helpers to actually get up on the bed to complete this transfer. Follow your facility policy.
5. Make sure the arms and legs of the resident are secure and protected during the transfer.

PERFORM:

6. On the count of three, the helpers should lift and move the resident to the bed all at once.

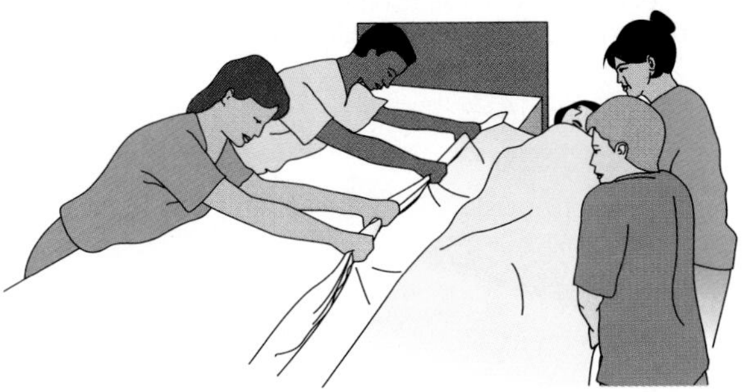

Figure 17-31.

7. The transfer sheet should then be removed by turning the resident from side to side.

FINISHING TOUCHES:

8. Carefully position the resident and make sure the resident is comfortable and that sheets are not wrinkled underneath. Secure the resident.

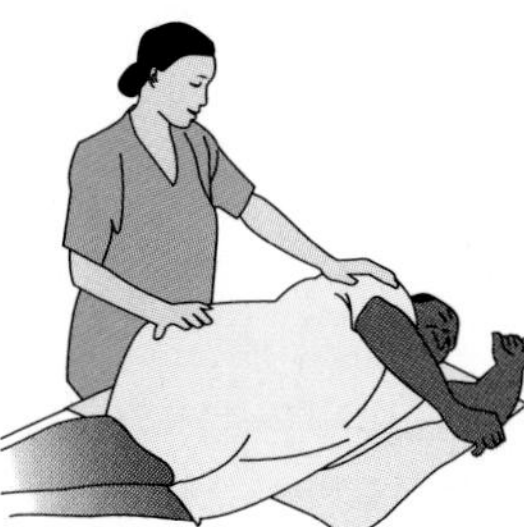

Figure 17-32.

9. **Perform the "5 Stars and 3 Rs."**

10. **Return the stretcher to the appropriate site for cleaning and wash hands.**

Transfer from Bed to Stretcher Using a Transfer Sheet: Four Co-Workers

Follow all standard and/or transmission-based precautions. Follow all rules for body mechanics.

Collect equipment:

- **transfer sheet**

1. **Perform the "5 Stars."**

PREPARE:

2. **Place stretcher solidly against the bed, lock stretcher, and bring bed height slightly above the height of the stretcher.**
3. **Two helpers should be on each side of the resident.**

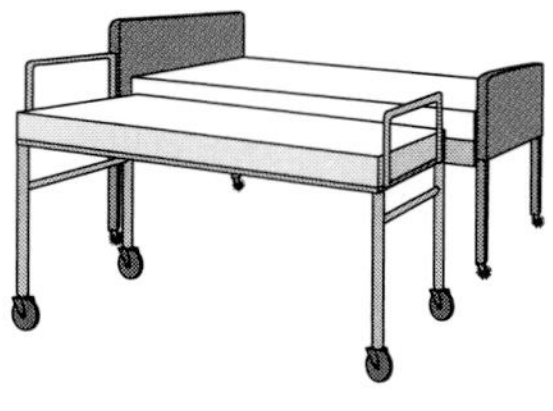

Figure 17-33.

4. **Each helper rolls the sides of the transfer sheet to better grip it, and prepares to move the resident. It may be your facility policy to allow some helpers to get on the bed to complete this transfer. Follow your facility policy.**
5. **Make sure the arms and legs of the resident are secure and protected during the transfer.**

PERFORM:

6. **On the count of three, the helpers should lift and move the resident to the stretcher all at one time.**

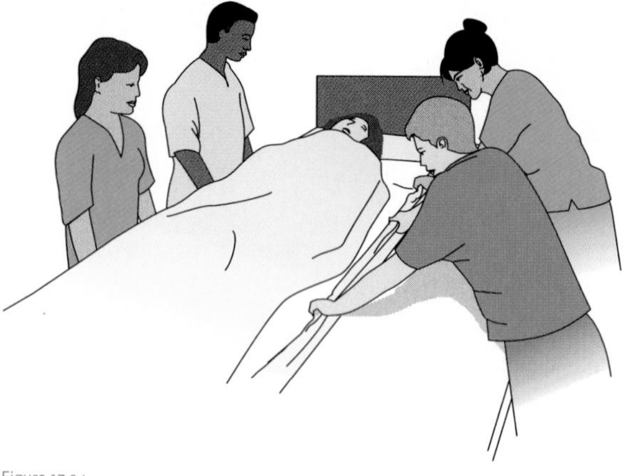

Figure 17-34.

FINISHING TOUCHES:

7. **Carefully position the resident in the stretcher and make sure the resident is comfortable. Place safety belts across the resident. Raise side rails on stretcher.**
8. **Bring resident to appropriate site and STAY with the resident! Resident should never be left alone on a stretcher.**
9. **Perform the "5 Stars and 3 Rs."**

Summary

The act of moving, lifting, and positioning residents is one that requires great skill and planning. Nursing assistants should make sure they are fully prepared when initiating one of these procedures, especially for the first time. It is vital for the resident's well-being as well as the safety of the staff that all health team members take great care and communicate with each other and the resident when performing the procedures detailed in this chapter.

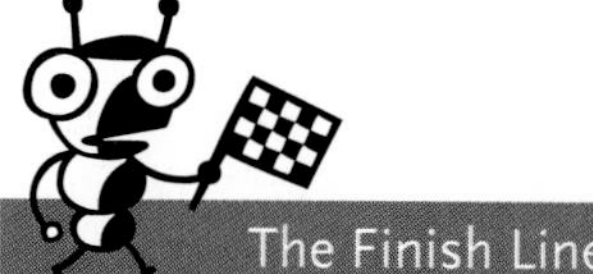

The Finish Line

What's Wrong With This Picture?

1. The 10 Rules for Proper Body Mechanics are listed below with three missing. Fill in the missing steps:

   Assess the load.

   Think ahead, plan, and communicate the move.

   Face what you are lifting.

   Begin in a squatting position and lift with your legs.

   Contract (tighten) your stomach muscles when beginning the lift.

   Do not twist.

   Push or pull when possible rather than lifting.

2. The procedure for logrolling a resident is listed below. Fill in the missing two steps:

1. **Perform the "5 Stars."**

PREPARE:

2. **Both co-workers stand on one side of the bed:**
   a. **One worker stands at the head and shoulders of the resident.**
   b. **One worker stands at the midsection of the resident.**

3. **Stand with feet spread apart about 12 inches and slightly bend the knees to protect your back.**

PERFORM:

4. **Place a pillow under the head to support the neck during the move.**
5. **Roll up the edges of the draw sheet next to the body toward the resident, fingers pointed downward to better grasp it.**

FINISHING TOUCHES:

6. **Carefully reposition the pillow under the head, back, and between the legs of the resident. Add pillows as needed.**
7. **Straighten all of the linens and make sure resident is comfortable.**
8. **Perform the "5 Stars and 3 Rs."**

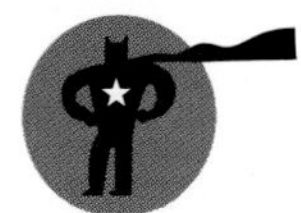

Star Student Central

1. Are you always careful with your muscles and joints when moving about at home and at work? Moving in a speedy fashion may cause you serious and long-lasting injury. For one full day, carefully observe the way you move. Examine whether you put the health of your muscles and joints at risk. Do you ever stretch to reach and grab something? Do your joints feel stiff frequently? Do you ever twist your neck when you are moving about? If you lift anything heavy, do you lift in a safe manner? Do some research and locate material that will educate you on the proper way to move your body. Share this material with your class.
2. Before you take on the responsibility of moving and transferring residents, it is a good idea to observe as many of these procedures as possible. Make the decision to lift a resident when you feel you are ready. Do not lift alone if you feel you are unable to handle a resident yourself.

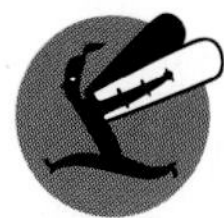

You Can Do It Corner!

1. How is the body helped to function by good body alignment? (LO 2)
2. For a resident with one weak side and one strong side, which side should do the transfer? Why? (LO 4)
3. Why should regular turning schedules always be maintained? (LO 3)
4. What steps can be taken to decrease the chance of rubbing and harming the skin during a mechanical lift transfer? (LO 4)
5. What are bony prominences? What can pressure on them cause? (LO 3)
6. Why should you try not to twist when you move? (LO 2)
7. When securing a gait belt, how much room should be left? (LO 4)
8. When moving a resident to the side of a bed with a lift sheet, why should you roll up the lift sheet? (LO 3)
9. During dangling, what should you do first if your resident feels faint during the procedure? (LO 3)
10. Why should you face what you are lifting? (LO 2)

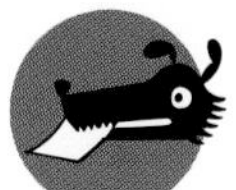

Star Student's Chapter Checklist

1. I have read my textbook chapter.
2. I have reviewed my own "Pocketful of Terms."
3. I have listened to my tutor tape.
4. I have reviewed and highlighted my class notes.
5. I have read and completed any handouts from this chapter.
6. I have completed "The Finish Line."
7. Star Time! Choose your reward!

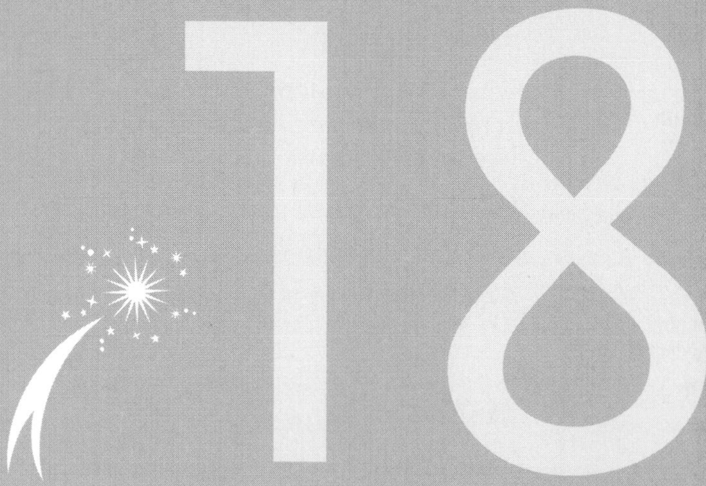

18

Your Introduction:

Restorative Care and Rehabilitation

Look Like a Star!

Look at the Learning Objectives and The Finish Line before you begin reading this chapter.

Look at your pocket calendar.
With your pencil, put a bracket (   ) around a study period every single day.

Look at your homework for this chapter.
Plug each piece of homework into a certain time slot.

Look at the Star Student's Chapter Checklist at the end of this chapter. Check off each item as it is completed.

"Rise, take up thy bed, and walk."

John V:8

"You cannot run away from a weakness. You must some time fight it out or perish..."

Robert Louis Stevenson, 1850-1894

Learning Objectives

1. Spell and define all STAR words.
2. Define the concepts of rehabilitation and restorative care and describe why promoting a resident's independence is important.
3. List and define eight activities of daily living and list ways exercise maintains normal body function.
4. Identify complications of bed rest for eight body systems.
5. Discuss the importance of regular ambulation.
6. Demonstrate the correct steps to assist a falling resident and identify the necessary follow-up.
7. Describe the purpose and use of canes, walkers, and crutches.
8. Identify nine types of equipment used to reduce the complications of bed rest.
9. Name the three types of range of motion exercises.

Successfully perform these Practical Procedures

Using a Cane

Using a Walker

Using Crutches

Performing Range of Motion Exercises

Using a Continuous Passive Motion (CPM) Machine

A View from the Past: Rehabilitation

In 1918, there were so many injured veterans returning from World War I that people in the United States developed an idea to bring an injured person to the point where he would have an opportunity to return to society. Following WWI, this idea of rehabilitation eventually grew. Facilities and programs were put into place, and when the thousands of victims of this war returned to the U.S.(many without arms or legs), they were able to begin their rehabilitation.

1 Spell and define all **STAR** words.

abduction: the movement of a body part away from the body.

activities of daily living (ADLs): activities that people perform on a daily basis such as dressing, eating, hygiene, and grooming.

adduction: the movement of a body part toward the body.

contractures: abnormal shortening of a muscle resulting in the disability of a limb.

dorsiflexion: bending backward, e.g. the toes pointed up.

extension: straightening of a body part.

flexion: bending a body part.

muscle atrophy: decrease in the size or wasting away of muscle tissues.

non-weight bearing (NWB): unable to support any weight on one or both legs.

partial weight bearing (PWB): able to support some weight on one or both legs.

passive range of motion (PROM): exercises used when residents do not have the ability to execute the movements on their own.

plantar flexion: foot drop; bending downward, e.g. the toes pointed down.

pronation: turning a body part downward, e.g. the face down or the palm down.

range of motion (ROM) exercises: exercises that move each joint through its full arc of motion.

rehabilitation: care directed by rehabilitation professionals (physical therapists, occupational therapists, speech therapists) to restore and maximize function.

restorative care: may follow rehabilitative care; carried out by nursing staff to maintain function and avoid loss of function.

rotation: the act of turning a joint.

supination: turning a body part upward, e.g. the face up or the palm up.

2 Define the concepts of rehabilitation and restorative care and describe why promoting a resident's independence is important.

Rehabilitation was still in its infancy during the time of World War II. The second world war was truly a springboard that allowed the concept of **rehabilitation** to grow into what it has become today: the true standard used to bring people to their highest level of functioning possible after an illness or injury. That level of functioning may be quite different for each person. For example, one person who has been injured, disabled, or is recovering from an illness may be rehabilitated to the point at which he is able to return to regular activities. Another person in need of rehabilitation may be brought to the point at which he has improved but is unable to resume all regular activities. The degree of rehabilitation possible depends upon many factors. Some of these factors include:

- exact time when rehabilitation actually began
- motivation of the injured person
- overall efforts of the staff and the family
- type of facility that admitted the person
- underlying disease process or injury

For rehabilitation to succeed, the entire staff of a facility joins together to return the person to the highest level of functioning possible. Every step of the care plan should be organized around the concept of rehabilitation.

In some cases, nursing assistants are hired directly by a patient who is disabled to help with rehabilitation. In this case, it is the patient who directs your work. If you are hired to do this, you must always make sure to be on time, dependable, and respectful.

Restorative care is a type of care that attempts to restore the person to the highest level of independence possible. A resident's independence may make

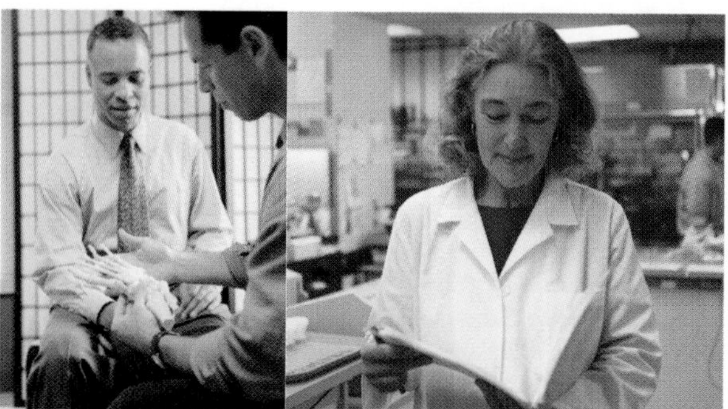

Figure 18-1. The physician and nurses will establish goals of care, which will include promoting independence in activities of daily living and restoring health to optimal condition.

the difference between a person's ability to take an active role in his or her day. It affects the resident's self-image positively and helps improve attitude.

Sometimes it will appear easier for you to do things for your resident rather than allowing the resident to accomplish a task independently. Your residents need to do as much for themselves as they can, regardless of how long it takes or how poorly they are able to do it. Although you think you could do it better or faster, be patient and encourage your resident to perform as much self-care as possible. Independence promotes self-esteem, as well as helping to speed recovery.

3 List and define eight activities of daily living and list ways exercise maintains normal body function.

A resident's day consists of many of the regular steps we all take to move through our days successfully. Some of these **activities of daily living** (ADLs) are listed below:

Activities of Daily Living (ADLs)

1. Bathing or showering
2. Dressing
3. Applying makeup and using personal hygiene products
4. Brushing teeth or cleaning dentures
5. Hair care and nail care
6. Toileting
7. Eating food and drinking fluids
8. Ambulating or moving about

The ability to perform the activities of daily living is of vital importance to every individual. When people are able to care for themselves, the burden on families and friends may decrease. When a person's ability to care for himself is compromised, the person's whole personal support structure of people may be affected. Lost hours on the job, along with a tremendous amount of stress on the family, may be a result of an inability to perform the ADLs.

Nursing staff members are responsible for restoring a person's ability to do as many of the ADLs as possible. When a person is able to perform the ADLs, she will have a much better chance of actively participating in daily activities. The care team helps to restore a resident's ability to do each and every ADL listed above. As pointed out before, each person will reach a different level of functioning when rehabilitation comes to an end. Rehabilitation is a skilled service that is a part of a facility's reimbursement for care. When the resident has met goals or his condition has stabilized, rehabilitation may no longer be needed. At that point, restorative care will continue to improve the resident's level of independence.

Nursing assistants are vital to the rehabilitation team. The process of rehabilitation revolves around each system of the body. One of the most important responsibilities of the nursing staff is to provide adequate exercise. Exercise affects each body system in some way. Some effects of exercise on each body system are outlined in the list below:

Integumentary: improves the quality and health of the skin

Cardiovascular: increases strength of the cardiac muscle and improves circulation

Respiratory: increases oxygen and reduces the chance of pneumonia

Musculoskeletal: increases blood flow to the muscles and improves strength

Nervous: improves relaxation and sleep

Endocrine: increases metabolic rate

Urinary: improves the elimination of liquid waste products

Gastrointestinal (GI): improves the elimination of solid waste products

4 Identify complications of bed rest for eight body systems.

When a person is unable to get adequate exercise, numerous complications may occur. The human body does not react well to long periods of time in bed. Complications that may occur with each body system when a person does not get enough exercise are outlined in the list below:

Integumentary: pressure sores and slow-healing wounds

Cardiovascular: blood clots, especially in the legs

Respiratory: pneumonia

Musculoskeletal: decrease in the size of muscles, known as **muscle atrophy** or **contractures**, the abnormal shortening of a muscle

Nervous System: depression or insomnia

Endocrine: weight gain

Urinary: kidney stones or infection

Gastrointestinal (GI): constipation

5 Discuss the importance of regular ambulation.

Ambulation means walking. Walking down to the dayroom for dinner, to the bathroom, to an activity like bingo, or to the barber or beauty shop are all examples of daily activities. The feeling of independence people may have when able to move about on their own cannot be underestimated. This type of independence may improve a person's self esteem and make each day more enjoyable.

Ambulation is important to maintain the health of many body systems. The strength of the heart muscle, the expansion of the lungs, and the ability of the body to eliminate solid and liquid wastes are all possible bonuses to getting enough exercise. Each facility may have schedules in place to ensure adequate ambulation. For example, residents' names and room numbers may be placed on a wall chart at regularly scheduled times to be followed by the staff. This helps make sure residents get enough exercise.

Residents may ambulate two, three, or possibly four times each day, for anywhere from ten to twenty minutes at a time. These scheduled walks help maintain the health of all of the body systems along with getting the resident out of the room and out among other residents, staff, and visitors.

Residents who ambulate independently still need to be encouraged to walk at regular intervals. We all know individuals who do not take the opportunity to exercise as often as they should. Residents, if not encouraged, may fall into the negative pattern of withdrawing to their rooms and not ambulating.

Making the decision to help a resident ambulate for the first time includes evaluating how much assistance he may need and the amount of time he may be able to sustain walking. It is a good idea to move very slowly when beginning an ambulation schedule. Here are some of the things a nurse or physical therapist will evaluate before taking a resident out for a first walk:

1. How many staff members should be present to help with the first walk?
2. Can the resident support full weight on both legs?
3. Can the resident walk short distances without feeling faint or dizzy?
4. Can the resident walk short distances without chest pain?
5. Can the resident walk short distances without shortness of breath?
6. Would it be safer to use a gait/transfer belt or other assistive device for this resident?

6 Demonstrate the correct steps to assist a falling resident and identify the necessary follow-up.

A resident who is weak or unsteady may fall unexpectedly. If you are not careful, this can cause you or your resident serious injury. Memorize the correct steps to take during falls and review them in your mind periodically to help prepare you for potential falls. This review will never take the place of a real fall; however, it can help prevent a mistake. This may ultimately protect your residents and you.

The most important words for you to remember when a resident falls are: "Cradle the head." If a resident falls and hits her head, a serious head injury may result. Although other areas of the body may also be seriously injured, the head must be protected first. Another serious injury that may occur is a broken hip. Common injuries among staff members are broken wrists or arms that result from trying to "catch" residents. You must understand it is not in anyone's best interest for you to try to "catch" someone, even though it may be your first instinct. "Catching" a resident is almost a guarantee that an injury will occur either to you or the resident.

Principal Steps

Assisting a Falling Resident

1. *If the resident is not wearing a gait belt, put your arms around the resident's waist.*

2. *Pull the resident close to you.*
3. *Immediately bend your knees and put one leg under the buttocks of the resident, if possible. This will depend on the resident's height.*
4. *Allow the resident to lower to the floor sliding down your leg.*
5. *After the resident has lowered to the floor, call for the nurse immediately. Do not try to help the resident get up until after the nurse arrives and assesses the situation. The nurse will ask you to assist in the completion of an incident report that will document the fall. It is important for you to give a complete description of the fall so that you and the resident are protected and future falls may be prevented.*

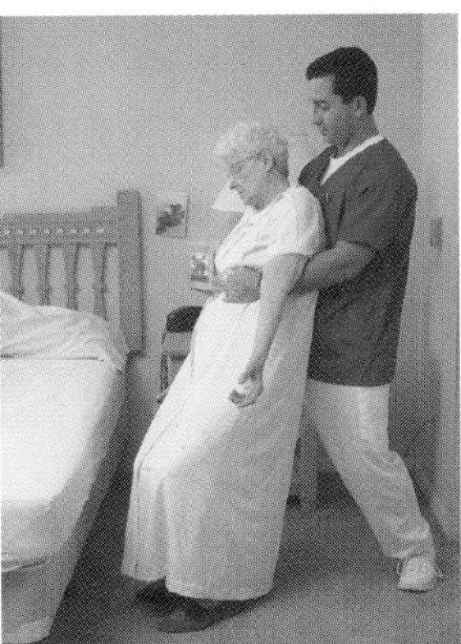

Figure 18-2.

7 Describe the purpose and use of canes, walkers, and crutches.

When residents are **non-weight bearing** or **partial-weight bearing**, they will benefit from using a device that helps support their weight. Canes, walkers, and crutches are types of equipment that can enable residents to move about on their own without a great deal of staff assistance or a wheelchair.

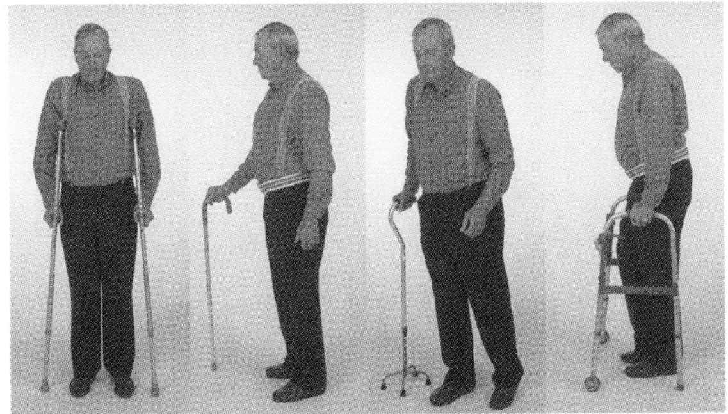

Figure 18-3. **Crutches, canes, or walkers may help residents who have difficulty walking.**

When using a cane or crutches and dealing with a resident with one weak leg and one strong leg, the approach is the same. The cane or set of crutches is moved first, then the weak leg, then the strong leg. When using a walker, the walker is moved first, then the weak leg, then the strong leg.

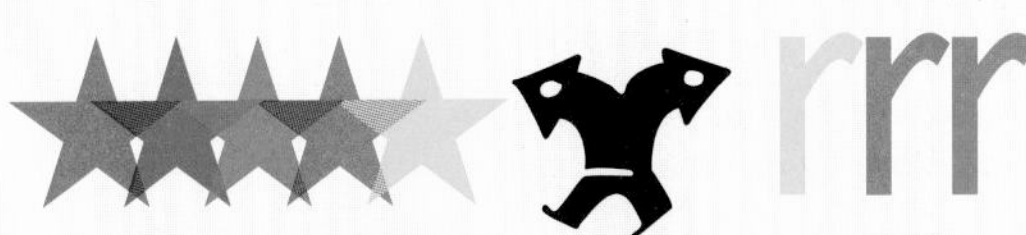

Beginning Steps

★ **RESPECT**
Knock first, ask and receive permission to enter a resident's room.

★ **INFECTION CONTROL**
Wash hands.

★ **COMMUNICATION**
Greet and identify the resident. Identify yourself. Explain the procedure, encouraging the resident to be as independent as possible throughout.

★ **BED SAFETY**
Lock bed wheels. Raise bed to safe working height. Lower one side rail if required.

★ **PRIVACY**
Provide for privacy by closing the door and covering the resident appropriately.

Ending Steps

★ **RESIDENT SAFETY AND COMFORT**
Secure the resident, lowering the bed, and raising the side rails if ordered. Check that the resident is comfortable and properly aligned.

★ **PRIVACY**
Remove any added privacy measures, such as a drape or a privacy screen.

★ **ESSENTIALS**
Place the call light, fresh beverage, and other items within reach.

★ **COURTESY**
Ask the resident if he or she needs anything else. Say thank you and goodbye.

★ **INFECTION CONTROL**
Wash hands.

r **Report** your care and any important observations to the nurse.

r **Record** your care and any important information/observations such as vital signs in the appropriate place.

r **Recheck** your resident for any changes as directed by the nurse!

Using a Cane

Follow all standard and/or transmission-based precautions. Follow all rules for body mechanics.

Collect equipment:
- cane

1. **Perform the "5 Stars."**

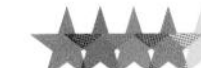

PREPARE:

2. **Carefully check cane for safety.**

Check to make sure cane is not bent or cracked and that cane tips are snugly in place.

3. Assist resident in putting on shoes or non-skid slippers and clothing or robe.
4. Bring resident to a sitting position at the side of the bed.
5. Have resident hold the cane with the strong hand or on side with stronger leg.

PERFORM:

6. Ask the resident to stand up by holding the cane four to six inches to the side of the strong foot.
7. The resident should move as follows: C-12-W-S
   a. Cane first, 12 inches or one stride forward

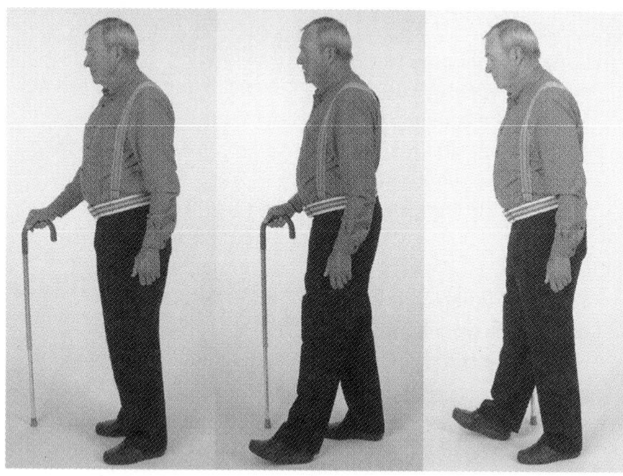

Figure 18-4.

   b. Weak (affected) leg forward same distance
   c. Strong (unaffected) leg forward either to cane or beyond if able
8. Repeat until the walk is completed.

FINISHING TOUCHES:

9. Return resident to the bed, chair, or wheelchair.
10. Carefully reposition the resident, straighten all of the linens if in bed, and make sure resident is comfortable.
11. Perform the "5 Stars and 3 Rs."

Using a Walker

Follow all standard and/or transmission-based precautions. Follow all rules for body mechanics.

Collect equipment:

- walker

1. Perform the "5 Stars."

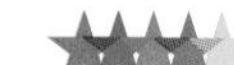

PREPARE:

2. Carefully check walker for safety.
   a. Check to make sure walker is not bent or cracked and that walker tips are snugly in place.
   b. Make sure the walker is set properly at the resident's height. This process is usually performed by a physical therapist. If you think that the height seems incorrect, report it to the nurse.
3. Assist resident in putting on shoes or non-skid slippers and clothing or robe.
4. Bring resident to a sitting position at the side of the bed.
5. Have resident hold the walker with both hands.

PERFORM:

6. Ask the resident to stand up by holding the walker, leaning slightly forward and pushing down on the walker's hand grips.
7. The resident should move as follows: W-6-W-S
   a. Walker first, 6 inches or one stride forward
   b. Weak (affected) leg forward same distance
   c. Strong (unaffected) leg forward
8. Repeat, being careful that neither the resident's nor your legs extend past the front of the walker.

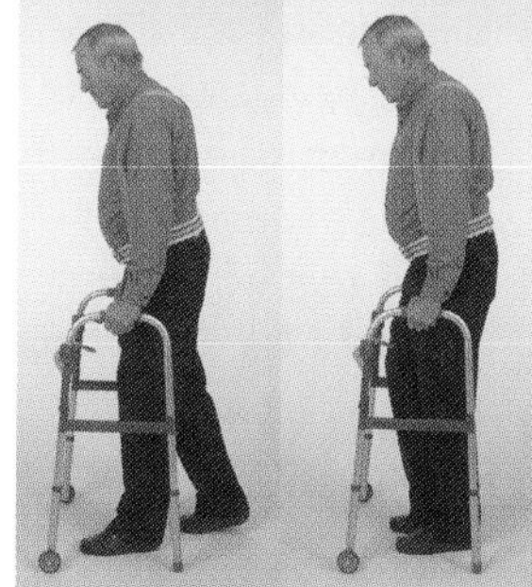

Figure 18-5.

FINISHING TOUCHES:

9. Return resident to the bed, chair, or wheelchair.
10. Carefully reposition the resident, straighten all of the linens if in bed, and make sure resident is comfortable.
11. Perform the "5 Stars and 3 Rs."

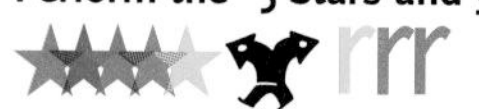

Using Crutches

Follow all standard and/or transmission-based precautions. Follow all rules for body mechanics.

Collect equipment:

- crutches

1. Perform the "5 Stars."

PREPARE:

2. Carefully check crutches for safety.
   a. Check to make sure they are not bent or cracked and that crutch tips are snugly in place.
   b. Make sure the crutches are set properly at the resident's height. Because crutch measurement is a complex process, it is usually performed by a physical therapist. If you think that the height seems incorrect, report it to the nurse.
3. Assist resident in putting on shoes or non-skid slippers and clothing or robe.
4. Bring resident to a sitting position at the side of the bed.
5. Assist resident to a standing position. Resident may push

down on the hand grips of crutches to stand.

6. Ask the resident to hold the crutches with both hands.

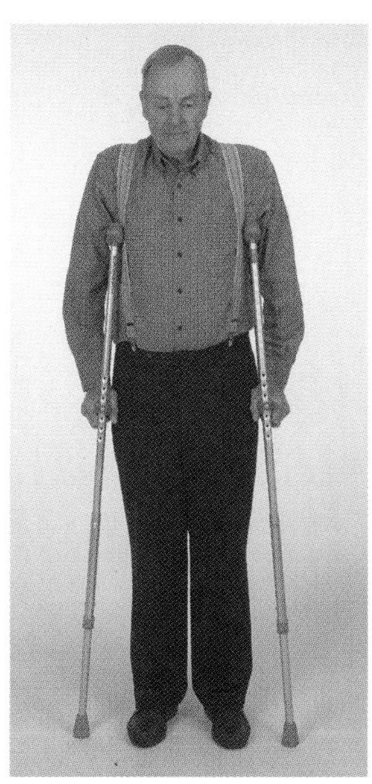

Figure 18-6.

PERFORM:

7. The resident should move as follows: C-6-W-S
   a. Crutches first, 6 inches or one stride forward
   b. Weak (affected) leg forward, toes even with crutch
   c. Strong leg (unaffected) forward either to crutches or beyond if able
8. Repeat until the move is completed.

FINISHING TOUCHES:

9. Return resident to the bed, chair, or wheelchair.
10. Carefully reposition the resident, straighten all of the linens if in bed, and make sure resident is comfortable.
11. Perform the "5 Stars and 3 Rs."

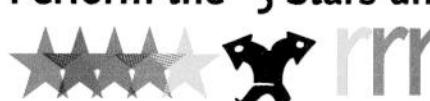

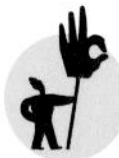

Canes, Walkers, and Crutches: Three Tips

CANE USE: C-12-W-S

C *= Cane 1st*
12 *= 12 inches*
W *= Weak leg*
S *= Strong leg*

WALKER USE: W-6-W-S

W *= Walker 1st*
6 *= 6 inches*
W *= Weak leg*
S *= Strong leg*

CRUTCH USE: C-6-W-S

C *= Crutches 1st*
6 *= 6 inches*
W *= Weak leg*
S *= Strong leg*

8 Identify nine types of equipment used to reduce the complications of bed rest.

There are many types of equipment available to help prevent complications that can occur during periods of bed rest. The following are examples of this type of equipment:

Abduction Wedge/Splint (hip wedge): keeps hips in proper position (abduction) after hip surgery

Anderson Frame (bed cradle): prevents **plantar flexion** (footdrop) and pressure sores

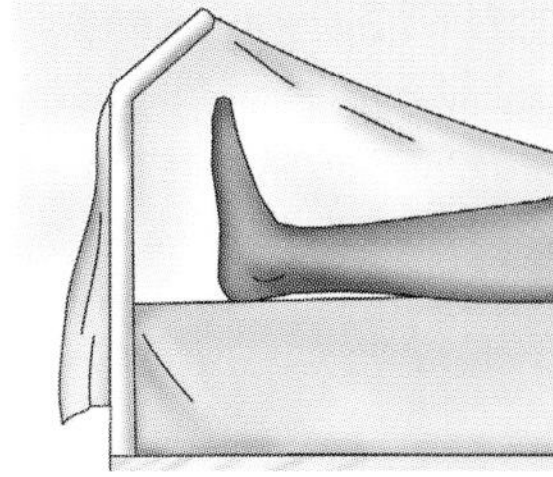

Figure 18-7. Bed cradles keep bed covers from pushing down on residents' feet.

Bed Board: prevents mattress from sagging and maintains good body alignment

Boot: protects the feet from falling into poor alignment

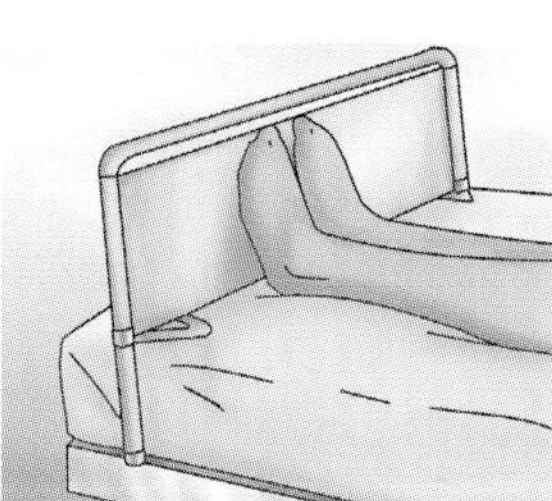

Figure 18-8. Footboards keep residents' feet flexed. Rolled blankets or pillows can also be used as footboards.

Finger Cushion: prevents contractures of the thumb or finger

Footboard: prevents footdrop (plantar flexion)

Handroll: prevents hand or wrist contractures

Trapeze: assists with movement while in bed; helps improve arm strength

Trochanter Roll: prevents hip and leg from moving into rotation

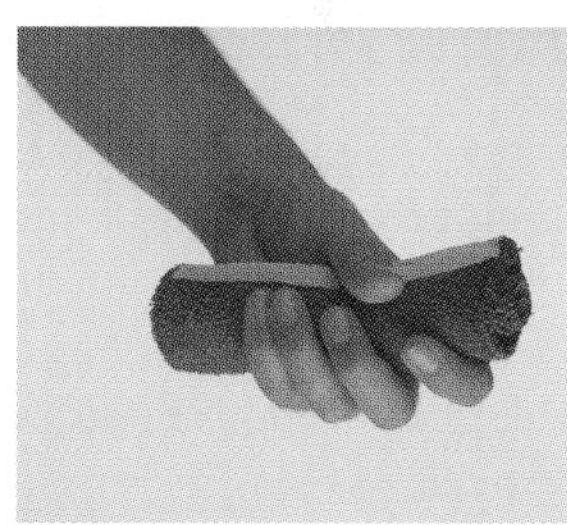

Figure 18-9. Handrolls keep the fingers from curling tightly.

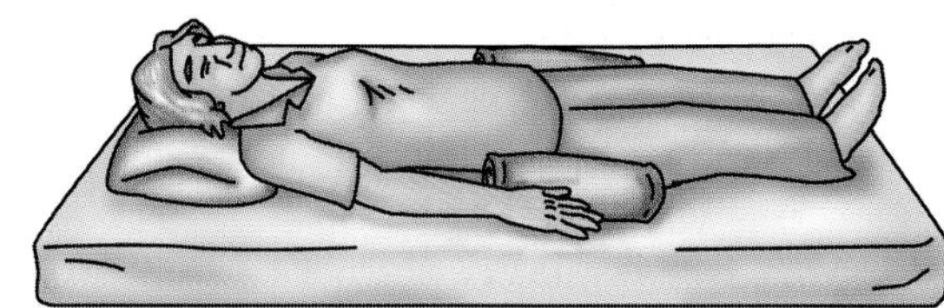

Figure 18-10. Trochanter rolls keep residents' hips from turning outward.

9 Name the three types of range of motion exercises.

The activities of daily living, as described in Learning Objective 3, will take a human body through its normal **range of motion** when a person is able to perform them independently. When a person has to be on bed rest for a length of time, the body experiences many changes due to lack of movement. Some examples of complications from bed rest for a period of time are outlined in Learning Objective 4. Encouraging residents to do as many ADLs as possible is very important for keeping muscles and bones strong. Nursing staff can also help residents maintain their normal range of motion by performing or assisting with range of motion exercises.

Range of motion exercises are best done by completing five movements per joint at least twice a day or more often, depending upon the doctor's orders and the nursing plan of care. When a joint is moved through its normal range of motion, it is moved without any pain. In other words, the old saying in sports of "no pain, no gain" is NOT used with these types of exercises. If a resident complains of any pain whatsoever, the exercises should stop and the nurse must be called. If a joint is moved incorrectly, it is also possible to cause injury to the joint. It is very important for nursing assistants to know the rules when performing range of motion exercises. The joint must be carefully supported throughout each of the exercises.

Residents may be able to participate fully or partially in these exercises. The three types of range of motion exercises are listed below.

AROM Active Range of Motion

Active range of motion is performed by the residents themselves. Usually, a nursing assistant will remind the resident at the time the exercises are due to be performed. The nursing assistant may then stand near the resident in order to answer questions or provide assistance.

PROM Passive Range of Motion

Passive range of motion is performed by the staff. A nursing assistant will take each joint through its normal range of motion gently, without causing pain.

AAROM Active-Assistive Range of Motion

Active-assistive range of motion is performed by the resident and the staff member jointly. The nursing staff will provide any help needed by the resident.

Range of motion exercises are not performed on the neck area in some facilities. When neck exercises are performed, it can sometimes cause injury to the fragile spinal column. Special neck exercises are usually performed by physical therapists.

Range of Motion Terms — Box 18-1

abduction: moving a body part away from the body.

adduction: moving a body toward the body.

extension: straightening a body part.

flexion: bending a body part.

dorsiflexion: bending backward.

pronation: turning downward.

rotation: turning the joint.

supination: turning upward.

"No pain, no gain" does not apply to residents!

Range of motion exercises are a vital part of keeping residents' muscles strong and healthy. Nursing assistants should be very sure they are skilled in the performance of these exercises before attempting them with a resident. Exercises are part of the resident's plan of care. Performing them in an overly-aggressive fashion may cause pain and possibly serious injury to your residents. In addition, nursing assistants should not perform range of motion exercises on the neck area because of the risk of spinal or neck injury. Causing unnecessary pain during the completion of these types of exercises is considered abuse.

Performing Range of Motion Exercises

Follow all standard and/or transmission-based precautions. Follow all rules for body mechanics.

Collect equipment:
- **bath blanket**

1. **Perform the "5 Stars."**

PREPARE:

2. **Adjust height of bed to a comfortable working height.**
3. **Place resident on his back with head on pillow.**
4. **Cover resident with bath blanket.**

PERFORM:

5. **As ordered, exercise the following joints of EACH arm or leg five times each (if possible) in this order:**

   a. *Shoulder*

   Place one hand above the elbow and the other hand around the wrist. Move the arm upward so that the upper arm is aligned with the side of the head (forward flexion). Move the arm downward to the side (extension). (Figure 18-11)

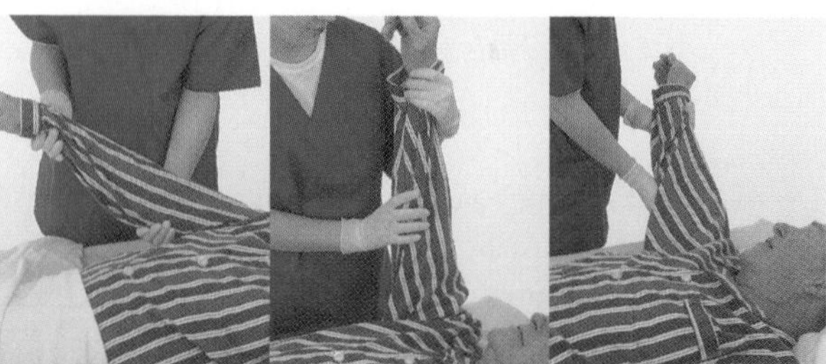

Figure 18-11.

Bring arm sideways away from the body to above the head (abduction) and back down (adduction). (Figure 18-12)

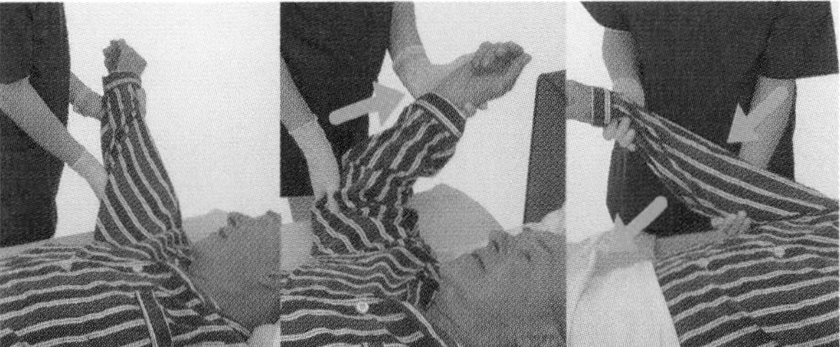

Figure 18-12.

Bend the elbow and position it at the same level as the shoulder. Move the forearm down toward the body (internal rotation). Now move the forearm toward the head (external rotation). (Figure 18-13)

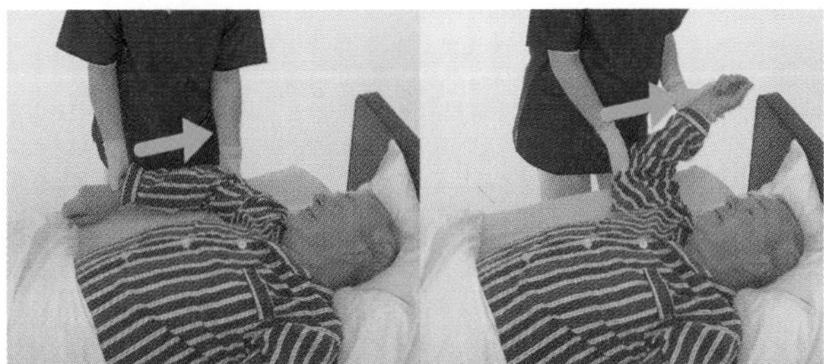

Figure 18-13.

b. *Elbow*

Hold the resident's wrist with one hand, the elbow with the other hand. Bend the elbow so that the hand touches the shoulder on that same side (flexion). Straighten the arm (extension). (Figure 18-14)

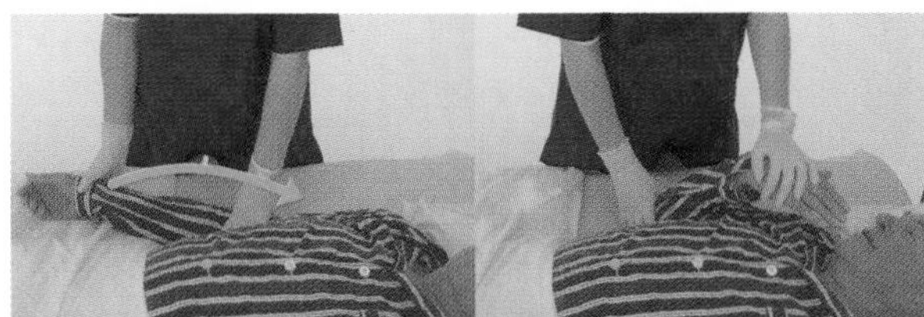

Figure 18-14.

c. *Wrist and forearm*

Hold the wrist with one hand and use the fingers of the other hand to help the joint through the motions. Bend the hand down (flexion); bend the hand backwards (extension). (Figure 18-15)

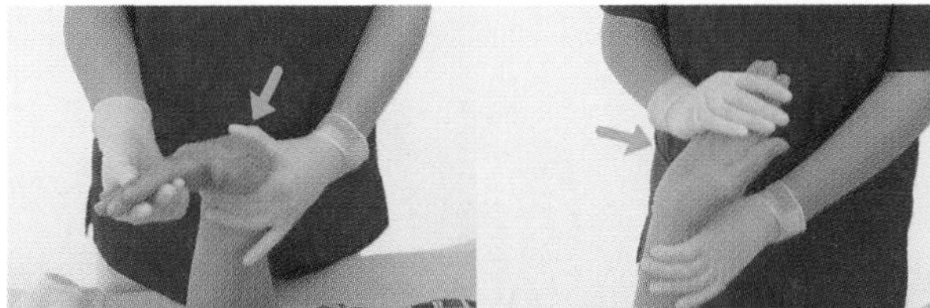

Figure 18-15.

Turn the hand in the direction of the thumb (radial flexion); turn the hand in the direction of the little finger (ulnar flexion). (Figure 18-16)

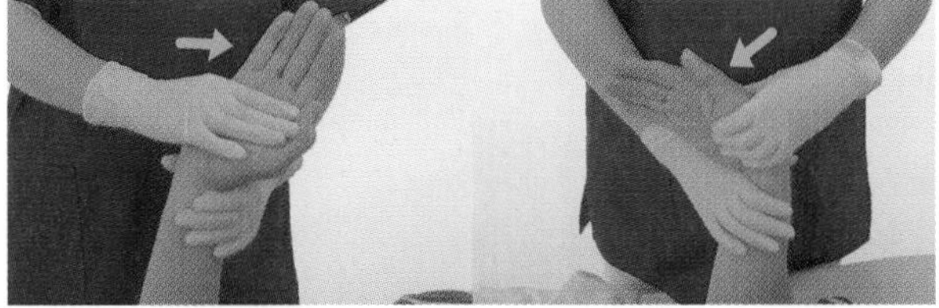

Figure 18-16.

Exercise the forearm by moving it so the palm is facing downward (pronation) and then the palm is facing upward (supination). (Figure 18-17)

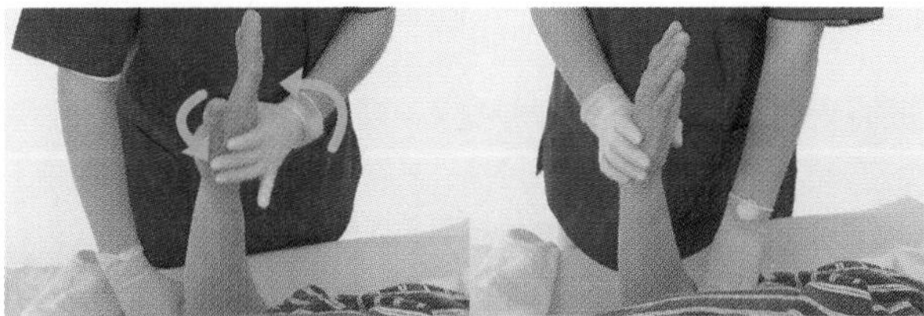

Figure 18-17.

d. *Thumb*

Move the thumb away from the index finger (abduction). Move the thumb back next to the index finger (adduction). (Figure 18-18)

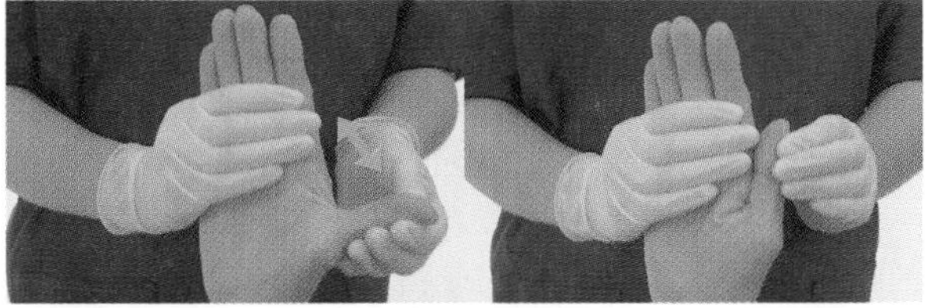

Figure 18-18.

Touch each fingertip with the thumb (opposition). (Figure 18-19)

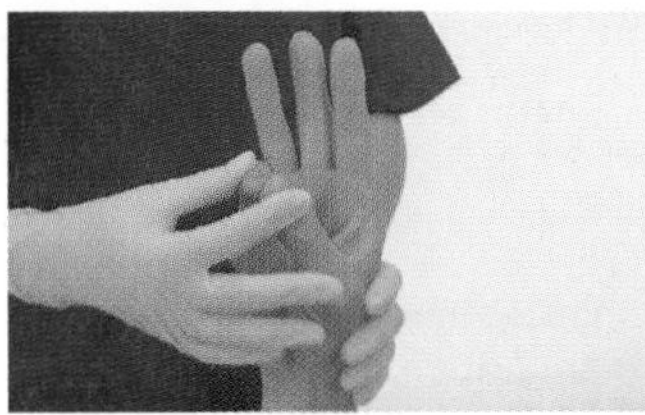

Figure 18-19.

Bend thumb into the palm (flexion) and out to the side (extension). (Figure 18-20)

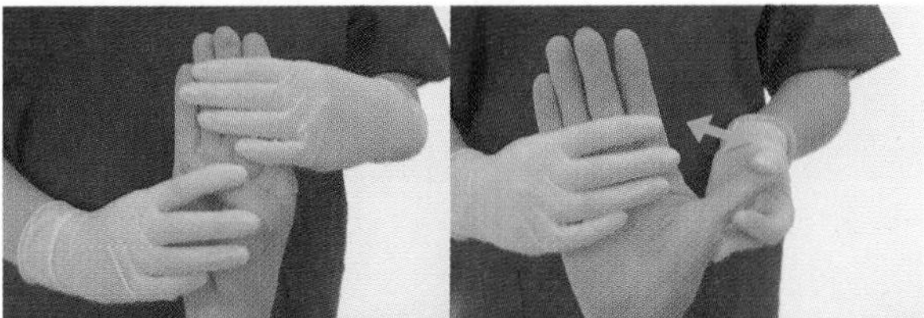

Figure 18-20.

e. *Fingers*

Make the hand into a fist (flexion). Straighten out the fist (extension). (Figure 18-21)

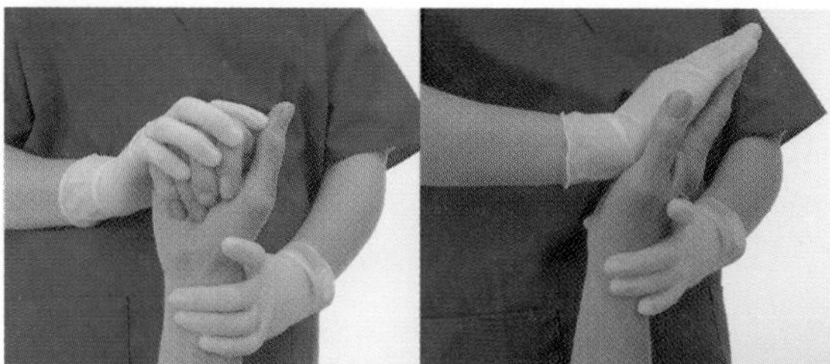

Figure 18-21.

Spread the fingers and the thumb far apart from each other (abduction). Bring the fingers next to each other (adduction). (Figure 18-22)

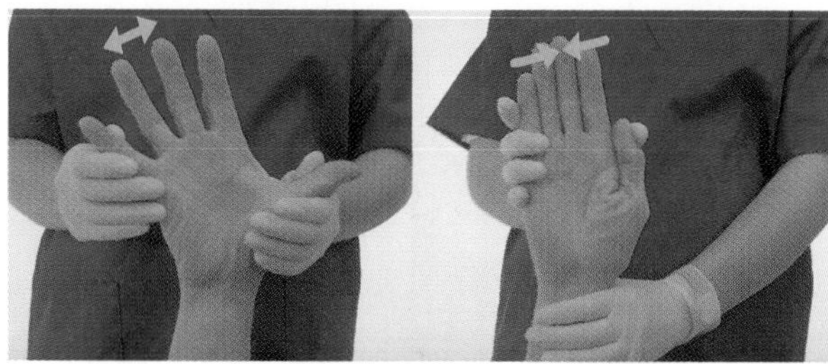

Figure 18-22.

f. *Hip*

Support the leg by placing one hand under the knee and one under the ankle. Straighten the leg and raise it gently upward. Move the leg away from the other leg (abduction). Move the leg toward the other leg (adduction). (Figure 18-23)

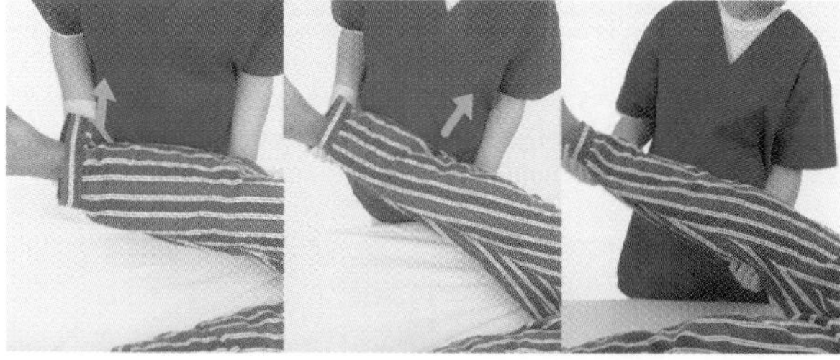

Figure 18-23.

Gently turn the leg inward (internal rotation), then turn the leg outward (external rotation). (Figure 18-24)

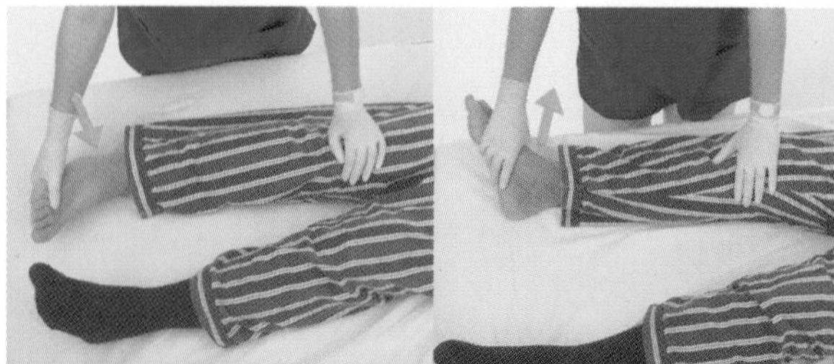

Figure 18-24.

g. *Knee*

Bend the leg at the knee (flexion). Straighten the leg (extension). (Figure 18-25)

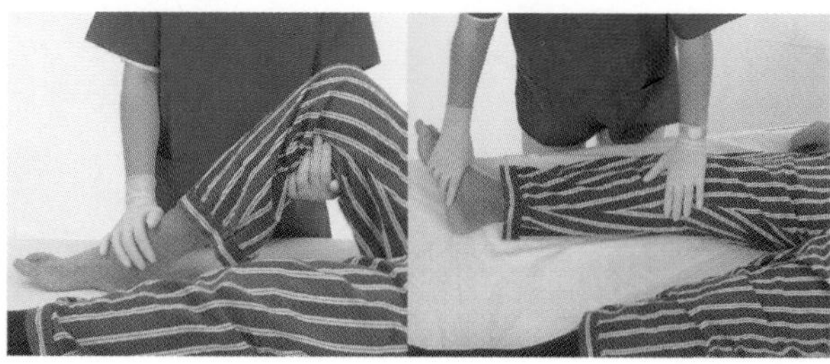

Figure 18-25.

h. *Ankle/foot*

Bend foot up toward the leg (dorsiflexion). Turn the foot down away from the leg (plantar flexion). (Figure 18-26)

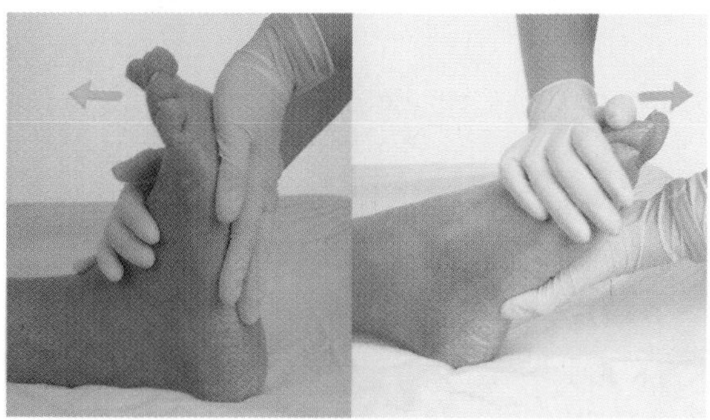

Figure 18-26.

Turn the inside of the foot inward toward the body (supination) and the sole of the foot so that it faces away from the body (pronation). (Figure 18-27)

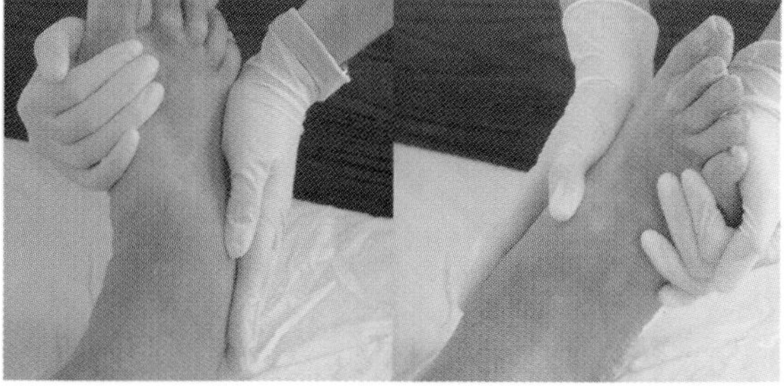

Figure 18-27.

i. *Toes*

Curl and straighten the toes (flexion and extension). (Figure 18-28)

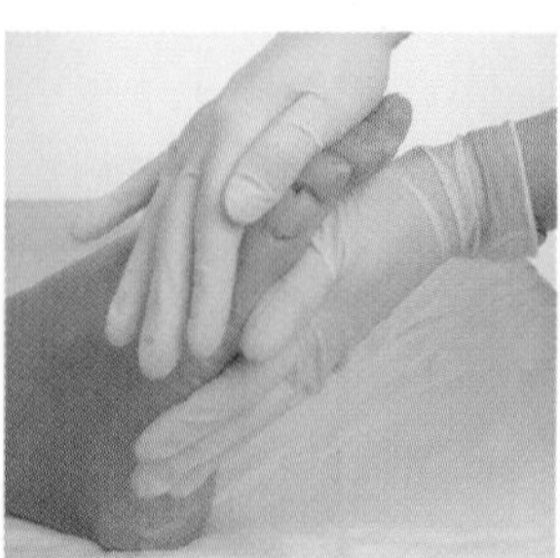

Figure 18-28.

Spread the toes apart (abduction). (Figure 18-29)

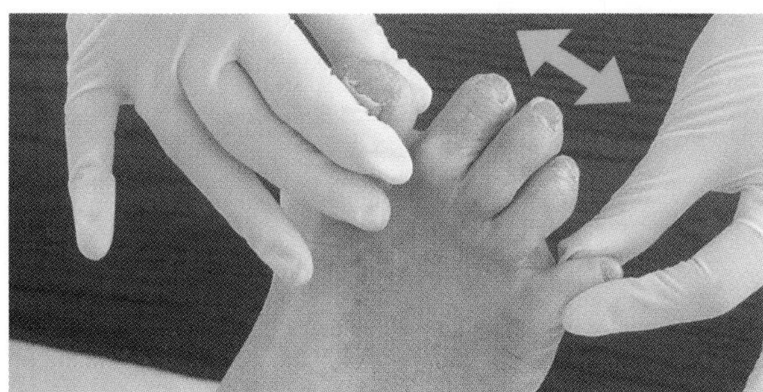

Figure 18-29.

FINISHING TOUCHES:

6. Carefully reposition resident, remove bath blanket, straighten all of the linens, and make sure resident is comfortable.
7. Perform the "5 Stars and 3 Rs."

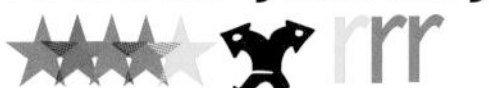

Using a Continuous Passive Motion (CPM) Machine

Follow all standard and/or transmission-based precautions. Follow all rules for body mechanics.

Collect equipment:
- sheepskin sling
- CPM machine with rate set ahead of time by the nurse

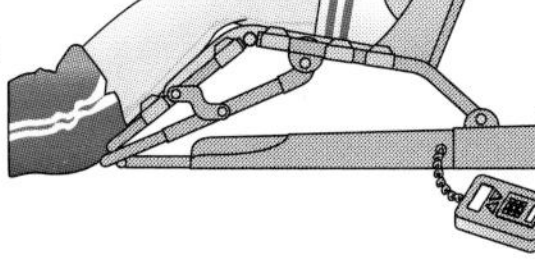

Figure 18-30.

1. Perform the "5 Stars."

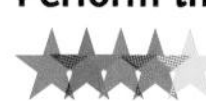

PREPARE:

2. Adjust height of bed to a comfortable working height.
3. Place the resident in flat or Semi-Fowler's position.
4. Secure the leg in the cradle of the CPM machine.
5. Attach straps or Velcro to keep the leg in place. Make sure straps are not too tight.

PERFORM:

6. Turn on the CPM machine.
7. Observe the resident for any problems.
8. Stay with the resident until the resident is comfortable with the movement of the machine.
9. SECURE RESIDENT, place signal light, and wash hands.

FINISHING TOUCHES:

10. Return to room after amount of time ordered for device to remain in place.
11. Wash hands.
12. While leg is extended, turn off machine.
13. Remove straps or Velcro and carefully remove leg from machine while supporting leg.
14. Remove CPM machine from the bed.
15. Carefully reposition resident, straighten all of the linens, and lower bed to its lowest position. Secure resident.
16. Perform the "5 Stars and 3 Rs."

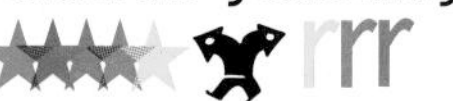

Summary

Restoring the resident to the highest level of functioning and maintaining the resident at that level is the primary goal of rehabilitation. It is important for nursing assistants to fully understand the positive aspects of exercise and all of the possible complications of bed rest. You must be skilled in the performance of range of motion exercises so that no harm comes to your residents during these exercises. In addition, you should be completely familiar with the use of special equipment so that you are prepared to assist residents with this equipment.

The Finish Line

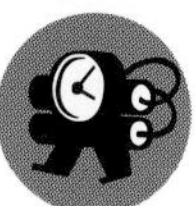

What's Wrong With This Picture?

Find the errors in this set of instructions for the use of a cane:

C-10-S-W

C Cane 1st

10 10 inches

S Strong leg

W Weak leg

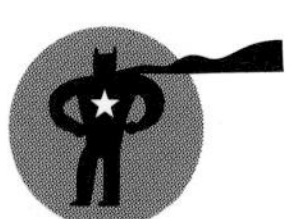

Star Student Central

1. Whether you are at home or work, you must always be on the lookout for safety risks. Have you ever almost fallen or fallen while getting up in the middle of the night to do something? It

can happen anywhere. Set up a regular habit to double-check your residents' rooms and the entire unit for any objects that may put them at risk for falls.

2. After becoming skilled with the use of a cane, sign up for a 5–10 minute time frame to use a cane during a break from class. Choose a weak side and practice the method described within this chapter.
3. After becoming skilled with the use of a walker, sign up for a 5–10 minute time frame to use a walker during a break from class. Follow the method shown within the chapter.

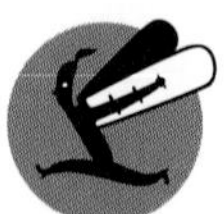

You Can Do It Corner!

1. Identify a possible integumentary, cardiovascular, respiratory, musculoskeletal, nervous, endocrine, and gastrointestinal complication of bed rest. (LO 4)
2. Identify two things that should be considered when preparing for a "first walk." (LO 5)
3. How many joint movements are normally completed per joint when doing range of motion? How many times a day might range of motion exercises be performed? (LO 9)
4. What is your primary concern when protecting a falling resident? (LO 6)
5. Identify three things you must double-check before assisting a resident to use a cane for a walk. (LO 7)
6. The degree of rehabilitation depends upon what five factors? (LO 2)
7. Identify what the following pieces of equipment help prevent: hip wedge, bed boards, bed cradles, boots, finger cushions, footboards, handrolls, trapeze, trochanter rolls. (LO 8)
8. Define the following terms: abduction, adduction, extension, flexion, dorsiflexion, pronation, rotation, and supination. (LO 9)
9. Should the weak or strong leg move first when using a cane, walker, or crutches? (LO 7)
10. List eight activities of daily living (ADLs). (LO 3)

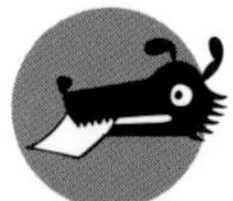

Star Student's Chapter Checklist

1. I have read my textbook chapter.
2. I have reviewed my own "Pocketful of Terms."
3. I have listened to my tutor tape.
4. I have reviewed and highlighted my class notes.
5. I have read and completed any handouts from this chapter.
6. I have completed "The Finish Line."
7. Star Time! Choose your reward!

19

Your Guide:
The Science of Skin Care

Look Like a Star!

Look at the Learning Objectives and The Finish Line before you begin reading this chapter.

Look at your pocket calendar.
With your pencil, put a bracket (   ) around a study period every single day.

Look at your homework for this chapter.
Plug each piece of homework into a certain time slot.

Look at the Star Student's Chapter Checklist at the end of this chapter. Check off each item as it is completed.

"To get the whole world out of bed and washed and dressed, and warmed, and fed...and back to bed again..."

John Masefield 1878-1967

"Cleanliness is a great virtue..."

Charles B. Fairbanks 1827-1859

Learning Objectives

1. Spell and define all STAR words.
2. Describe morning, afternoon, and evening care of residents.
3. Summarize "The 5 Basic Steps to Quality Skin Care."
4. Describe four stages of pressure sores and nine signs to observe.
5. Identify five risk factors for pressure sores on the Norton Scale.
6. Identify six important areas in prevention and care of pressure sores.
7. Name four kinds of baths and identify the type of resident best suited to each.
8. Summarize your role in resident safety during a bath.
9. List the order in which body parts are washed during a partial or complete bed bath.
10. Name important observations to make while bathing and the two groups into which they are divided.
11. Identify the legal implications for performing male or female peri-care.
12. Explain how to perform a safe and effective back massage.

Successfully perform these Practical Procedures

Giving Male or Female Peri-Care

The Complete Bed Bath

The Partial or Set-up Bath

The Tub Bath

The Shower

Giving a Back Massage

Public Health and Hygiene

During the fifth century, many people lived in tiny homes with little ventilation. Since there was no way to keep the streets clean, they were covered in filth. People generally wore sandals while walking outside, so they had to wash their feet before entering their homes. Bathing was done in public as well as in the home. Public baths were shared by the people of the community. In later centuries, public baths were still used, but less regularly due to the spread of diseases.

1 Spell and define all STAR words.

before-breakfast care: personal care done before breakfast.

afternoon care: personal care done before dinner.

after-breakfast care: personal care done after breakfast.

axilla: underarm or armpit area.

bed bath: bath given to a resident in bed.

decubitus ulcer: pressure sore or bedsore.

evening care: personal care done before bedtime.

partial bath: bath performed at the bedside or in a bathroom consisting of bathing only certain parts of the body.

perineal care: cleansing of the genital and rectal areas; also called peri-care.

pressure points: areas of the body that bear much of the body weight; points where skin breakdown is likely to occur when residents are not frequently repositioned.

pressure sore or ulcer: break or opening in the skin due to a reduction in blood flow.

shearing: pressure from sliding skin across another surface.

2 Describe morning, afternoon, and evening care of residents.

The types of care you will provide for your residents on a daily basis will depend upon what shift or shifts you work at the facility. Care varies a bit depending upon the time of day. Generally, certain responsibilities are designated for certain shifts. Bathing usually occurs during morning care; however, it can be done during evening care depending upon residents' preferences and facility policy.

Before-Breakfast Care

Bathing: In bed, shower, tub, shower room, or in bathroom
Toileting: Bathroom break or incontinent brief change; wash resident's hands
Oral care: Mouth care or denture care
Dressing: Robe and slippers or clothes
Grooming: Varies depending upon breakfast site
Unit care: Prepare overbed table for breakfast if served in room.

After-Breakfast Care

Toileting: Bathroom break or incontinent brief change; wash resident's hands
Oral care: Mouth care or denture care
Skin care: back massage
Dressing: Changing resident's gown or pajamas
Grooming: Shaving, hair care, nail care, makeup
Unit care: Making the bed and tidying room, providing fluids

Afternoon Care

Toileting: Bathroom break or change incontinent brief; wash resident's hands
Oral care: Mouth care or denture care after lunch
Unit care: Changing linens; passing fresh drinking water

Evening Care

Toileting: Bathroom break or incontinent brief change; wash resident's hands
Oral care: Mouth care or denture care after dinner
Skin care: Back massage; bathing, if resident prefers this time
Dressing: Undressing; changing resident's gown or pajamas
Grooming: Hair care before bed; wash face and remove makeup
Unit care: Bedmaking and tidying room, providing fluids

3 Summarize "The 5 Basic Steps to Quality Skin Care."

Understanding the importance of good skin care is the first step to giving outstanding resident care. Giving each and every resident quality skin care is one of the primary responsibilities of a nursing assistant. When skin care is lacking, all sorts of problems occur. Residents can develop dry, itchy skin and serious sores. Potentially dangerous problems on the body can be missed due to a lack of observation.

Box 19-1 identifies the five Steps to Quality Skin Care. Memorize these steps so that they come naturally to you every shift you work. The comfort of your residents depends upon how well you know and understand these steps.

The Five Basic Steps to Quality Skin Care
Box 19-1

1. Skin Condition
   Check skin often. Report skin problems promptly.
2. Skin Care Tips
   Clean skin gently. Use lukewarm water for bathing. Rinse often and thoroughly. Dry skin thoroughly. Do not use soap on the face. Use mild soap on the body. Lotion skin often.
3. Equipment Tips
   Change linen or pads as necessary. Make sure there are no wrinkles in bed linens or in pads on chairs. Use pillows to prevent skin from rubbing together.
4. Position Change
   Follow positioning orders for each resident. Change position at least every one or two hours in bed. Change position at least every 15-30 minutes in a chair.
5. Use of Massage
   Massage back daily, if allowed.

4 Describe four stages of pressure sores and nine signs to observe.

A **pressure sore** is an ulcer resulting from skin deterioration (break-up) from pressure and shearing (pressure from sliding skin across another surface). Eventually blood does not circulate properly and sores or ulcers form, swell, and may become infected, causing damage to underlying tissue. Pressure sores are also referred to as **decubitus ulcers**, bed sores, and pressure ulcers.

There are four stages of pressure sores:

Stage 1: Area where skin is intact but there is redness that is not relieved within 15 to 30 minutes after removing pressure.

Stage 2: Partial skin loss involving epidermis and/or dermis. The ulcer is superficial and looks like a blister or a shallow crater.

Stage 3: Full skin loss involving damage or death of tissue that may extend down to but not through the fibrous tissue that covers muscle. The ulcer looks like a deep crater.

Stage 4: Full skin loss with extensive destruction, tissue death, damage to muscle, bone, or supporting structures.

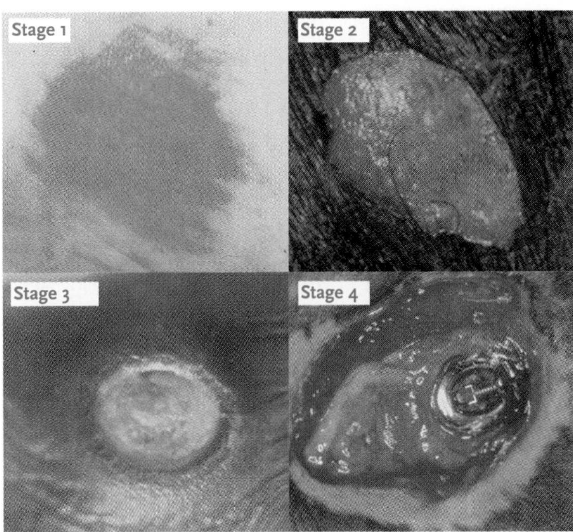

Figure 19-1. Pressure sores are categorized by Stage 1 through Stage 4.

When a resident is confined to bed for long periods of time, pressure on a body part reduces circulation of blood to the area. The risk of skin breaking down increases at pressure points. **Pressure points** are areas of the body that bear much of the body's weight. Common sites for pressure sores are heels, elbows, and the sacrum, the lower part of the spinal column.

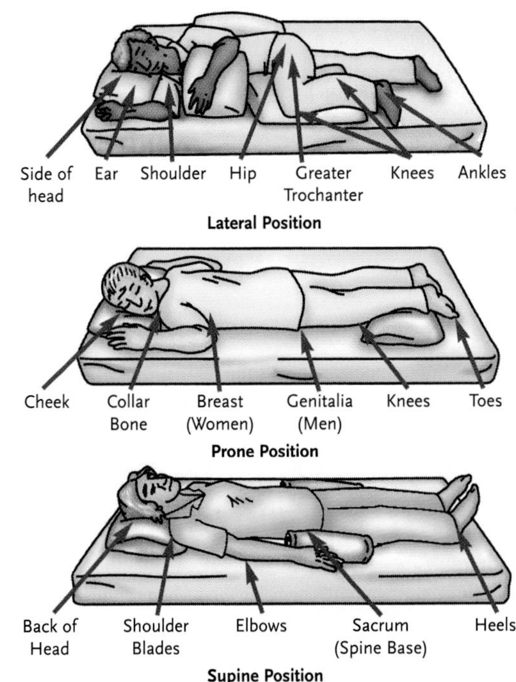

Figure 19-2. Pressure sore danger zones.

The signs and symptoms of pressure sores include the following:

- warm, reddened areas on the skin that do not go away when pressure is relieved
- skin that is cyanotic (a bluish color)

- dry, cracked, flaking, or torn skin
- blisters or sores on the skin
- rashes
- itching
- swelling
- wounds or ulcers on the skin
- any wetness on the skin

Pressure sores are a common problem in long-term care. No one is in a better position than you to observe the early stages of pressure sores. Each time you provide personal care, such as bathing, toileting, and repositioning, inspect your resident's skin carefully. If you observe any of these signs, notify the nurse immediately.

5 Identify five risk factors for pressure sores on the Norton Scale.

Nurses are trained to do risk assessment of pressure sores on each person admitted to care. Even though nursing assistants do not assess for risk of pressure sores, you play a major role. Your observations of change in any of these factors must be reported. Communicating your skilled observations can make the difference in early detection and prevention.

The Norton Scale is a simple tool for assessing the risk for pressure sores. It takes into consideration the following five factors:

1. physical condition
2. mental condition
3. activities
4. mobility
5. incontinence

Each of these categories has four sub-categories, which are rated from 1 to 4 by risk (with 1 being the greatest risk). The numbers are added and a total score of all five gives a final risk rating of low risk, medium risk, or high risk.

6 Identify six important areas in prevention and care of pressure sores.

Skin care, Protection, and Hygiene

Skin care, protection and hygiene are the most important measures in prevention and care of a pressure sore. The following should be considered in a good skin care, protection, and hygiene program:

- Avoid dry skin by rinsing off all soap during the bath and using moisturizing creams and lotions.
- Restore blood supply to bony areas by relieving pressure.
- DO NOT massage reddened or bony areas, as this may actually contribute to tissue breakdown. You may gently massage around bony prominences to help improve circulation.
- Keep residents clean and dry from incontinence, perspiration and drainage. Always wear gloves and follow standard precautions when dealing with incontinence.
- Use draw sheets to avoid skin injury due to friction of skin dragging over sheets.
- Observe the skin for new ulcer areas.
- Report any breaks in the skin.
- Always check the diabetic's feet for open sores caused by rubbing shoes (diabetics have poor sensation in their feet).
- Avoid **shearing**, or tearing of skin on the elderly person whose skin is thin and fragile. Handle residents carefully and keep your nails short.

Five Risk Factors on the Norton Scale — Box 19-2

Physical Condition	Mental Condition	Activity	Mobility	Incontinence	Total Score
Good 4	Alert 4	Ambulant 4	Full 4	None 4	20
Fair 3	Apathetic 3	Walk/help 3	Slightly Limited 3	Occasional 3	15
Poor 2	Confused 2	Chairbound 2	Very Limited 2	Usually/urine 2	10
Very Bad 1	Stupor 1	Bed 1	Immobile 1	Both 1	5

High-Risk Individual 5-10

Medium-Risk Individual 11-14

Low-Risk Individual 15-20

- Always keep the bed linens dry and free from wrinkles, which could irritate the skin.
- Assist the resident in applying creams and ointments as ordered by the physician. Be sure the skin is not left wet or damp.
- Use powders to absorb wetness, but not enough to clump or crumble.
- Offer a back massage daily; give special attention to the sacral area, which is prone to pressure sores. Always use this time to observe the skin carefully for warm, red, or blanched areas.

Activity

Inactivity is a major problem for residents at higher risk for skin breakdown. Unless otherwise ordered, you should encourage residents at risk of skin breakdown to be as active as safely possible. ADLs, or activities of daily living, should be designed to increase activity. For example, if the resident can go from bed to a chair by the sink for bathing, the activity of getting there can be beneficial.

Lack of activity can also cause or contribute to difficulties with maintaining good nutrition. Appetite can be increased with even a little additional activity or moderate exercise. The inactive resident is more likely to be "blue" or depressed because of a feeling of dependence. If at all possible, nursing assistants should be the motivating force to encourage activity.

Circulation

Impaired circulation to extremities and pressure points is a major cause of pressure sores. When the blood supply is poor, the tissues do not receive adequate oxygen, and cells are destroyed. Major medical conditions such as diabetes and heart disease can cause poor circulation, as can pressure on the tissue. Once a breakdown of tissue occurs, healing is slowed because of the same poor circulation.

Other disease situations that impair circulation are venous ulcers, anemia, renal failure, spinal injuries, stroke, and neurological impairment.

Pressure Relief

Turning the resident frequently is an important aspect of pressure relief. Turning every two hours and positioning the resident correctly and comfortably are the first measures of pressure relief. In addition, some pressure-relieving devices were listed in Chapter 18.

Nutrition

Poor nutrition and inadequate fluid intake increase a resident's risk of developing pressure sores because poorly-nourished tissue breaks down more easily than healthy tissue. Inadequate nutrition also contributes to poor healing and reduces the body's resistance to infection.

There are a number of factors which contribute to poor nutritional status of residents in your care:

- Swallowing difficulties due to strokes and neurological diseases
- Poor absorption of food due to intestinal disease
- Dental problems, mouth sores, and lesions
- Decreased appetite due to disease or medication
- Loneliness
- Depression
- Reduced income
- Inability to buy and prepare food
- Inactivity

Certain nutrients play different roles in wound healing. Protein, vitamins A and C, zinc, and iron are all essential for assisting the body to heal. A resident with pressure sores may be on a high-calorie, high-protein diet. If the resident is gaining weight and the pressure sore is healing, nutrition is probably adequate.

The following are general guidelines to maximize calorie, protein, vitamin, and mineral intake:

- Eating small, frequent meals of high calorie, high protein foods
- Serving food when the resident is most hungry
- Offering nutritious beverages instead of sodas, tea, or coffee

Prevention of New Ulcer Sites

Pressure sores can be prevented if risk assessments are done and risk factors are considered. All healthcare team members should be well-educated in skin assessment, skin care, positioning, and use of supportive devices. You must provide excellent care, and members of the care team must communicate well, especially if there are changes in the condition of a resident with a pressure sore.

Other skills in caring for a resident with skin impairments include the following:

- Providing range of motion (ROM) exercises and ambulation to increase circulation

- Observing and reporting drainage
- Maintaining a clean, safe, and dry environment
- Offering nutrition and fluids
- Taking temperature, pulse, and respirations (TPRs)

7 Name four kinds of baths and identify the type of resident best suited to each.

There are four basic types of baths you may be asked to give a resident. These are a **partial** or set-up bath, a shower, a tub bath, or a complete **bed bath**. No matter what bath you give, make sure all soap residue is removed. The decision on which bath to give a specific resident rests first with the doctor, then with the resident's preference. For example, a doctor may write an order for "no shower" until a wound has healed. Certain residents are confined to bed, which prevents them from getting up for a tub bath or a shower. Some residents do not shower for personal reasons; they may simply prefer a tub bath because they have always taken baths at home.

Some nursing homes do not have showers installed in the bathrooms; they only have bathtubs. When the doctor has given the choice of bathing to the nursing service, the nursing staff must choose, based on the resident's preferences and abilities, the best bath to give each resident each day. The choice may change from day to day due to staffing levels and the condition of the residents. Discuss residents' preferences and decisions regarding bathing with the charge nurse prior to providing the care.

Each style of bathing is best suited to certain types of residents.

1. **Partial Bath (set-up)**

Suited to a resident who:
- is older, and has dryer, fragile, more sensitive skin; should not have daily full baths
- is unable to get up to take a shower or tub bath
- wishes to get cleaned up before breakfast or another meal and plans on taking a shower or bath later in the day

2. **Shower**

Suited to a resident who:
- prefers to shower and is able to stand and shower
- is able to sit in a shower chair

3. **Tub Bath**

Suited to a resident who:
- is able to transfer into and out of a tub and wishes to take a tub bath
- has a doctor's order for a special bath using an additive—a substance added to another substance changing its effect—to the tub water

4. **Complete Bed Bath**

Suited to a resident who:
- is unable to get out of bed and shower or bathe and requires a full bath

8 Summarize your role in resident safety during a bath.

Nursing assistants should think of safety first during bathing. Many people do not consider the risk to the resident and staff member bathing the resident. Consider the following examples:

1. A 72-year-old male resident is placed in a shower chair. Halfway through the shower, the NA asks the resident to stand briefly in order to fully bathe the perineal area. The resident has a doctor's order not to put any weight on the right leg. However, the nursing assistant has forgotten this order. When the resident stands up, he is unable to support his full weight and starts to fall in the shower. The nursing assistant, without thinking, tries to "catch" the resident, fracturing her arm.
2. An 84-year-old resident is ready for a tub bath. She has been transferring successfully to the tub with two staff members helping her. Today, the unit has less staff and a nursing assistant tries to transfer the resident alone. The resident falls and hits her head, which results in a concussion.

When bathing residents, you should constantly remain alert to the possibility of accidents. When staff members let their guard down even for a few seconds, it can cause a resident or staff member to be seriously injured. You must assess your ability to complete a bed bath, shower, or tub bath alone. Ask yourself the following question before beginning the actual bathing process, "Do I believe I can handle this resident safely by myself?" If the answer is no, ask for help.

9 List the order in which body parts are washed during a partial or complete bed bath.

When you are bathing a person, it is very important that you follow a specific order on the body so that

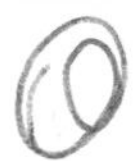

you reduce the risk of transferring microorganisms from a dirty body area to a clean body area. The best way to remember the order of a bath is to look at the following bathing wheel.

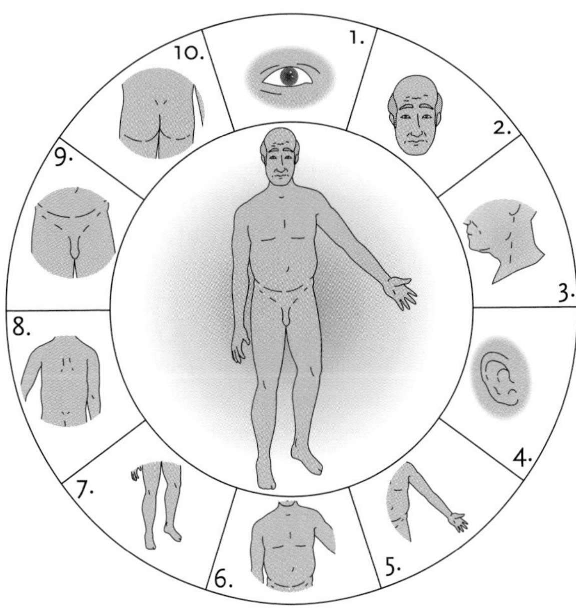

Figure 19-3. **The Bathing Wheel.**

The Bathing Wheel

Correct order of body parts:

1. eyes

2. face

3. neck

4. ears

5. arms and **axilla** (axillae)

6. chest and abdomen

7. legs and feet

8. back

9. perineal area

10. buttocks

The parts of the body have corresponding numbers in the illustration that show the exact order to complete a bed bath. The wheel outlines bathing in the "clean to dirty" method. You would bathe the face before bathing the buttocks. This order of bathing is vital to prevent the transfer of microorganisms from a dirty area to a clean area of the body.

10 Name important observations to make while bathing and the two groups into which they are divided.

In Chapter 6, the "Basic Observations At A Glance" identified general observations to look for when caring for your residents. During the bath, you will have a great opportunity to observe your residents in more detail. Following are observations you might make about areas of the body bathed. These observations are divided into two groups, Visible Signs and Resident Complaints, to separate objective data from subjective data. Objective data is information based on what you see, hear, touch, or smell. Subjective data is information you cannot or did not observe, but that the resident reported to you.

You should be careful to look for these possible signs in both males and females. Many more possibilities exist; these are simply examples. Observations to make about the eyes, face, neck, ears, arms, axillae, chest, abdomen, legs, feet, back, perineal area, and buttocks include the following:

Visible signs:

- yellow color in the whites of the eyes
- red collection of blood in the white of an eye
- change in the size of one or both pupils
- any color drainage from the eye(s)
- foul smell around the eye area
- difference in appearance of one eye from the other
- bruises, cuts, scratches, or bumps around the eyes
- drooping on one side of the face
- pale or blue-tinged skin (cyanosis)
- rashes
- bruises, cuts, scratches, or bleeding
- foul smells
- funny-colored or odd-looking moles or spots, especially red, white, dark brown, gray, or black
- lumps or bumps
- noticeable presence of ear wax
- drainage coming from the nipples or back
- weight loss
- reddened or open areas on hips or any other areas, especially around pressure points
- poor condition of fingernails or toenails

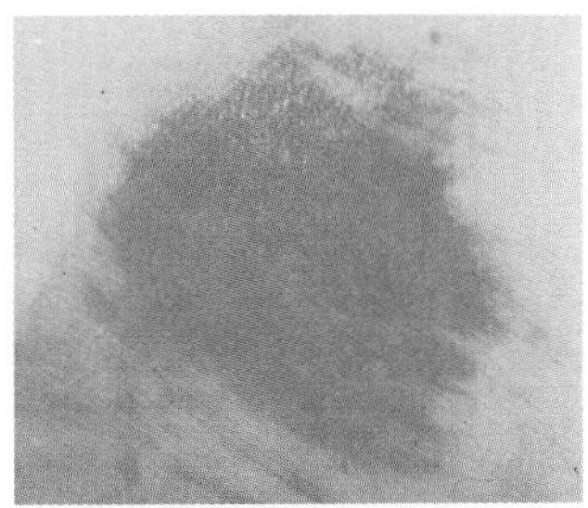

Figure 19-4. **Watch for any reddened or open areas on the body.**

- swelling of knuckles or feet and legs (edema); rings that will not come off, shoes too tight
- discolored or swollen groin

Resident complaints:

- Resident complains of a change in vision.
- Resident complains of pain, discomfort, numbness or tingling, or itching.
- Resident complains of a change in the ability to hear.
- Resident complains of a stiff neck.

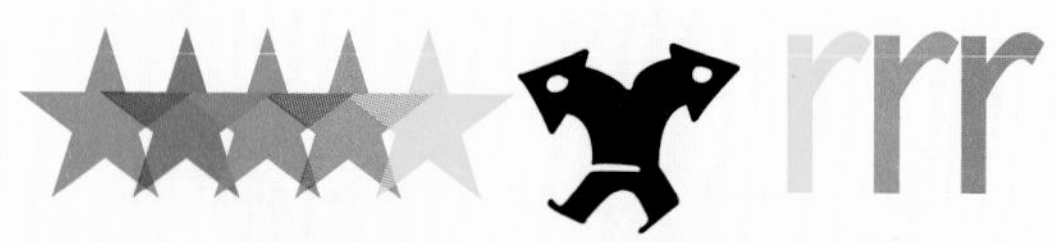

Beginning Steps

★ RESPECT
Knock first, ask and receive permission to enter a resident's room.

★ INFECTION CONTROL
Wash hands.

★ COMMUNICATION
Greet and identify the resident. Identify yourself. Explain the procedure, encouraging the resident to be as independent as possible throughout.

★ BED SAFETY
Lock bed wheels. Raise bed to safe working height. Lower one side rail if required.

★ PRIVACY
Provide for privacy by closing the door and covering the resident appropriately.

Ending Steps

★ RESIDENT SAFETY AND COMFORT
Secure the resident, lowering the bed, and raising the side rails if ordered. Check that the resident is comfortable and properly aligned.

★ PRIVACY
Remove any added privacy measures, such as a drape or a privacy screen.

★ ESSENTIALS
Place the call light, fresh beverage, and other items within reach.

★ COURTESY
Ask the resident if he or she needs anything else. Say thank you and goodbye.

★ INFECTION CONTROL
Wash hands.

Report your care and any important observations to the nurse.

Record your care and any important information/observations such as vital signs in the appropriate place.

Recheck your resident for any changes as directed by the nurse!

11 Identify the legal implications for performing male or female peri-care.

The performance of **perineal care** on a resident (care and cleaning of the genital and rectal areas of the body) carries some risks. When performing perineal care on any resident, it is very important to gain the resident's consent for the procedure, if this is possible. Gaining consent may be as simple as asking permission to go further, or you may have to explain what you are going to do in more detail to the resident and possibly the resident's family. When there is a language barrier, stop and think. Make sure you have explained the procedure completely so that the person fully understands it. It may be necessary to obtain the services of an interpreter or a translator in order to make sure the resident fully understands the procedure. Remember that if the resident does not fully understand the procedure, he or she may not give an informed consent.

Does your resident really understand the procedure?

Mrs. Cvenic is a resident from "the old country" as she calls it. That phrase is one of the few English phrases she knows well. When a new male nursing assistant comes in to bathe her, she does not realize what this staff member is going to do to her. When the nursing assistant explains the procedure to her, it sounds like a jumble of words she cannot understand. The resident smiles anyway and nods her head and tries to be agreeable. Then, during the bath, the nursing assistant lifts up her gown and tries to separate her legs, and Mrs. Cvenic starts to scream. People run down the hallway to her room to see what is the matter.

This example shows how a situation can easily get out of control if the staff member does not make sure the resident fully understands the procedure. If the nursing assistant had STOPPED and thought about what to do when it did not seem the resident understood what he was saying, he could have found an interpreter and avoided this difficult situation. Not taking the time to ensure residents' understanding of procedures can be considered abuse.

Making a Mitt

When bathing a resident, making a mitt with a washcloth will help make the procedure easier. See Figure 19-5 to learn how to make a mitt for bathing.

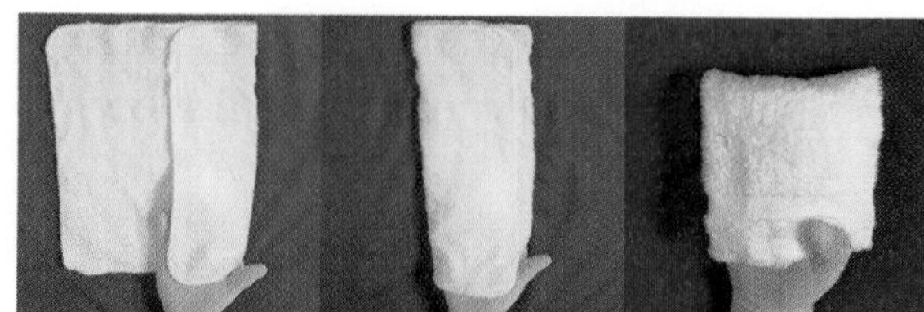

Figure 19-5.

Giving Male or Female Peri-Care

Follow all standard and/or transmission-based precautions. Follow all rules for body mechanics.

Collect equipment:
- gloves • soap dish • soap • basin with lukewarm water
- washcloths or wipes • bath blanket • face towel
- bath towels • bath thermometer if available

1. Perform the "5 Stars."

PREPARE:

2. Cover the resident with the bath blanket. Add tiny amount of soap to water and swirl water around. Check water temperature. Temperature should be about 105 to 109 degrees Fahrenheit.

PERFORM:

3. Give the resident the washcloth and towel and allow the resident to bathe himself to the extent possible. SECURE THE RESIDENT if your facility allows you to leave the room at this time.
4. Ask resident to press call button when in need of your assistance to complete the bath. Wash hands and leave the room.
5. Re-enter the room and wash hands when call button is pressed.
6. Apply gloves and assist resident by completing the peri-care. The following guidelines should be used when performing male and female peri-care.

Male Peri-Care

7. Ask resident to open his legs and flex knees, if possible. If he is not able to flex his knees, help him spread his legs as much as possible.
8. Wet the washcloth or wipes. If using washcloth, make a mitt with it.
9. Retract the foreskin if he is uncircumcised by gently pushing skin toward the base. Grasp the penis. The cleaning should be done in a circular motion towards the base of the penis. Start at the urethral opening and work outward. Repeat as necessary. Use a different part of the washcloth each time. Rinse the area with another clean washcloth. If resident has foreskin, allow it to return to normal position. Clean the shaft of the penis with firm downward strokes. Rinse area. Clean the scrotum and rinse and dry entire area completely.

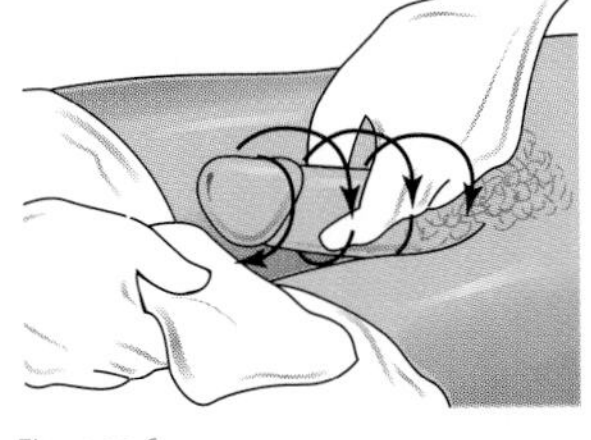

Figure 19-6.

10. Using another clean washcloth, turn the resident to the side and clean the rectal area. Rinse and dry when finished. Carefully wipe from the front side of the body to the back side of the body. Return the resident to his back.

FINISHING TOUCHES:

11. Remove bath blanket, change gown or pajamas if needed, and cover resident.
12. Clean up equipment and dispose of any disposable supplies or linen in appropriate place. Check to see if sheets on bed are dry and wrinkle-free. Secure the resident.
13. Perform the "5 Stars and 3 Rs."

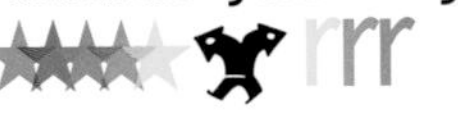

Female Peri-Care

7. Ask resident to open her legs and flex knees, if possible. If she is not able to flex her knees, help her spread her legs as much as possible.
8. Wet the washcloth, or wipes. If using washcloth, make a mitt with it.
9. Using one hand, separate the labia. With the other hand, clean the female perineal area moving washcloth from the front of the body to the back of the body. Repeat this, using a different part of the washcloth each time, on both sides of the labia until the area is clean. Use more than one washcloth if needed. Finish with the center of the labia.

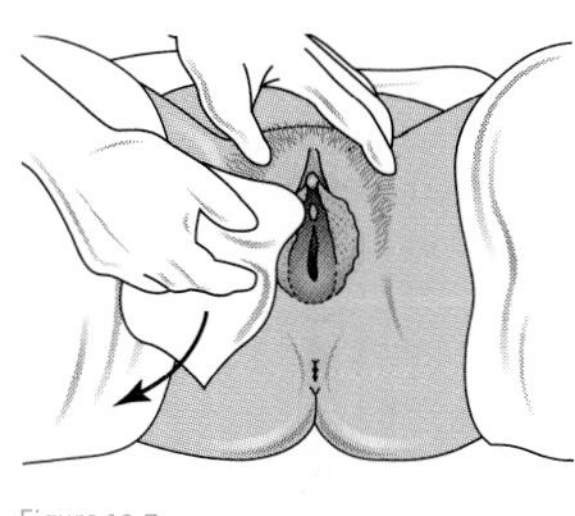

Figure 19-7.

10. Rinse the perineum with a clean washcloth. Separate the labia. Stroke downward from the front of the body to the back of the body. Repeat as necessary, using a different part of the washcloth each time. Dry entire perineal area.
11. Turn the resident to the side and using another clean washcloth, clean the rectal area. Carefully wipe from the front side of the body to the back side of the body. Rinse and dry when finished. Return resident to her back.

FINISHING TOUCHES:

12. Remove bath blanket, change gown or pajamas if needed, and cover resident.
13. Clean up equipment and dispose of any disposable supplies or linen in appropriate place. Check to see if sheets on bed are dry and wrinkle-free. Secure the resident.
14. Perform the "5 Stars and 3 Rs."

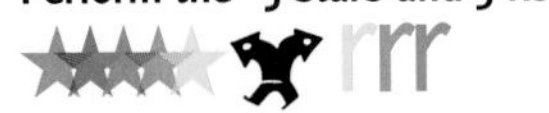

The Complete Bed Bath

Follow all standard and/or transmission-based precautions. Follow all rules for body mechanics.

Collect equipment:
- gloves • soap dish • soap • bath thermometer • face towel
- basin with lukewarm water • wash cloths • bath blanket
- two large bath towels • gown or pajamas or nightgown
- lotion • powder if allowed • deodorant or antiperspirant

Prevent chills by closing windows and doors prior to beginning procedure.

Soap should only be used when deemed acceptable by your charge nurse/care team. An elderly resident's skin may be too fragile and easily broken to use a drying agent such as soap. Check with your supervisor for the facility-approved cleansing agent.

Oral hygiene, nail care, hair care, and makeup application are separate procedures and will be treated as such. These procedures are outlined in Chapter 21.

1. Perform the "5 Stars."

PREPARE:

2. Apply gloves and begin the bath.

PERFORM:

The following body parts should be washed in a complete bed bath in this order:
1. eyes
2. face
3. neck
4. ears
5. arms and axillae
6. chest and abdomen
7. legs and feet
8. back
9. perineal area
10. buttocks

3. Remove top linen by first placing bath blanket over resident, then pulling out top sheet from FOB.

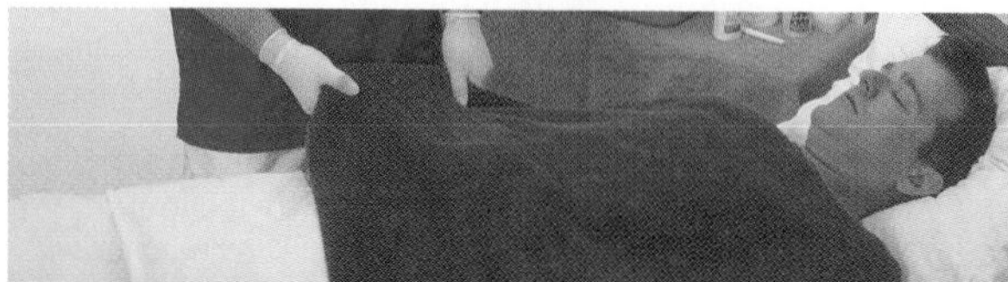

Figure 19-8.

4. Ask resident to hold bath blanket and remove gown, pajamas, or nightgown carefully.

5. Pick up washcloth and form mitt.

6. EYES:
Towel Placement: Under chin
Soap: none
Direction: Inner to outer canthus (corner) (Use different parts of the washcloth/mitt for each eye.)
Follow-up: Rinse and dry thoroughly.

7. FACE:
Towel: Under chin
Soap: none
Direction: Top to bottom with nose and mouth last.
Follow-up: Rinse and dry thoroughly.

Figure 19-9.

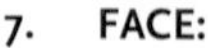

8. NECK and EARS:
Towel: Under chin
Soap: Swirled in water
Direction: Neck, then one ear at a time.
Follow-up: Rinse and dry.

9. FAR ARM:
Towel: Under far arm
Soap: Optional
Direction: Start with the shoulder, then arm, hand, and axilla.
Follow-up: Rinse and dry thoroughly.

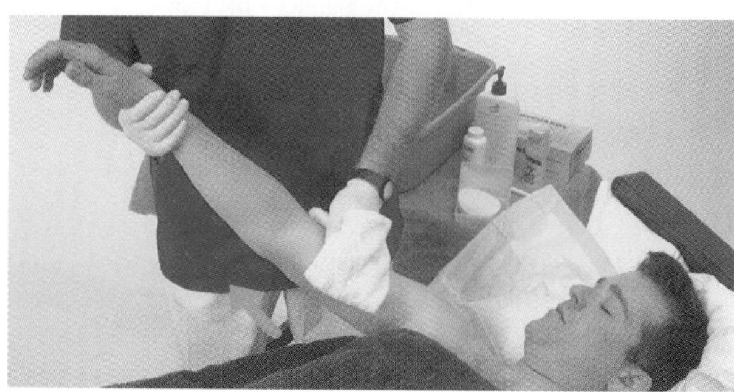

Figure 19-10.

10. NEAR ARM:
Repeat 9 exactly for the near arm.

11. CHEST and ABDOMEN:
Towel: Across chest horizontally, then across abdomen
Soap: Optional
Direction: Chest, then under breasts, abdomen and navel, including any skin folds on the abdomen.
Follow-up: Rinse and dry thoroughly.

12. FAR LEG:
Towel: Under far leg.
Soap: Optional
Direction: Wash far leg, then foot, carefully washing toes.

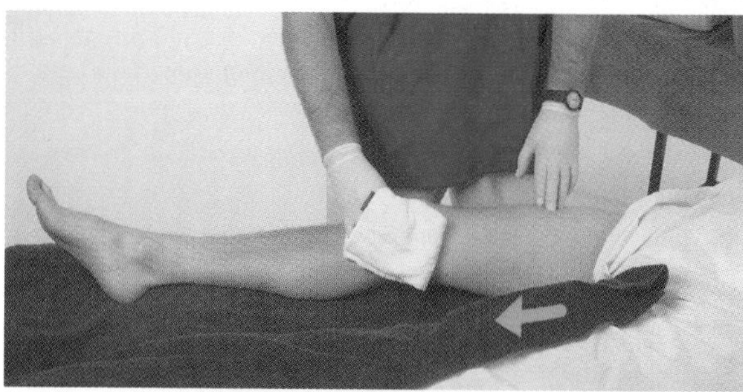

Figure 19-11.

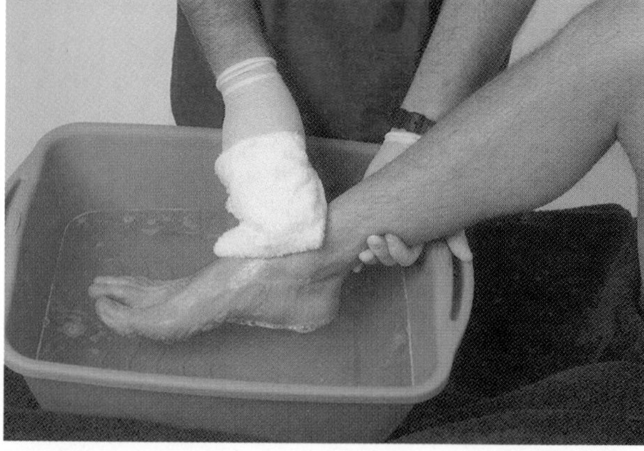

Figure 19-12.

Follow-up: Rinse and dry foot and toes thoroughly.

13. NEAR LEG:
Repeat 12 exactly for the near leg.

14. BACK:
Towel: Under back
Soap: Optional
Direction: Resident turned to side away from you. Wash back from top to bottom with firm strokes.

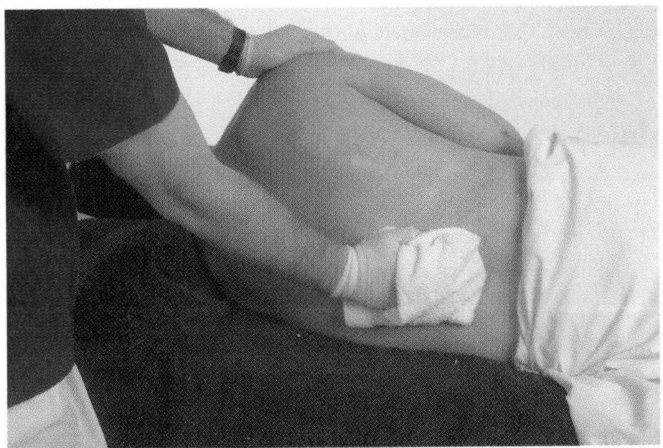

Figure 19-13.

Follow-up: Rinse and dry back thoroughly. Back massage optional now. (See Learning Objective 12.)

15. SECURE THE RESIDENT and raise the side rail. Get a clean basin of lukewarm water and return to the bedside. Lower side rail.

16. PERINEAL AREA and BUTTOCKS:
Towel: Over perineal area; use clean washcloth
Soap: Small amount
Direction: Resident returned to back. Complete male or female perineal care following the proper procedure. Both the vulva and the rectal area or the penis and the rectal area should be done at this time.
Follow-up: Rinse and dry entire perineal area thoroughly.

17. Help resident with the use of personal items such as deodorant or lotion.

FINISHING TOUCHES:

18. Assist resident to put on gown, pajamas, or clothing.

19. SECURE THE RESIDENT. Clean up equipment and dispose of any disposable supplies in appropriate place.

20. Perform the "5 Stars and 3 Rs."

The Partial or Set-Up Bath

Follow all standard and/or transmission-based precautions. Follow all rules for body mechanics.

Collect equipment:
- gloves • soap dish • soap • bath thermometer • face towel
- basin with lukewarm water • wash cloths • bath blanket
- two large bath towels • gown or pajamas or nightgown
- lotion • powder if allowed • deodorant or antiperspirant

Prevent chills by closing windows and doors prior to beginning procedure.

Oral hygiene, nail care, hair care, and makeup application are separate procedures and will be treated as such. These procedures are outlined in Chapter 21.

1. Perform the "5 Stars."

PREPARE:

2. Raise head of the bed so that resident is sitting up, or sit resident to the side of the bed.

PERFORM:

3. Give the resident the washcloth and towel and allow the resident to bathe himself to the extent possible. SECURE THE RESIDENT if your facility allows you to leave the room at this time.

4. Ask resident to press call button when in need of your assistance to complete the bath. Wash hands and leave the room.

5. Re-enter the room and wash hands when call button is pressed.

6. Apply gloves and assist resident by completing the bath. The following body parts should be washed in a partial bath, in this order:
   1. face, neck, and ears
   2. hands
   3. axillae
   4. back
   5. perineal area
   6. buttocks
   7. Offer resident a back massage, if allowed.
   8. Help resident with the use of personal items such as deodorant or lotion.

FINISHING TOUCHES:

7. Assist resident to put on gown, pajamas, nightgown, or clothing.

8. SECURE THE RESIDENT. Clean up equipment and dispose of any disposable supplies or linen in appropriate place.

9. Perform the "5 Stars and 3 Rs."

The Tub Bath

Follow all standard and/or transmission-based precautions. Follow all rules for body mechanics.

Collect equipment:
- two pairs of gloves; one standard pair and one pair heavy-duty • soap dish • soap • wash cloths • two large bath towels • bath thermometer if available • face towel • lotion
- robe and clean gown, pajamas, or nightgown
- powder if allowed • deodorant or antiperspirant

To save time, check tub room for cleanliness and pre-fill the tub with warm water and prepare the tub by placing bath mat, etc. in tub before bringing resident to the room.

1. Perform the "5 Stars."

PREPARE:

2. Assist resident to tub room by walking or by wheelchair.
3. Place "In Use" sign on door to tub room, if available.
4. Check temperature of the water and security of bath mat.
5. Carefully transfer the resident to the tub, holding on to him the entire time.
6. Stay with the resident for the entire bath.

PERFORM:

7. Encourage independence by allowing the resident to bathe himself to the fullest extent possible.
8. Apply gloves and assist resident as needed in completing the bath. The following body parts should be washed, in this order:

   1. eyes
   2. face
   3. neck
   4. ears
   5. arms and axillae
   6. chest and abdomen
   7. legs and feet
   8. back (with back massage optional)
   9. perineal area
   10. buttocks

   Drain water and carefully assist the resident out of tub to safe area. Wrap resident in a towel. Provide her with another towel for drying herself. Offer assistance in drying hard-to-reach places.

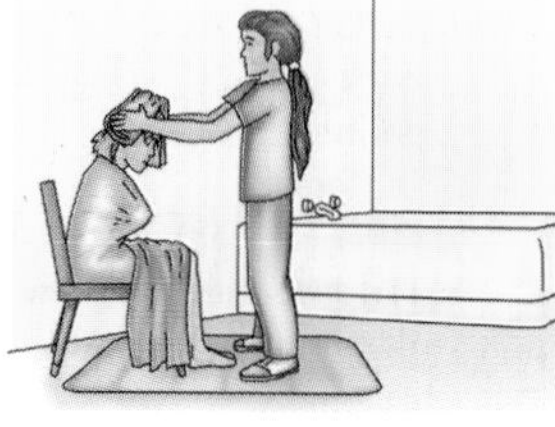

Figure 19-14.

9. Help resident with the use of personal items such as deodorant or lotion.

FINISHING TOUCHES:

10. Assist resident to put on gown, pajamas, nightgown, robe, or clothing.
11. Return the resident to room or other area. Secure resident.
12. Perform the "5 Stars and 3 Rs."

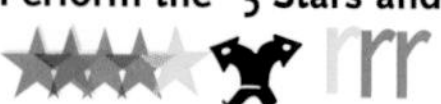

13. Return to tub room and clean room. Using heavy-duty gloves, if facility policy, thoroughly clean tub and other areas and dispose of any disposable supplies and linen in appropriate place.

The Shower

Follow all standard and/or transmission-based precautions. Follow all rules for body mechanics.

Collect equipment:

• two pairs of gloves; one standard pair and one pair heavy-duty • soap dish • soap • wash cloths • two large bath towels • bath thermometer if available • face towel • lotion • robe and clean gown, pajamas, or nightgown • powder if allowed • deodorant or antiperspirant

1. Perform the "5 Stars."

PREPARE:

2. Assist the resident to the shower room by walking or by wheelchair.
3. Place "In Use" sign on door to shower room, if available.
4. Check the temperature of the water and security of bath mat, if used.
5. Carefully transfer the resident to the shower, holding on to her the entire time.
6. Stay with the resident for the entire shower.

PERFORM:

7. Encourage independence by allowing the resident to bathe herself to the fullest extent possible.
8. Apply gloves and assist resident in completing the shower. The following body parts should be washed, in this order:

   1. eyes
   2. face
   3. neck
   4. ears
   5. arms and axillae
   6. chest and abdomen
   7. legs and feet
   8. back (with back massage optional)
   9. perineal area
   10. buttocks

9. Assist resident out of shower to a safe area. Wrap resident in a towel. Provide her with another towel for drying herself. Offer assistance in drying hard-to-reach places. Help resident with the use of personal items such as deodorant or lotion.

FINISHING TOUCHES:

10. Assist resident to put on gown, pajamas, nightgown, robe, or clothing.
11. Return the resident to room or other area. Secure resident.
12. Perform the "5 Stars and 3 Rs."

13. Return to tub room and clean room. Using heavy-duty gloves, if facility policy, thoroughly clean tub and other areas and dispose of any disposable supplies and linen in appropriate place.

12 Explain how to perform a safe and effective back massage.

Back massages are helpful in relaxing tired, tense muscles and improving the circulation. Residents sometimes request a back massage prior to going to bed in the evening. Back massages may also be a part of the partial or complete bed bath, or possibly a tub bath or a shower. Sometimes back massages should not be given for certain reasons. For example, a spinal injury may be further aggravated with a back rub. It is extremely important that you check with the nurse in charge prior to giving back massages to residents. If you forget, you may put your resident at risk.

The Risks of Blood Clots with Massages

When performing a back massage on a resident or a family member or friend, you should be aware of one possible risk. Giving a massage can cause a blood clot to break free inside a vein. The greatest risk of this happening is inside the veins of the lower legs. People with poor circulation and pregnant women are at greater risk for blood clots. It is best for you to not massage any part of the legs when performing a massage.

Giving a Back Massage

Follow all standard and/or transmission-based precautions. Follow all rules for body mechanics.

Collect equipment:
- **gloves • basin of warm water • large bath towel**
- **gown, pajamas or nightgown • lotion.**

1. **Perform the "5 Stars."**

PREPARE:

2. **Make sure the back massage is safe for this resident. Put lotion bottle into warm water to warm, if desired.**
3. **Apply gloves only if needed and turn resident to the side (lateral) or abdomen (prone position) and make comfortable.**

PERFORM:

4. **Pour lotion into hand, rub between hands to warm lotion slightly, and let resident know that you are ready to apply lotion to the back.**

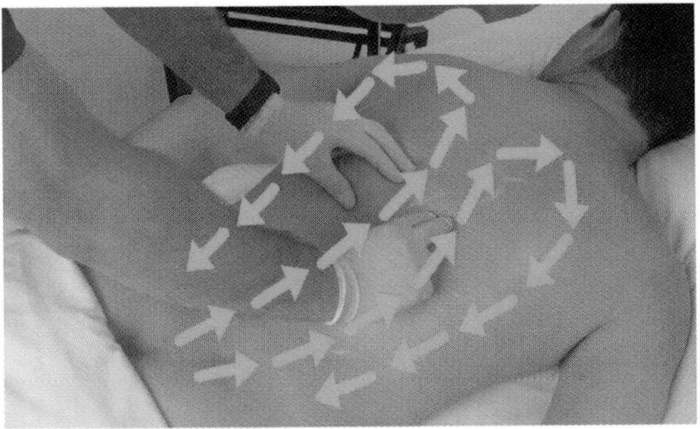

Figure 19-15.

5. **Rub back using long, smooth, firm strokes, starting at the buttocks and moving in the direction of the shoulders.**
6. **Move then to massage the arms, then return to the back and rub downward, back in the direction of the buttocks. (See Figure 19-15.)**
7. **Continue until the resident asks you to stop or about two to three minutes have passed. You may massage for a few extra minutes if the resident requests. Remember to observe for signs of skin breakdown. Massage around, but not directly on, an area where a pressure sore may be developing.**

FINISHING TOUCHES:

8. **Using bath towel, make sure entire back is dry.**
9. **Assist resident to put on gown, pajamas, nightgown, or clothing. Secure the resident.**
10. **Perform the "5 Stars and 3 Rs."**

Summary

Cleanliness is an important part of a person's health and well-being. Nursing assistants should strive to keep residents clean and fresh throughout each day. The correct steps for bathing must be carefully followed in order to not transfer dangerous microorganisms from one area of the body to another. Privacy concerns need to be taken into account during bathing and especially perineal care. Keeping the body clean enables a person to look better and feel better. This may ultimately improve a resident's attitude and self-esteem.

Bathing offers you the best opportunity to observe and report any sign of skin breakdown. Becoming familiar with signs of pressure sores will help you prevent this common problem.

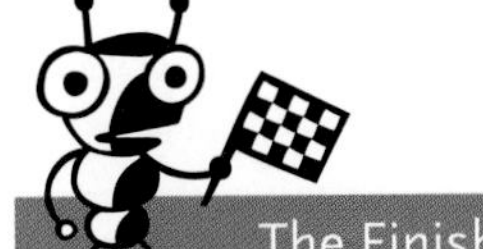

The Finish Line

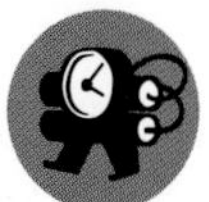

What's Wrong With This Picture?

This is a listing of the order of body parts that have to be washed for the partial bath. The order is incorrect. Fix the list so that it is correct.

1. perineal area

2. face
3. buttocks
4. eyes
5. arms and axilla (axillae)
6. chest and abdomen
7. legs and feet
8. neck
9. ears
10. back

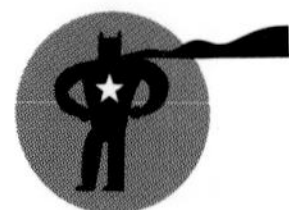

Star Student Central

1. The ability to recognize unusual or odd-looking areas on your resident's skin during skin care begins with YOU. Be able to identify unusual spots or areas on yourself as well. Stand in front of a full-length mirror and look at your entire body. Look closely at all of the moles on your body. Note any spots that seem to be an unusual color, especially red, white, dark brown, gray, or black, or any areas that have an odd feeling when touched with your fingertips. Also note whether any spots or moles have changed in color or size, or moles that seem to have spread. Any change in color or size of a mole could mean a problem. If you find any spots or moles that you are concerned about, call for an appointment with your healthcare provider.
2. Make an appointment with a specialist called a dermatologist. Ask the dermatologist for educational handouts about good skin care while you are there. Look specifically for pamphlets on moles and possible changes that may occur and look for photos inside the pamphlets that show examples of cancerous moles. Share them with your class.

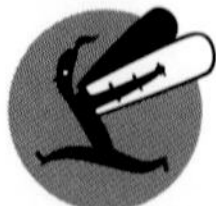

You Can Do It Corner!

1. As far as safety is concerned, what should you assess before giving a resident a bath? (LO 8)
2. Why might bathing be done on a resident in the evening rather than the morning? (LO 2)
3. List the order in which body parts are washed during a complete bed bath. (LO 9)
4. List the five steps to quality skin care. (LO 3)
5. What are the six areas in prevention and care of pressure sores? (LO 6)
6. While washing the neck, you note a raised area to the side of the neck. When you look at the neck, one side seems to be bigger than the other side. What would you do? Why might this be important? (LO 10)
7. What happens to a pressure sore during each of the four stages? (LO 4)
8. Define objective and subjective data. If a resident complains of pain when her right ear is washed, is it objective or subjective data? (LO 10)
9. A resident who should not have daily full baths is best suited to what type of bath? (LO 7)
10. According to the Norton Scale, what are the five risk factors for pressure sores? (LO 5)
11. How are back massages helpful for residents? (LO 12)
12. Why might you need an interpreter when discussing peri-care? (LO 11)

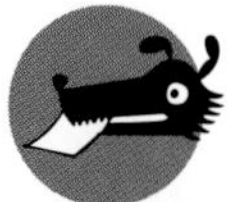

Star Student's Chapter Checklist

1. I have read my textbook chapter.
2. I have reviewed my own "Pocketful of Terms."
3. I have listened to my tutor tape.
4. I have reviewed and highlighted my class notes.
5. I have read and completed any handouts from this chapter.
6. I have completed "The Finish Line."
7. Star Time! Choose your reward!

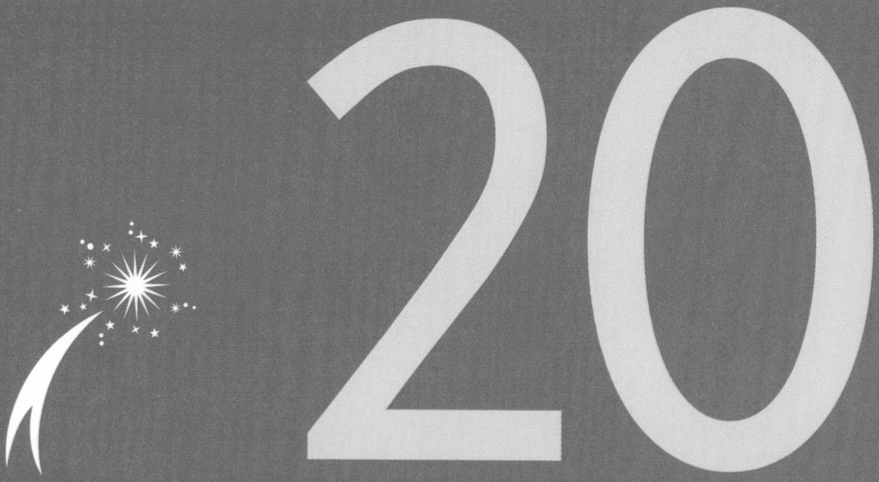

20

Your Guide:

Oral Hygiene and Specialized Care of the Unconscious Resident

Look Like a Star!

Look at the Learning Objectives and The Finish Line before you begin reading this chapter.

**Look at your pocket calendar.
With your pencil, put a bracket (   ) around a study period every single day.**

**Look at your homework for this chapter.
Plug each piece of homework into a certain time slot.**

Look at the Star Student's Chapter Checklist at the end of this chapter. Check off each item as it is completed.

"Bid them wash their faces/And keep their teeth clean."

William Shakespeare, 1564-1616

"Every tooth in a man's head is more valuable than a diamond."

Miguel de Cervantes, 1547-1616

Learning Objectives

1. **Spell and define all STAR words.**
2. **Summarize the importance of excellent oral hygiene and list seven areas to observe and report.**
3. **Explain four questions that help determine the type of oral care to be given.**
4. **Identify eight types of supplies used during oral care.**
5. **Describe four types of dental appliances that replace natural teeth and explain the importance of quality denture care.**
6. **Identify the risks of performing mouth care for unconscious residents.**
7. **Describe five steps to ensure quality eye care for an unconscious resident.**

Successfully perform these Practical Procedures

Assisting with Brushing Teeth

Brushing Teeth

Flossing Teeth

Denture Care

Mouth Care for the Unconscious Resident

Eye Care for the Unconscious Resident

Dentistry in its Infancy

The art of dentistry was once not governed as it is today, by licensing agencies and medical boards. Anyone who wished to work with teeth could do so. People sometimes practiced "dentistry" on the street corners. Louis XIV of France recognized that dentists were professionals in 1699. Dentists were then required to complete two years of school. Pierre Fauchard, 1678-1761, collected and put together a large amount of research about dentistry. He had a firm belief that dentists should receive special training. He wrote *The Surgeon Dentist* (1728), which was considered the authority on dentistry for many years.

1 Spell and define all STAR words.

aspiration: a potentially dangerous situation where a person inhales fluid, food, or an object into the airway and the lungs.

bridge: a type of dental appliance that replaces as few as one or two teeth.

canthus: inner aspect of the eye area where the lids come together closest to the nose.

decay: a gradual deterioration to an inferior state; also called dental caries.

dentures: artificial teeth.

floss: waxed or unwaxed thread used to clean and remove plaque from between the teeth and under the gums.

gingivitis: inflammation of the gums.

halitosis: bad or foul-smelling breath.

oral hygiene: procedures done in order to keep the mouths of residents clean and fresh.

periodontic: branch of dentistry that studies the areas supporting the teeth, such as the gums.

plaque: a substance on the teeth that can turn into hard deposits called tartar if allowed to remain on the teeth too long.

sordes: crusts common on the lips, gums, and teeth of people who are unconscious; crusts containing microorganisms, mucous, and food.

tartar: hard deposits of plaque filled with dead bacteria; can cause gum disease and loose teeth.

unconscious: lacking awareness of the environment, resulting from an injury or disease process.

2 Summarize the importance of excellent oral hygiene and list seven areas to observe and report.

Oral hygiene or oral care means keeping residents' mouths clean and fresh. It is an extremely important responsibility of every nursing assistant. When a person's mouth is not fresh, it affects his interactions with others. People may shy away from a person with foul-smelling breath, known as **halitosis**. In addition to bad breath, serious problems, such as gum disease, can occur when proper oral care is not done. An unhealthy mouth can also lead to a poor appetite and weight loss. These things are big problems in nursing homes. It is the responsibility of each nursing assistant to provide excellent oral hygiene to all residents during each shift. Oral care may be necessary every one to two hours on some residents. For other residents, twice a day is sufficient.

Plaque is a substance that forms in a brief period of time if a resident does not receive adequate oral hygiene. This plaque can turn into hard deposits called **tartar** if left on the teeth too long. Tartar is filled with bacteria and may ultimately cause gum disease and loose teeth if it is not removed by a dentist or a dental hygienist. Dental plaque and tartar may cause health problems other than gum disease. See the Textbook Tip on gum disease in this chapter.

Gingivitis is an inflammation of the gums. This can lead to **periodontal** disease when the areas supporting the teeth, such as the gums, become diseased.

Nursing assistants also have a duty to observe the inside and outside of the mouth along with the teeth during oral care. Sometimes a problem found inside the mouth is a sign that a bigger problem exists elsewhere in the body. For example, a person with unusually fruity breath, similar to a lemon or a lime, may have a disease called diabetes mellitus. When people have difficulty managing their diabetes, they will sometimes develop fruity-smelling breath. You may be the first staff member to note the fruity breath during oral care, and this information helps the nurse provide prompt care for the problem.

Another problem that a resident may have is a sore throat or strep throat. If a nursing assistant notices halitosis and connects it to the resident's complaint of a sore throat, this enables the nurse to provide faster treatment for the problem. Quicker access to treatment often prevents complications of strep throat, such as scarlet fever or rheumatic fever. These illnesses can cause heart problems if left untreated.

During oral hygiene, these are observations to note and report:

Lips: dry, red, cracked, or bleeding lips; cold sores on the lips

Gums: red, irritated, swollen, or bleeding gums

Teeth: cracked, chipped, or broken teeth; loose teeth; partials, bridges, or dentures; teeth with blackened areas that might show **decay**; poorly-fitting dentures

Mouth: yellow-filled or red sores, such as canker sores inside the mouth; white spots inside the mouth; areas of pus or infection

Tongue: a red or swollen tongue; tongue coated with a white substance; bumps on the tongue

Breath: bad breath or halitosis; fruity-smelling breath

Drinking, sucking, or swallowing ability: change in the person's ability to drink, suck on a straw, or swallow; gagging or choking; reports of any mouth pain

Many of these observations could be serious and should be reported immediately to the nurse-in-charge. For example, a broken tooth or teeth may be due to a resident being hit by someone. Pus inside the mouth or white patches might need prompt treatment. If you feel the observation is an emergency of some kind, remember this:

★ *"Don't Delay. Report Right Away!"*

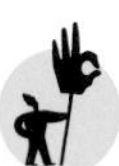

Gum Disease and Heart Attacks: Is there a link?

A link may exist between gum disease and the risk of having a heart attack. The incidence of heart disease may be higher in people with gum disease. Some studies point to a link between a type of bacteria found in plaque that develops on the teeth and gums. The bacteria could cause blood clots to form. If a blood clot develops and moves into your bloodstream, it may cause a heart attack or a stroke. It is a good investment in your health and the health of your family to have regular dental checkups and cleanings each year. Most dentists recommend cleaning at least twice every year with a dental exam at least yearly.

3 Explain four questions that help determine the type of oral care to be given.

Residents require different kinds of care for their mouths, teeth, and gums. This care is dependent upon the following assessment:

1. Is the resident alert, confused, or **unconscious**?
2. Does the resident have his own teeth, bridges or partials, dentures, or a combination?
3. How much oral care can the resident do himself?
4. Does the resident prefer certain products?

Determining the answers to these questions can help you plan your care.

For example, you have eight residents, and they all need to be set up for breakfast. You would first determine the number that need help with their oral care. If four out of the eight require assistance with oral care, you would set up the four independent residents so that they perform their own oral care, and secure those residents. Then you would focus on the four who need more of your assistance.

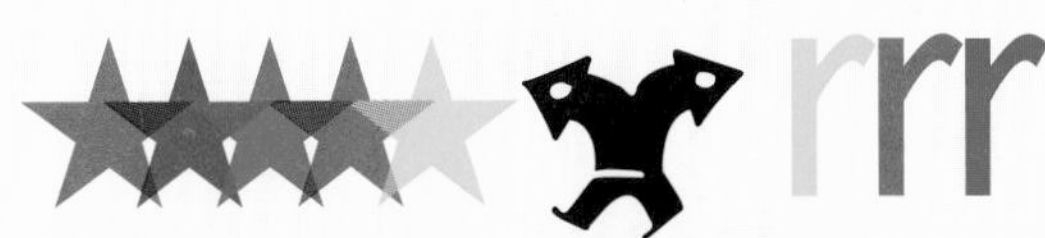

Beginning Steps

★ **RESPECT**
Knock first, ask and receive permission to enter a resident's room.

★ **INFECTION CONTROL**
Wash hands.

★ **COMMUNICATION**
Greet and identify the resident. Identify yourself. Explain the procedure, encouraging the resident to be as independent as possible throughout.

★ **BED SAFETY**
Lock bed wheels. Raise bed to safe working height. Lower one side rail if required.

★ **PRIVACY**
Provide for privacy by closing the door and covering the resident appropriately.

Ending Steps

★ **RESIDENT SAFETY AND COMFORT**
Secure the resident, lowering the bed, and raising the side rails if ordered. Check that the resident is comfortable and properly aligned.

★ **PRIVACY**
Remove any added privacy measures, such as a drape or a privacy screen.

★ **ESSENTIALS**
Place the call light, fresh beverage, and other items within reach.

★ **COURTESY**
Ask the resident if he or she needs anything else. Say thank you and goodbye.

★ **INFECTION CONTROL**
Wash hands.

Report your care and any important observations to the nurse.

Record your care and any important information/observations such as vital signs in the appropriate place.

Recheck your resident for any changes as directed by the nurse!

4 Identify eight types of supplies used during oral care.

Once you have determined the type of oral care you must provide to your residents, it is important for you to be familiar with the supplies available. Types of supplies and equipment available for oral hygiene include the following:

- toothbrush
- dental **floss**
- aqua or pink spongy foam on a stick
- toothpaste
- mouthwash

- denture cleaner
- lubricant
- gauze pads

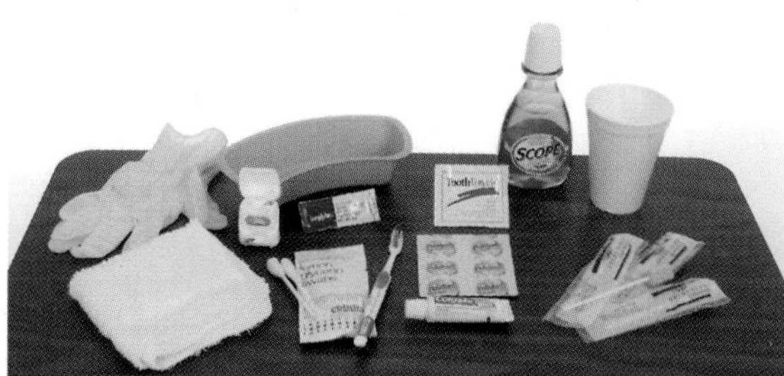

Figure 20-1. **Supplies needed for oral care.**

Assisting with Brushing Teeth

Follow all standard and/or transmission-based precautions. Follow all rules for body mechanics.

Collect equipment:
• two pairs of disposable gloves • glass of water and straw • small towel • kidney (emesis) basin • lip lubricant • toothbrush • toothpaste or other cleaning agent

Make sure trash container is next to the bed.

1. **Perform the "5 Stars."**

PREPARE:

2. **Sit the resident up in bed comfortably, using pillows if needed.**
3. **Place the towel under the resident's mouth and chin.**
4. **Put on gloves and wet toothbrush. Put a pea-sized amount of toothpaste on the toothbrush.**

PERFORM:

5. **Assist the resident to brush the teeth and tongue. Provide as much help as is needed.**
6. **Allow the resident to rinse the mouth completely and spit the water into the emesis (kidney) basin.**
7. **Wipe mouth and add lubricant to the lips, if desired.**

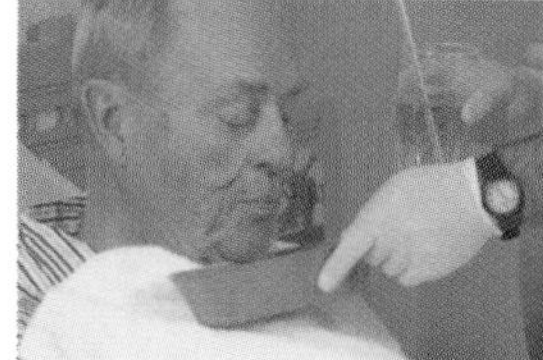

Figure 20-2.

FINISHING TOUCHES:

8. **SECURE THE RESIDENT. Position the resident comfortably and replace linen over the resident.**
9. **Clean up the entire area, disposing of trash and linen, cleaning out basin, and then removing gloves and disposing of them.**
10. **Perform the "5 Stars and 3 Rs."**

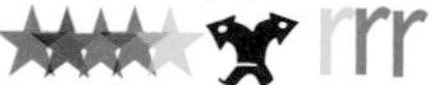

Brushing Teeth

Follow all standard and/or transmission-based precautions. Follow all rules for body mechanics.

Collect equipment:
• two pairs of disposable gloves • glass of water and straw • small towel • kidney (emesis) basin • lip lubricant • toothbrush • toothpaste or other cleaning agent

Make sure trash container is next to the bed.

1. **Perform the "5 Stars."**

PREPARE:

2. **Sit the resident up in bed comfortably, using pillows if needed.**
3. **Place the towel under the resident's mouth and chin.**
4. **Put on gloves and wet toothbrush. Put a pea-sized amount of toothpaste on the toothbrush.**

PERFORM:

5. **Brush the resident's teeth and tongue.**
6. **Ask the resident to rinse her mouth completely and spit the water into the kidney basin. Dry the mouth completely using the towel.**
7. **Add lubricant to the lips, if desired.**

FINISHING TOUCHES:

8. **SECURE THE RESIDENT. Position the resident comfortably and replace linen over the resident.**
9. **Clean up the entire area, disposing of trash and linen, cleaning out basin, and then removing gloves and disposing of them.**
10. **Perform the "5 Stars and 3 Rs."**

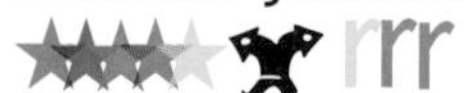

Flossing Teeth

Follow all standard and/or transmission-based precautions. Follow all rules for body mechanics.

Collect equipment:
• two pairs of disposable gloves
• enough dental floss to complete the entire mouth (approximately 18 inches) • glass of water, kidney (emesis) basin • a small towel

Make sure trash container is next to the bed.

1. **Perform the "5 Stars."**

PREPARE:

2. **Sit the resident up in bed comfortably, using pillows if needed, or position the resident comfortably on his back.**
3. **Place the towel under the resident's mouth and chin.**
4. **Put on gloves and wrap the ends of the floss around your gloved index (first) fingers.**

PERFORM:

5. Floss all of the resident's teeth.

   a. Change to a new area of floss between teeth.

   b. Discard floss and pull out a new strand when needed.

   c. Give water to rinse when necessary.

   d. Ask resident to spit into kidney basin.

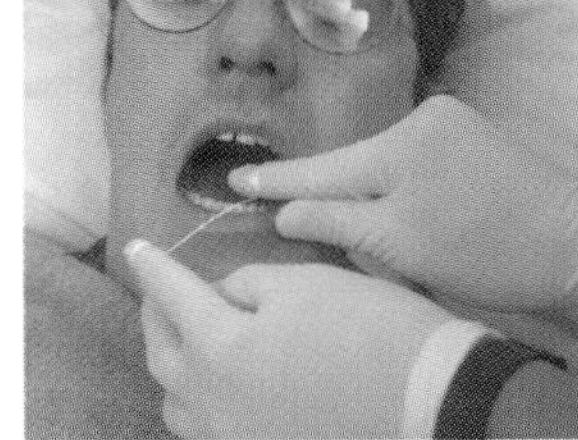

Figure 20-3.

6. Ask the resident to rinse the mouth completely and spit the water into the kidney basin. Dry the mouth completely.

7. Add lubricant to the lips, if desired.

FINISHING TOUCHES:

8. SECURE THE RESIDENT. Position the resident comfortably and replace linen over the resident.

9. Clean up the entire area, disposing of trash and linen and cleaning out basin. Remove gloves and dispose of them.

10. Perform the "5 Stars and 3 Rs."

5 Describe four types of dental appliances that replace natural teeth and explain the importance of quality denture care.

There are different types of dentures, or artificial teeth, that replace teeth that have been removed. They include the following:

- full set of dentures
- top or bottom set of dentures
- partial plate
- bridge

Dentures are artificial teeth held together by a type of plate. A **bridge** is a dental appliance that replaces as few as one or two teeth. Bridges may be permanently placed in the mouth or attached by a clasp, so that it may be removed for cleaning. A resident may refer to a bridge as a "partial."

Dentures and bridges are the resident's teeth and are very important. They are expensive pieces of equipment and time-consuming for a denture specialist to make. All staff must be extremely careful when working with any dental appliance to avoid damaging it. Remember, if a resident's dentures break, he or she cannot eat. Handle residents' dentures and bridges with care.

When cleaning dentures, gloves must always be used to prevent transfer of blood or microorganisms from the resident to you or from your hands to the resident's teeth and mouth. The type of cleaning products will depend on the resident's likes and dislikes or facility policy. After cleaning dentures, they must always be placed in a special cup filled with cool water so that they do not dry out and warp. Dentures dry out and crack if left uncovered. When dentures are in a denture container for the night, some residents may ask that a cleaning product be added to the cool water for storage.

Denture Care

Follow all standard and/or transmission-based precautions. Follow all rules for body mechanics.

Collect equipment:

- two pairs of disposable gloves • gauze squares
- denture cleaner and denture cup or glass • mouthwash
- special brush or toothbrush for cleaning
- two small towels • kidney (emesis) basin

1. Perform the "5 Stars."

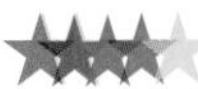

PREPARE:

2. Sit the resident up in bed comfortably using pillows, if needed, or position the resident comfortably on the back.

3. Place the towel under the resident's mouth and chin.

4. Put on gloves and open gauze squares or ask resident to remove dentures and place in basin.

5. SECURE THE RESIDENT. Take the basin to the sink. Line the sink with a towel to protect the dentures from breaking should they be dropped.

PERFORM:

6. Clean the dentures using warm water and either toothpaste and a toothbrush or denture cleanser and a denture brush.

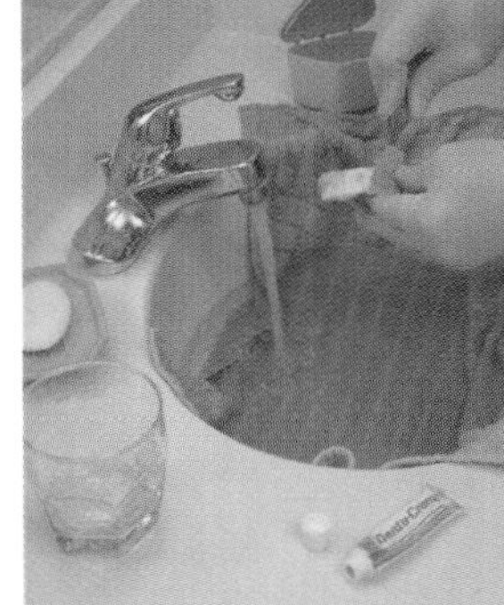

Figure 20-4.

7. Place dentures in a clean denture cup or a glass and cover with water so that no part of the dentures float above the water.

8. Ask resident if he would like to clean his mouth. Offer mouthwash and ask resident to spit into basin.

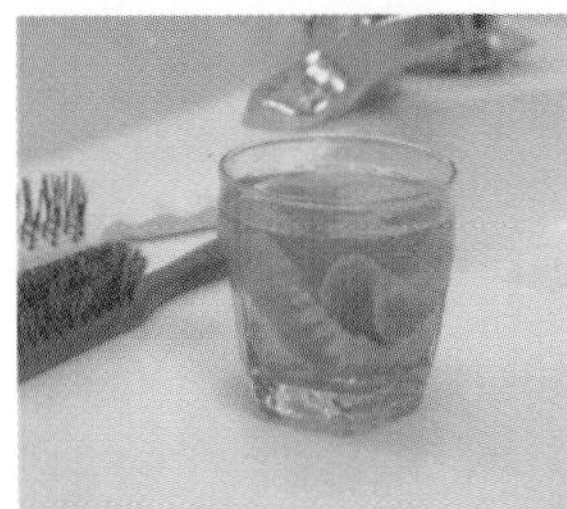

Figure 20-5.

9. If dentures are to be stored, place cup with dentures in a safe place. If dentures are to be placed back in the mouth, either allow resident to reinsert them or assist resident to reinsert dentures, making sure they are secure inside the mouth. Make sure you note how well the dentures fit.
10. Add lubricant to the lips, if desired.

FINISHING TOUCHES:

11. SECURE THE RESIDENT. Position the resident comfortably and replace linen over the resident.
12. Clean up the entire area, disposing of trash and linen, cleaning out basin, and then removing gloves and disposing of them.
13. Perform the "5 Stars and 3 Rs."

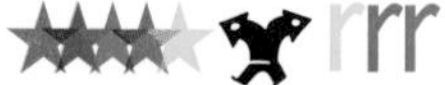

6 Identify the risks of performing mouth care for unconscious residents.

Oral care must be done frequently when a person is unconscious. Residents in this situation can no longer take care of their teeth and mouths, so the staff must take over this care completely. When residents are unconscious, they may not have enough saliva inside their mouths due to lack of oral fluids, breathing through the mouth, or oxygen therapy, which can dry out the mouth.

Unconscious mouth care requires the use of special supplies. Swabs with a mixture of lemon juice and glycerine are traditionally used to soothe the gums, but may further dry the gums if used too often. Padded tongue blades are used to separate the upper and lower teeth.

Crusts called **sordes** are common on the lips, gums, and teeth of people who are unconscious. These contain microorganisms, mucous, and food. Quality mouth care removes sordes and prevents them from developing.

The primary risk to the residents during unconscious mouth care is aspiration. **Aspiration** is the inhaling of food or fluid into the airway and the lungs. This risk can be prevented using extreme caution during this type of special mouth care. Preventing any fluids from going into the resident's airway during mouth care is the best way to prevent aspiration. This can be done by making sure your unconscious residents are always turned on their sides before beginning oral care. In addition, only swabs soaked in tiny amounts of fluid should be used to clean the mouth.

What if your resident can hear everything you say?

When caring for unconscious residents, staff may forget that the person in the bed may still be able to hear. Nursing assistants and all staff must make sure they do not behave in an inappropriate fashion when providing care for unconscious residents. Sometimes, unconscious or comatose people "wake up" and relate many of the things they heard while they were unconscious. Limit your discussions to appropriate subjects and do not talk about anything personal or say hurtful things. This may be considered abuse.

Mouth Care for the Unconscious Resident

Follow all standard and/or transmission-based precautions. Follow all rules for body mechanics.

Collect equipment:
- two pairs of disposable gloves • padded tongue blade
- cotton swabs or Toothettes, special commercial swabs
- lemon glycerine swabs • toothbrush • small towel
- glass of water and straw • kidney (emesis) basin
- lip lubricant • toothpaste or other cleaning agent

Make sure trash container is next to the bed.

1. Perform the "5 Stars."

Remember to speak to unconscious residents in the same manner as you would a conscious resident. Always assume they can hear every word.

PREPARE:

2. Turn the resident to the side of the bed and position comfortably using pillows, if needed.
3. Place the towel or Chux (absorbent pads) and the kidney (emesis) basin under the resident's mouth and chin.
4. Put on gloves. Pick up the padded tongue blade and insert it into the resident's mouth to separate the upper and lower teeth.

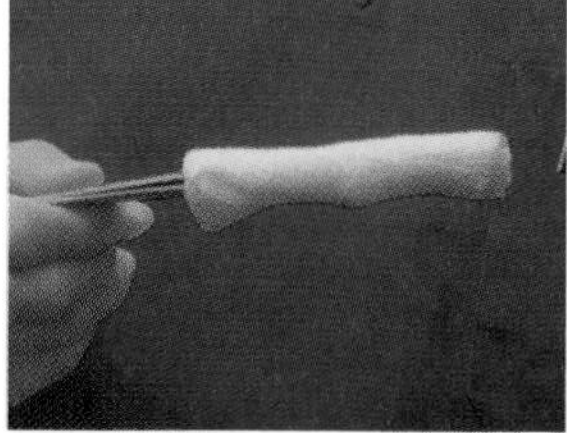

Figure 20-6. To make a padded tongue blade, place two wooden tongue blades together and wrap the upper portion with gauze. Tape the gauze in place.

PERFORM:

5. Using cotton swabs dipped in tiny amounts of water or mouthwash, clean the resident's teeth, gums, and tongue. Use fresh swabs when needed.
6. Swab again using the lemon glyercine swabs.
7. Dry the mouth completely using the towel.

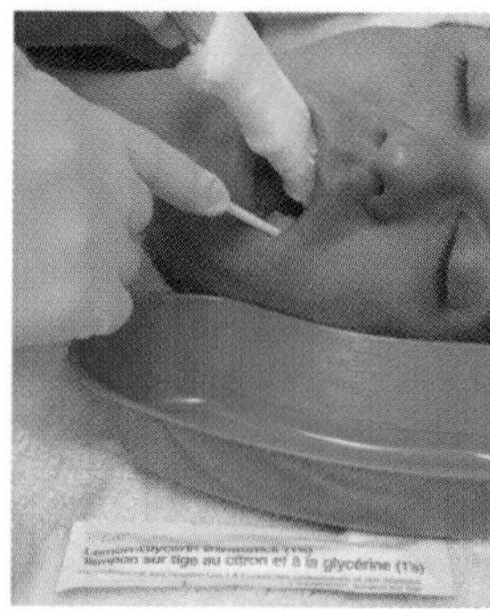

Figure 20-7.

8. Add lubricant to the lips.

FINISHING TOUCHES:

9. SECURE THE RESIDENT. Position the resident comfortably and replace linen over the resident.
10. Clean up the entire area, disposing of trash and linen, and clean basin.
11. Perform the "5 Stars and 3 Rs."

7 Describe five steps to ensure quality eye care for an unconscious resident.

An unconscious resident's eyes require special care because it is difficult for his or her eyes to remain moist. The air causes the eyes of an unconscious resident to dry out and require added moisture. Nurses take certain steps to ensure that the eyes remain moist. You can assist the nurse in this effort by doing the following during regular care:

1. During bathing, use gloves and clean supplies, such as washcloths and towels. If using a washcloth, rinse the washcloth thoroughly before cleansing the opposite eye. If using cotton balls, always use one cotton ball per eye and then dispose of it so that you do not transfer microorganisms. Do not use the same cotton ball to clean both eyes!
2. Wipe from the inner aspect or **canthus** (near the nose) to the outer canthus of the eye. This prevents harmful deposits from being pushed into a special duct at the inner corner of the eye.
3. Follow all instructions from the nurse regarding placing moist compresses on the eyes. Compresses using any special solution have to be applied by the nurse. You may be asked to apply compresses using plain water. More detailed information on hot and cold compresses can be found in Chapter 24.
4. Follow the nurse's instructions regarding putting any type of simple lubricant on the eyelids. Special lubricants may have to be applied.
5. Eye pads, if used, must be changed periodically. However, this is usually done by a nurse.

Eye Care for the Unconscious Resident

Follow all standard and/or transmission-based precautions. Follow all rules for body mechanics.

Collect equipment:
- two pairs of disposable gloves• washcloths • towel
- cotton balls • gauze pads
- non-medicated eye-area lubricant • water
- kidney (emesis) basin • wash basin

1. Perform the "5 Stars."

Remember to speak to unconscious residents in the same manner as you would a conscious resident. Always assume they can hear every word that you say.

PREPARE:

2. Position the resident comfortably using pillows, if needed.
3. Place the towel or Chux and the kidney (emesis) basin under the resident's chin.

PERFORM:

4. Put on gloves and do one of the following per the nurse's instructions:
   a. Dip washcloth into water and clean eyes, moving from inner canthus to outer canthus of the eye. Rinse washcloth completely before changing to other eye.
   b. Dip cotton balls into water and clean one eye at a time from the inner canthus to the outer canthus, disposing of each cotton ball as you use it. Use different cotton balls for each eye.
   c. If requested by the nurse, apply moist compresses to the eyes using gauze squares dipped lightly in water. Follow nurse's instructions for time period for compresses.
5. Dry the eye area completely using the towel.
6. Add lubricant to the eyelid area if instructed.

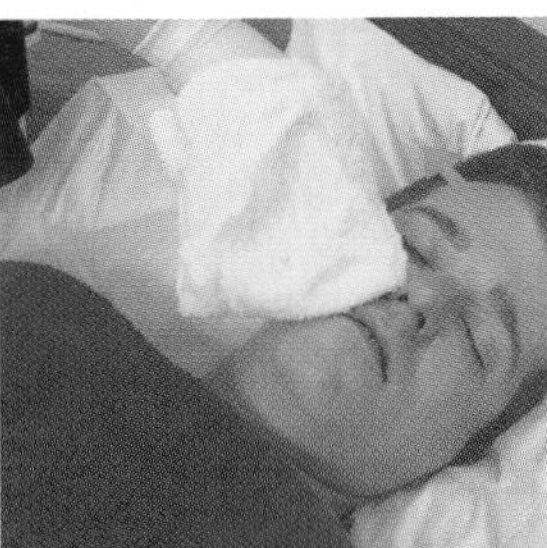

Figure 20-8.

FINISHING TOUCHES:

7. SECURE THE RESIDENT. Position the resident comfortably and replace linen over the resident.
8. Clean up the entire area, disposing of trash and linen, cleaning out basin, and then removing gloves and disposing of them.
9. Perform the "5 Stars and 3 Rs."

Summary

Quality mouth care is a very important part of the care given to residents daily. When bacteria gather inside the mouth, many problems can occur. Keeping a resident's mouth, teeth, and gums healthy is a big part of maintaining overall health.

The quality of the daily care of unconscious residents must be no different than the care of conscious residents. Unconscious residents deserve the same respect and attention as do alert residents. Making sure unconscious residents are well taken care of is a responsibility of all nursing staff.

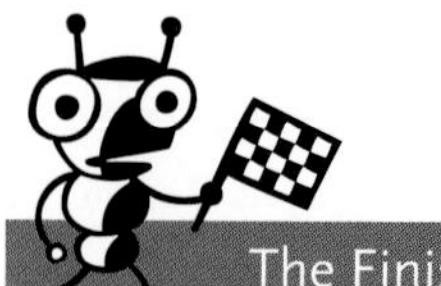

The Finish Line

What's Wrong With This Picture?

1. Look at the equipment listed for the Practical Procedure: Assisting with Brushing Teeth. Two important pieces of equipment are missing. List the missing pieces of equipment.

Collect equipment:
• two pairs of disposable gloves • glass of water and straw • small towel • toothbrush • toothpaste or other cleaning agent

2. Look at the equipment listed for the Practical Procedure: Denture Care shown below. One important piece of equipment is missing. List the missing piece of equipment.

Collect equipment:
• two pairs of disposable gloves
• denture cleaner and denture cup • gauze squares
• kidney (emesis) basin • mouthwash
• special brush or toothbrush for cleaning

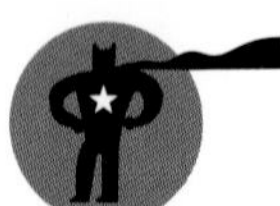

Star Student Central

1. You are an important part of the healthcare team and your own health is of supreme importance. If you are not healthy, you cannot be there for your residents.

   If you do not see a dentist regularly, make an appointment today with your dentist. If you do not have a dentist, shop around by asking trusted friends, family members, your doctor or pediatrician. Many communities have dental clinics or schools of denistry or dental hygiene that offer free or low-cost dental care. In some states, there is a web site to check the record of physicians and dentists. If possible, locate the web site and examine the record of each dentist to check for possible complaints from other consumers.

2. Do you have a relative, friend, or neighbor who has dentures? Ask this person to allow you to watch one day during morning or evening denture care. Then ask whether you may perform the denture care yourself the next time. Remember, you must use quality disposable gloves in order to perform this procedure. Always wear gloves, even if the person is a close friend or family member.

3. During your next visit to the dentist's office, ask whether they have any educational handouts regarding quality oral hygiene. Gather all available pamphlets and share these with your class, supervisor, or fellow employees. You may be able to place some pamphlets up on an employee bulletin board at your facility.

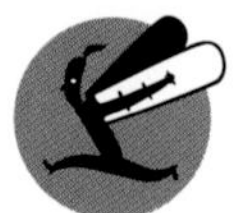

You Can Do It Corner!

1. Identify the difference between plaque and tartar. (LO 2)
2. Why is it so important for dentures to be completely covered with water when placed inside a denture container? (LO 5)
3. If you are not cautious during unconscious mouth care, what can happen? (LO 6)
4. List four questions to assess the type of oral care needed by residents. (LO 3)
5. During unconscious eye care, why is it important to use different cotton balls when moving from eye to eye? When cleaning the eyes, what is the proper direction to move in? Why? (LO 7)
6. What are eight types of supplies used for oral care? (LO 4)

7. Identify two observations you might make about each of the following: lips; gums; tongue; mouth; teeth; breath; and drinking, sucking, or swallowing ability. (LO 2)

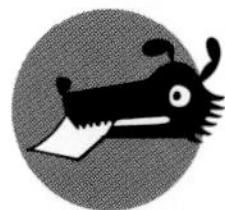

Star Student's Chapter Checklist

1. I have read my textbook chapter.
2. I have reviewed my own "Pocketful of Terms."
3. I have listened to my tutor tape.
4. I have reviewed and highlighted my class notes.
5. I have read and completed any handouts from this chapter.
6. I have completed "The Finish Line."
7. Star Time! Choose your reward!

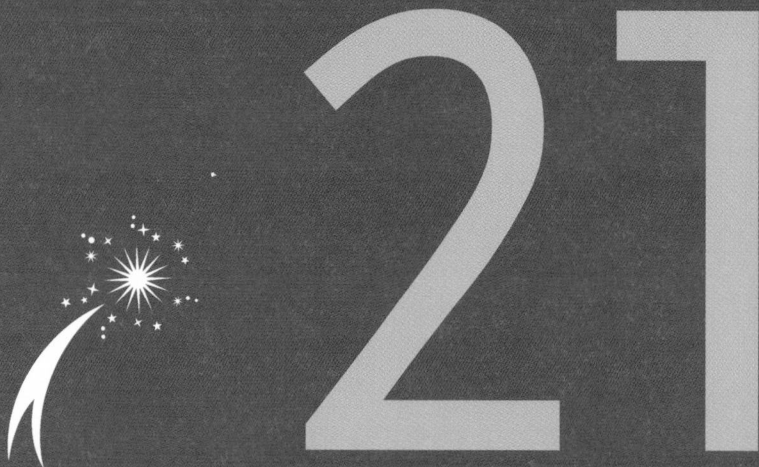

21

Your Guide:

Expert Grooming and Dressing Skills

Look Like a Star!

Look at the Learning Objectives and The Finish Line before you begin reading this chapter.

Look at your pocket calendar.
With your pencil, put a bracket ( ) around a study period every single day.

Look at your homework for this chapter.
Plug each piece of homework into a certain time slot.

Look at the Star Student's Chapter Checklist at the end of this chapter. Check off each item as it is completed.

"Any man may be in good spirits and good temper when he's well dressed."

Charles Dickens, 1812-1870

"Tis not a lip or eye we beauty call/But the joint force and full result of all."

Alexander Pope, 1688-1744

Learning Objectives

1. **Spell and define all STAR words.**
2. **Explain the importance of proper grooming and its effects on self-esteem.**
3. **Identify two shaving methods and ways to keep yourself and your resident safe during a shave.**
4. **Explain why your role in nail care is limited and discuss the proper care of feet.**
5. **Describe quality hair care and explain why gentleness is important.**
6. **Discuss the use of cosmetics and body care products and their effect on self-esteem.**
7. **Explain the importance of care of residents' clothing and why independent dressing and undressing should be encouraged.**
8. **Describe how to ensure a resident's dignity when wearing a facility gown and identify the gown used on a resident with an IV.**
9. **Identify nine assistive devices used in dressing residents.**

Successfully perform these Practical Procedures

Shaving a Male Resident

Shaving a Female Resident

Expert Nail Care

Safe Foot Care

Shampooing in Bed

Combing or Brushing Hair

Dressing a Resident or Changing Clothing

Undressing a Resident

Putting on and Removing a Gown on a Resident with an IV

Ancient Cosmetics

The earliest record of cosmetics comes from the 1st Dynasty of Egypt, 2920-2770 B.C. Searches of tombs from this time period have identified scented oils inside jars sealed in the tombs. Egyptian women decorated their eyes, adding dark green color under the eyes and using kohl, a substance sometimes made from soot or antimony, to darken lashes and the upper lids.

In the 1st century A.D., many Romans used cosmetics. Some of the cosmetics used by the Romans were kohl on eyelashes and eyelids, complexion-lightening chalk on the face, and rouge. The Romans also used substances to remove body hair. When the Crusaders came to the Middle East, they saw the use of cosmetics and brought them all over Europe during their travels.

1 Spell and define all STAR words.

cosmetics: products to enhance beauty or cleanse and improve the skin.

grooming: to care for the appearance of a person.

necrotic tissue: tissue that is no longer living.

necrosis: tissue death.

podiatrist: health professional trained in the examination and treatment of the feet.

orange sticks: sticks made of wood to clean under the nails.

2 Explain the importance of proper grooming and its effects on self-esteem.

Grooming means to care for the appearance of a person. Good grooming affects the way residents feel about themselves, as well as how they look to other residents, staff, and visitors. A well-groomed person is likely to feel better physically, because she is clean and neatly dressed. As a result, she may feel better emotionally as well, improving her overall attitude and making her much less likely to become unhappy or depressed.

Proper grooming is also important for health reasons. For example, if a resident does not bathe regularly, dirt and sweat gather on areas of the body. Bacteria multiplies on these areas and can cause an infection.

We all have routines for personal care and preferences for how we want this care to be done. These routines remain important even when we are elderly, sick, or disabled. Learn and follow your resident's individual preferences. Let your residents make as many choices as possible. Encourage them to do what they can do for themselves.

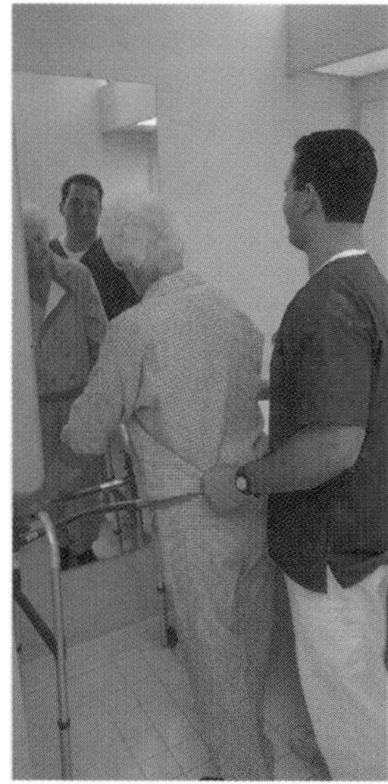

Figure 21-1. A well-groomed appearance helps people of all ages feel good about themselves.

3 Identify two shaving methods and ways to keep yourself and your resident safe during a shave.

Shaving is a very important part of some people's daily grooming routine. When people shave on a regular basis, they tend to feel more comfortable. Razor stubble on a man's face can be scratchy and uncomfortable. Women may feel uncomfortable when they do not shave their legs and underarms on a regular basis. However, keep in mind that some residents will not want to be shaved. Respect personal preferences regarding shaving.

Shaving requires extreme caution due to the risk of bleeding and bloodborne diseases. As always, when you help residents shave, follow standard precautions. You must always wear gloves when preparing, performing, and completing a shave. All shaving utensils must be handled, cleaned, and stored very carefully to prevent any transfer of bloodborne diseases between residents, or between residents and team members.

There are two methods of shaving that are utilized for most residents—shaving with a disposable razor or an electric razor. The method will usually depend upon the personal preferences of the resident or the resident's family. When shaving a resident with an electric razor, you must still wear gloves. Electric razors may cause skin tears and bleeding. Always shave in the direction of the hair growth. If you shave against the hair growth, you may shave too closely and nick the skin, causing a cut. This increases the chance of infection from microorganisms entering the cut.

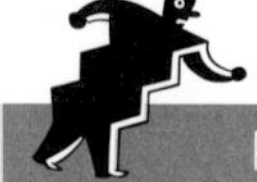

Principal Steps

Shaving Residents

1. *Always wear gloves when using either disposable or electric razors.*
2. *Soften hair first with a warm cloth.*
3. *Always shave in the direction of the hair growth.*
4. *Use shaving products like aftershave only with resident's permission.*
5. *Carefully discard any disposable shaving products in the biohazard container.*

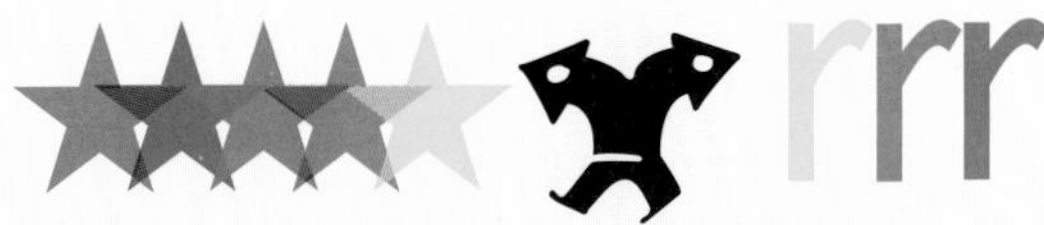

Beginning Steps

★ RESPECT
Knock first, ask and receive permission to enter a resident's room.

★ INFECTION CONTROL
Wash hands.

★ COMMUNICATION
Greet and identify the resident. Identify yourself. Explain the procedure, encouraging the resident to be as independent as possible throughout.

★ BED SAFETY
Lock bed wheels. Raise bed to safe working height. Lower one side rail if required.

★ PRIVACY
Provide for privacy by closing the door and covering the resident appropriately.

Ending Steps

★ RESIDENT SAFETY AND COMFORT
Secure the resident, lowering the bed, and raising the side rails if ordered. Check that the resident is comfortable and properly aligned.

★ PRIVACY
Remove any added privacy measures, such as a drape or a privacy screen.

★ ESSENTIALS
Place the call light, fresh beverage, and other items within reach.

★ COURTESY
Ask the resident if he or she needs anything else. Say thank you and goodbye.

★ INFECTION CONTROL
Wash hands.

r **Report** your care and any important observations to the nurse.

r **Record** your care and any important information/observations such as vital signs in the appropriate place.

r **Recheck** your resident for any changes as directed by the nurse!

Shaving a Male Resident

Follow all standard and/or transmission-based precautions. Follow all rules for body mechanics.

Collect equipment:
• two pairs of disposable gloves • washcloths • towel
• kidney basin (emesis) • shaving cream • electric razor or disposable razor • after-shave products (optional)
• wash basin with warm water

1. Perform the "5 Stars."

PREPARE:

2. Position the resident either sitting to the side of the bed or with the HOB in semi-Fowler's position.
3. Place a towel over the chest of the resident.
4. Apply gloves.
5. Place washcloth in warm water and apply to area to be shaved. Leave in place for three to five minutes.

PERFORM:

Do not shave any facial hair that the resident wishes to keep.

6. Shave the resident.
   a. Follow this procedure for electric razors. Electric razors work better on dry skin.
   - Apply pre-shave if desired, or pat the skin dry.
   - Turn on razor.
   - Shave in the direction of the hair growth. Some electric razors work best using a circular motion.

   b. Follow this procedure for disposable razors:
   - Apply shaving cream in a circular motion to area to be shaved. This lifts the whiskers away from the skin.
   - Wet razor and shave in the direction of hair growth, rinsing razor often. Keep area taut—pulled or drawn tight—to reduce the risk of cuts.
   - Clean off remaining shaving cream with warm washcloth.
   - Pat dry the shaved area with towel.

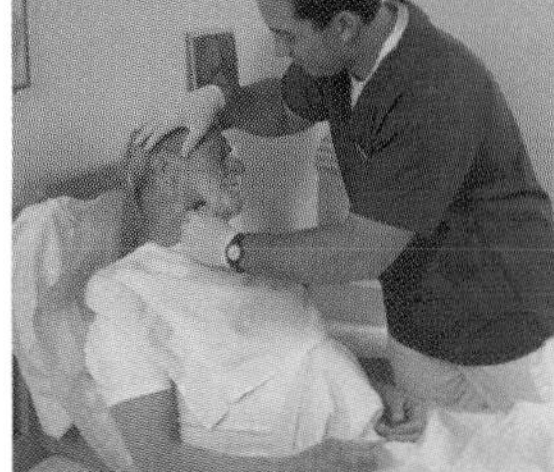

Figure 21-2.

FINISHING TOUCHES:

7. Apply after-shave if desired.
8. SECURE THE RESIDENT.
9. Dispose of razors in biohazard containers and shaving supplies in appropriate spot.
10. Remove gloves.
11. Perform the "5 Stars and 3 Rs."

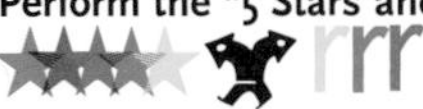

Shaving a Female Resident

Follow all standard and/or transmission-based precautions. Follow all rules for body mechanics.

Collect equipment:
• two pairs of disposable gloves • washcloths • towel
• kidney basin (emesis) • shaving cream • electric razor or disposable razor • after-shave products (optional)
• wash basin with warm water

1. Perform the "5 Stars."

PREPARE:

2. Position the resident with HOB in semi-Fowler's position.
3. Place a towel under the area to be shaved.
4. Apply gloves.
5. Place washcloth in warm water and apply to area to be shaved. Leave in place for three to five minutes.

PERFORM:

6. Shave the resident.

 a. Follow this procedure for electric razors:

 - Apply pre-shave if desired or pat the skin dry.
 - Turn on razor.
 - Shave in the direction of the hair growth.
 - Apply lotion or other cosmetics, if desired.

 b. Follow this procedure for disposable razors:

 - Apply shaving cream in a circular motion to area to be shaved.
 - Wet razor and shave in the direction of hair growth, rinsing razor often. Keep area taut—pulled or drawn tight—to reduce the risk of cuts.
 - Clean off remaining shaving cream with warm washcloth.
 - Pat the shaved area dry with towel.
 - Apply lotion or other cosmetics, if desired.

FINISHING TOUCHES:

7. SECURE THE RESIDENT.
8. Dispose of shaving supplies.
9. Remove gloves.
10. Perform the "5 Stars and 3 Rs."

 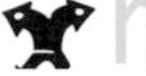

4 Explain why your role in nail care is limited and discuss the proper care of feet.

Good grooming includes quality nail care. When fingernails are dirty, they present a poor impression to others. They also collect and hide microorganisms under the nails. In addition, nails can easily scratch residents, visitors, and staff members. It is important that you always keep nails clean and short. In most places, it is not the responsibility of nursing assistants to trim fingernails or toenails.

When you trim nails of any kind, it is very easy to "nick" the surrounding skin of the nail. Many parents know they have to be extremely careful when trimming a baby's nails. Older people are at a similar risk of being "nicked." Nicking is extremely dangerous with the elderly because they may have poor blood circulation. Accidentally clipping the surrounding skin can cause a sore that heals very slowly or does not heal at all. If this happens, the skin in that area may die and eventually have to be removed. The process of tissue death is called **necrosis**, and skin that dies is referred to as **necrotic tissue**.

If you are allowed and are asked to trim fingernails, you must take great care not to nick the surrounding skin. Soaking fingernails first before cutting makes nails easier to trim. However, soaking nails can also cause you to cut more off than is necessary, so you must be very careful after soaking. Do not trim any resident's toenails. If you decide residents need their toenails trimmed, notify the nurse. The nurse may set up an appointment with a foot doctor, or a **podiatrist**, who will come in and trim the nails.

Washing and cleaning the fingernails and toenails is a part of the bathing process. Some facilities have sticks made of wood called **orange sticks** to clean under the nails. If a stick is used to clean under the nails, staff must be very gentle to make sure they do not injure the resident in any way with the stick.

Emery boards are used to file the nails. They can be used on both fingernails and toenails. It is a good idea to ask first whether you can file a resident's nails. Nail files can tear fragile skin around the nail. Diabetic residents and other people with poor circulation can be harmed by nail files.

Quality foot care is extremely important and should be a part of the daily care of residents. Keeping the feet clean and dry helps prevent complications that occur when feet develop sores, cracked or dry skin, or ingrown nails. Nursing assistants may be the first staff members who observe and report early problems with the feet.

Foot Care Tips — Box 21-1

During the daily care of the feet, observe and report:

- excessive dryness of the skin of the feet
- breaks or tears in the skin
- ingrown nails
- reddened areas on the feet
- drainage or bleeding
- change in color of the skin or nails, especially black
- soft, fragile heels
- corns and blisters

Expert Nail Care

Follow all standard and/or transmission-based precautions. Follow all rules for body mechanics.

Collect equipment:

- washcloths • towel • kidney basin (emesis)
- wash basin with warm water • orange stick • nail file
- unscented lotion

1. Perform the "5 Stars."

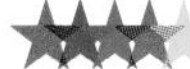

PREPARE:

2. Position the resident with the HOB in semi-Fowler's position or sitting to the side of the bed.
3. Place the overbed table with the towel and kidney basin on it over the resident.

PERFORM:

4. Place the hands in the kidney basin of warm water for five to ten minutes. Wash and rinse the resident's hands.
5. Dry the resident's hands and your own.
6. Use the orange stick to gently and carefully clean under the nails.
7. Use emery board to shape nails and file edges smooth.
8. Apply unscented lotion, if desired.

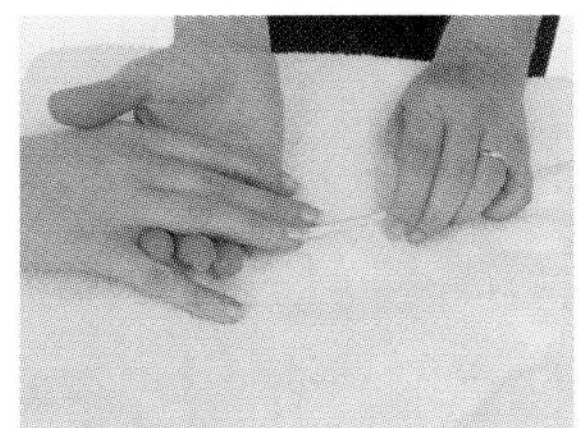

Figure 21-3.

FINISHING TOUCHES:

9. SECURE THE RESIDENT.
10. Dispose of nail care supplies. Wash and rinse basin.
11. Perform the "5 Stars and 3 Rs."

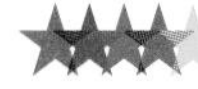  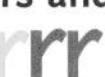

Safe Foot Care

Follow all standard and/or transmission-based precautions. Follow all rules for body mechanics.

Collect equipment:

- two pairs of disposable gloves • washcloths • towel
- kidney basin (emesis) • wash basin with warm water
- orange stick • nail file • unscented lotion

1. Perform the "5 Stars."

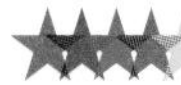

PREPARE:

2. Position the resident with the HOB in semi-Fowler's position or sitting to the side of the bed.
3. Apply gloves.

PERFORM:

4. Place the feet in the basin of warm water for five to ten minutes. Wash and rinse feet. Smooth any rough areas with a washcloth.
5. Dry resident's feet.
6. Use the orange stick to gently and carefully clean under the toenails.

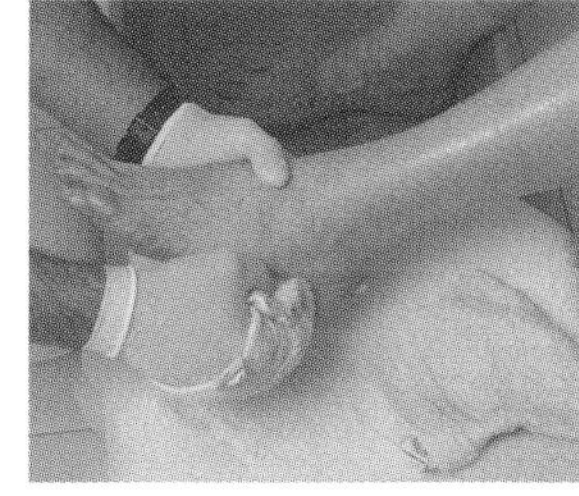

Figure 21-4.

7. Use nail file to shape nails and file edges smooth.
8. Apply unscented lotion, if desired. Do not apply lotion or powder of any kind between the toes. Observe for signs of problems.

FINISHING TOUCHES:

9. SECURE THE RESIDENT.
10. Dispose of nail care supplies. Wash and rinse basin.
11. Remove gloves.
12. Perform the "5 Stars and 3 Rs."

5 Describe quality hair care and explain why gentleness is important.

Daily hair care affects the way residents look and feel about themselves. It is important for nursing staff to keep hair clean and styled in an attractive manner. It is also important for staff to allow residents to choose their own hairstyles. Use hair ornaments only as requested by residents. Do not comb or brush any residents' hair into a childish style.

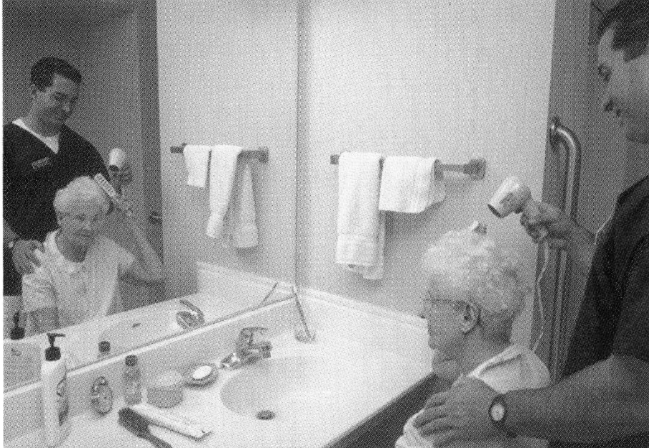

Figure 21-5. **Allowing residents to choose their own hairstyle is important in helping maintain independence.**

Nursing assistants should never cut a resident's hair for any reason. Hair cutting should be left to professional hairstylists. Many places have a hairstylist available to residents during certain days of the month. Nursing assistants may sign up residents for hair appointments, or residents may have regular hair appointments with a stylist. It is vital for nursing assistants to plan for the appointment ahead of time and be careful not to miss it. Residents tend to look forward to their hair appointments.

It is extremely important for residents' hair to be handled gently and carefully. The hair sometimes becomes thinner as people get older. Pieces of hair can be pulled out of the head while using a comb or a brush on a resident. The skin on residents' heads is also very fragile and should not be treated roughly during hair care.

Shampooing in Bed

Follow all standard and/or transmission-based precautions. Follow all rules for body mechanics.

Collect equipment:
• two pairs of disposable gloves • disposable bed protector • washcloths • towel • wash basin with warm water • comb, brush, or hair pick • shampoo • conditioner • pitcher • shampoo trough

Dry shampoos are available when a wet shampoo cannot be used.

1. **Perform the "5 Stars."**

PREPARE:

2. **Position the resident with the HOB in flat position.**
3. **Apply gloves.**
4. **Place disposable bed protector under the head of the resident, shampoo trough over the bed protector, and the bath towel across the shoulders of the resident.**

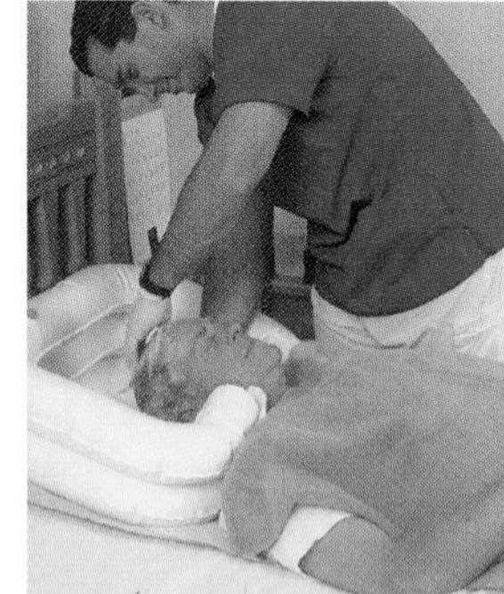

Figure 21-6.

PERFORM:

5. **Cover the eyes of the resident with one washcloth.**
6. **Completely wet the hair and apply a tiny amount of shampoo.**
7. **Lather hair and massage the scalp to help stimulate the circulation.**
8. **Rinse the hair thoroughly.**
9. **Towel-dry the hair.**
10. **Finish drying the hair using drying method of choice. If using electric blow dryer, use a cool setting. Take great care not to burn the resident's head or face.**

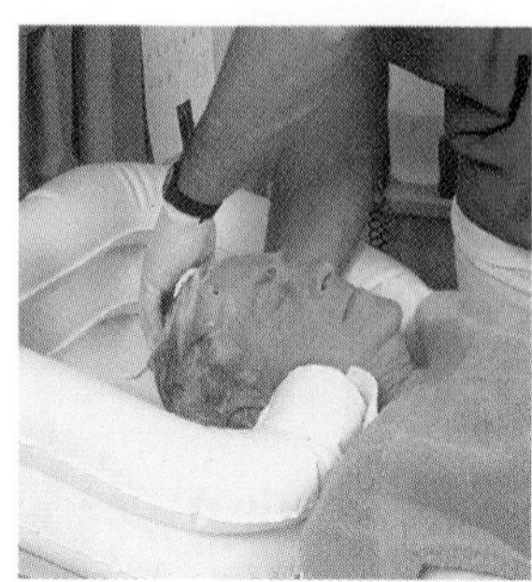

Figure 21-7.

11. **Style hair according to resident's preference.**

FINISHING TOUCHES:

12. **SECURE THE RESIDENT!**
13. **Dispose of shampoo supplies. Rinse and replace equipment.**
14. **Remove gloves.**
15. **Perform the "5 Stars and 3 Rs."**

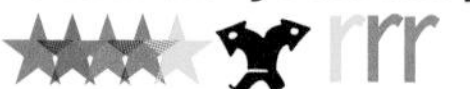

Combing or Brushing Hair

Follow all standard and/or transmission-based precautions. Follow all rules for body mechanics.

Collect equipment:
• comb, brush, or hair pick • towel • mirror
• hair lotion or oil if needed
• detangler or leave-in conditioner if the hair is tangled
• accessories, such as barrettes, bobby pins, small combs, depending on the resident's style preference

1. **Perform the "5 Stars."**

PREPARE:

2. **If the resident is confined to bed, raise the head of the bed, use a backrest, or use pillows to raise the resident's head and shoulders. Place the towel under the resident's head. If the resident is ambulatory, provide a comfortable chair. Place the towel around the resident's shoulders.**

PERFORM:

3. **Gently brush two-inch sections of hair at a time. Brush from roots to ends.**
4. **If the hair is tangled, work on the tangles first. Put a small amount of detangler or leave-in conditioner on the tangle. Hold the lock of hair just above the tangle so you don't pull at the scalp, and gently comb or brush through the tangle.**

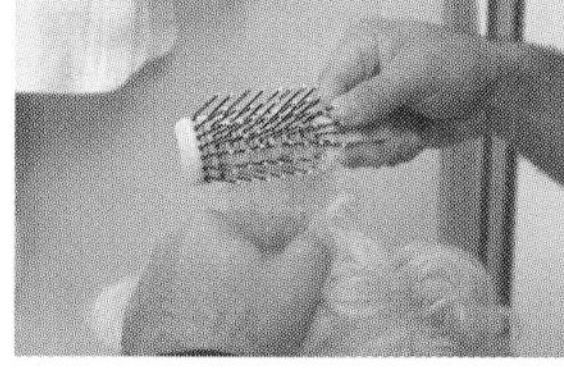

Figure 21-8.

5. **Residents who have dry, brittle hair may require a special treatment with oil or hair lotion. Residents whose hair is tightly curled may use a comb with large teeth, or a pick.**
6. **Style the hair according to the resident's preferences.**

FINISHING TOUCHES:

7. **Remove towel and shake excess hair into the trash. Place soiled towel in facility approved container. Store supplies.**
8. **Perform the "5 Stars and 3 Rs."**

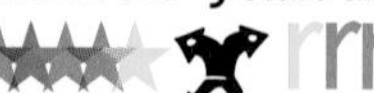

6 Discuss the use of cosmetics and body care products and their effect on self-esteem.

Skin care is a very important part of overall daily care of your residents. There are products that residents will use or that you may choose for your residents that can enhance or improve the health of the skin. Some of these products, with precautions, are listed here.

Skin-Care Products

Be sure to ask residents if they prefer hypoallergenic products, which are less likely to cause an allergic reaction. They are usually unscented and contain no artificial colors.

Talc Powder: May cause talc-induced pneumonia when inhaled, especially with elderly

Cornstarch: May be chosen over talc powder for residents; can be used in between skin folds to help skin stay dry and reduce moist areas

Body Oil: May cause risk of falls in bathing areas due to slipperiness

Body Lotion: Usually improves the quality of the skin and helps prevent cracks and dryness that may cause skin tears; avoid using between toes

Cosmetics are preparations used to enhance beauty or cleanse and improve the skin. They are usually used by women, although some men use certain kinds of cosmetics.

Allowing extra time in residents' routines for the application of makeup may improve their sense of self-esteem. The application of makeup should be based upon a resident's personal preferences. Family may also wish to be involved in the application of makeup or the choice of cosmetics. The type and the amount of makeup applied depends upon the needs of each resident.

Drawing stares or maintaining independence—which is more important?

When an alert, visually-impaired resident applies too much makeup or fragrance, nursing assistants can gently step in. For example, if lipstick is applied to the skin around the lips because the resident cannot see well enough, it would be considerate of you to step in and help.

If the resident refuses assistance, the staff will at least know that they offered it. The resident's independence is always a priority and of utmost importance. The failure of staff to properly groom residents according to their wishes can be considered abuse or neglect.

7 Explain the importance of care of residents' clothing and why independent dressing and undressing should be encouraged.

Staff must treat resident clothing as they would treat their own or their family's clothing—with great care. Residents may have clothing that is very important to them. For example, a sweater that was a gift from a son or a dress that was a present from a late husband may be a favorite piece of clothing. Staff members must use care when they put clothing on and remove clothing from residents. A rip or tear in a prized piece of clothing may be difficult to mend.

Residents should be encouraged to be as independent as possible when dressing and undressing. Additional time is needed when residents dress themselves. Dressing and undressing allows residents to use very important muscles. The daily use of muscles can increase muscle strength, stimulate circulation, and increase resident self-esteem because of the ability to dress oneself. Being able to choose their own clothing promotes dignity and respect. Remember that clothes should fit properly and that both shoes should be on and the laces tied, even on residents who are not ambulatory.

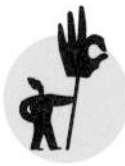

POW

Dressing and undressing residents is an important part of daily care. When a resident has one side of the body that is weaker than the other side, nursing assistants should begin with the affected or weaker side of the body to reduce the risk of injury. The following acronym may be used to help you remember this important step:

POW
Put
On
Weak

In health care, the weaker side is the "affected side" because it is the side affected by a disease or disability. Never refer to the affected side as the "bad side."

Undressing a Resident

Follow all standard and/or transmission-based precautions. Follow all rules for body mechanics.

Collect equipment
- bath blanket
- nightclothes or other clothing

1. Perform the "5 Stars."

PREPARE:

2. Position the resident in the best position for undressing.
3. Encourage resident to do that which she is able to do.

PERFORM:

4. Cover resident with bath blanket to ensure privacy at all times.
5. Remove, or assist in removing, shirt, blouse, or dress using the stronger side. Remove arms one at a time, supporting weaker limbs.
6. Remove, or assist in removing, slacks, using the stronger side. Remove legs one at a time, supporting weaker limbs.
7. Remove underclothing, if desired, pulling off one leg at a time and turning side to side or asking resident to lift buttocks. Always support weaker limbs.
8. Put on nightclothes or other clothing following the dressing procedure.

FINISHING TOUCHES:

9. Remove the bath blanket, and SECURE THE RESIDENT.
10. Place old clothing in appropriate hamper.
11. Perform the "5 Stars and 3 Rs."

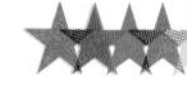 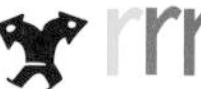

Dressing a Resident or Changing Clothing

Follow all standard and/or transmission-based precautions. Follow all rules for body mechanics.

Collect equipment:
- bath blanket
- clothing

1. Perform the "5 Stars."

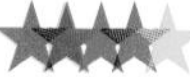

PREPARE:

2. Position the resident in the best position for dressing.
3. Encourage resident to do that which he is able to do.

PERFORM:

4. Cover resident with bath blanket to ensure privacy at all times.
5. Remove, or assist in removing, old clothing or gown.
6. Put on underclothing first. Pull, or assist in pulling, underwear on, lifting one leg at a time and turning from side to side as needed or asking resident to lift buttocks. Always support weaker limbs.
7. Apply, or assist in applying, a woman's bra carefully, making sure breasts are positioned inside the cups. The straps should be checked to make sure they are not twisted.
8. If wearing pants, put on by lifting one leg at a time and turning from side to side as needed or asking resident to lift buttocks. Always support weaker limbs.
9. If wearing a shirt or blouse, put on one sleeve at a time using the acronym POW (put on weak side). If wearing a pullover or a dress, pull over the head and put on one sleeve at a time using the acronym POW (put on weak side). Always support weaker limbs.

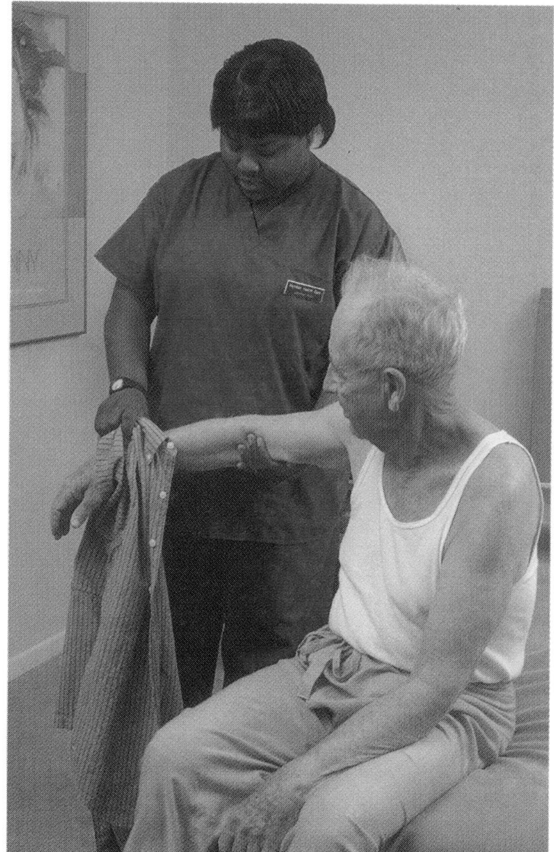

Figure 21-9.

10. If the resident cannot hold his arm up to put on one sleeve at a time, put your hand inside the sleeve. By taking his hand in yours, you can slip the sleeve up his arm. Do this for both arms.

FINISHING TOUCHES:

11. Remove the bath blanket, and SECURE THE RESIDENT.
12. Place old clothing in appropriate hamper.
13. Perform the "5 Stars and 3 Rs."

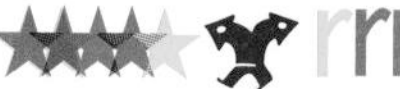

8 Describe how to ensure a resident's dignity when wearing a facility gown and identify the gown used on a resident with an IV.

For anyone who has ever lived in or visited a facility, the hospital gown may be one of the most dreaded things. Just as you would not want your backside exposed while walking down a hallway, neither will your residents. Always make sure that you cover residents completely so that they will not be exposed to anyone. This includes other staff members, other residents, and visitors. Adding a robe or a second gown to cover the back of the facility gown is vital to maintaining your residents' dignity.

When using intravenous lines (IVs), it is important to choose facility gowns that will allow staff members to apply and remove these gowns easily. There are two types of facility gowns, gowns that tie or have an adhesive in the back and gowns that have snaps. The snap-opening styles are used with IVs to make the process of applying and removing IVs easier.

Putting on and Removing a Gown on a Resident with an IV

Follow all standard and/or transmission-based precautions. Follow all rules for body mechanics.

Collect equipment:
- **bath blanket**
- **gown**

1. **Perform the "5 Stars."**

PREPARE:

2. **Position the resident in the best position for changing the gown.**

PERFORM:

3. **Cover resident with bath blanket to ensure privacy at all times.**
4. **Remove or assist in removing gown, using the strong side. In this case, the strong side is the side without the IV.**
5. **Pull off the gown carefully, sliding it over the tubing, then lifting the IV bag or bottle off the hook and pulling the gown over the bag or bottle.**
6. **Always keep the bag or bottle above the IV site on the body.**

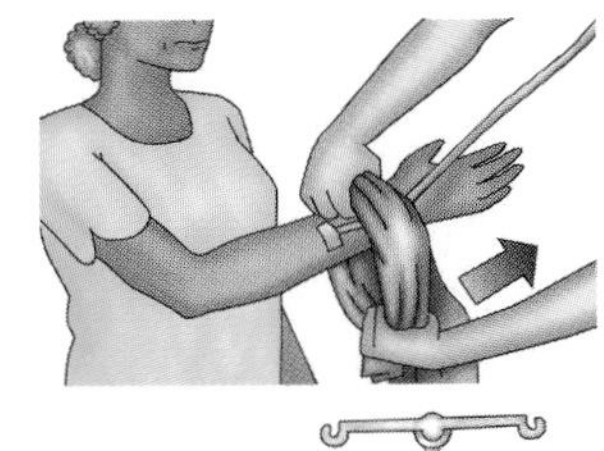

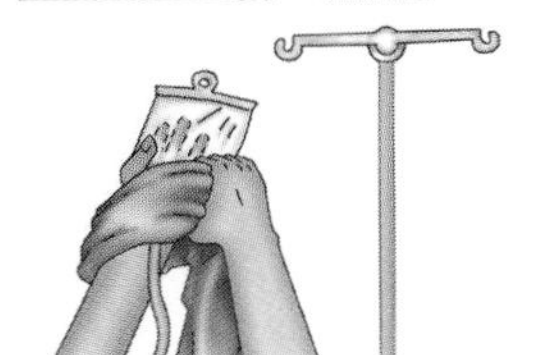

Figure 21-10.

7. **Pick up clean gown and slide the correct arm opening over the bag or bottle, then over the tubing and the resident's IV arm. Use the POW (put on weak side) acronym; in this case the weak side is the side WITH the IV.**
8. **Now assist in pulling the other side on, adjust gown comfortably, and snap the snaps or tie the strings.**

FINISHING TOUCHES:

9. **Remove the bath blanket, and SECURE THE RESIDENT.**
10. **Place used gown in appropriate hamper.**
11. **Perform the "5 Stars and 3 Rs."**

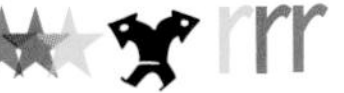

The nurse may want to check the IV.

9 Identify nine assistive devices used in dressing residents.

Residents want to maintain independence in their activities of daily living, such as dressing and grooming. There are devices to help them remain independent while dressing. Some of these devices are listed in Box 21-2 and shown in Figure 21-11.

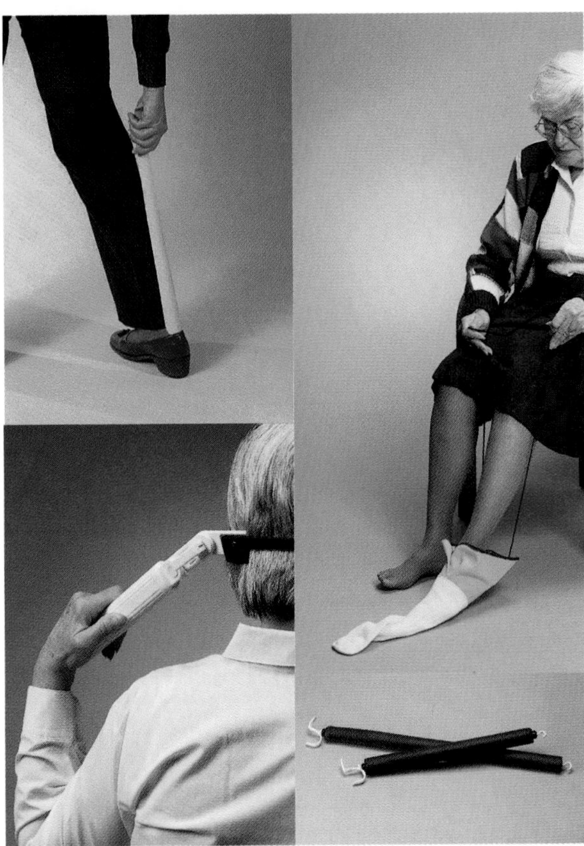

Figure 21-11. **Dressing and grooming aids.**

Devices to Promote Independence with Dressing/Undressing

Box 21-2

Shoehorn

Sock Puller

Pantyhose Aid

Button-hook/Zipper Puller

Dressing Stick

Elastic Shoelaces

Shoelace Lock

Pant Clips

Trouser Pull

Summary

The art of grooming is an important part of nursing assistant responsibilities. When residents look good and appear clean and neat, they feel good about themselves and leave a good impression with everyone who visits their facility. Nursing assistants should take the time to perform good grooming techniques on all of their residents each and every day.

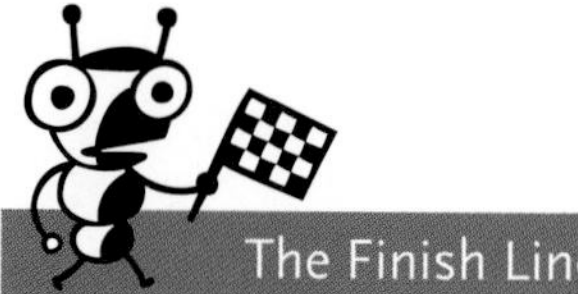

The Finish Line

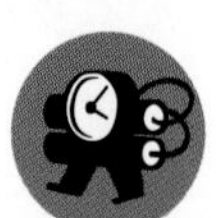

What's Wrong With This Picture?

1. Look at the equipment listed for the Practical Procedure: Shaving a Male Resident, shown below. One important piece of equipment is missing. List the missing piece of equipment.

Collect equipment:
- **washcloths • towel • kidney basin (emesis)**
- **shaving cream • electric razor or disposable razor**
- **after-shave products (optional)**
- **wash basin with warm water**

2. Look at the Principal Steps: Shaving Residents shown below. One important step is missing. List the missing step.

Always wear gloves when using either disposable or electric razors.

Soften hair first with a warm cloth.

Use shaving products like aftershave only with resident's permission.

Carefully discard any disposable shaving products in the biohazard container.

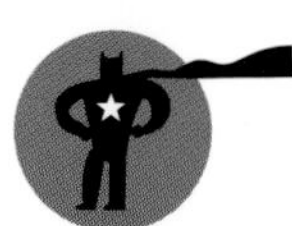

Star Student Central

1. Shaving a male can be a challenging procedure if you have never done so before. After receiving instructions and following careful review of the procedure, find a willing friend or relative who will allow you to perform a facial shave using a new disposable razor. To complete a shave, you must have a pair of disposable gloves and a new disposable razor of the person's choice. You must wear gloves no matter who the willing person might be. Follow the procedure very carefully. Afterward, ask the person to sign a short note evaluating the shave and return the note to your instructor.
2. Dressing and undressing people can be a challenge. After reviewing dressing procedures, ask a friend to allow you to practice dressing the person with a shirt that buttons in the front and a pair of slacks that zip. Pretend that the person has one weak side and follow the procedure.

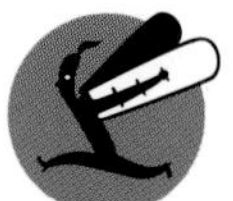

You Can Do It Corner!

1. Why is it important to follow the resident's preferences regarding grooming? (LO 2)
2. Why is nicking a resident's skin during nail care so dangerous? (LO 4)
3. Why should you encourage a resident's independence while dressing and undressing? (LO 7)
4. Why should you shave in the direction of the hair growth? (LO 3)

5. What should you add to a facility gown to preserve a resident's dignity? (LO 8)
6. What is the difference between using talc and cornstarch powder for your residents? (LO 6)
7. When assisting with dressing a resident, what side of the body should you begin with? What is the acronym you can use to help you remember this step? (LO 7)
8. Why should you always wear gloves when shaving a resident? (LO 3)
9. What are nine assistive devices used for help with dressing? (LO 9)
10. Why should a resident's hair be handled gently? (LO 5)

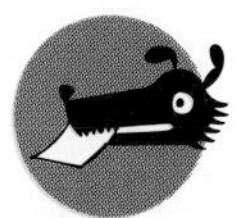

Star Student's Chapter Checklist

1. I have read my textbook chapter.
2. I have reviewed my own "Pocketful of Terms."
3. I have listened to my tutor tape.
4. I have reviewed and highlighted my class notes.
5. I have read and completed any handouts from this chapter.
6. I have completed "The Finish Line."
7. Star Time! Choose your reward!

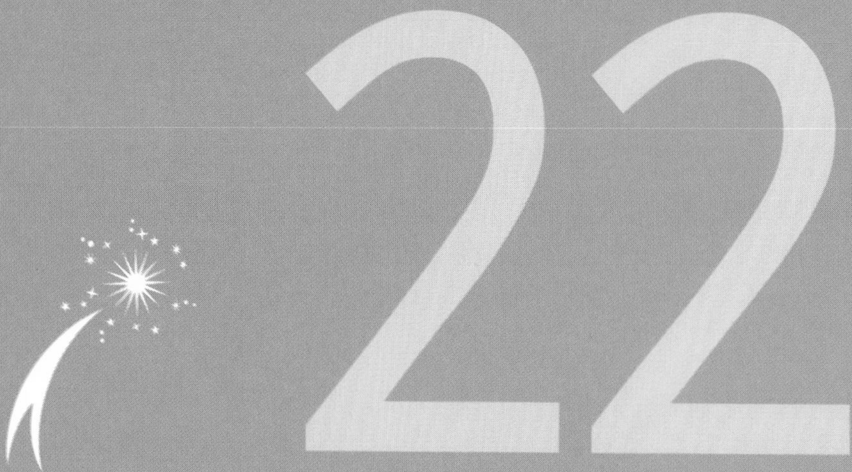

22

Your Guide: Basic Nutrition and Fluid Balance

Look Like a Star!

Look at the Learning Objectives **and** The Finish Line **before you begin reading this chapter.**

Look at your pocket calendar.
With your pencil, put a bracket (   ) around a study period every single day.

Look at your homework for this chapter.
Plug each piece of homework into a certain time slot.

Look at the Star Student's Chapter Checklist **at the end of this chapter. Check off each item as it is completed.**

"In general, mankind, since the improvement of cookery, eats twice as much as it requires."

Benjamin Franklin, 1706-1790

"One should eat to live, not live to eat."

Moliere, 1622-1673

Learning Objectives

1. **Spell and define all STAR words.**
2. **Identify six nutrients necessary for good nutrition.**
3. **Identify the six divisions of the Food Guide Pyramid.**
4. **Explain why special diets may not be ordered for residents and list nine signs that indicate a risk for unintended weight loss.**
5. **Explain the importance of following diet orders and identify special diets.**
6. **Describe three steps to prevent errors in passing meal trays.**
7. **List ten guidelines for preventing aspiration.**
8. **State two reasons certain residents must eat all of their snacks/nourishment.**
9. **Describe and practice a common method used to track nutritional intake.**
10. **Demonstrate converting ounces (oz.) to cubic centimeters (cc).**
11. **Demonstrate charting a resident's daily liquid nutrition.**
12. **Explain the importance of fluid balance and list signs of edema and dehydration.**
13. **Name six types of residents who may have fluid restrictions.**

Successfully perform these Practical Procedures

Preparing Residents for Meals

Serving Meal Trays to Resident Rooms and Dayrooms

Feeding a Resident

Measuring and Recording Intake

Passing Fresh Water

Pernicious Anemia: The Vanquishing of a Formerly Fatal Disease

A Nobel Prize was awarded to George Richards Minot, William Parry Murphy, and George Whipple for discovering that a serious and fatal disease called pernicious anemia could actually be cured. Minot worked for many years and finally found that with a simple change in diet, adding a large amount of liver, the disease could be cured. The three men eventually proved the disease was caused by a lack of Vitamin B12. Today many people live long lives with this disease by simply taking periodic shots of B12.

1 Spell and define all **STAR** words.

aspiration: a potentially dangerous situation where a person takes fluid, food, or an object into the airway and the lungs; may cause pneumonia or death.

D.A.T.: diet as tolerated.

dehydration: condition which occurs when a person does not have enough fluid in the body.

edema: swelling of body tissues, especially the feet and ankles, due to the accumulation of fluids.

fluid restriction: orders that require fluids to be carefully measured and limited to maintain proper fluid balance.

Food Guide Pyramid: a guide developed by the U.S. Department of Agriculture recommending foods and quantities people should eat from each food group in a day.

metabolism: the process of utilizing all nutrients that enter the body to provide energy, growth, and maintenance of vital functions.

nutrients: substances in food that are metabolized and absorbed to feed our bodies.

2 Identify six nutrients necessary for good nutrition.

The human body cannot survive without food and water. Good health requires a daily amount of each of the main nutrients for each of the cells, tissues, organs, and systems to continue to function in optimal condition. A **nutrient** is something in food that enables the body to use energy for metabolism. **Metabolism** is the process of utilizing all nutrients that enter the body to provide energy, growth, and maintenance of our vital functions. There are six primary nutrients required for optimum health:

1. **Water**: Water is needed by every cell in the body. It is needed to move oxygen and other nutrients into the cells and to remove the waste products from each cell. Water is the main "ingredient" in our blood.
2. **Fats**: Fats protect our organs and help keep us warm. Fat serves as insulation for our body, much like the insulation in a house. Fat also provides the flavor in many foods. Fat contains many calories and may also add cholesterol to our diet. Thus, fat must be used sparingly.
3. **Carbohydrates**: Carbohydrates supply the body with the vital energy it needs to make it through each day. Carbohydrates also add much-needed fiber to diets, which helps with bowel elimination.
4. **Proteins**: Proteins are needed by every cell in the body. They help the body grow new tissue during tissue repair and provide additional energy.
5. **Vitamins**: Vitamins are very important to the

Source and Function of Essential Minerals Box-22-1

MINERAL	SOURCE	FUNCTION
Iron	egg yolks, green leafy vegetables, breads, cereals, and organ meats	necessary for the red blood cells to carry oxygen; helps in the formation of enzymes
Sodium	almost all foods and table salt	important for maintaining fluid balance (helps the body retain water)
Potassium	fruits and vegetables, cereals, coffee, and meats	essential for nerve and heart function and muscle contraction
Calcium	milk and milk products such as cheese, ice cream, and yogurt; green leafy vegetables such as collards, kale, mustard, dandelion, and turnip greens; and canned fish with soft bones, such as salmon	important for the formation of teeth and bones, the clotting of blood, muscle contraction, and heart and nerve function
Phosphorus	milk, milk products, meat, fish, poultry, nuts, and eggs	needed for the formation of bones and teeth and nerve and heart function; important for the body's utilization of proteins, fats, and carbohydrates

normal functioning of the body.

6. **Minerals**: Minerals help the body function normally. Many minerals are needed daily by the body. Some minerals keep bones and teeth strong while others help maintain fluid balance. Normal cardiac, muscular, and nervous system functions are aided by certain minerals.

3 Identify the six divisions of the Food Guide Pyramid.

The **Food Guide Pyramid** is divided into six different categories. Foods close to the bottom of the pyramid should make up most of our diet. Foods closer to the top should be eaten in smaller quantities.

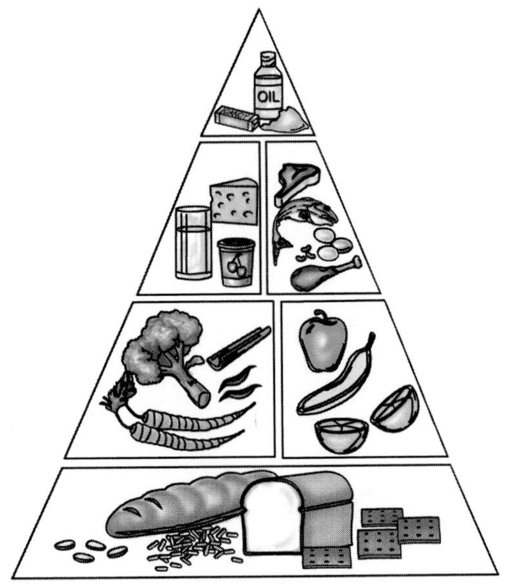

Figure 22-1. The Food Guide Pyramid was created by the U.S. Department of Agriculture to show the six food groups and how, together, they form a healthy diet.

1. **Grains, including cereals, bread, rice, and pasta**: Breads and other foods in this group provide the body with energy. The Food Guide Pyramid recommends eating between six and eleven servings from this group each day. Examples of one serving include one slice of bread, one cup of dry cereal, or 1/2 cup of cooked pasta or rice.

2. **Fruits**: Fruits provide very little calories or fat and are good sources of carbohydrates, fiber, and vitamins, especially vitamin C. The Food Guide Pyramid recommends eating two to four servings from this group each day. One serving from this group could include one medium-sized apple, orange, banana, 3/4 cup of juice, or 1/4 cup of raisins.

3. **Vegetables:** Vegetables are low in fat and calories and a great source of vitamins and fiber. The Food Guide Pyramid recommends eating three to five servings from this group each day. One serving from this group consists of 1/2 cup cooked or chopped vegetables or 3/4 cup of vegetable juice.

4. **Milk and milk products**: Milk and milk products, such as yogurt and cheese, provide calcium, protein, and vitamins. The Food Guide Pyramid recommends two to three servings from this group each day. A serving of milk equals one cup. Other serving sizes include one cup of yogurt, two cups of cottage cheese, or one-and-a-half ounces of cheese.

5. **Meat, poultry, fish, eggs, dry beans, and nuts**: Meat and other foods at this level provide protein, minerals and vitamins. The Food Guide Pyramid recommends eating two to three servings from this group each day. One serving from this group equals three ounces of cooked meat, one egg, or 1/2 cup cooked dry beans.

6. **Fats:** Fats, oils, and sweets should be eaten sparingly as these foods may be high in fat and calories and very low in protein. The best kind of fats to use in a healthy diet are vegetable oils, including olive oils, canola oil, and corn oil.

Scurvy: The Scourge of the Early Sea Traveler

Scurvy was a terrible problem for people who had to travel by sea for long periods of time. It caused bleeding gums, loosened teeth, joint pain, weakness, and hemorrhages from mucous membranes. In 1747, James Lind was able to identify a cure for the dreaded scurvy. He found that simply by giving people citrus juice, such as from lemons, he could successfully treat the disease. Vitamin C, also known as ascorbic acid, was the cure.

4 Explain why special diets may not be ordered for residents and list nine signs that indicate a risk for unintended weight loss.

When a resident enters a facility, a diet order is generally written by the physician. The order is based upon overall health and any specific disorders.

Poor nutrition, unhealthy weight loss and **dehydration** are big problems among the elderly, in and out of nursing homes. Responding to this problem, many providers are rethinking special diets for some patients or residents. For example, if an unappetizing diet is leading to unhealthy weight loss, the resident may be better off on a less strict diet that he will eat. If you notice food going uneaten or if a resident complains about the food, report it. Report any weight loss you notice, no matter how small.

Warning signs that your residents are at risk for unintended weight loss include the following:

- needs help eating or drinking
- eats less than 70% of meals or snacks served
- has mouth pain
- has dentures that do not fit properly
- has a hard time chewing or swallowing
- coughs or chokes while eating
- is sad, cries, or withdraws from others
- is confused, wanders, or paces
- has diabetes, chronic obstructive pulmonary disease (COPD), cancer, HIV/AIDS, or other chronic diseases

If you notice any of these these signs, report it immediately to your supervisor.

5 Explain the importance of following diet orders and identify special diets.

Residents who have orders for specific diets require additional care and supervision. Nursing assistants need to follow the diet order carefully in order to prevent complications from allowing a food or fluid not on the diet. When a resident is on a sodium-restricted diet, make sure there is no salt on the tray and that salt shakers and salt packets cannot be accessed by the resident.

The information that follows identifies many types of facility diets and gives additional helpful information regarding each type of diet.

A. Advancing Diets (due to illness or surgery)

Clear Liquid Diet: fluids that you can see through, such as clear soups

Full Liquid Diet: fluids that you cannot see through, such as milk

Soft Diet: food that may be easily chewed, such as mashed potatoes

D.A.T. (Diet as tolerated): food the resident is able to keep down and tolerate well

Regular, House, or General Diet: any food may be served

B. Specific Diets

Bland Diet: no spicy foods; used for ulcers

High Residue: high in fiber and grains; used for bowel elimination

Low Residue: low in fiber, grains, seeds; used for bowel disorders

High Calorie: increase in calories; for anorexia

Low Calorie: decrease in calories; for weight loss

High Protein: high protein foods, meats; used for tissue repair and wound healing, such as burns

Low Fat/Low Cholesterol: limited cholesterol and fat; used for heart disease and artery problems

Low Sodium: salt restriction; used for heart or kidney disease

High Potassium: increased potassium; residents on diuretics (water pills); used for hypertension

Diabetic: provides a balance of all nutrients; used for diabetes

Fluid Restricted: limits fluids in 24-hour period; for heart or kidney disease

Residents with swallowing difficulties may require thickened foods and fluids to reduce the risks of choking. Sometimes food or fluids are frozen and carefully fed to residents. Again, always report problems with any resident's diet, including how much they did not eat.

Family members have to be educated about the risks of bringing in food or fluids not on the diet order. Sometimes family may choose to do this anyway, despite a nurse's request not to do so. If you see this behavior, remember you have a responsibility for the health and well-being of all of your residents. Report this situation to the nurse-in-charge so that she may handle the problem.

It was the lead container, not the apple juice!

Sometimes the culprit in a severe illness proves to be the method of food preparation. In the town of Devonshire in the 18th century, George Baker (1722-1809) identified the cause of the "Devonshire Colic." He noted that the people drank apple juice that had been made inside containers that were lined with lead, causing the illness.

6 Describe three steps to prevent errors in passing meal trays.

Diet trays come to facility units at specific times. Usually breakfast arrives between 7:00 and 8:00 a.m., lunch between 11:30 a.m. and 12:30 p.m., and dinner between 5:30 and 6:30 p.m.

Nursing assistants' responsibilities for passing diet trays depend upon the shift they work. When diet trays are passed, there is always a chance of human error. Nursing assistants can prevent diet tray errors by following a few simple steps:

1. Check with the nurse or ward (unit) clerk for any special orders. Special orders consist of residents being placed on nothing by mouth (NPO) or a change in diet or fluid order.
2. Identify the resident to make sure it is the right person.
3. If the resident is alert, ask her if the food looks correct.

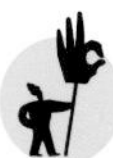

Ask before you pass!

Ask nurses and ward clerks before you pass trays to everyone on the unit! Always find out any special diet orders and names of residents who are NPO.

7 List ten guidelines for preventing aspiration.

Elderly residents frequently choke on food or drink. This is called **aspiration**. If this material flows into the lungs, it can cause pneumonia or death. To ensure the safety and well-being of all of your residents, it is vital that you follow certain guidelines to prevent aspiration.

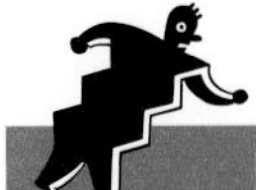

Principal Steps

Preventing Aspiration

1. *Place residents in proper position (usually high-Fowler's) for eating and drinking all fluids.*
2. *Feed residents slowly.*
3. *Food must be fed in tiny pieces or in small spoons of pureed food. It is best to give a solid then a liquid, then repeat.*
4. *Food must be placed into the non-paralyzed side of the mouth, if one side is paralyzed.*
5. *Residents should stay in Fowler's position for about 30 minutes after eating or drinking.*
6. *Make sure resident actually swallows food after each bite. Do not put your fingers inside the mouth.*
7. *Never leave anything dangerous near a resident that might be swallowed.*
8. *Explain to all visitors and volunteers the risks of aspiration with certain residents.*
9. *Watch residents who choke easily during eating and drinking.*
10. *If any signs of choking or aspiration occur such as: coughing, gagging, clutching throat, cyanosis, unconsciousness, shortness of breath, or dyspnea, or if resident complains of chest pain or tightness in the chest,* ★ *"Don't Delay. Report Right Away!"*

Residents who have had a stroke or a cerebrovascular accident (CVA) will need extra time and patience with eating and drinking. Stroke residents should have food and/or drink put in the unaffected side of the mouth to help prevent choking and aspiration. (See also Star Kare: Aspiration Safety and the CVA Resident in Chapter 27.)

Take time when feeding your residents.

When nursing staff or family feed residents, the time allotted may seem very short. The time frame allowed for the meal is not always what it should be to ensure safety of all residents. Feeding residents too quickly encourages choking and aspiration. When you are feeding residents or supervising others in the process of feeding, make sure you encourage slow, methodical feeding. Never allow a resident to be rushed. Do not appear to be in a hurry when you feed anyone. People can tell when you are in a hurry. Feeding residents too fast may be considered abuse.

8 State two reasons certain residents must eat all of their snacks/nourishment.

Residents are usually fed three meals a day along with additional snacks or nourishment. Sometimes the snacks are required by special diets. For example, a diabetic needs all of her snack to maintain her blood sugar while on insulin injections. Another resident who is losing too much weight will need to eat all of his snacks to maintain a healthy weight. Due to disease and the problem of unintended weight loss, encourage residents to eat all of their snacks. If a resident does not finish the snack, a family member eats it, or you find it in the trash, notify the nurse.

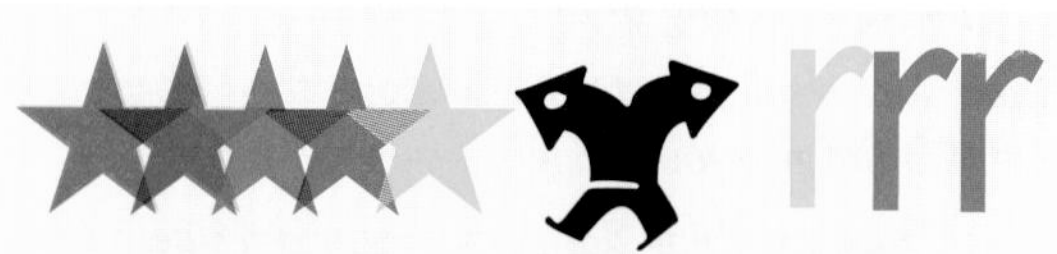

Beginning Steps

★ RESPECT
Knock first, ask and receive permission to enter a resident's room.

★ INFECTION CONTROL
Wash hands.

★ COMMUNICATION
Greet and identify the resident. Identify yourself. Explain the procedure, encouraging the resident to be as independent as possible throughout.

★ BED SAFETY
Lock bed wheels. Raise bed to safe working height. Lower one side rail if required.

★ PRIVACY
Provide for privacy by closing the door and covering the resident appropriately.

Ending Steps

★ RESIDENT SAFETY AND COMFORT
Secure the resident, lowering the bed, and raising the side rails if ordered. Check that the resident is comfortable and properly aligned.

★ PRIVACY
Remove any added privacy measures, such as a drape or a privacy screen.

★ ESSENTIALS
Place the call light, fresh beverage, and other items within reach.

★ COURTESY
Ask the resident if he or she needs anything else. Say thank you and goodbye.

★ INFECTION CONTROL
Wash hands.

r **Report** your care and any important observations to the nurse.

r **Record** your care and any important information/observations such as vital signs in the appropriate place.

r **Recheck** your resident for any changes as directed by the nurse!

Preparing Residents for Meals

Follow all standard and/or transmission-based precautions. Follow all rules for body mechanics.

Collect equipment:
- two pairs of disposable gloves
- soap • basin with warm water • washcloth • towel
- mouth care equipment • robe and slippers or clothing

1. Perform the "5 Stars."

PREPARE:

2. Apply gloves.

PERFORM:

3. Perform oral hygiene or help resident as needed. Assist in the insertion of dentures if worn.
4. Help resident use the bathroom or bedpan. Wash resident's hands. Remove gloves, discard, and wash your hands.
5. Resident may choose his or her preferred eating place.
   a. FOR DAYROOM:
      Assist resident in dressing in appropriate clothing.
      Assist resident to stand or sit in wheelchair.
      Help ambulate or wheel resident to the dayroom and seat safely and comfortably. If resident has a special chair, section, or seating preference, honor it.
      Transfer resident from wheelchair to regular chair if appropriate.
      Place napkin per resident's preference.
      Use clothing protectors only if the resident agrees.
   b. FOR ROOM/MEAL IN BED:
      Raise HOB to high-Fowler's position.
      Place towel or napkin over chest.
      Clear overbed table and place at proper height .
      Place signal light in reach. Secure the resident.

FINISHING TOUCHES:

6. Perform the "5 Stars and 3 Rs."

 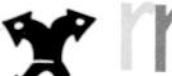

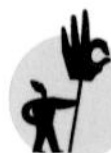

Help make dining rooms pleasant for everyone!

Because unintended weight loss is such a serious problem, dining rooms should be monitored for things that negatively affect appetite. Some of these include unnecessary noise level, odors, and ostomy or other drainage bags. Reduce noise or provide soothing music while residents are dining. Eliminate odors by making sure residents are clean and well groomed before they dine. Respectfully cover drainage bags.

Serving Meal Trays to Resident Rooms and Dayrooms

Follow all standard and/or transmission-based precautions. Follow all rules for body mechanics.

Collect equipment:
- two pairs of disposable gloves • diet trays with diet cards
- mouth care equipment • notepad and pen

Check with nurse or ward clerk for any special orders!

1. **Perform the "5 Stars."**

PREPARE:

2. **Make sure all residents are prepared for the meal.**

PERFORM:

3. **Carefully lift one tray and go to resident's room or dayroom spot. Before you place tray in front of resident, identify the resident and match ID to name and diet on the diet card.**
4. **Place tray on overbed table or on table in the dayroom. Remove items from tray, if facility policy, and set up on overbed table.**
5. **Open food containers and milk cartons, pour coffee or tea, cut meat or other food, add spices as desired, and make sure everything needed is near resident.**
6. **SECURE THE RESIDENT and leave room or dayroom area.**
7. **Continue passing trays in this fashion until all residents are served.**
8. **Check on all residents continuously to provide any necessary assistance.**
9. **When meals have been completed, begin the process of removing trays and placing each tray in server.**
10. **As you remove each diet tray do the following for each resident:**
    a. **Measure the intake, as needed, for each resident on intake and output. (See Learning Objective 11.)**
    b. **Document the intake and how well each resident ate in your notes.**
    c. **Apply gloves and perform oral hygiene in a private area or wipe resident's face and hands as indicated.**
    d. **Make resident comfortable and secure whether in dayroom, bed, or chair.**

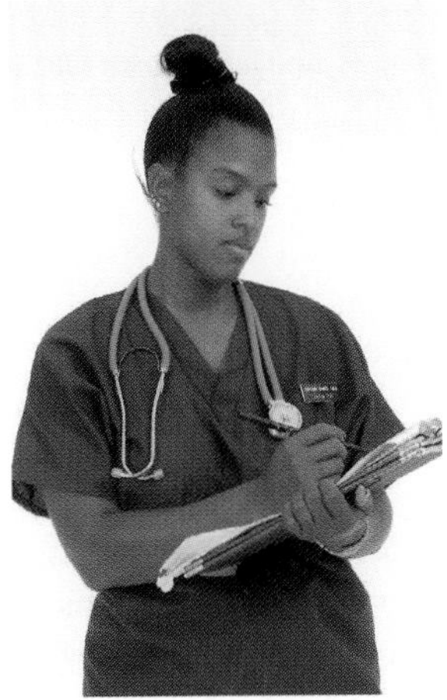

Figure 22-2.

FINISHING TOUCHES:

11. **Perform the "5 Stars and 3 Rs."**

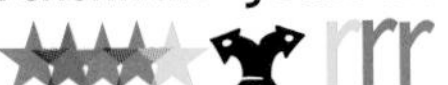

When assisting residents with feeding, remember to promote independence by encouraging them to do whatever they can for themselves. For example, if a resident can hold and use a napkin and can hold and eat finger foods, she should.

Independence with eating positively affects self-esteem. It is very difficult when a person has to start depending on another person for assistance with a basic need such as this. Always empathize with your residents.

While assisting with feeding, make sure you take time to talk and be social. Meal time should be a pleasant experience.

Feeding a Resident

Follow all standard and/or transmission-based precautions. Follow all rules for body mechanics.

Collect equipment:
- **two pairs of disposable gloves • soap**
- **basin with warm water • washcloth • clothing protector (towel) • mouth care equipment • robe and slippers or clothing**

Check with nurse or ward clerk for any special orders!

1. **Perform the "5 Stars."**

PREPARE:

2. **Clear overbed table and place it at the proper height over resident.**
3. **Bring tray into room, match ID with diet card, and place on overbed table or dayroom table.**
4. **Raise HOB to high-Fowler's position.**
5. **Place clothing protector, such as towel or napkin, over chest.**
6. **Prepare food as desired.**
7. **Review all food and drink on the tray.**

PERFORM:

8. **Offer food as resident requests. Give small spoonfuls or bites to resident.**
9. **Encourage fluids. Use straw if desired.**
10. **Allow enough time to swallow food.**

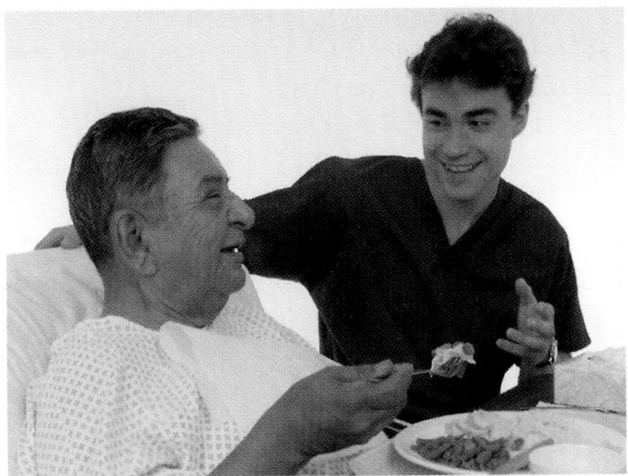

Figure 22-3. **Be professional and pleasant when feeding a resident. Never rush a resident while eating.**

FINISHING TOUCHES:

11. **Clean resident's mouth and nose area after eating.**
12. **Remove clothing protector.**
13. **Measure intake and percentage of food eaten and document in notepad.**
14. **Apply gloves.**
15. **Perform oral hygiene as needed.**
16. **SECURE THE RESIDENT. Remove tray and place on server.**
17. **Remove gloves.**
18. **Perform the "5 Stars and 3 Rs."**

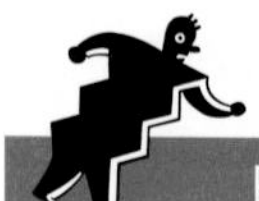

Principal Steps

Serving a Blind Resident

1. *Place tray in directly in front of the blind resident at a good height for eating.*
2. *Review placement of food and drinks on the tray. Placement of food is identified using the face of a clock.*
3. *Allow for as much independence as possible while providing any support and assistance needed during meals.*
4. *Check back frequently and respond promptly to any call button asking for assistance.*
5. *If any signs of choking or aspiration occur, such as: coughing, gagging, clutching throat, cyanosis, unconsciousness, shortness of breath, or dyspnea, or if resident complains of chest pain or tightness in the chest,*
   ★ *"Don't Delay. Report Right Away!"*

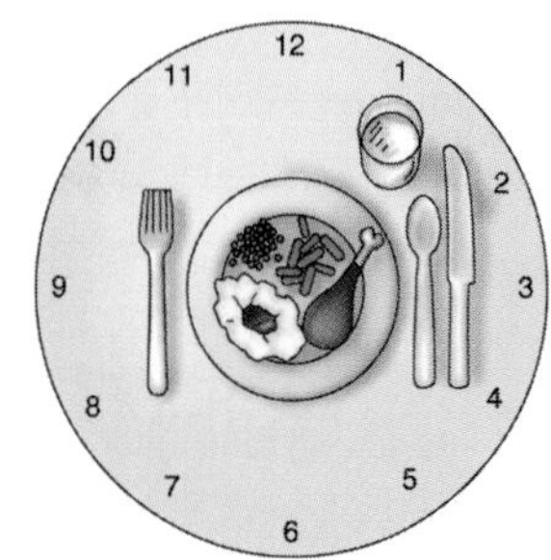

Figure 22-4. **Use the face of an imaginary clock as a guide to explain the position of food in front of your resident.**

9 Describe and practice a common method used to track nutritional intake.

The percentage method is often used by facilities to add and record food intake. For you to record percentages, it is important to understand percentages. If you need to review percentages, refer to Chapter 1.

Facilities often use menus that list the percentage of total calories each item served represents. A dietitian calculates these percentages. It is important to accurately record how much of the meal the resident ate. To do this, observe how much of each item was consumed. Then, adjust the percentage of total calories the item provided. Finally, add the adjusted percentages for a total percentage consumed.

For example, egg, juice, toast, and milk is on a resident's breakfast tray. The egg is worth 20% of calories needed for her breakfast. If she finishes half of the egg, you would write that she consumed 10% of the total breakfast. If the juice is worth 15%, and she consumed all of the juice, then you would record the full 15% toward the total calories consumed.

Many facilities ask that the nurse be notified if a resident eats 70% of his meal or less. Follow your facility's policy about this.

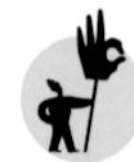

Chicken Soup and the Common Cold

Have you ever wondered if it is true that chicken soup may help the common cold? Chicken soup has been found to have an ingredient that may do just that. The next time someone you know has a cold, you get a can of chicken soup and see if the person feels better. Sometimes the oldest and simplest remedies turn out to be the best!

10 Demonstrate converting ounces (oz.) to cubic centimeters (cc).

When residents are on special diets or have special problems, you may measure their intake and output (I & O). I & O is a method for staff to add and record all of the food and fluids the resident takes in and eliminates during a 24-hour time period. When you add a resident's intake of food and fluids, most facilities use cubic centimeters to record it. Cubic centimeters are units of measurement in the metric system. A cubic centimeter is equal to one milliliter (ml), which is 1/1000 of a liter. An ounce equals 30 cubic centimeters. You multiply the number of ounces by 30 to get the number of cubic centimeters. Containers, called graduates, measure fluid in cubic centimeters and may also measure in ounces. It is very important for you to memorize the conversion of ounces to cubic centimeters.

Conversion Table: Ounces (oz.) to Cubic Centimeters (cc)

Box-22-2

1 oz.= 30 cc	5 oz.= 150 cc
2 oz.= 60 cc	6 oz.= 180 cc
3 oz.= 90 cc	7 oz.= 210 cc
4 oz.= 120 cc	8 oz.= 240 cc

When output is measured, the output containers are also usually measured in cubic centimeters. Output is recorded at the end of each shift and anytime in between as needed. Examples of output are urine, diarrhea, suction material, and wound drainage.

11 Demonstrate charting a resident's daily liquid nutrition.

Intake and output is measured at the end of each shift and throughout the shift when water, juices, or other food and fluids are consumed. This is done by asking the resident (if alert), all visitors, volunteers, and staff members to document what the resident eats and drinks. When you are ready to record intake and output, special forms are used for this purpose. They usually have a listing of all the containers used at the facility and the corresponding amount of ounces or cubic centimeters the containers hold. At the end of each meal or snack, add all intake for all residents on the I & O form.

Intake & Output Record

Client Name: ____________ HCA Name: ____________
Address: ____________ Record Date: ____________

Intake			**Output**		
Time	Type	Amount	Time	Urine Amount	Incontinent Episode

Output	Time	Approximate Amount
Vomiting		
Heavy Perspiration		
Diarrhea		

Figure 22-5. Your facility should provide you with an Intake and Output (I & O) sheet.

Recording Intake and Output

Breakfast Tray

The resident ate and drank the following:

1 bowl soup	160 cc
1 cup coffee	120 cc
1 carton milk	240 cc
Total intake	520 cc

Day Shift

7 a.m. void or urinate x 1	Output measured= 325 cc
9 a.m. void or urinate x 1	Output measured= 400 cc
11:30 a.m. void or urinate x 1	Output measured= 200 cc
2:00 p.m. void or urinate x 1	Output measured= 250 cc
Total output	1175 cc

Figure 22-5 shows a sample I & O form.

Measuring and Recording Intake

Follow all standard and/or transmission-based precautions. Follow all rules for body mechanics.

Collect equipment:
- **notepad** • **pen**

PREPARE:

1. **Perform the "5 Stars."**

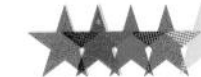

PERFORM:

2. **Look at each liquid on the tray and determine what percentage of the liquid the resident ate or drank.**
3. **Document the number of cubic centimeters (cc) of each item. Do not forget to include:**

   creamed cereals
   soup
   flavored frozen ice sticks
   ice cream, ice milk, or sherbet
   coffee, tea, or milk
   juices, sodas, or water

FINISHING TOUCHES:

4. **Perform the "5 Stars and 3 Rs."**

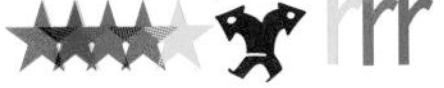

12 Explain the importance of fluid balance and list signs of edema and dehydration.

Human beings maintain the health of every living cell by balancing the amount of fluid and nutrition taken into the body and eliminated from the body. This is sometimes called fluid balance. There are two fluid imbalances that may occur. The first type of imbalance is when the intake of fluid is greater than the output of fluid. When this happens, signs of edema may be noted. **Edema** is the swelling of body tissues, especially the feet and ankles, due to an accumulation of excess fluid. Other signs to observe and report are weight gain, a reduction in urine output, shortness of breath, and elevated pulse rate. A **fluid restriction** may be ordered for this resident.

The other fluid imbalance is called dehydration. Dehydration occurs when the amount of fluid in the body becomes dangerously low. As mentioned previously, dehydration is a major problem. Several recent reports found that a large percentage of nursing home residents are dehydrated. A "force fluids" (FF) order may be written for a resident who is at risk of being dehydrated.

Warning signs that your residents are at risk for dehydration include the following:

- drinks less than six cups of liquids per day
- needs help drinking from a cup or glass
- has dry mouth, cracked lips, sunken eyes, and/or dark urine
- has trouble swallowing liquids
- frequent vomiting, diarrhea, or fever
- is easily confused or tired

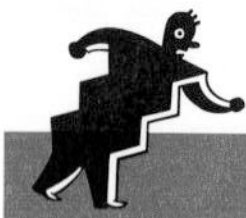

Principal Steps

Preventing Dehydration

1. *Post schedules for offering fluids.*
2. *Observe residents carefully for signs and symptoms of dehydration.*
3. *Encourage residents to drink fluids every time you see them.*
4. *Remind all staff, visitors and volunteers of the importance of following the schedule.*
5. *Report changes in fluid balance promptly!*
6. *Report any of the following:*

- *eyes that look sunken in the head*
- *resident not drinking water or other fluids*
- *fever or other change in vital signs, such as drop in blood pressure or irregular heartbeat*
- *dry skin and mucous membranes, such as the lips, mouth and throat*
- *decrease in urinary output, dark urine, or signs of urinary tract infection*
- *constipation or weight loss*
- *weakness, dizziness, or confusion*

It is very important for all staff members to follow set schedules for fluid intake for all residents. It is quite common for dehydration to occur in facilities. One method of encouraging fluids is the acronym outlined below:

POURR

Post a regular schedule for offering fluids to residents.

Observe residents carefully for signs and symptoms of dehydration.

Use other kinds of fluids, such as flavored frozen ice sticks, to improve fluid balance and increase fluid intake.

Remind all staff, visitors, and volunteers p.r.n. of the importance of following the schedule.

Report changes in fluid balance or any signs and symptoms of dehydration promptly!

Passing Fresh Water

Follow all standard and/or transmission-based precautions. Follow all rules for body mechanics.

Collect equipment:
• cart • ice container with ice cubes • ice scoop
• cups • water pitcher sheaths (if used in facility)
• straws • paper towels

1. **Wash your hands.**

PREPARE:

2. **Prepare the cart. Make sure you have all of your equipment. Fill all pitcher sheaths three-fourths full of water.**
3. **Check and make a list of all residents who are NPO or on fluid restrictions.**

PERFORM:

4. **Go to each room. Identify each resident. Empty water pitcher into the sink. If sheath system is used, remove inner sheath and discard.**
5. **Refill pitcher or get new sheath of water and ice if desired. If ice bucket is used, return to ice machine when empty to refill. If used, place new sheath in water pitcher.**
6. **Replace pitcher on overbed table in room. Add cups, straws, and paper towels as needed.**

7. Fill clean cup with water if desired by resident.
8. Leave overbed table within reach of resident if resident is in room.
9. Wash your hands.
10. Repeat above procedure with all residents in your area.

FINISHING TOUCHES:

11. When finished, empty and clean cart.
12. Perform the "5 Stars and 3 Rs."

13 Name six types of residents who may have fluid restrictions.

Fluid restrictions are ordered when the amount of fluid must be carefully measured and limited due to certain reasons and disorders. Two examples are heart and kidney disease. Other reasons for fluid restrictions include:

- resident is post-op (surgery)
- illness, such as a gastrointestinal (GI) illness
- special test ordered
- feeding done through a special tube

Summary

Nutrition and hydration are two of the most important aspects of your residents' daily lives. Good nutrition and hydration can vastly improve the quality of life. It is vital to carefully observe the intake of food and fluids for all of your residents. Report signs of dehydration before the condition worsens. Observing for signs of any fluid imbalance is also important. Watching for signs of weight loss or gain is a nursing assistant's duty, as well.

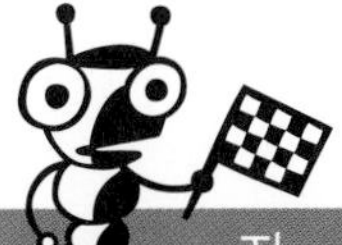

The Finish Line

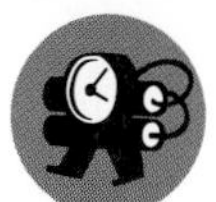

What's Wrong With This Picture?

1. Look at the equipment listed for the Practical Procedure: Passing Fresh Water. One important piece of equipment is missing. List the missing piece of equipment.

Collect equipment:
- cart • ice container with ice cubes • ice scoop • cups
- water pitcher sheaths • straws • paper towels

2. Look at the equipment listed for the Practical Procedure "Preparing Residents for Meals," shown below. One important piece of equipment is missing. List the missing piece of equipment.

Collect equipment:
- two pairs of disposable gloves
- soap • basin with warm water • washcloth • towel
- robe and slippers or clothing

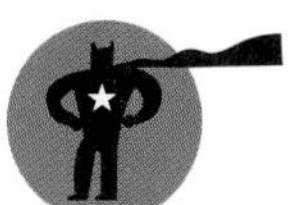

Star Student Central

1. Do you have any history of heart disease in your family? Many families do. See a local dietician and ask for information about a heart-friendly diet. Share this information with your class.
2. Go to as many fast food restaurants as you can and ask for nutrition information about all of the things on the menu. Bring the information back and share with your class. You might be surprised to find out how much fat and how many calories are in an average fast food meal.

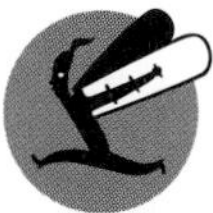

You Can Do It Corner!

1. You have a cup that holds 8 ounces. Convert the ounces (oz.) into cubic centimeters (cc). (LO 10)
2. What is the first step you should take to prevent errors when passing meal trays? (LO 6)
3. List a reason that a doctor would not order a special diet for a resident. (LO 4)
4. List seven signs to observe and report about dehydration. (LO 12)
5. Explain why the following specific diets could be ordered for residents: low sodium, low calorie, high residue, high protein, and low fat. (LO 5)
6. Name four reasons a resident may have a fluid restriction. (LO 13)

7. Discuss two reasons that residents should eat all of their snacks. (LO 8)

8. List the six groups on the Food Guide Pyramid in the order of foods that should be eaten most to foods that should be eaten least. (LO 3)

9. What is aspiration? List eight ways you can help prevent aspiration. (LO 7)

10. List six primary nutrients and the function of each. (LO 2)

11. Which of the following would you include in your documentation of intake of fluids: water, frozen ice stick, apple juice, coffee, potatoes, ice cubes? (LO 11)

12. Create percentages for each food item. Then assign correct percentages to document how much the resident ate. Total them when you've finished. Would you need to report this to the nurse? (LO 9)

    Sandwich: resident ate all

    Cup of soup: resident ate one-half

    Water: resident drank all

    Salad: resident ate one-half

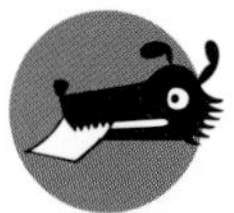

Star Student's Chapter Checklist

1. I have read my textbook chapter.
2. I have reviewed my own "Pocketful of Terms."
3. I have listened to my tutor tape.
4. I have reviewed and highlighted my class notes.
5. I have read and completed any handouts from this chapter.
6. I have completed "The Finish Line."
7. Star Time! Choose your reward!

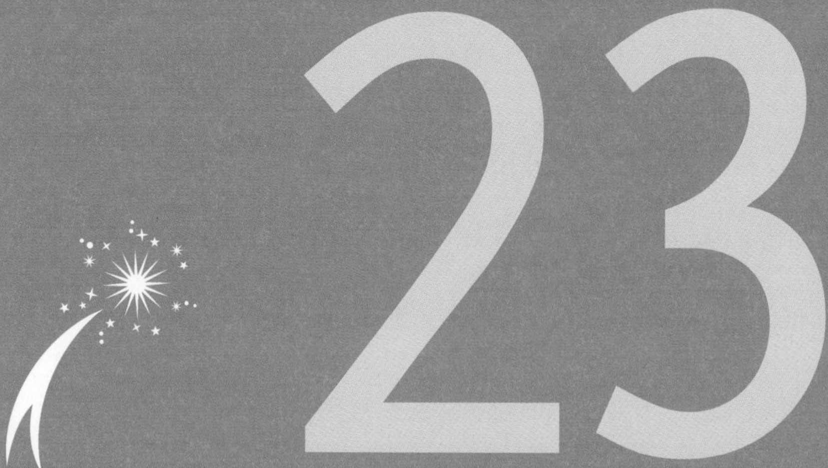

Your Guide: Urinary and Bowel Elimination

Look Like a Star!

Look at the Learning Objectives and The Finish Line before you begin reading this chapter.

Look at your pocket calendar.
With your pencil, put a bracket ( ) around a study period every single day.

Look at your homework for this chapter.
Plug each piece of homework into a certain time slot.

Look at the Star Student's Chapter Checklist at the end of this chapter. Check off each item as it is completed.

"A man's body is like a pot, which does not disclose what is inside. Only when the pot is poured, do we see its contents."

Jane Yolen, 1939-present from *The Pot Child*

". . . unconscious gratitude for a good digestion."

Friedrich Wilhelm Nietzsche, 1844-1900

Learning Objectives

1. Spell and define all STAR words.
2. List qualities of urine and stool and identify four characteristics of normal urination and bowel elimination.
3. List ten factors that affect urinary and bowel elimination and problems that can occur with both.
4. List and describe the use of supplies for assisting with urinary and bowel elimination.
5. Explain the process of accurately collecting and measuring urine and stool and discuss the "5 Rights" of specimen collection.
6. Describe the life-saving potential of correctly testing for occult blood in the stool.
7. List four reasons incontinence occurs and identify five steps to prevent incontinence.
8. Explain three reasons for using a straight catheter or a Foley catheter and describe the importance of quality catheter care.
9. Describe care of a resident using a condom catheter and a leg bag.
10. State three reasons an enema is ordered and explain three safety precautions when giving an enema.
11. Describe the use of a Harris flush or rectal tube.
12. Discuss two positions that help reduce gas inside the intestines.
13. Explain nine guidelines for assisting with urinary or bowel retraining.

Successfully perform these Practical Procedures

Helping a Resident Use a Bedpan

Assisting a Male Resident with a Urinal

Helping a Resident Use a Commode

Collecting a Routine Urine Specimen

Collecting a Clean-Catch or Midstream Specimen

24-Hour Urine Specimen Collection

Collecting a Stool Specimen

Testing a Stool Specimen for Occult Blood

Changing Adult Incontinent Pads

Performing Basic Urinary Catheter Care

Emptying a Urinary Catheter Drainage Bag and Measuring Output

Giving a Cleansing Enema

Giving a Commercial Enema

Giving the Harris Flush

Positioning a Rectal Tube

Privies over the Centuries

Sewage disposal was not unprovided for in the 14th century, though far from adequate. Privies . . . and public latrines existed, though they did not replace open street sewers. Castles and wealthy townhouses had privies built . . . with a hole in the bottom allowing the deposit to fall into a river or a ditch . . . Townhouses away from the riverbank had cesspools in the backyard . . . they frequently seeped into wells and other water sources . . . The 15th and later centuries preferred to ignore human elimination.

from *A Distant Mirror*
by Barbara Tuchman

1 Spell and define all STAR words.

anuria: absence of urine or a very small amount of urine (under 100 cc) in a 24-hour period.

bedpan: piece of equipment, usually plastic, used to collect urine and feces.

bowel elimination: the process of releasing or emptying the colon or large intestine of stool or feces.

bowel obstruction: potentially life-threatening situation when stool forms an obstruction or a block in the colon.

catheter: tube used to remove or add fluid into body openings.

clean-catch urine specimen: a urine specimen collected midstream after the perineal area is cleaned.

commode: chair containing a bedpan or bucket used to collect urine and feces.

condom catheter: external catheter made of a condom and a tube attached to a drainage bag; also called Texas catheter.

constipation: the difficult and often painful elimination of a hard, dry stool (bowel movement).

diarrhea: the frequent elimination of liquid or semiliquid feces.

dysuria: painful or difficult urination.

enema: the introduction of fluid into the colon through the rectum to cleanse the colon of feces.

fecal impaction: inability to pass stool because it has formed into a large mass, usually toward the lower part of the colon.

feces: solid waste products eliminated by the colon; stool; bowel movement.

flatulence, flatus: excessive amount of gas formation in the digestive tract.

Foley catheter: catheter inserted into the bladder.

graduate: measuring container with markings for ounces (oz.) and cubic centimeters (cc).

Harris flush: special type of enema given to remove flatulence; also called a return-flow enema.

"hat": specimen pan, usually plastic, used to collect and measure urine and stool from the toilet.

Hemoccult: test performed to check for occult blood in the stool.

incontinence: the inability to control the bladder or bowels.

leg bag: small catheter drainage bag attached to the leg.

midstream: a urine specimen taken after urination begins.

nocturia: frequent urination during the night.

nocturnal enuresis: bedwetting during the night.

occult blood: hidden blood found in specimen using a microscope or special chemical test.

oliguria: reduced amount of urine formation.

polyuria: increased amount of urine formation.

rectal tube: tube placed inside the rectum for the purpose of eliminating flatulence.

Sims' position: position on the left side with the right knee bent toward the chest; often called the enema position.

specimen: sample of something.

stool: feces, bowel movement.

straight catheter: catheter tube placed in the bladder temporarily to obtain a specimen of urine for laboratory examination or to empty the bladder when the resident cannot void on his or her own.

twenty-four-hour specimen: urine collected over a 24-hour time period and kept on ice or in a specimen refrigerator; the first specimen is discarded.

urinal: container, usually plastic, to collect urine from males.

urinary retention: when urine is retained in the body.

urgency: the need to urinate or have a bowel movement right away.

urination: the process of emptying the bladder; also called voiding.

2 List qualities of urine and stool and identify four characteristics of normal urination and bowel elimination.

Urination is the physical process of releasing or emptying the bladder of urine. Urine consists of waste products removed from the blood. Humans must urinate several times daily. There may be a slight difference in the number of times different people urinate. Regular urination is vital to keep the urinary system, including the kidneys, ureters, bladder, and urethra healthy.

Urine will normally be light, pale yellow or amber in color and should be clear or transparent. It has a faint smell, and the amount that should be produced per day is approximately 1500 cc.

Bowel elimination is the physical process of releasing or emptying the colon or large intestine of stool or feces. **Feces**, or **stool**, are solid waste products eliminated by the colon. The time and frequency of bowel movements varies with each individual from one or two per day to several a week. Regular bowel movements are vital to keeping the gastrointestinal system healthy.

Stool is normally brown in color, and its consistency is soft, moist, and formed (not loose). The amount of stool produced per day varies depending upon the food eaten.

The Four A's of Normal Urination and Bowel Elimination

1. **Absence of Pain:** Pain, burning, or pressure should not occur when urinating. Bowel movements should not be painful.
2. **Absence of Accidents:** Accidents should not occur except the rare occasions when unable to find a bathroom in time (such as when traveling by vehicle).
3. **Absence of Abnormal:** No blood, pus, or mucous should be in urine or stool. Urine should not have protein or glucose present.
4. **Adequate Amount:** The amount of normal production of urine and stool varies with the age of the person and the amount and type of liquids and food consumed. Adults should produce about 1500 cc of urine per day. Elderly adults may produce 1500 cc or less per day. It is especially important for elderly people to have regular bowel movements to prevent serious problems like obstructions.

3 List ten factors that affect urinary and bowel elimination and problems that can occur with both.

There are many things that affect normal urination and bowel elimination and may end up causing problems. Factors are listed below, with examples that outline specific problems:

Growth and development: Aging can change the amount of urination and the regularity of bowel movements.

Disorders: Certain disorders may affect urine and stool production. Diabetes mellitus may cause nocturia and polyuria. Cystic fibrosis may increase the amount of stool.

Pregnancy: Pregnancy may cause polyuria and constipation.

Anxiety: Nervousness may increase urination and cause more frequent bowel movements.

Fluid intake: A decrease in fluids may decrease urine production and cause constipation. The body's ability to remove wastes in the stool may be affected. When wastes build up, infections can occur.

Fluid output: Increased sweating during strenuous exercise, for example, may decrease urine production.

Types of foods chosen: Foods high in caffeine increase urine production. Chocolate can increase frequency of bowel movements or cause diarrhea.

Medications: Certain medications cause urine production to increase or decrease and cause diarrhea or constipation.

Exercise: Exercise helps maintain adequate urine production and regular bowel movements.

Work/sleep schedule: People in jobs where bathroom breaks are limited can develop problems with urination and bowel elimination. Shift change may disrupt their ability to urinate and have bowel movements on a regular schedule.

Types of Urination Problems

Anuria: absence of urine or a very small amount of urine, under 100 cc, in a 24-hour period.

Dysuria: painful or difficult urination.

Nocturia: waking up in the night to urinate.

Nocturnal Enuresis: nighttime accidental urination; "bedwetting."

Oliguria: small amount of urine; usually below 400 cc in 24-hour period.

Polyuria: eliminating a large amount of urine.

Urinary Retention: the collection of urine in the bladder, causing the inability to urinate or preventing the release of urine.

Urinary Urgency: the feeling of needing to urinate right away.

Urinary Incontinence: the inability to control the bladder.

Types of Bowel Elimination Problems

Bowel Incontinence: inability to control the passage of bowel movements.

Bowel Obstruction: potentially life-threatening situation when stool forms an obstruction in the colon, may require surgery to remove obstruction.

Bowel Urgency: the feeling of needing to have a bowel movement right away.

Constipation: passage of dry, hard stool or no stool for a period of time.

Diarrhea: passage of liquid or semi-liquid feces; may have an increase in frequency of bowel movements.

Fecal Impaction: inability to pass stool because it has formed into a large mass, usually toward the lower part of the colon.

4 List and describe the use of supplies for assisting with urinary and bowel elimination.

The supplies used for assisting residents with urinary and bowel elimination are:

- bathroom tissue
- **urinal**
- **bedpan**
- cornstarch powder
- bedpan cover/disposable pad
- **commode**
- "**hat**" or collection device

Remember, any time you risk contact with a body fluid, wear the appropriate PPE, including gloves.

When using a bedpan for the collection of urine or stool, there are a few simple steps that may make this procedure easier, safer, and less embarrassing for everyone involved. Placing a bedpan under a resident may be easier if you spread a small amount of cornstarch powder on the edges of the pan. However, you cannot use powder when collecting a specimen.

Use great caution in removing the bedpan from the bed. It must be held as still as possible to avoid spilling the contents. A bedpan cover or disposable pad is used to cover the contents while transferring the bedpan into the resident's bathroom.

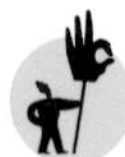

"Please hold the sauce"

When you stand in front of the kitchen sink and clean dishes and pans covered with spaghetti sauce, it is easy to get the sauce all over your clothes and your face and arms if you are not careful.

Cleaning bedpans can be just as tricky. Always be careful when spraying a bedpan with any sprayer device. If you hold the bedpan facing you, you could spray the contents of the bedpan all over you! You do not want any microorganisms from urine or stool to get inside of you. Wear protective PPE when cleaning this type of equipment.

There are two kinds of bedpans: standard pans and fracture bedpans. The fracture pan is placed from the side or the foot of the bed and used for very small or thin people or those who cannot lift their buttocks.

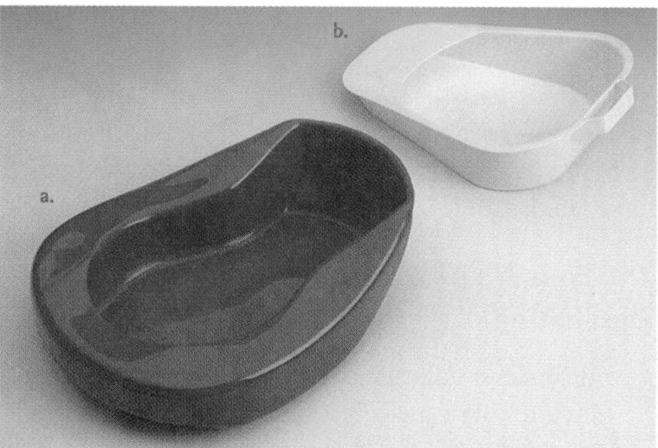

Figure 23-1. **a) Standard pan and b) fracture pan.**

Men use a urinal to void. It is usually made of plastic and has a cover. Urinals may be hung on the side of the bed after use to be picked up by a staff member, emptied, and cleaned. A device for cleaning the bedpan or urinal may be attached to the toilet in the resident's bathroom. If this is the case, a faucet-like piece will spray water when the toilet is flushed. Other types of water sprayers may be attached to the side of the toilet. It is important to clean the bedpan immediately after use to avoid strong odors. This reduces embarrassment to the resident or to others.

Bedside commodes are often used for people who find it difficult to walk to the bathroom. This equipment may or may not have wheels. It is important to lock the wheels of a bedside commode before moving the resident into or out of the commode. Commodes are made either with a bedpan or a buck-

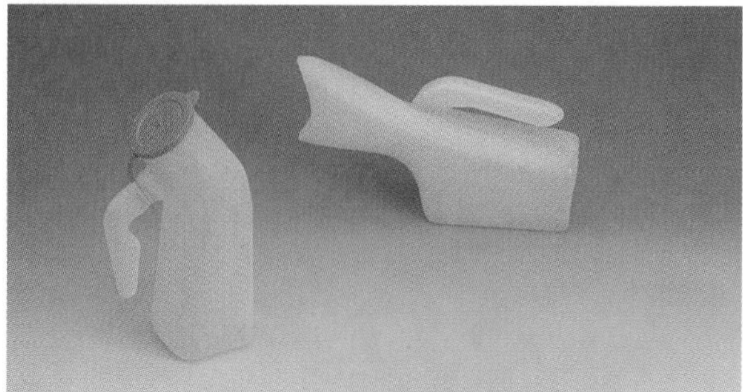

Figure 23-2. **Urinals.**

et that slides underneath the chair. The bedpan or bucket must be cleaned after each use.

A plastic collection container called a "hat" is sometimes inserted into a toilet to collect and measure urine or stool. Hats should be labeled and must be cleaned after each use.

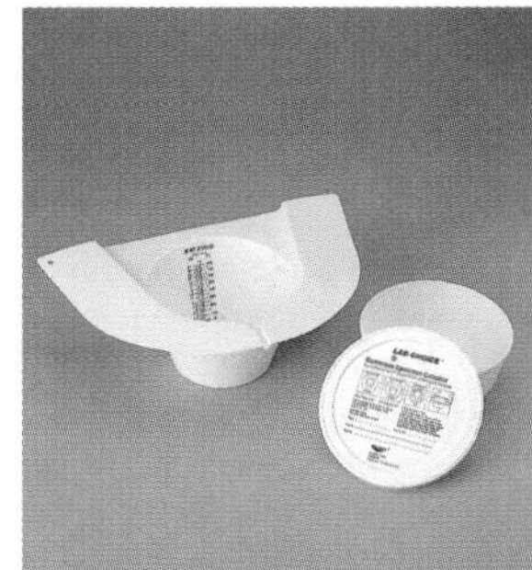

Figure 23-3. A "hat" is a container that is placed under the toilet seat to collect specimens for residents who use the toilet rather than a bedpan or portable commode.

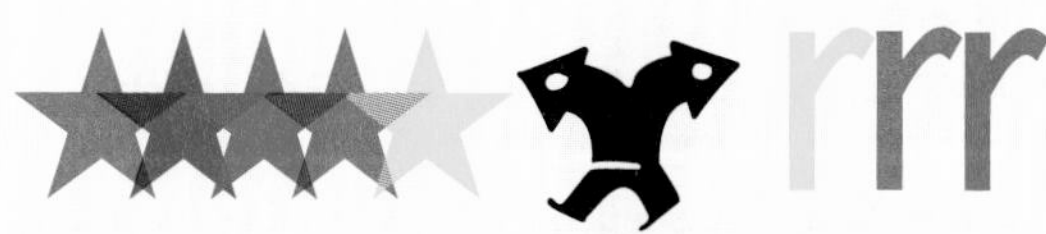

Beginning Steps

★ RESPECT
Knock first, ask and receive permission to enter a resident's room.

★ INFECTION CONTROL
Wash hands.

★ COMMUNICATION
Greet and identify the resident. Identify yourself. Explain the procedure, encouraging the resident to be as independent as possible throughout.

★ BED SAFETY
Lock bed wheels. Raise bed to safe working height. Lower one side rail if required.

★ PRIVACY
Provide for privacy by closing the door and covering the resident appropriately.

Ending Steps

★ RESIDENT SAFETY AND COMFORT
Secure the resident, lowering the bed, and raising the side rails if ordered. Check that the resident is comfortable and properly aligned.

★ PRIVACY
Remove any added privacy measures, such as a drape or a privacy screen.

★ ESSENTIALS
Place the call light, fresh beverage, and other items within reach.

★ COURTESY
Ask the resident if he or she needs anything else. Say thank you and goodbye.

★ INFECTION CONTROL
Wash hands.

r **Report** your care and any important observations to the nurse.

r **Record** your care and any important information/observations such as vital signs in the appropriate place.

r **Recheck** your resident for any changes as directed by the nurse!

Helping a Resident Use a Bedpan

Follow all standard and/or transmission-based precautions. Follow all rules for body mechanics.

Collect equipment:
- two pairs of disposable gloves • disposable bed protector
- bedpan and cover • cornstarch powder • toilet tissue
- washcloth or wipes • wash basin of warm water
- towel • disposable plastic bag

1. Perform the "5 Stars."

2. Apply gloves.

PREPARE:

3. Ensuring privacy, remove bed linen and lift gown or pull down pajamas.
4. Turn resident to side, and place the bed protector underneath resident. (Figure 23-4)

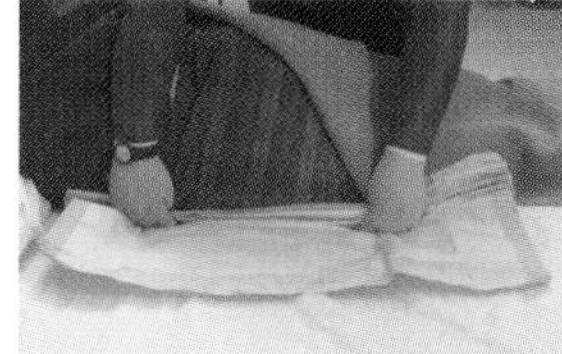

Figure 23-4.

5. Optional: Unless collecting a specimen, prepare bedpan by sprinkling cornstarch powder over the plastic rim. Place bedpan, choosing one of the following methods:

Method 1:

a. Return resident to his back. Ask him to bend his knees and raise his buttocks by pressing the bottom of the feet against the bed.
b. Count to three and gently slide the bedpan under his buttocks and center it.

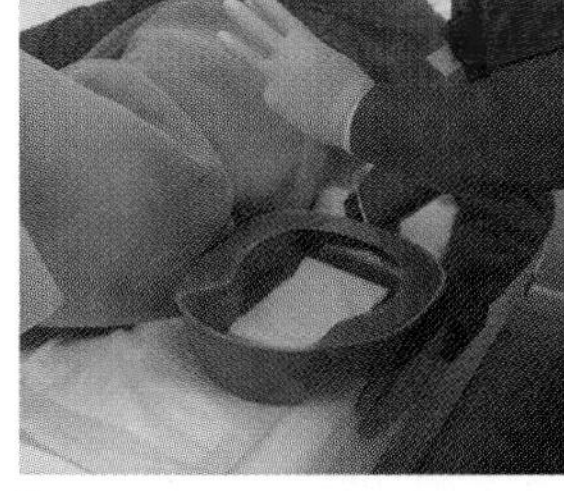

Figure 23-5.

Method 2:

a. With the resident turned to his side, position the bedpan against his buttocks.
b. Roll the resident onto his back and center the bedpan.

6. Cover the resident and place toilet tissue in reach.
7. Raise the HOB to a comfortable position.

PERFORM:

8. Allow resident to use bedpan. If a sample is not being collected, the toilet tissue can be discarded in the bedpan.

   Leave the resident if asked to do so. If you stay, give the resident privacy. You can stand behind the other side of the privacy curtain if there is one. If you leave, you must SECURE THE RESIDENT by raising the side rails and lowering the bed. Place the call light within reach of the resident, remove and discard gloves, and wash hands before leaving the room.
9. Return to the bedside (wash hands again if you left the room).

10. Lower the side rail and raise the bed.
11. Put on gloves.
12. CAREFULLY remove the bedpan, cover it, and place on facility-approved spot. Never place it on the overbed table.
13. Help resident to clean perineal area by using disposable wipes or washcloth and basin of water. Always clean from front to back.
14. Place the following inside the plastic bag: wipes (or return washcloth to wash basin), disposable bed protector, and your used gloves.
15. Replace gown or pajamas and cover the resident.
16. SECURE THE RESIDENT.

FINISHING TOUCHES:

17. Apply gloves.
18. In two completely separate steps, pick up wash basin first and later bedpan, bring to appropriate area, and do the following steps:
    - discard washcloth and towel in appropriate area
    - clean, disinfect, and dry wash basin
    - check urine and/or stool for color, odor, amount, and character
    - measure urine or stool if ordered
    - collect specimen if ordered
    - clean, disinfect, and dry bedpan
19. Remove gloves and discard. Wash your hands.
20. Return to bedside. Return wash basin and bedpan to storage. Assist resident in cleaning hands. Secure resident.
21. Perform the "5 Stars and 3 Rs."

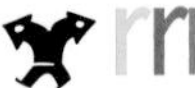
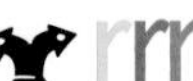

22. If specimen is obtained, bring specimen to appropriate spot and plastic bag to biohazard container and discard.

Assisting a Male Resident with a Urinal

Follow all standard and/or transmission-based precautions. Follow all rules for body mechanics.

Collect equipment:
• two pairs of disposable gloves • disposable bed protector • urinal • toilet tissue • washcloth or wipes • wash basin of warm water • towel • disposable plastic bag

1. Perform the "5 Stars."

2. Apply gloves.

PREPARE:

3. Ensuring privacy, remove bed linen and lift gown or pull down pajamas.
4. Place bed protector under resident.
5. Raise the HOB if desired. Place urinal between the legs so that the penis is inside the urinal.
6. Cover the resident and place toilet tissue in reach.

PERFORM:

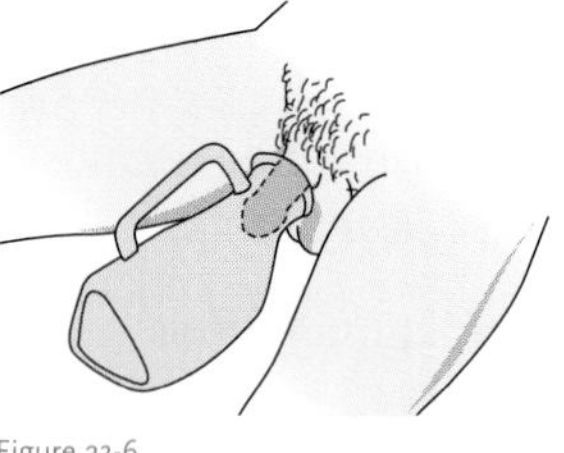

Figure 23-6.

7. Allow resident to use the urinal.

   Leave the resident if asked to do so. If you stay, give the resident privacy. You can stand behind the other side of the privacy curtain if there is one. If you leave, you must SECURE THE RESIDENT by raising the side rails and lowering the bed. Place the call light within reach of the resident, remove and discard gloves, and wash hands before leaving the room.
8. Return to the bedside (wash hands if you have left the room).
9. Lower the side rail and raise the bed.
10. Put on gloves.
11. CAREFULLY remove the urinal, cover, and hang on side rail or place in other appropriate spot.
12. Help resident to clean perineal area by using disposable wipes or washcloth and basin of water. Cleaning should be done in a circular motion towards the base of the penis. Start at the urethral opening and work outward.
13. Place the following inside the plastic bag:
    - wipes (or return washcloth to wash basin)
    - disposable bed protector
    - your used gloves
14. Replace gown or pajamas and cover the resident.
15. SECURE THE RESIDENT.

FINISHING TOUCHES:

16. Apply second pair of gloves.
17. In two completely separate steps, pick up wash basin and urinal, bring to appropriate area, and do these steps:
    - check urine for color, odor, amount, and character
    - discard washcloth and towel in appropriate area
    - clean, disinfect, and dry wash basin
    - measure urine if ordered
    - collect specimen if ordered
    - clean, disinfect, and dry urinal
18. Remove gloves and discard. Wash your hands.
19. Return to bedside. Return wash basin and urinal to storage. Assist resident in cleaning hands. Secure resident.
20. Perform the "5 Stars and 3 Rs."

21. If specimen is obtained, bring specimen to appropriate site and plastic bag to biohazard container and discard.

Helping a Resident Use a Commode

Follow all standard and/or transmission-based precautions. Follow all rules for body mechanics.

Collect equipment:

- two pairs of disposable gloves • disposable bed protector
- commode with bucket or bedpan in place
- washcloth or wipes • wash basin of warm water
- towel • disposable plastic bag • toilet tissue

1. Perform the "5 Stars."

PREPARE:

2. Apply gloves.
3. Lock wheels on commode and raise the lid. (Most commodes have wheels that can be locked for resident safety.)

PERFORM:

4. Raise the HOB to a comfortable position.
5. Place slippers on the resident.
6. Carefully transfer the resident to the commode using proper procedure and SECURE THE RESIDENT by making sure she is sitting in the center of the chair.
7. If the resident agrees, you should stay with her while she uses the commode. Allow resident to use commode. Offer toilet tissue or clean perineal area. Place tissue inside bedpan if not measuring urine. If on I & O, place toilet tissue inside plastic bag. Using wipes or washcloth, clean resident's hands.
8. Remove gloves and place inside plastic bag.

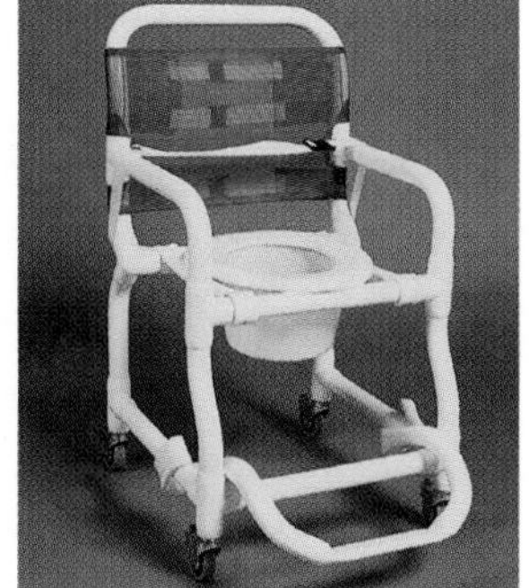

Figure 23-7. A portable commode can be used for residents who can get out of bed but may not be able to move to the bathroom easily.

9. Transfer resident back to bed, replace linen and make resident comfortable, and SECURE THE RESIDENT.

FINISHING TOUCHES:

10. Apply gloves.
11. In two completely separate steps, pick up wash basin and bucket or bedpan, bring to appropriate area, and do the following steps, as necessary:
    - discard washcloth and towel in appropriate area
    - clean, disinfect, and dry wash basin
    - check urine or stool for color, odor, amount, and character
    - measure urine or stool if ordered
    - collect specimen if ordered
    - clean, disinfect, and dry urinal
12. Return wash basin to bedside storage and bucket/bedpan to commode. Assist resident with cleaning hands.
13. Remove gloves and discard. Wash hands, and return to the bedside.
14. Perform the "5 Stars and 3 Rs."

15. If specimen is obtained, bring specimen to appropriate spot and plastic bag to biohazard container and discard.

---

5 Explain the process of accurately collecting and measuring urine and stool and discuss the "5 Rights" of specimen collection.

When a **specimen** of urine or stool is required, the first step is to inform an alert resident that the doctor has ordered the specimen. Because bowel movements are not usually as frequent as urination, the resident should be prepared to give a specimen the next time he or she has a bowel movement. The following instructions should be given to the resident prior to the collection of a specimen:

- Show the resident the correct container to use.
- Remind the resident not to place bathroom tissue in the specimen container, and to keep menstrual blood out of the specimen container. If you are collecting a urine specimen, also remind the resident to keep stool out of the container, and vice versa.
- Request that the resident notify a staff member right away when specimen is available.

The "5 Rights" for specimen collection are:

Do you have the right:

- resident?
- specimen/lab slip?
- container?
- date/time?
- storage and delivery?

Asking the wrong resident for a specimen wastes time and money. Make sure you have the right resident and look at the lab slip to double-check the type of specimen needed. Ask the nurse for information regarding the right container and correct method.

Urine or stool that cannot be sent to the lab immediately may need to be placed in a special refrigerator used strictly for specimens. Never place a specimen inside a refrigerator used for food.

There are many different types of urine specimens. A **24-hour specimen** is collected over a full day's time. A **clean-catch specimen** is a specimen that is collected after a special cleaning process of the perineal area is completed. The procedures that follow explain each type of collection.

Collecting a Routine Urine Specimen

Follow all standard and/or transmission-based precautions. Follow all rules for body mechanics.

Collect equipment:

- two pairs of disposable gloves • bedpan and cover
- toilet tissue • bed protector • labeled specimen container
- laboratory requisition slip • plastic bag (to transport specimen)

1. Perform the "5 Stars."

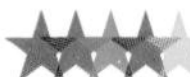

PREPARE:

2. Apply gloves.

PERFORM:

3. Help the resident onto the bedpan (or onto the commode or to the bathroom).
4. Request that the resident not place toilet tissue into the container.
5. Ask the resident to urinate into the specimen container or into the bedpan or commode, or "hat." A specimen container should be at least one-half full, if possible.
6. Use toilet tissue to clean perineal area and place tissue in bed protector or in toilet, not in "hat." Cover bedpan if used.
7. SECURE THE RESIDENT.
8. Bring covered bedpan to bathroom and pour urine into the specimen container or pour urine from hat into specimen container.
9. Carefully apply lid without touching the inside of the lid or container and place inside plastic transport bag.

FINISHING TOUCHES:

10. Clean and replace bedpan or "hat" in storage area.
11. Remove gloves and discard. Wash hands.
12. Perform the "5 Stars and 3 Rs."

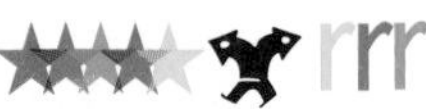

13. Bring disposable bag with specimen container inside to appropriate area.

Collecting a Clean-Catch or Midstream Specimen

Follow all standard and/or transmission-based precautions. Follow all rules for body mechanics.

Collect equipment:

- two pairs of disposable gloves • bedpan and cover
- toilet tissue • bed protector• labeled specimen container
- plastic bag for specimen • laboratory requisition slip
- clean-catch kit • one plastic bag for trash

1. Perform the "5 Stars."

PREPARE:

2. Apply gloves.
3. If in bed, place disposable bed protector on bed underneath resident.

PERFORM:

4. Help the resident onto the bedpan (or onto the commode or to the bathroom).
5. Request that the resident not place toilet tissue into the container.
6. Open the clean-catch kit. Open the wipes and then, using one gloved hand, clean the penis or perineal area in the following manner:

   Male: Clean the penis in a circular motion, beginning at the tip of the penis, moving outward from the urethra towards the base.

   Female: Clean the vulva from front to back with the wipes or other material, beginning with the outer labia and ending with the inner labia and then the urinary opening (the meatus).
7. For uncircumcised men, keep the foreskin retracted until the specimen is collected. For women, keep the labia open until the specimen is collected.
8. This specimen is called **midstream** because the initial and last urine are not included in the sample. Direct the resident to urinate in the following manner:

   FIRST into the toilet, bedpan, or "hat"

   SECOND into the specimen container

   LAST into the toilet or bedpan again
9. Carefully apply lid without touching the inside of the lid or container and place inside plastic transport bag.
10. Use toilet tissue to clean perineal area and place tissue in toilet or bedpan. Remove gloves.
11. Place the following inside the plastic bag:
    - disposable bed protector
    - your used gloves
12. SECURE THE RESIDENT and wash hands.

FINISHING TOUCHES:

13. Apply gloves, bring bedpan to bathroom, and clean it.
14. Clean, disinfect, and replace bedpan or "hat" in storage area.
15. Remove gloves and discard. Wash hands.
16 Perform the "5 Stars and 3 Rs."

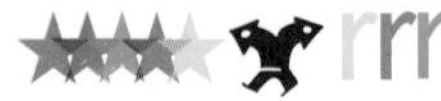

17. Bring disposable bag with specimen container inside to appropriate area.

24-Hour Urine Specimen Collection

Follow all standard and/or transmission-based precautions. Follow all rules for body mechanics.

Collect equipment:

- two pairs of disposable gloves • bedpan and cover

• toilet tissue • labeled 24-hour urine specimen container
• bed protector • plastic bag • laboratory requisition slip

A large sign is usually posted with the 24-hour start and end time and hung in or by the resident's room.

1. Perform the "5 Stars."

2. Apply gloves.

PREPARE:

3. Help the resident onto the bedpan (or onto the commode or to the bathroom).
4. Use toilet tissue to clean perineal area and place tissue on bed protector.

PERFORM:

5. Discard the FIRST urine of the collection. It is not included in the specimen.
6. Request that the resident save all urine from now on for the next 24 hours.
7. Request that resident save all urine in a bedpan, urinal, or commode and press the call light immediately after urinating. Request that resident not place toilet tissue into the container.
8. Each time urine is collected, pour it into the specimen container and return container to refrigerator or ice bucket. Be cautious so that you do not allow any urine to spill.
9. At the end of the 24-hour period of time, ask the resident to urinate. Pour urine into the 24-hour specimen container and cap container.

FINISHING TOUCHES:

10. Each time you collect a specimen, clean and replace bedpan in storage area. Remove gloves and discard.
11. Perform the "5 Stars and 3 Rs."

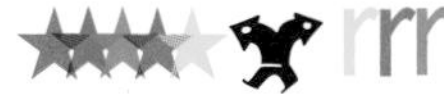

12. When 24-hour time period is over, bring the specimen containers to the lab immediately.

Collecting a Stool Specimen

Follow all standard and/or transmission-based precautions. Follow all rules for body mechanics.

Collect equipment:
• two pairs of disposable gloves • bedpan and cover
• toilet tissue • bed protector• specimen container
• tongue depressors • laboratory requisition slip
• plastic transport bag

1. Perform the "5 Stars."

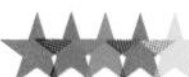

PREPARE:

2. Apply gloves.
3. Help the resident onto the bedpan (or onto the commode or to the bathroom). Ask the resident to have a bowel movement in the specimen container.
4. Request that resident not place toilet tissue into the container. Remind resident not to urinate in the sample.
5. Use toilet tissue to clean rectal area and place tissue inside a bed protector. Provide any peri-care necessary. Remove gloves and discard.
6. Cover and SECURE THE RESIDENT.

PERFORM:

7. Apply gloves. Cover and bring bedpan to bathroom. Use a tongue depressor to take two tablespoons of feces from the bedpan and place this feces into the specimen container. Apply lid and place inside plastic bag.

FINISHING TOUCHES:

8. Place tongue depressor inside disposable bag.
9. Clean and replace bedpan in storage area.
10. Assist the resident with handwashing. Secure the resident. Remove gloves and discard. Wash hands.
11. Perform the "5 Stars and 3 Rs."

12. Bring disposable bag with specimen container inside to appropriate area.

---

6 Describe the life-saving potential of correctly testing for occult blood in the stool.

Hidden or **occult blood** is found inside the stool through the use of a microscope or special chemical test. This may be a sign of a serious physical problem, such as cancer. The collecting and testing of stool to check for occult blood is now a common procedure. The **Hemoccult** test checks for occult blood in the stool. Many people use the Hemoccult 3-step card collection as a part of their annual physical exam. This test is potentially life-saving because early detection helps in treating many disorders successfully. Because of this, it is important to perform this procedure exactly as instructed.

Testing a Stool Specimen for Occult Blood

Follow all standard and/or transmission-based precautions. Follow all rules for body mechanics.

Collect equipment:
• two pairs of disposable gloves • specimen container
• tongue depressors
• disposable plastic bag
• paper towel
• testing card/package

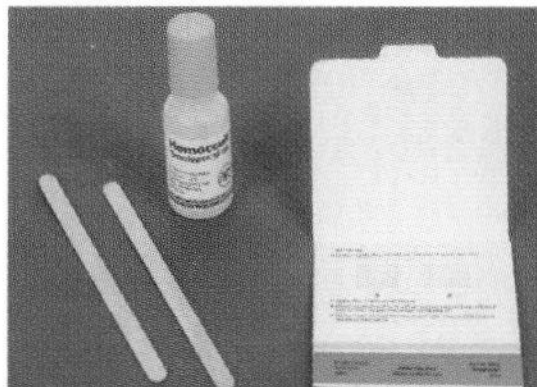

Figure 23-8.

PREPARE:

1. Check expiration date of testing card/package.

Read all of the instructions.

2. Apply gloves.
3. Collect the stool specimen, following proper procedure. Bring specimen to appropriate testing site.
4. Open the testing card.

PERFORM:

5. Pick up a tongue depressor and obtain small amount of feces from specimen container.
6. Using tongue depressor, smear a small amount of feces onto one square. See Figure 23-9.

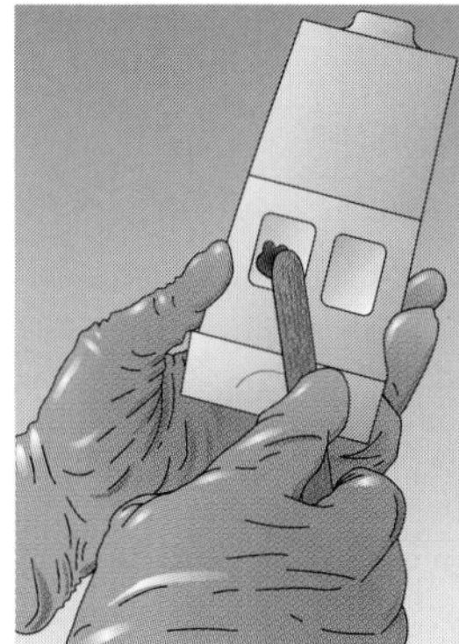
Figure 23-9.

7. Flip tongue depressor, and using depressor, smear small amount of feces onto second square.
8. Close the testing card and turn over to other side.
9. Open the flap on the other side.
10. Open developer and drop two drops of developer onto each square or follow specific instructions.
11. Wait the appropriate amount of time as listed in instructions.
12. Observe the squares for any color changes. In some test kits, the color blue is the color that would appear if blood exists in the stool.

FINISHING TOUCHES:

13. Place tongue depressor inside disposable bag.
14. Empty, clean, and replace bedpan in storage area.
15. Assist the resident with handwashing. Secure the resident. Remove gloves and discard. Wash hands.
16. Perform the "5 Stars and 3 Rs."

 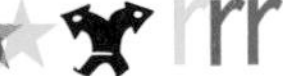

17. Bring disposable bag with tongue depressor to appropriate area and place in biohazard container.

7 List four reasons incontinence occurs and identify five steps to prevent incontinence.

Incontinence is the inability to control the bladder or bowels. Incontinence can occur in residents who are confined to bed, ill, paralyzed, or who have circulatory or nervous system diseases or injuries. For example, after a stroke, a person's ability to control urination or bowel movements may decrease, depending upon the kind of brain damage caused by the stroke. Incontinence is **not** a normal part of aging.

Whatever the reason for incontinence, it is important for nursing assistants to act professionally when handling incontinence. Never show anger or frustration toward residents who are incontinent. By observing your residents, you can help prevent occasional accidents. Being familiar with residents' daily routines can help prevent the embarrassment, shame, and frustration that occur with the loss of control. Take the following steps to help prevent incontinence:

Five Steps to Prevent Incontinence

1. **Routines:** Know your residents' daily routines and urinary and bowel habits. Know their physical signs, such as holding the lower abdomen, which might indicate the need to urinate. Abdominal cramping might mean they need to have a bowel movement. Give your residents the opportunity to have a bowel movement around the same time each day.

2. **Call Lights:** Answer call lights promptly to prevent avoidable accidents.

3. **Diet:** Be cautious with residents' diets. Residents who drink fluids heavily close to bedtime may be at greater risk for nighttime incontinence. However, due to the serious problem of dehydration, you should never limit a resident's fluids without a doctor's order. Help residents choose foods that will not cause loose stools or gas.

4. **Exercise:** Walking can stimulate the circulation and the need to go to the bathroom. Make sure daily walks occur close to a bathroom.

5. **Briefs:** If you know your resident is prone to accidents, offer an incontinent brief, especially when the resident goes anywhere for an activity or appointment. Do not delay changing a wet or soiled incontinent brief. Always refer to incontinence products as briefs or pads; never call them diapers.

Changing Adult Incontinent Pads

Follow all standard and/or transmission-based precautions. Follow all rules for body mechanics.

Collect equipment:
• two pairs of disposable gloves • disposable bed protector • incontinent brief • washcloth or wipes • towel • basin one-half full of warm water • disposable plastic bag

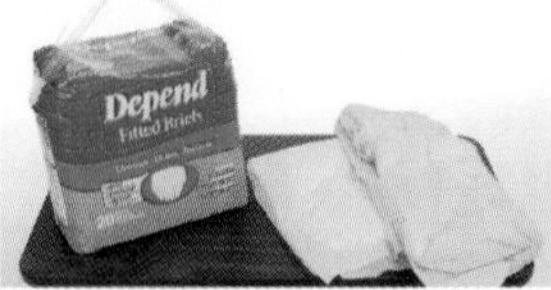

Figure 23-10. A type of incontinent pad.

1. Perform the "5 Stars."

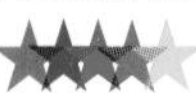

PREPARE:

2. Apply gloves.
3. Ensuring privacy, remove bed linen and lift gown or pull down pajamas.
4. Turn resident to side, place bed protector under resident.

PERFORM:

5. Undo incontinent brief, carefully remove it, by turning the resident gently from side to side. Place in disposable bag. Clean resident with disposable wipes or washcloth. Place wipes inside disposable plastic bag or return washcloth to basin.
6. Remove gloves and discard. Wash hands. Apply a second clean pair of gloves.
7. Replace with fresh brief by turning resident from side to side. Take care not to pull too hard on brief, which might cause it to tear. Use cornstarch powder if instructed to do so.
8. Remove adhesive protector from back of brief and attach strips to front of brief. Do not wrap too tightly.

FINISHING TOUCHES:

9. Replace gown or pajamas and secure resident.
10. Pick up wash basin, bring to appropriate area, and do the following steps:
   - discard washcloth and towel in appropriate area
   - clean, disinfect, and dry wash basin
11. Remove gloves and discard. Wash your hands.
12. Return to bedside and return wash basin and bedpan to storage area by bedside. Assist resident in cleaning hands.
13. Perform the "5 Stars and 3 Rs."

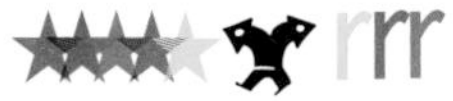

No shortcuts with resident care!

Residents sometimes become incontinent in bed. Do not take a "short-cut" when changing residents' linen after incontinence. Just removing a disposable pad and replacing it with a clean one without changing the wet bed linen lying underneath the pads may be considered abuse or neglect. This type of shortcut should never be performed. Always remove all wet linen and disposable pads and replace them with clean linen and clean pads when a resident is incontinent.

8 Explain three reasons for using a straight catheter or a Foley catheter and describe the importance of quality catheter care.

Residents who are unable to pass urine in a normal fashion may require a doctor's order for a urinary catheter. A **catheter** is a tube that removes urine from the bladder through the urethra. Some residents need a **straight catheter**. This type of a catheter does not remain inside the resident; it is removed immediately after the urine is drained. Two reasons a straight catheter is necessary include a doctor requiring a "clean" specimen from inside the bladder and a resident's inability to release urine independently.

Other residents require placement of a catheter that remains inside the urethra and bladder for a period of time. This type of a catheter is called a **Foley**, retention, or indwelling catheter. Foleys are ordered to allow the skin to heal during a period of incontinence or for placement during and after surgery.

Foley catheters are usually inserted by nurses. It is vital that all nursing staff take excellent care of Foley catheters. Nursing assistants must follow strict guidelines regarding catheter care. If any mistakes are made, serious complications may occur. Residents may get serious infections due to poor catheter care. These infections can move from the bladder to the kidneys. This can be life-threatening.

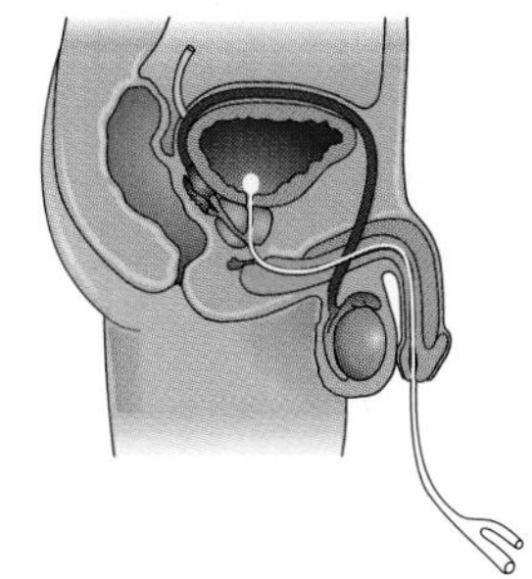

Figure 23-11. **Foley catheter (male).**

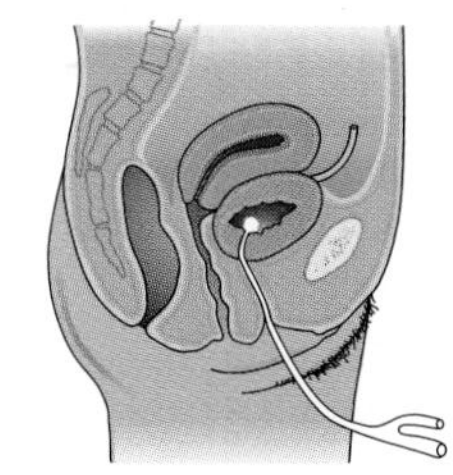

Figure 23-12. **Foley catheter (female).**

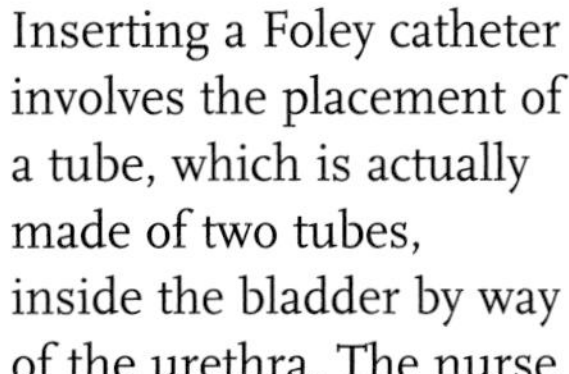

Inserting a Foley catheter involves the placement of a tube, which is actually made of two tubes, inside the bladder by way of the urethra. The nurse chooses the size of the tube and inserts it into the bladder using sterile technique. The catheter remains inside the bladder because of a tiny balloon at the tip of the catheter that rests inside the bladder. The nurse inflates the tiny balloon by inserting or injecting a small amount of sterile water into the tube. This water blows up the balloon and stays inside of the balloon until the nurse withdraws it when the catheter is removed.

The catheter tubing connects to a bag that collects urine draining out of the bladder. This bag is emptied into a container, called a **graduate**, with markings for ounces and cubic centimeters. The emptying of bags is completed by the nursing staff at the end of each shift and as necessary. You must be careful when emptying catheter bags. Always wear disposable gloves and open and close the clamp without touching the tip of the clamp to any other object. Touching the tip could transfer microorganisms to the inside of the tubing, and they could move up into the bladder, causing an infection.

When residents move about with a catheter drainage bag, the bag must hang below the level of the bladder. The flow of urine back into the bladder from a drainage bag can have serious consequences. Bacteria grow rapidly in these bags, and when bacteria travels back to the bladder, infections may occur.

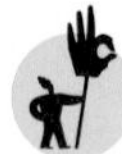

Observe and report catheter problems!

Catheters can be very dangerous! If you ever find problems like these with any catheter,

★ *"Don't Delay. Report Right Away!"*

- *The catheter is leaking.*
- *The catheter tubing has become disconnected.*
- *Bag has moved above level of bladder.*

Performing Basic Urinary Catheter Care

Follow all standard and/or transmission-based precautions. Follow all rules for body mechanics.

Collect equipment:

- **two pairs of disposable gloves • disposable bed protector**
- **antiseptic wipes or solution • washcloth**
- **wash basin of warm water • towel • disposable plastic bag**

NOTE: Following the proper procedure, provide perineal care *before* providing catheter care. The perineal area must be clean in order to ensure that microorganisms are not transferred to the catheter.

1. Perform the "5 Stars."

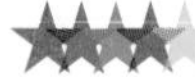

PREPARE:

2. Apply gloves.

3. Ensuring privacy, remove bed linen and lift gown or pull down pajamas as necessary to expose catheter.

4. Turn resident to side, place bed protector under resident, and return to back.

PERFORM:

5. Pour antiseptic solution onto part of the washcloth or use the wipes to clean the entire area around the catheter. For female residents, carefully separate the labia and wash one side, then the other, and then the center. Wipe once, and use a clean wipe or a different part of the washcloth each time. If using a washcloth, rinse it frequently. For male residents, retract the foreskin, if uncircumcised, and wash the penis from the urethra outward in a circular motion. Use a clean wipe or different part of the washcloth for each cleaning stroke. Return the foreskin, if uncircumcised, to its proper position.

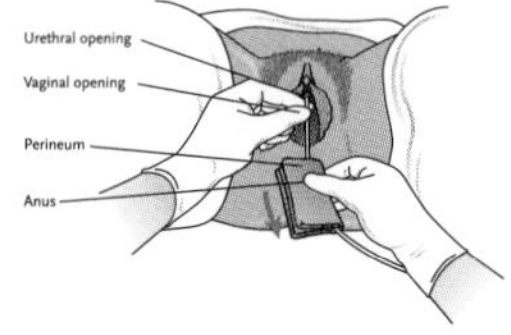

Figure 23-13.

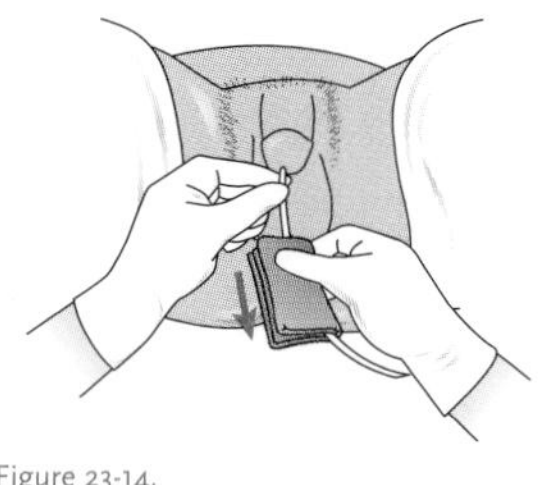

Figure 23-14.

6. Using a clean wipe or clean part of the washcloth with antiseptic solution, clean the catheter tubing, starting at the body, and moving OUTWARD from the body about four inches.

7. Observe for any bleeding, sores, or leakage around the catheter.

8. Check that the catheter and tubing are free from kinks and twists and that it is securely taped to the leg.

9. Place the following inside the plastic bag:

- **wipes (or return washcloth to wash basin)**
- **disposable bed protector**
- **your used gloves**

10. Wash hands.

11. Replace gown or pajamas and cover the resident.

12. SECURE THE RESIDENT.

FINISHING TOUCHES:

13. Apply gloves.

14. Pick up wash basin, bring to appropriate area, and do the following steps:

- **discard washcloth and towel in appropriate area**
- **clean, disinfect, and dry wash basin**

15. Return to bedside and return wash basin to storage area.

16. Bring plastic bag to biohazard container and discard. Remove and discard gloves.

17. Perform the "5 Stars and 3 Rs."

9 Describe care of a resident using a condom catheter and a leg bag.

Condom catheters, often called external or Texas catheters, are sometimes ordered for men who require catheters. This style of catheter is placed outside of the body over the penis and is then attached to the tubing that drains into the bag. The condom is held in place by special catheter tape or a catheter holder strap so that it stays on the body. Care must be taken so that the tape does not irritate the skin or interfere with circulation. Urine drains through the condom into the tubing, then into the drainage bag.

Some residents use smaller bags to collect the urine, called **leg bags**. These bags attach to the leg. This type of drainage bag is also emptied at the end of each shift and as necessary. Care must also be taken when attaching a leg bag. The band that wraps around the leg must not be so tight that it affects circulation in the leg or causes any harm to the skin.

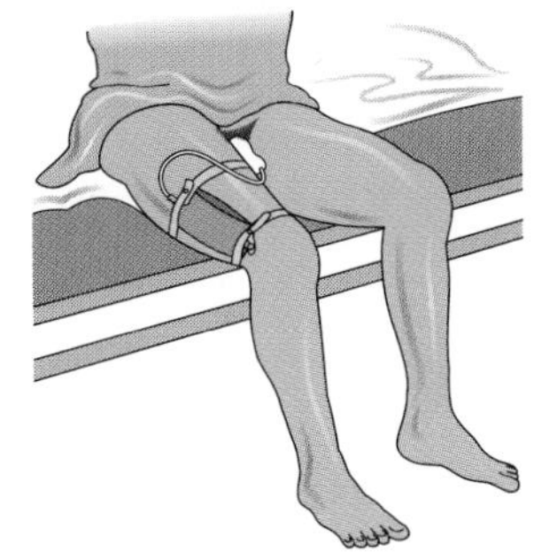

Figure 23-15. **External or condom catheter (male).**

The nurse will usually attach the indwelling catheter to the leg bag. You are normally responsible for emptying urine from leg bags.

Principal Steps

Condom Catheter Application

1. *Wear gloves during care.*
2. *Provide perineal care.*
3. *Roll the condom over the penis, leaving a one-inch space between the penis and the end of the condom.*
4. *Apply the special catheter tape spirally around the condom and penis. Do not completely encircle the penis or it can interfere with circulation.*
5. *Attach the catheter to tubing and bag.*
6. *Check back often to make sure that circulation is not cut off and that urine is flowing properly.*

Sheath
Tape
1 inch
Catheter

Figure 23-16.

Emptying a Urinary Catheter Drainage Bag and Measuring Output

Follow all standard and/or transmission-based precautions. Follow all rules for body mechanics.

Collect equipment:
- **two pairs of disposable gloves • alcohol wipes**
- **graduated measuring container • pen**
- **notepad or I & O sheet**

1. **Perform the "5 Stars."**

PREPARE:

2. **Apply gloves.**
3. **Place paper towel on the floor and put graduate on it.**

PERFORM:

4. **Open the drain or spout on the bag, carefully allowing all urine to drain into the graduate. Do not let spout touch sides of graduate.**
5. **After urine has drained, close spout. Wipe drain or spout with an alcohol wipe, and replace in the holder on the bag.**

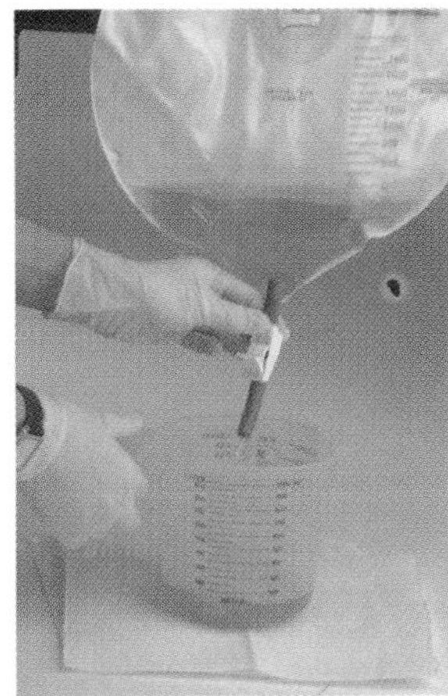

Figure 23-17.

6. **SECURE RESIDENT.**
7. **Pick up graduate, bring into bathroom and set down on paper towel. Measure urine on flat surface at eye level. Record amount of urine on pad or on I & O form.**
8. **Clean, disinfect, and dry graduate.**
9. **Remove gloves and discard. Wash your hands.**
10. **Return graduate to storage site.**

FINISHING TOUCHES:

11. **Perform the "5 Stars and 3 Rs."**

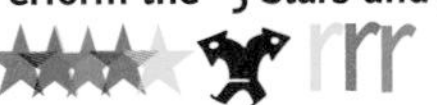

10 State three reasons an enema is ordered and explain three safety precautions when giving an enema.

As people age, normal habits of bowel elimination change. Digestion takes longer and is less efficient. Body waste moves more slowly through the intestines. Constipation, the inability to have a bowel movement, may occur.

An **enema** is given to a resident when help is needed eliminating stool from the colon. A specific amount of water flows inside of the colon in order to help remove stool. Some facilities allow nursing assistants to give enemas. If you are allowed to give enemas at your facility, it is extremely important that you carefully follow the procedural steps for giving enemas.

Enemas are ordered for three primary reasons:

1. Preparation for a diagnostic test
2. Preparation for surgery
3. To remove stool that a resident cannot eliminate on his or her own

Doctors or other healthcare providers will write an enema order for a specific amount of fluid to be introduced into the colon. Cleansing enemas are given in one of four different styles:

- Tap Water Enema (TWE): 500-1000 cc water with nothing added to water
- Soap Suds Enema (SSE): 500-1000 cc water with 5 cc of mild castile soap added to the water
- Saline Enema: 500-1000 cc water with two teaspoons (tsp) of salt added to the water
- Commercial Enemas: 120 cc solution; may have oil or other additive

Safety is one of the most important aspects of the enema procedure. Serious problems occur when mistakes are made while giving an enema. There are three major safety steps to remember when preparing for an enema:

1. You must remove the air from the enema tubing before the tube is inserted inside the resident's body. Allowing a small amount of water to flow into a bedpan will allow the air to escape. Water temperature must be approximately 105 F.
2. You must measure the distance from the rectal area to the bottom of the enema bag. The bottom of the enema bag must be not more than 12 inches above the rectal opening. (Figure 23-18)

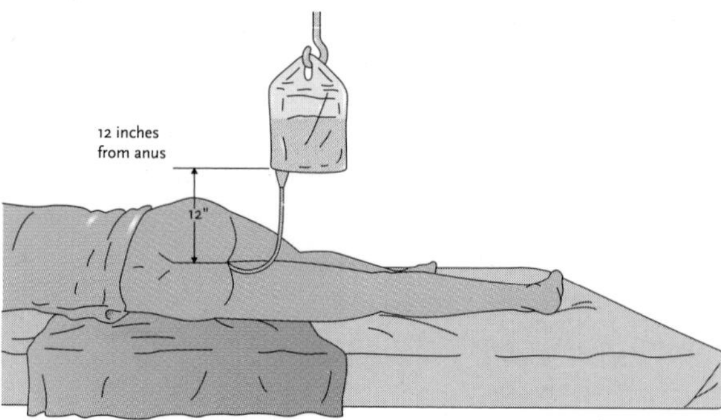

Figure 23-18.

3. The resident must be in the left **Sims' position** during the enema. Because of the way the human body is made, the person must be positioned on the left side so that the enema water does not have to flow against gravity.

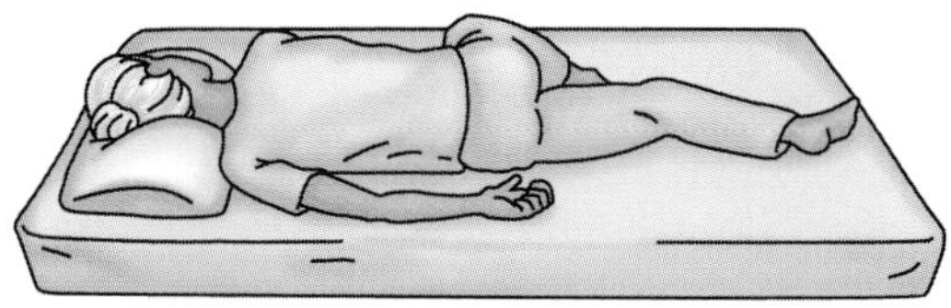

Figure 23-19. **The left Sims' position.**

It is vital to make sure before you open the clamp that you have completed all three safety checks.

Safety First with Enemas!

Giving an enema can be dangerous. Take great care to follow the safety rules "to the letter." When these safety steps are not taken seriously, the resident can suffer complications. Intentionally skipping the safety steps may be considered abuse.

Giving a Cleansing Enema

Follow all standard and/or transmission-based precautions. Follow all rules for body mechanics.

Collect equipment:

- **measuring tape • two pairs disposable gloves • IV pole**
- **washcloths or wipes • castile soap packet or two tsp salt**
- **disposable enema kit or enema bucket, tubing, and clamp**
- **bedpan with cover • toilet tissue • bed protector**
- **bath blanket or drape • towel • lubricating jelly**

This step may be done outside of the resident's room in some facilities.

1. **Prepare the enema solution as instructed by the nurse.**

   Fill bag or bucket with 500-1000 cc of warm water (105 F) if tap water enema (TWE). If soapsuds enema (SSE), add 5 cc of castile soap and mix. If saline enema, add two teaspoons of salt and mix.
2. **RELEASE THE AIR. Unclamp tubing and allow a little water to run through tubing into bedpan to release all of the air inside of the tube.**
3. **Re-clamp the tubing, hang on IV pole, and bring to bedside of resident.**
4. **Perform the "5 Stars."**

PREPARE:

5. **Apply gloves.**
6. **Take off pants, if worn, and underwear. Position the resident in the left Sims' position and cover with bath blanket or drape, exposing only the buttocks. (Figure 23-20)**
7. **Place bed protector under resident.**
8. **Measure the distance from the bottom of the enema bag to the rectal opening. The distance should be NOT MORE than 12 inches.**

PERFORM:

9. **Lubricate tip of tubing if not pre-lubricated.**

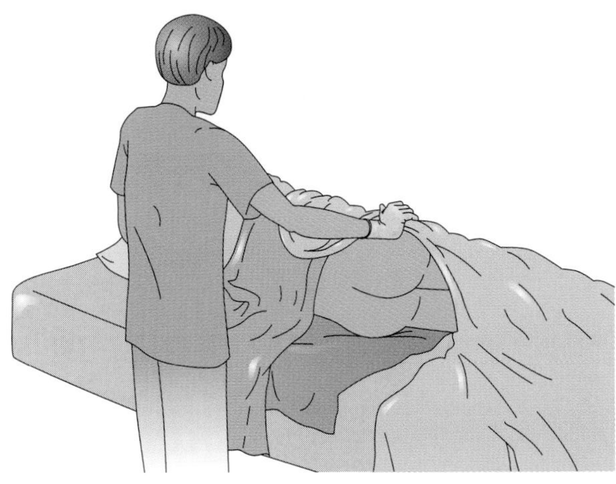

Figure 23-20.

10. Place one hand on the upper buttock and lift to expose rectal opening. Using other hand, get ready to insert the tubing into the anus.
11. Tell the resident when he exhales (breathes out), you will be inserting the tip of the enema.
12. Ask the resident to take a deep breath and then to exhale (breathe out). Insert the tip of the enema slowly and carefully two to four inches into the rectum. STOP THE INSERTION IF YOU FEEL RESISTANCE OR IF THE RESIDENT COMPLAINS OF ANY PAIN. If this happens, discontinue and report to the nurse.

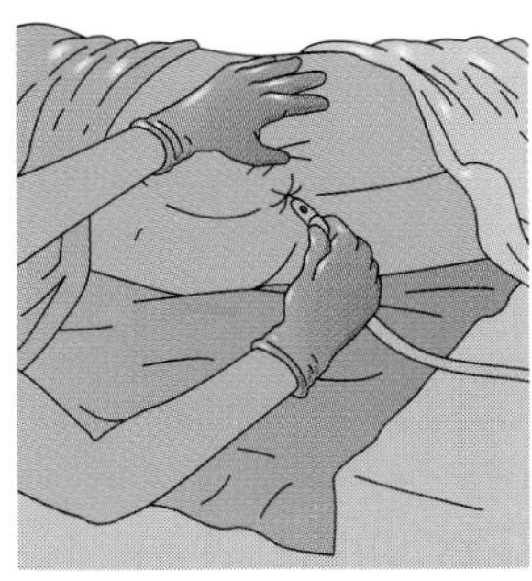

Figure 23-21.

13. Unclamp the tubing and allow the solution to begin running into the rectum slowly. Continue enema telling the resident to take slow deep breaths which will help relieve cramping. If the resident complains of any pain, discontinue and report this to the nurse.
14. Allow almost all of the water to run into the rectum. Stop solution by clamping slowly before the bag is empty.
15. Request resident to try to hold solution inside as long as possible.
16. Gently remove the tip of the enema, and carefully place tip inside the bucket or bag.
17. Place toilet tissue against rectal opening.

FINISHING TOUCHES:

18. Assist the resident in using bedpan, commode, or to the bathroom following proper procedure. Check stool for color, odor, consistency, and amount.
19. Remove gloves and discard. Wash hands.
20. Apply gloves. Assist resident with washing hands. Secure resident.
21. Dispose of enema supplies.
22. Remove gloves.
23. Perform the "5 Stars and 3 Rs."

Giving a Commercial Enema

Follow all standard and/or transmission-based precautions. Follow all rules for body mechanics.

Collect equipment:

- two pairs disposable gloves
- standard or oil retention commercial enema kit
- washcloths or wipes• bedpan with cover
- toilet tissue • bed protector• bath blanket or drape
- towel • lubricating jelly

Warm commercial enema under warm running water or in bowl of warm water.

1. Perform the "5 Stars."

PREPARE:

2. Apply gloves.
3. Take off pants, if worn, and underwear. Position the resident in the left Sims' position and cover with bath blanket or drape, exposing only the buttocks.
4. Place bed protector under resident.

PERFORM:

5. Lubricate tip if not pre-lubricated.
6. Place one hand on the upper buttock and lift to expose rectal opening. Using other hand, get ready to insert the tubing into the anus.
7. Tell the resident when he exhales (breathes out), you will be inserting the tip of the enema.
8. Ask the resident to take a deep breath and then to exhale (breathe out). Insert the tip of the enema carefully about one and a half inches into the rectum. STOP THE INSERTION IF YOU FEEL RESISTANCE OR RESIDENT COMPLAINS OF ANY PAIN. If this happens, discontinue and report to the nurse.
9. Slowly squeeze and roll the enema container so that the solution runs inside the resident. Continue enema telling the resident to take slow deep breaths which will help relieve cramping. Do not release the pressure on the bottle until almost all of the solution is in. If resident complains of any pain, discontinue and report this to the nurse.
10. Allow almost all of the water in the commercial enema to run into the rectum. Stop solution by clamping before the container is empty.
11. Ask resident to try to hold solution inside as long as possible. When an oil retention enema is used, ask the resident to wait and hold at least 30 to 60 minutes.
12. Gently remove the tip of the enema, and carefully place tip inside the box upside down.
13. Place toilet tissue against rectal opening.

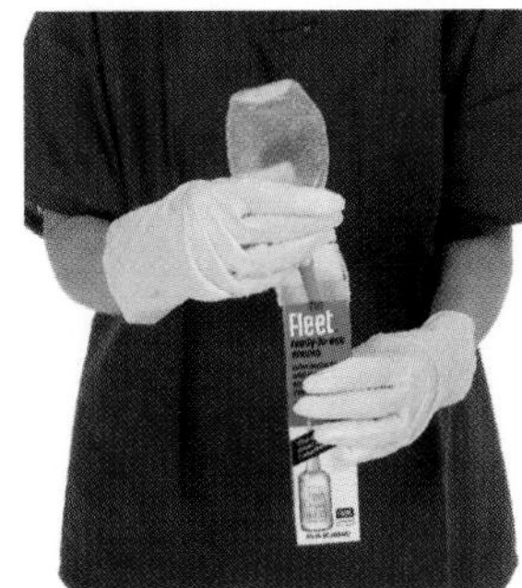

Figure 23-22.

FINISHING TOUCHES:

14. Assist the resident in using bedpan, commode, or to the bathroom following proper procedure. Check stool for color, odor, consistency, and amount.
15. Remove gloves and discard. Wash hands.
16. Apply gloves. Assist resident with washing hands. Secure resident.
17. Dispose of enema supplies.
18. Remove gloves and discard.
19. Perform the "5 Stars and 3 Rs."

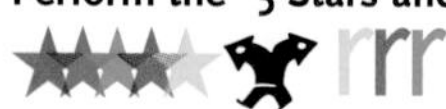

11 Describe the use of a Harris flush or rectal tube.

Flatus or **flatulence** is air or gas bubbles eliminated from the GI, or digestive, tract. Flatulence can be embarrassing for many residents. This occurs when too much air or gas gathers inside the digestive tract.

There are two primary methods used in health care for the relief of flatus: the rectal tube and the Harris flush. A **Harris flush**, also called a return-flow enema or a colonic irrigation, is a special type of enema that reduces gas. A **rectal tube** is placed inside the rectum to reduce gas. When too much gas develops in the body, it can cause severe cramping. Some people have compared the pain from cramping to that of passing kidney stones or having a baby.

Giving the Harris Flush

Follow all standard and/or transmission-based precautions. Follow all rules for body mechanics.

Collect equipment:
- measuring tape • two pairs of disposable gloves
- IV pole • towel • lubricating jelly
- disposable enema kit or enema bucket, tubing, or clamp
- bedpan with cover • toilet tissue • bed protector
- bath blanket or drape • washcloths or wipes

This step may be done outside of the resident's room in some facilities.

1. Prepare the enema solution. Fill bag or bucket with 100 to 200 cc of warm water.
2. Perform the "5 Stars."

PREPARE:

3. Apply gloves.
4. Take off pants, if worn, and underwear. Position the resident in the left Sims' position and cover with bath blanket or drape, exposing only the buttocks.
5. Place bed protector under resident.
6. Measure the distance from the bottom of the enema bag to the rectal opening. The distance should be NOT MORE than 12 inches.

PERFORM:

7. Lubricate tip if not pre-lubricated.
8. Place one hand on the upper buttock and lift to expose rectal opening. Using other hand, get ready to insert the tubing into the anus.
9. Tell the resident when he exhales (breathes out), you will be inserting the tip of the enema.
10. Ask the resident to take a deep breath and then exhale (breathe out). Insert the tip of the enema slowly and carefully two to four inches into the rectum. STOP THE INSERTION IF YOU FEEL RESISTANCE OR IF THE RESIDENT COMPLAINS OF ANY PAIN. If this happens, discontinue and report to the nurse.
11. Allow about 100 cc of the solution to run inside the resident's rectum.
12. Lower the enema bag so that the solution can run back out into the bag. This process should be repeated as ordered or instructed by the nurse. As the solution returns to the bag, flatus and feces may run back into the bag. Continue the process of the flush unless resident complains of pain.
13. Replace the fluid in the bag with fresh water if the bag collects too much feces.
14. Return to bedside and continue flush unless resident complains of pain.
15. Stop solution by clamping the tubing. Gently remove the tip of the tubing and place tip inside the bag.
16. Place toilet tissue against rectal opening.

FINISHING TOUCHES:

17. Assist the resident in using bedpan, commode, or to the bathroom following proper procedure. Check stool for color, odor, consistency, and amount.
18. Remove gloves and discard. Wash hands.
19. Apply gloves. Assist resident with washing hands. Secure resident.
20. Dispose of enema supplies.
21. Remove gloves and discard.
22. Perform the "5 Stars and 3 Rs."

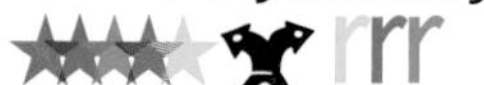

Positioning a Rectal Tube

Follow all standard and/or transmission-based precautions. Follow all rules for body mechanics.

Collect equipment:
- two pairs disposable gloves • toilet tissue • bed protector
- rectal tube • bath blanket or drape • towel
- washcloths or wipes • adhesive tape

1. Perform the "5 Stars."

PREPARE:

2. Apply gloves.
3. Take off pants, if worn, and underwear. Position the resident in the left Sims' position and cover with bath blanket or drape, exposing only the buttocks.
4. Place bed protector under resident.

PERFORM:

5. Lubricate tip if not pre-lubricated.
6. Place one hand on the upper buttock and lift to expose rectal opening. Using other hand, get ready to insert the tubing into the anus.
7. Tell the resident when he exhales (breathes out), you will be inserting the tip of the rectal tube.
8. Ask the resident to take a deep breath and then to exhale (breathe out). Insert the tip of the rectal tube carefully about two inches into the rectum. STOP THE INSERTION IF YOU FEEL RESISTANCE OR IF THE RESIDENT COMPLAINS OF ANY PAIN. If this happens, discontinue and report to the nurse.
9. Secure the tube with a small piece of adhesive tape to the buttocks.
10. Place the flatus tube bag inside the bed protector, wrap, and secure.
11. Cover and SECURE THE RESIDENT. Raise side rails and lower bed. Remove gloves and wash hands. You may leave the resident with the rectal tube in place for as long as 20 minutes.

FINISHING TOUCHES:

12. Return to room, wash hands, and apply clean gloves. Raise bed and lower side rail.
13. Remove the rectal tube and place it inside bed protector.
14. Use toilet tissue to clean rectal area and place tissue inside bed protector.
15. Remove bed protector and bath blanket. Secure resident.
16. Dispose of enema supplies. Remove gloves and discard. Wash hands.
17. Perform the "5 Stars and 3 Rs."

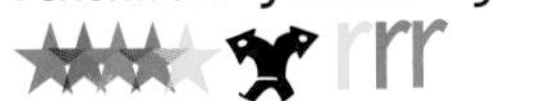

12 Discuss two positions that help reduce gas inside the intestines.

When people develop flatus, they may experience severe discomfort due to the cramping that often develops inside the abdomen. Some of the causes for this type of cramping are things like tests, surgery, or certain types of foods. In addition, some residents experience cramping on a daily basis due to physical characteristics.

There are two positions used to help reduce gas in residents. These are:

1. Side-lying or lateral position, usually the left side
2. Flat or supine position

The side-lying position allows flatus or gas to escape due to gravity. Make the resident comfortable in the side-lying position. Placing the resident in this position for at least 20 minutes usually assists in elimination of gas.

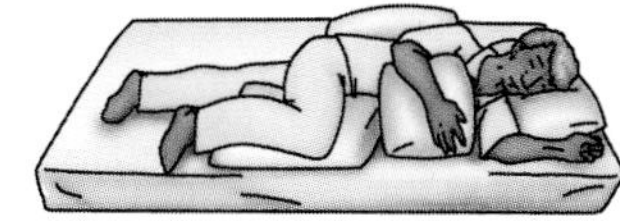

Figure 23-23. Side-lying position.

The flat or supine position is used with residents who have returned to a long-term care facility following some type of surgery. Placing the resident in the supine position allows gas that was forced inside the abdomen due to the surgery to help escape more quickly.

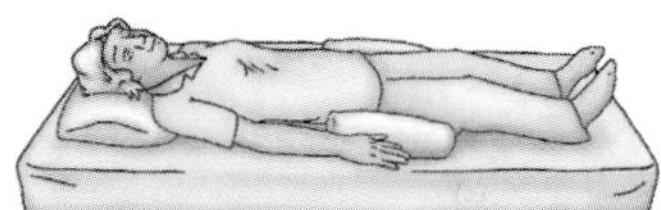

Figure 23-24. Flat position

When your resident complains of severe cramping, take this complaint very seriously. Serious discomfort such as this can lead to unexpected complications if not handled promptly. Stress in one area of the body may cause stress in another area.

13 Explain nine guidelines for assisting with urinary or bowel retraining.

Residents who have had an illness, injury, or a period of inactivity may need assistance in re-establishing a regular routine and normal urinary and bowel function. You play a big part in helping these functions return to normal. Retraining is the process of assisting residents to regain control of their bowel and bladder. Retraining is started after physical reasons for incontinence have been ruled out by a physician. Having a history of the residents' habits before beginning is important. For urinary retraining, the idea is to expand the bladder by gradually increasing the time between voiding. Facilities plan, chart, and implement this with all the caregivers in various ways. Make certain you understand and follow the procedures for this at your facility.

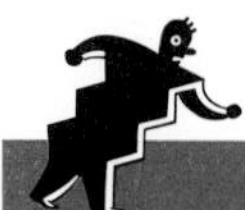

Principal Steps

Assisting with Urinary or Bowel Retraining

1. *Always act professionally when handling incontinence or helping to re-establish routines. Incontinence is difficult enough for residents without them having to worry about your reactions.*
2. *Follow the plan consistently.*
3. *Offer a bedpan or a trip to the bathroom before beginning long procedures or bathing.*
4. *As discussed earlier, observe your residents' elimination habits to help predict when a trip to the bathroom or a bedpan will be necessary. Observe and record times of incontinence to help establish a routine.*
5. *Encourage fluids throughout the day. Offer a bedpan or a trip to the bathroom about 30 minutes after fluids are taken.*
6. *If ordered, encourage your resident to eat foods high in fiber.*
7. *If a resident has difficulty urinating once he or she is on a commode or toilet, try running water from the tap. You can also suggest that he or she leans slightly forward to put pressure on the bladder.*
8. *If attempts or accomplishments are made, offer positive words and encouragement.*
9. *Never show frustration or anger toward residents who are incontinent. Not only is that abusive behavior, but your negative reactions will only make the problem worse. Patience with any setbacks is necessary if the effort is to be successful.*

Summary

The process of elimination requires efficient handling by nursing assistants. Residents require a great deal of privacy with elimination, and nursing assistants must make sure privacy needs are met. All standard and transmission-based precautions must be met when performing elimination procedures.

It is important that you make careful observations when performing these procedures. Potentially serious physical problems can be discovered during this process. Steps can then be taken to prevent complications. Careful observation of elimination helps to ensure a resident's health and well-being.

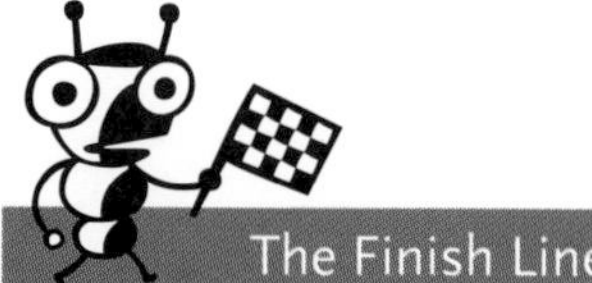

The Finish Line

What's Wrong With This Picture?

Some definitions of urination and bowel elimination problems are incorrectly listed. Write the correct definition for each problem.

Anuria: painful or difficult urination.
Dysuria: the waking up in the night to urinate.
Fecal Impaction: inability to control the passage of bowel movements.
Oliguria: small amount of urine; usually below 400 cc in 24-hour period.
Bowel Urgency: when stool forms an obstruction or a block in the colon, may require surgery to remove obstruction.
Nocturia: the collection of urine in the bladder causing the inability to urinate or preventing the release of urine.

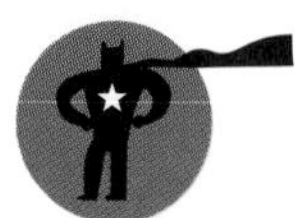

Star Student Central

1. Do you drink enough fluids, including water, every day? Keep track of what you drink for two days, including things like soup, soda, juices, and especially water. Eight eight-ounce glasses of water are suggested for good health.
2. Make an appointment with your doctor or healthcare provider to be tested for blood in your stool. Do not forget to call for results; some offices no longer call people with test results.

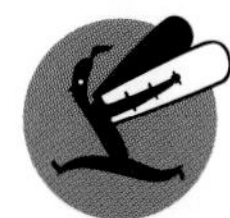

You Can Do It Corner!

1. When giving enemas, what should the distance be from the bottom of the bag to the rectal opening? (LO 10)
2. What are the two positions that can help reduce gas in the intestines? (LO 12)
3. List the "four As" of normal urination and bowel elimination. (LO 2)
4. What could you use to assist with the smooth placement of a bedpan under a resident? (LO 4)
5. List and describe nine factors affecting urinary and bowel elimination. (LO 3)
6. What is a midstream specimen? (LO 5)
7. List five steps to prevent incontinence. (LO 7)
8. What is a "hat"? What does it do? (LO 4)
9. What are two problems that may occur with the tape on a condom catheter? (LO 9)
10. What are the "5 Rights" of specimen collection? (LO 5)
11. What is the difference between a Foley and a straight catheter? (LO 8)
12. Why is testing for occult blood so important? (LO 6)
13. Describe the three safety steps when giving an enema. (LO 10)
14. When should you replace the fluid in the bag during a Harris flush? (LO 11)
15. List the seven guidelines for assisting with urinary or bowel retraining. (LO 13)
16. How should you always refer to incontinence products? (LO 7)

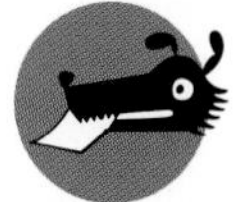

Star Student's Chapter Checklist

1. I have read my textbook chapter.
2. I have reviewed my own "Pocketful of Terms."
3. I have listened to my tutor tape.
4. I have reviewed and highlighted my class notes.
5. I have read and completed any handouts from this chapter.
6. I have completed "The Finish Line."
7. Star Time! Choose your reward!

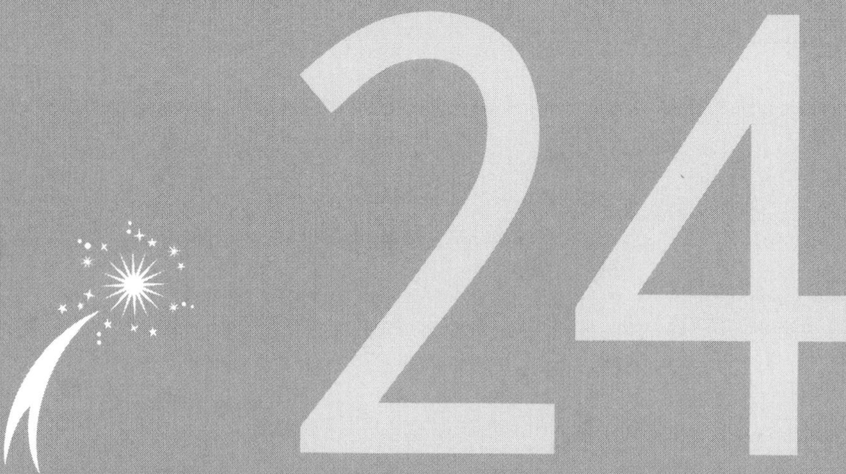

Specialized Care: The Integumentary System

Look Like a Star!

Look at the Learning Objectives and The Finish Line before you begin reading this chapter.

Look at your pocket calendar.
With your pencil, put a bracket (   ) around a study period every single day.

Look at your homework for this chapter.
Plug each piece of homework into a certain time slot.

Look at the Star Student's Chapter Checklist at the end of this chapter. Check off each item as it is completed.

"Beauty's but skin deep."

John Davies, 1565-1618

"Men should be judged, not by their tint of skin. . . But by the quality of thought they think."

Laurence Hope 1865-1904

Learning Objectives

1. **Spell and define all STAR words.**
2. **Summarize the changes that occur in the skin during normal aging.**
3. **Name four common disorders of the integumentary system.**
4. **Describe the benefits and the risks of hot and cold applications.**
5. **Describe care of a resident with a burn.**
6. **Describe care of the resident with a pressure sore.**
7. **Discuss safety precautions used to prevent damage to a dressing site during care.**
8. **Identify the differences between sterile and non-sterile dressings.**

Successfully perform these Practical Procedures

Applying Warm Compresses (Moist)

Administering Warm Soaks (Moist)

Assisting with a Sitz Bath (Moist)

Using an Aquamatic Pad (Dry)

Applying an Ice Bag (Moist)

Giving a Cold Sponge Bath (Moist)

Assisting the Nurse with Non-Sterile Dressing Care

Applying Sterile Gloves

Assisting the Nurse with Sterile Dressing Care

The Field of Dermatology in its Infancy

Ferdinand Hebra [1816-1880] was one of the first doctors to specialize in the diseases of the skin. He founded a division of dermatology. One of the discoveries he made concerned the disease known as scabies, a disorder that causes intense itching. Hebra noted that when the itch- mite parasite was destroyed, scabies was then cured. He also made the important discovery that scabies was contagious and that people could actually pass it from one person to another.

1 Spell and define all **STAR** words.

chemotherapy: the use of a chemical agent that can destroy or inhibit the growth of cancerous cells; may kill both normal and abnormal cells; used as a treatment for certain cancerous tumors.

contact dermatitis: inflammation or swelling of the skin due to contact with an irritant.

decubitus ulcer: break or opening in the skin due to a reduction in blood flow; pressure sore.

dermatologist: a doctor who specializes in care of the diseases of the skin.

first-degree burn: burn involving the epidermis.

malignant: describing a tumor that is cancerous, involving many organs, and spreading.

malignant melanoma: most serious form of skin cancer.

melanocyte: a special cell in the epidermis layer of the skin that produces melanin, a pigment giving color to the skin, hair, and the eyes.

pressure sore or ulcer: break or opening in the skin due to a reduction in blood flow; decubitus ulcer.

radiation therapy: a treatment used for certain types of cancers which may kill normal and abnormal cells.

second-degree burn: burn involving the epidermis and the dermis.

shearing: pressure from sliding skin across another surface.

third-degree burn: burn involving the epidermis, dermis, tissue, and possibly muscle and bone.

wart: rough, hard bump on the skin that may be white, yellow, brown, or black; caused by a virus and very contagious.

2 Summarize the changes that occur in the skin during normal aging.

As the skin ages, the amount of collagen decreases, and the elastic fibers lose elasticity, causing wrinkles. Hair and nail growth slows. Dry skin may occur because the oil glands decrease in size. Skin becomes thinner and more fragile. Gray hair is due to a decrease in the number of certain **melanocytes**. Age or "liver" spots may develop due to the increase in the size of another kind of melanocyte.

3 Name four common disorders of the integumentary system.

1. Contact Dermatitis

Contact dermatitis occurs when the skin in an area (e.g., the hands) begins to break down due to exposure to an irritating agent. For example, teachers sometimes develop a contact dermatitis to chalk after writing on the blackboard for a long time. There may be redness, itching, and skin lesions or breakdown.

CAUSE: Exposure of the skin to an agent that irritates it.

CURE/TREATMENT: Topical steroid creams and soothing or drying lotions prescribed by a **dermatologist** (a physician specializing in conditions of the skin) may help cure contact dermatitis. Avoiding the irritant is important.

The Risks of Steroid Creams

Sometimes residents have special steroid creams that are applied by the nurse on areas of the skin. It is very important for the nurse to wear gloves when applying a steroid cream. Residents should not apply this type of cream themselves. They also should not touch the area where the steroid cream has been applied for a period of time determined by the nurse. You must be careful about touching skin areas that have steroid cream on them.

The STAR KARE METHOD will be used for some disorders in the disorder sections in Chapters 24 through 34. Based on the acronym "KARE," this method teaches you to know the resident's plan of care, and how to assist the resident and nurse with specific types of care. It also includes the observations that should be made with each disorder, as well as serving as a reminder to promote and encourage residents' progress and independence.

KNOW
ASSIST
REPORT/RECORD/RECHECK
ENCOURAGE

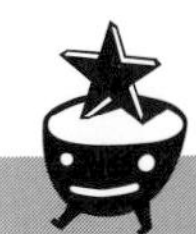

Star K.A.R.E.

Contact Dermatitis

***KNOW** your resident's care plan.*
***ASSIST** the resident/nurse.*

- *Help nurses determine the cause of the dermatitis.*
- *Reduce or eliminate exposure to agent causing dermatitis.*
- *Follow orders limiting harsh soaps and other products in area of dermatitis.*
- *Monitor vital signs carefully, especially temperature.*

***REPORT** observations.*
***RECORD** data.*
***RECHECK** resident as needed.*

If the following occurs:

- *worsening of dermatitis, severe itching, or pain*
- *signs of infection such as warmth, redness, swelling in area*
- *change in vital signs, especially fever*

★ *"Don't Delay. Report Right Away!"*

***ENCOURAGE** resident's independence and progress.*

2. Fungal Infections

Fungal infections, called tinea, occur anywhere on the body. They are most common in very moist areas such as the toes, under the breasts, and the groin area. Red, scaly patches, as well as itchy, raw, painful symptoms may occur. Jock itch is an example of a type of fungal infection in men and can spread from the groin area to the thighs.

If you're caring for a resident with a fungal infection, report any skin abrasions, flaking, redness, sores, or itching to the nurse.

CAUSE: Perspiration usually causes tinea to occur. Tinea can worsen in the summer, when we perspire too much, or when our body is too moist. Tight-fitting clothing may also cause tinea.

CURE/TREATMENT: Topical antifungal creams and antifungal drugs may help cure fungal infections.

3. Warts

Warts are quite common and are very contagious. Warts are caused by a virus that invades the skin, usually through a cut or tear in the skin. A wart is a rough, hard bump. The bump or bumps may be spongy-looking with red, yellow, brown, or black spots. They may spread to other areas of the body if not treated.

CAUSE: A virus causes warts. Children and people with weakened immune systems may be more prone to catching the wart virus.

CURE/TREATMENT: The doctor may prescribe medications to break down the wart. Sometimes, the wart is removed with a laser or a special instrument. It is important to wash hands frequently to try to prevent the spread of warts to other parts of the body.

4. Skin Cancer

Skin cancer is becoming more and more common in the United States, especially in the sunny areas. There are three kinds of skin cancer: malignant melanoma, squamous cell carcinoma, and basal cell carcinoma. **Malignant melanoma** is the worst form of skin cancer and can be fatal if left untreated. This means that a tiny spot of cancer on the arm, leg, face, or anywhere else could kill you or your residents if you do nothing about it.

CAUSE: One cause of the increasing rate of skin cancer may be the fact that people tanned in the 1960s and the 1970s. At that time sunscreens were not readily available or encouraged by doctors. Sometimes it can take many years for skin cancer to develop from the damage that was done in the past by the sun.

CURE/TREATMENT: If skin cancer is caught in the early stages, when it is still superficial, there is a much higher rate of recovery. Once diagnosis has been made, a larger area of skin is usually removed to make sure no cancerous cells remain beneath the skin surface. If the cancerous cells have spread to surrounding areas, further treatment may be necessary. Surgery may be performed and followed up with **chemotherapy** and **radiation therapy**.

Some tips on preventing skin cancer include:

- reducing or eliminating exposure to the sun and never allowing sunburn to occur
- wearing sunscreen, even on cloudy days
- wearing protective clothing, such as hats and long sleeves
- not risking sun exposure between the hours of about 10:00 a.m. and 3:00 p.m.

The ABCD's of Skin Cancer — Box 24-1

Every time you perform care for your residents, from toileting to bathing, examine their skin. Report any changes in their skin to the nurse right away. Watch for the following with moles:

A • Asymmetry (one half of the mole does not match the other half)

B • Border irregularity (the edges of the mole are blurred or ragged)

C • Color variation (shades of other colors, such as red, white, black, or brown may be seen)

D • Diameter: The mole is over six millimeters in size—the size of an eraser on a pencil.

Observing Residents' Skin: It is a Daily Duty!

How carefully do you look at the skin of your residents during bathing and dressing? LOOK at your residents' skin often! This is the only way to know how your residents' skin looks every day. Pressure sores, skin cancer, and contagious skin diseases, if caught early, could cause residents much less pain and misery.

Remember:

You alone see the skin of your residents on a regular basis.

You alone have the ability to report a tiny problem before it may become quite serious.

Do not allow one life to slip through your fingers!

Pressure sores are discussed in detail in Chapter 19 on skin care and will be further discussed in Learning Objective 6 in this chapter.

4 Describe the benefits and the risks of hot and cold applications.

Applications of heat or cold often have beneficial effects on an injury, an infection, or a fever. Some facilities do not allow nursing assistants to apply hot and cold applications. If your facility does allow this practice, make sure you carefully follow the order and the instructions of the nurse when performing one of these procedures. Hot or cold applications can be either moist or dry. Procedures will identify which are moist or dry.

When the body is exposed to hot or cold applications, it responds in different ways. Heat helps reduce pain and swelling, increases waste removal from the area, and increases blood flow to the application area. Increased blood flow brings more oxygen and nutrients to the tissues for healing. However, there are risks associated with hot applications. Heat can cause burns, make bleeding worse, and cause confusion, dizziness, or fainting due to a reduction of blood to the brain.

Cold applications are helpful in reducing bleeding and pain, preventing swelling, and bringing down high temperatures. Risks of cold applications include skin becoming cyanotic or pale, and chills and shivering. Lack of blood flow to the application area may damage tissue.

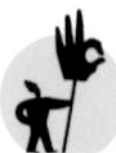

Hot Opens, Cold Closes

When using hot and cold applications, it is helpful to remember what happens with each kind of application. The following tip may help you remember the difference in the body's response to hot and cold:

Hot Opens (blood vessels) and Cold Closes (blood vessels)

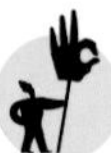

The 20-minute Rule

Hot and cold applications should not be applied for too long a period of time. When either a hot or a cold application is applied for too long, amazingly, the OPPOSITE effect occurs from what we desire. This means that if you leave an ice bag on for longer than 20 minutes, the blood vessels may actually start to open up again. This could increase bleeding and swelling at the injury site. So, remember to limit a hot or cold application to 20 minutes at a time, and then wait an hour before placing the application back on the skin. This allows the skin to rest for a period of time.

Remember, if the resident has non-intact skin or open sores, wear gloves when applying hot or cold applications. You should always wear gloves when assisting with a sitz bath. A sitz bath is a warm soak of the perineal area to clean perineal wounds and reduce inflammation and pain.

Applying Warm Compresses (Moist)

Follow all standard and/or transmission-based precautions. Follow all rules for body mechanics.

Collect equipment:

- **disposable bed protector • tape • towel**
- **compresses or washcloths • disposable plastic bag**
- **basin full of warm water, approximately 115°F**

1. **Perform the "5 Stars."**

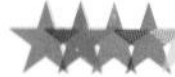

PREPARE:

2. **Ensuring privacy, adjust bed linen and clothing to only expose compress area.**
3. **Place bed protector under compress area.**
4. **Prepare compress supplies on clean, flat, dry surface.**

PERFORM:

5. Expose compress area.

6. Apply compress and wrap in plastic or towel as desired. Tape if desired.

7. Look at the time. Return and check every five minutes for signs of redness or blisters. Remove the compress if you find these signs or if the resident complains of pain or numbness.

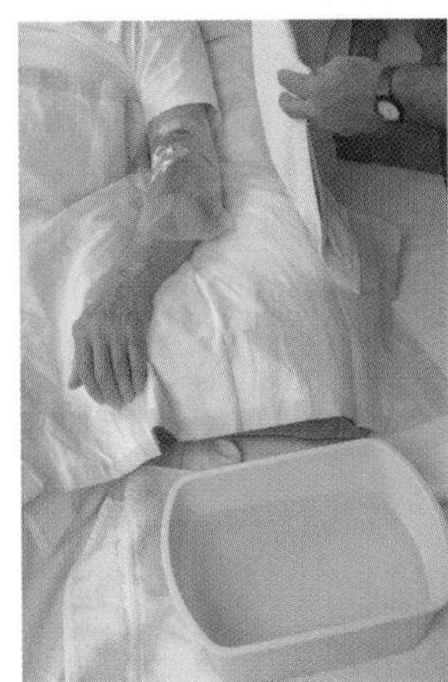
Figure 24-1.

8. Change compress as needed.

9. Return and remove compress after 20 minutes.

10. Replace clothing and linen and cover the resident.

11. SECURE THE RESIDENT.

12. Dispose of supplies.

FINISHING TOUCHES:

13. Perform the "5 Stars and 3 Rs."

Administering Warm Soaks (Moist)

Follow all standard and/or transmission-based precautions. Follow all rules for body mechanics.

Collect equipment:
- disposable bed protector • bath thermometer
- basin with warm water, approximately 100°F • two towels

1. Perform the "5 Stars."

PREPARE:

2. Ensuring privacy, remove bed linen and position comfortably for soak.

PERFORM:

3. Check water temperature with bath thermometer.

4. Place body part carefully in hot soak. Pad the edge of the basin with a towel if needed.

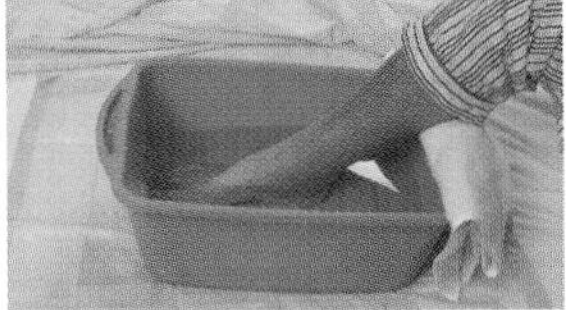
Figure 24-2.

5. Look at the time. Return and check every five minutes for signs of redness or blisters. Remove the body part from the soak if you find these signs or if the resident complains of pain or numbness.

6. Top off soak with warm water as needed.

7. Return and remove body part after 20 minutes. Use the second towel to dry the resident.

8. Replace clothing and linen and cover the resident.

9. SECURE THE RESIDENT.

10. Dispose of supplies.

FINISHING TOUCHES:

11. Perform the "5 Stars and 3 Rs."

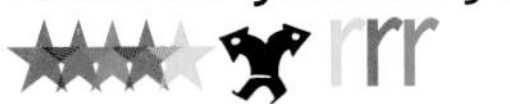

Assisting with a Sitz Bath (Moist)

Follow all standard and/or transmission-based precautions. Follow all rules for body mechanics.

Collect equipment:
- two pairs of disposable gloves • disposable sitz bath kit
- two towels • bath thermometer

1. Perform the "5 Stars."

PREPARE:

2. Apply gloves.

3. Set up sitz bath on toilet seat in bathroom. Fill the sitz bath two-thirds full with hot water. Water temperature should be approximately 100°F–104°F. Check water temperature with bath thermometer.

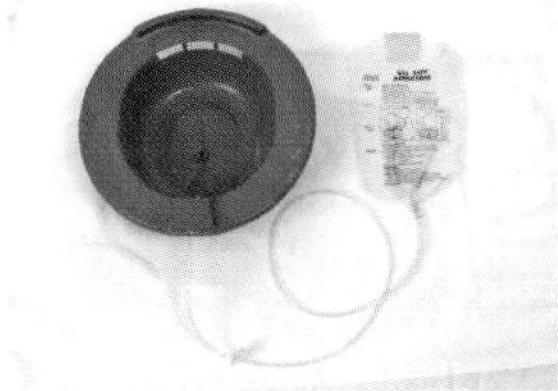

Figure 24-3.

4. Ensuring privacy, remove pants, and assist in seating the resident comfortably on the sitz bath.

PERFORM:

5. Unclamp tubing and allow sitz bath to begin. A valve on the tubing connected to the bag allows the resident or you to add hot water to water in the sitz bath.

6. You may be required to stay with the resident during the bath for safety reasons. If you leave the room, check on the resident every five minutes to make sure she is not faint or dizzy due to blood rushing to the perineal area.

7. Remove from sitz bath after 20 minutes or when ordered. Provide towels and assistance in drying resident.

8. Assist resident in returning to bed and replacing clothing and linen. Cover and secure the resident.

9. Dispose of supplies and remove gloves.

FINISHING TOUCHES:

10. Perform the "5 Stars and 3 Rs."

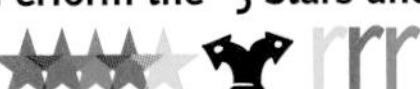

Using an Aquamatic Pad (Dry)

Follow all standard and/or transmission-based precautions. Follow all rules for body mechanics.

Collect equipment:
- Aquamatic pad and control unit • cover or pillowcase

Unit should already be properly filled with water by the nurse or Central Supply.

1. Perform the "5 Stars."

PREPARE:

2. Ensuring privacy, adjust bed linen to only expose area for hot pad.
3. Place the pad in the cover. Do not pin the pad. Turn pad on and allow to heat.

PERFORM:

4. Carefully place aquamatic pad in appropriate spot.
5. Place main unit on clean, flat, dry surface so that it is even in height with pad on bed. Make sure the tubing is not hanging below the level of the bed.

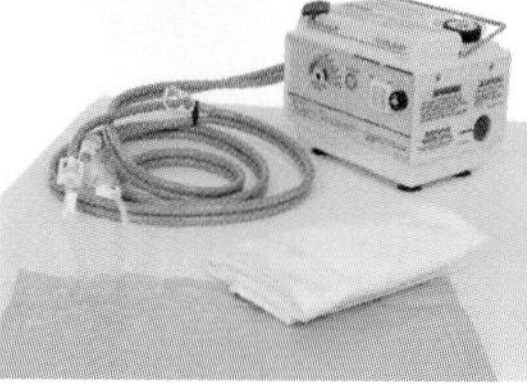

Figure 24-4.

6. Secure resident in comfortable spot with pad in place.
7. Look at the time. Return and check every five minutes for signs of redness or blisters. Remove the pad if you find these signs or if the resident complains of pain or numbness.
8. Return and remove pad after 20 minutes.
9. Replace gown or pajamas and cover the resident.
10. SECURE THE RESIDENT.
11. Dispose of supplies.

FINISHING TOUCHES:

12. Perform the "5 Stars and 3 Rs."

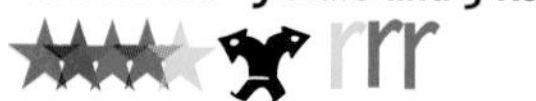

Applying an Ice Bag (Dry)

Follow all standard and/or transmission-based precautions. Follow all rules for body mechanics.

Collect equipment:
- disposable bed protector • two towels
- ice bag two-thirds full of crushed ice • flannel cover

Crushed ice molds better to the skin than ice cubes.

1. Perform the "5 Stars."

PREPARE:

2. Ensuring privacy, adjust bed linen and lift gown or pull down pajamas to only expose area to be treated.
3. Place bed protector under area to be treated.

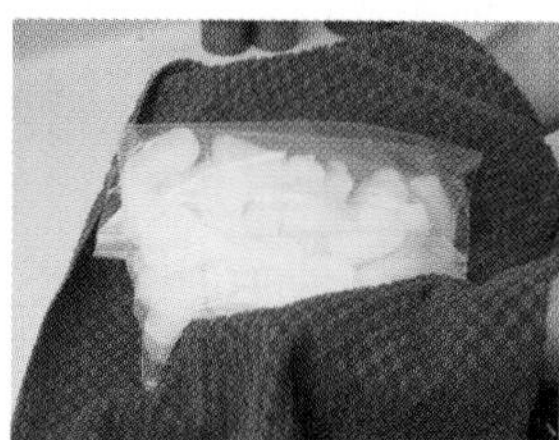

Figure 24-5.

PERFORM:

4. Wrap ice bag in flannel cover or towel (Figure 24-5).
5. Apply ice bag to the area.
6. Look at the time. Return and check every five minutes for signs of blisters or pale, white, or gray skin. Remove the bag if you find these signs or if the resident complains of pain or numbness.
7. Return and remove ice bag after 20 minutes.
8. Replace clothing and linen and cover the resident.
9. SECURE THE RESIDENT.
10. Dispose of supplies.

FINISHING TOUCHES:

11. Perform the "5 Stars and 3 Rs."

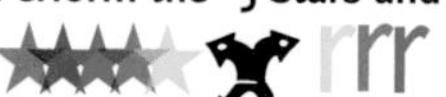

Giving a Cold Sponge Bath (Moist)

Follow all standard and/or transmission-based precautions. Follow all rules for body mechanics.

Collect equipment:
- two pairs of disposable gloves • disposable bed protectors
- flannel covers or washcloths • extra washcloths
- bath basin two-thirds full of water • ice chips
- ice bags two-thirds full of ice chips • towels
- equipment for vital signs

1. Perform the "5 Stars."

PREPARE:

2. Apply gloves.

PERFORM:

3. Take baseline set of vital signs.
4. Ensuring privacy, remove bed linen.
5. Pad bed with disposable bed protectors.

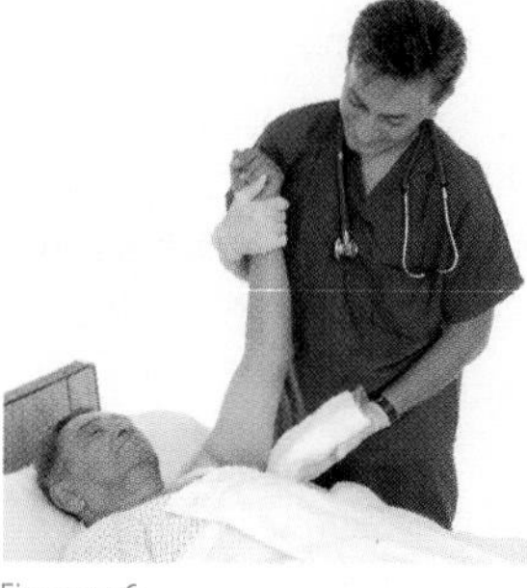

Figure 24-6.

6. Only expose areas for ice bags to be placed. Keep the rest of the body covered to avoid chills. Some spots for the ice bags are underarms and the groin. Make sure all ice bags are covered.
7. Place basin nearby on flat surface and wet washcloth.
8. Pad area under top of body with towels. Sponge each arm, then the chest and abdomen.

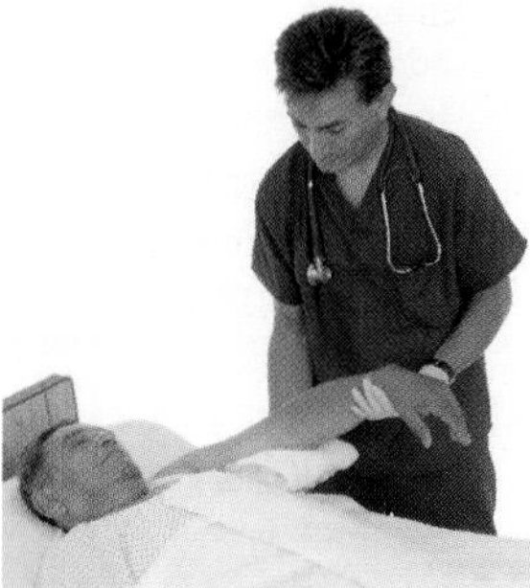

Figure 24-7.

Dry by patting areas if directed to do so.

9. Take a second set of vital signs. Check the sponged skin for signs of blisters or pale, white, or gray skin. Stop bath if resident complains of numbness or pain or if directed to do so by the nurse.

10. Pad area under bottom half of the body with towels. Sponge each leg, then the back. Dry by patting areas if directed to do so.

11. Take a third set of vital signs. Check the sponged skin for signs of blisters or pale, white, or gray skin. Stop bath if resident complains of numbness or pain or if directed to do so by the nurse.

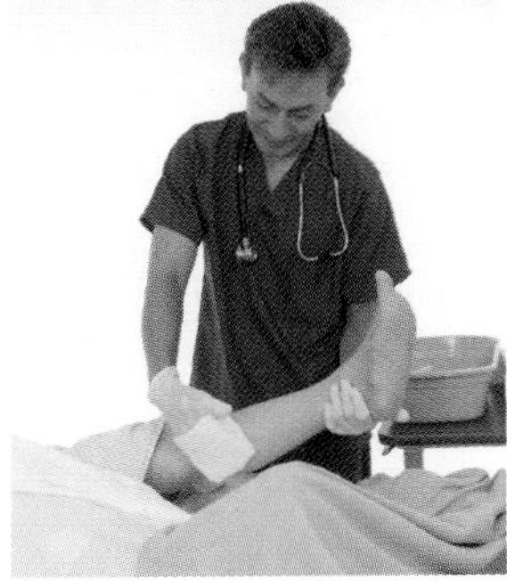

Figure 24-8.

12. Remove the ice bags. Dry all skin completely.

13. Remove all towels and bed protectors, apply clean gown, and change linen as needed.

14. Replace clothing and linen and cover the resident.

15. SECURE THE RESIDENT.

16. Dispose of supplies and remove gloves.

FINISHING TOUCHES:

17. Perform the "5 Stars and 3 Rs."

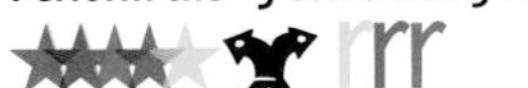

5 Describe care of a resident with a burn.

When caring for a resident with burns, be very careful not to cause any additional pain. This can only be accomplished with a solid understanding of how to plan for your resident's care ahead of time. For example, prior to care it may be necessary for you to arrange a time with the nurse to have the resident's pain medication given. That way, it takes effect before you begin the care.

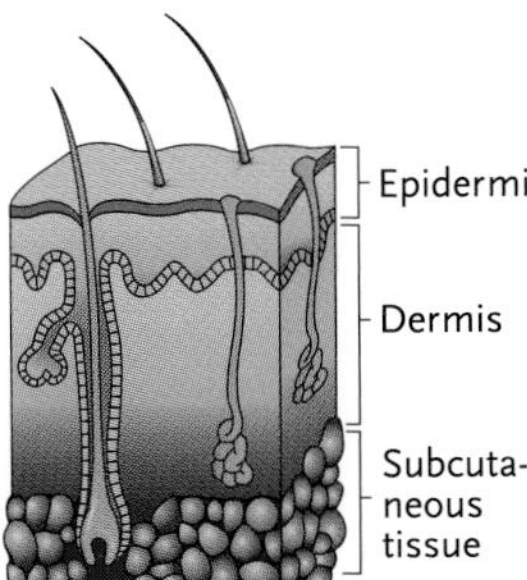

Figure 24-9.

When caring for a resident with burns, you may be asked to assist the nurse with dressing care. It is important to have a thorough understanding of the care required for burns before you attempt to assist. You may attend an in-service or special training in order to work with people who have burns.

When a burn occurs, there is a varying degree of skin damage. The different degrees of burns follow:

Degree	Layer of Skin Involved	Damage
First Degree	Epidermis (Outer layer)	Usually none or minor
Second Degree	Dermis (Deeper layer)	Some skin damage and scarring
Third Degree	Epidermis, dermis, and underlying tissue	Serious scarring; muscle and bone may be affected

Star K.A.R.E.

Caring for a Burn

***KNOW** your resident's care plan.*
***ASSIST** the resident/nurse.*

- *Notify the nurse at least 30 minutes prior to care in case pain medication should be given.*
- *Take great care when moving and positioning resident to reduce pain and chance of damaging dressing.*
- *Use any special protective devices, such as pads or special mattresses or beds, as ordered.*
- *Follow instructions regarding I & O measurement.*
- *Follow diet order carefully and encourage fluids and eating tray/nourishments.*

***REPORT** observations*
***RECORD** data*
***RECHECK** resident as needed.*

- *If the following occurs:*
  - *pus or other fluid around burn areas*
  - *blood in IV tubing*
  - *pain*
  - *decrease in appetite or I & O*

★ *"Don't Delay. Report Right Away!"*

***ENCOURAGE** resident's progress.*

- *Provide support; burns can be very painful and disturbing.*

6 Describe care of the resident with a pressure sore.

A **pressure sore** is an ulcer resulting from skin deterioration (breaking up) from pressure and **shearing** (pressure from sliding skin across another surface). Eventually, blood does not circulate properly and sores or ulcers form, swell, and may become infected, causing damage to underlying tissue. Pressure sores are also referred to as **decubitus ulcers**, bed sores, and pressure ulcers.

Pressure sores are a common problem in long-term care. If they are caught early enough, a break or tear in the skin can heal fairly quickly without other complications. One complication is poor circulation. If a cut or skin tear is not treated in the early stages, the cut may turn into a pressure sore.

Because you are in the best position to observe for signs of pressure sores, inspect your resident's skin every time you provide care. If you observe any of these signs, notify the nurse immediately.

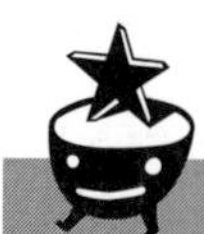

Star K.A.R.E.

Caring for a Pressure Sore

KNOW your resident's care plan.
ASSIST the resident/nurse.

- *Change position as ordered, but at least every two hours.*
- *Avoid rubbing skin against linen or other surfaces, which causes shearing, or tearing of skin..*
- *Ask every resident in a wheelchair or any other chair to change position frequently. Follow facility policy on the frequency of this practice.*
- *Perform range of motion exercises as ordered.*
- *Offer backrubs daily if allowed.*
- *Keep linen dry and free of wrinkles and lumps of any kind.*
- *Use special pads or other equipment or devices to help reduce pressure as ordered.*
- *Use pillows to separate skin surfaces.*
- *Follow diet and fluid order carefully and encourage fluids.*
- *Perform excellent skin care all through the day and night and clean and dry skin immediately after each episode of incontinence.*
- *Use lukewarm water to bathe residents.*
- *Take great care when touching resident's skin; the resident's skin can tear very easily.*
- *Prevent irritation to any area on the skin; wearing anything foreign, such as an oxygen delivery device or an armboard for an IV, can irritate and cause sores.*
- *Never get the pressure sore area or dressing site wet.*
- *Use lubricants as ordered on unbroken skin.*
- *Use powder as directed in creases and folds of skin.*
- *Follow directions when using ANY cream, lotion, soap, or other cosmetic or product on skin that has a pressure sore.*

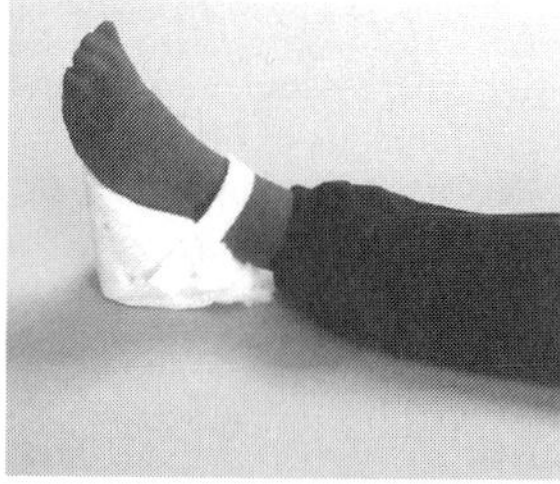

Figure 24-10. Heel and elbow protectors made of foam and sheepskin may be used.

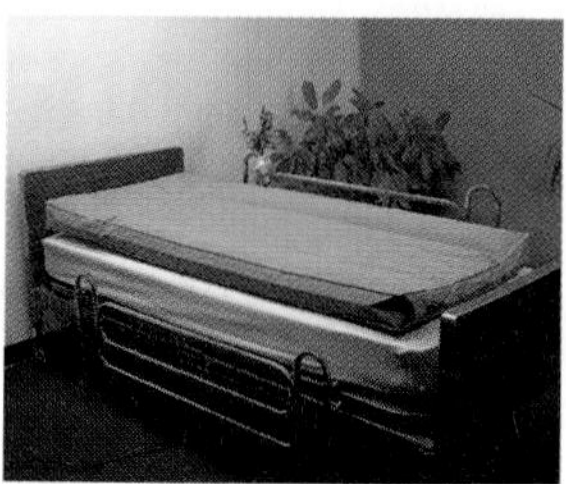

Figure 24-11. Flotation pads are made of a gel-like substance encased in heavy plastic.

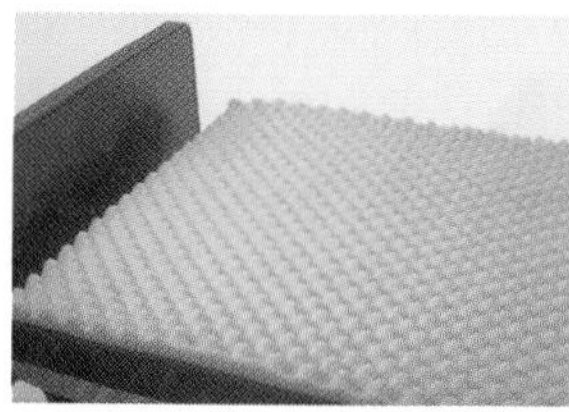

Figure 24-12. An egg crate mattress is made of foam and looks like an egg carton. It is placed on top of a regular mattress to distribute weight more evenly.

REPORT observations
RECORD data
RECHECK resident as needed.

If the following occurs:

- *warm, reddened areas on the skin that do not go away when pressure is relieved*
- *skin that is cyanotic (a bluish color)*
- *dry, cracked, flaking, or torn skin*
- *blisters or sores on the skin*
- *rashes*
- *itching*
- *swelling*
- *new wounds or ulcers on the skin*
- *any wetness on the skin*

★ *"Don't Delay. Report Right Away!"*

ENCOURAGE resident's progress.

- *Encourage fluids and good nutrition.*
- *Encourage movement to increase circulation.*

7 Discuss safety precautions used to prevent damage to a dressing site during care.

Open wounds increase a resident's risk for infection. The intact or closed skin surface cannot easily be invaded by dangerous microorganisms. Open cuts or breaks in the skin may be a "port" for bacteria and other microorganisms to sneak into the body. It is very important to follow instructions carefully when caring for residents who have any kind of open wound. Residents and staff members can accidentally poke or jab wounds with furniture, utensils, fingernails, and other objects.

Sometimes dressings are used to cover and protect wounds from the many dangers around them. Wounds are also covered to prevent residents and visitors from becoming uncomfortable with the site of a wound, especially at the time when it looks its worst. There are three main things for you to remember. Take care not to:

- further damage the wound area
- damage the dressing or tape
- cause pain to the resident

Never hesitate to point out to a nurse or doctor how fragile a resident's skin really is!

Have you ever seen anyone remove a dressing or a bandage too quickly, causing pain? If this is done to an elderly person, it may not only cause pain, but the entire piece of skin may come off with the dressing! An elderly person's skin is extremely fragile, and the removal of dressings and tape must be done carefully. Do not hesitate to remind someone about this.

8 Identify the differences between sterile and non-sterile dressings.

Sterile dressings are required when a resident's wound is fresh, and the healing process has recently begun. They are also required when there is a greater risk of an infection occurring.

Non-sterile dressings are utilized when the wound has healed for a period of time or when the risk of infection is not as high. Nursing assistants may be asked to assist with sterile and non-sterile dressings. It is important for you to know the correct methods to perform each procedure. Sterile gloves will be used for sterile dressing care, and usually, non-sterile gloves will be used for non-sterile dressing care. A sterile field—the area that is kept sterile—is created with sterile dressing care.

Nursing assistants must make sure not to contaminate the sterile field and the sterile gloves. If any part of the sterile field becomes contaminated, the entire process must be started again. This can cause the resident great pain, discomfort, and emotional upset.

The History of the Rubber Glove

William Halsted developed rubber gloves to protect the hands of his nurse (and future wife) in the early 20th century. A student suggested the surgeons adopt them. The gloves were very thick, though, and many surgeons would not wear them. Some surgeons actually wore cloth gloves over the rubber. Over the years, gradually, rubber gloves became thinner and easier to wear. Today's gloves are usually latex.

Assisting the Nurse with Non-Sterile Dressing Care

Follow all standard and/or transmission-based precautions. Follow all rules for body mechanics.

Collect equipment:

• two pairs of disposable gloves • disposable bed protector • tape • non-sterile dressings • disposable plastic bag

1. **Perform the "5 Stars."**

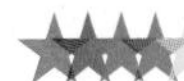

Ask if resident has any latex or tape allergies.

PREPARE:

2. **Apply gloves.**
3. **Ensuring privacy, remove bed linen and lift gown or pull down pajamas to only expose dressing area.**
4. **Turn resident to side, place bed protector under resident and return to back.**
5. **Prepare dressing supplies on clean, flat, dry surface.**

PERFORM:

6. **Assist the nurse as he carefully removes the tape and the old dressing and places it in the plastic bag.**
7. **Wait until nurse inspects and/or measures the wound.**

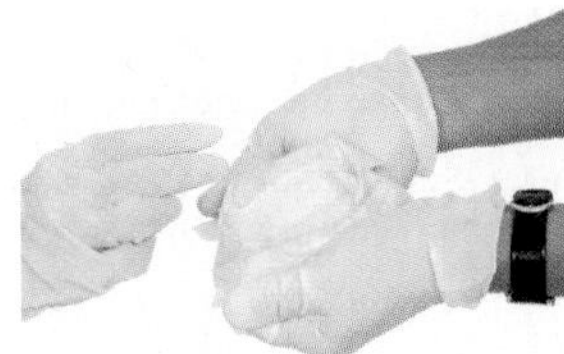

Figure 24-13.

8. **Assist the nurse as he applies a clean, dry dressing.**
9. **Replace clothing and cover the resident.**
10. **Dispose of supplies and remove gloves.**

FINISHING TOUCHES:

11. **Perform the "5 Stars and 3 Rs."**

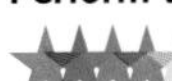 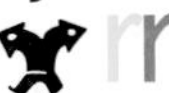

Applying Sterile Gloves

Follow all standard and/or transmission-based precautions. Follow all rules for body mechanics.

Collect equipment:
- **two pairs of sterile gloves in your size**

(Make sure you are not allergic to latex or to the powder inside most sterile gloves.)

PREPARE:

1. **Wash your hands.**
2. **Prepare gloves on clean, flat, dry surface.**

PERFORM:

3. **Remove outer wrapper from gloves and place inner wrapper on clean, dry, flat surface. The word LEFT should be on your left side and the word RIGHT should be on your right side.**
4. **Slowly and carefully open the inner wrapper, being cautious only to touch the small flaps of the wrapper.**
5. **The gloves will be placed palm-side up with cuffs in place. Pick up the first glove by the bottom end of the cuff.**
6. **Slip your fingers into the glove. If you make a mistake and fingers are not in their places, do not try to fix the fingers at this point. If you touch one of the sterile gloves on the outside, it is contaminated. You will then have to start over. Wait to fix it until the second glove is on your other hand.**

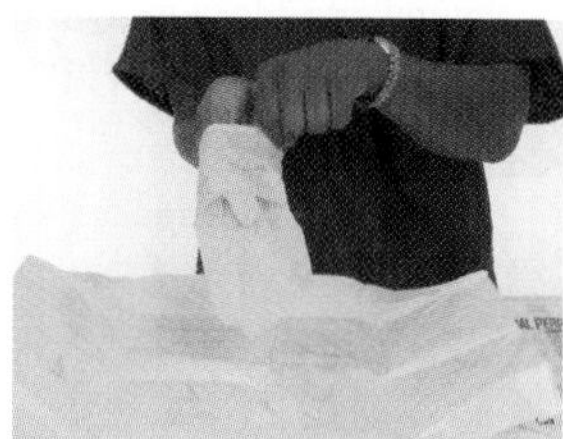

Figure 24-14.

7. **Slip your gloved hand into the second glove in the area under the cuff.**
8. **Slowly slip the fingers of your ungloved hand into the second glove, and pull it completely over your hand and wrist.**

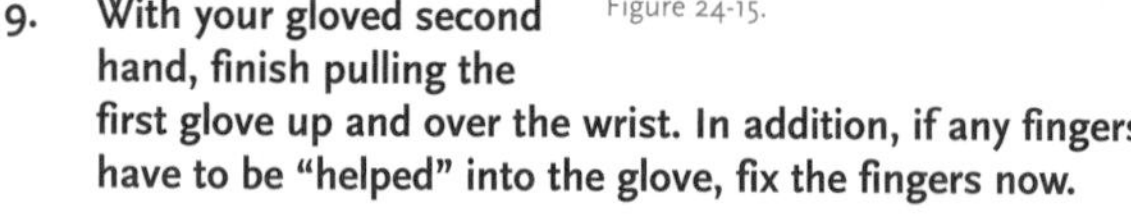

Figure 24-15.

9. **With your gloved second hand, finish pulling the first glove up and over the wrist. In addition, if any fingers have to be "helped" into the glove, fix the fingers now.**
10. **If either glove has a tear in it, STOP and start again with the second set of sterile gloves.**
11. **Always keep your gloved hands above the level of your waist at all times during the procedure.**
12. **Perform the sterile procedure.**

Assisting the Nurse with Sterile Dressing Care

Follow all standard and/or transmission-based precautions. Follow all rules for body mechanics.

Collect equipment:
- **two pairs of gloves, one sterile and one clean**
- **disposable bed protector • tape, sterile dressings**
- **disposable plastic bag**

1. **Perform the "5 Stars."**

Ask if resident has any latex or tape allergies.

PREPARE:

2. **Apply gloves.**
3. **Ensuring privacy, adjust bed linen and clothing to only expose dressing area.**
4. **Turn resident to side, place bed protector under resident, and return resident to back.**
5. **Assist in the preparation of dressing supplies on clean, flat, dry surface. This becomes the sterile field.**

PERFORM:

6. **Assist the nurse as she carefully removes the tape and the old sterile dressing and places it in the plastic bag.**
7. **Wait until nurse inspects and/or measures the wound.**
8. **Assist the nurse to apply a clean, dry, sterile dressing.**
   a. **Put on sterile gloves using sterile technique.**
   b. **Open sterile packages as needed following sterile technique.**
   c. **Dispose of any supplies as needed.**
9. **Replace clothing and linen and cover the resident.**
10. **Secure resident.**
11. **Dispose of supplies and remove gloves.**

FINISHING TOUCHES:

12. **Perform the "5 Stars and 3 Rs."**

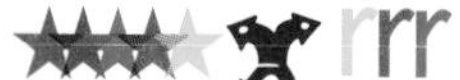

Summary

The integumentary system is the largest organ in the body: the skin. The skin acts as a barrier to the outside world. If that barrier is broken, all of the dangerous microorganisms that lurk out in the world are able to get inside the body. Changes in the skin can alert us to problems inside the body. Good, healthy skin may make people look and feel better about themselves. It is important to carefully observe the skin to watch for any changes that put the residents at risk, especially with pressure sores.

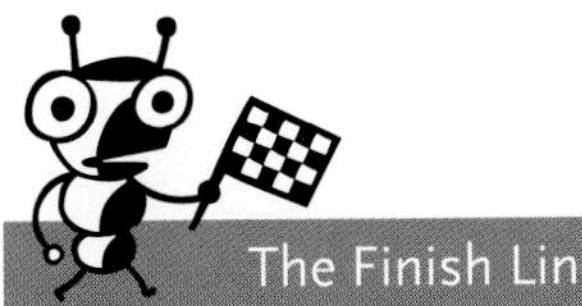

The Finish Line

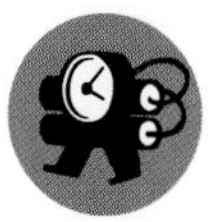

What's Wrong With This Picture?

1. Look at the equipment listed for Assisting the Nurse with Sterile Dressing Care, shown below. List the missing piece of equipment.

Collect equipment:
- **two pairs of gloves, one sterile and one clean**
- **disposable bed protector • sterile dressings**
- **disposable plastic bag**

2. Look at the equipment listed for Applying Warm Compresses, shown below. List the missing piece of equipment.

Collect equipment:
- **basin full of warm water • tape**
- **compresses or washcloths • towel • disposable plastic bag**

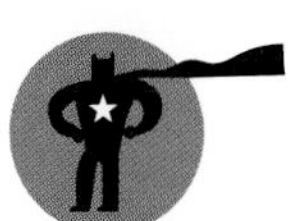

Star Student Central

1. Find out if your area has a Shriner's Hospital. These hospitals provide free care for children who have serious illnesses or injuries such as burns. Make an appointment to visit and tour a Shriner's Hospital with your group. It may be a truly inspirational experience.
2. Go to your **dermatologist** or family practice physician and ask for pamphlets on the risk of skin cancer, especially malignant melanoma. This information can be shared with your class, your family, and your friends.

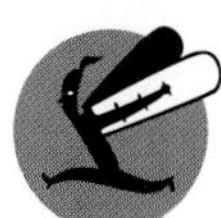

You Can Do It Corner!

1. Identify three risks of both hot and cold applications and the suggested length of time for each. (LO 4)
2. Explain what you would do if the fingers of the first hand get "messed up" when inserting them into a sterile glove. (LO 8)
3. What are three things to remember when trying to prevent damage to a dressing site? (LO 7)
4. What are four signs and symptoms to observe with moles? (LO 3)
5. Name five normal changes of aging that occur with the integumentary system. (LO 2)
6. What are four things to observe and report while caring for resident with a burn? (LO 5)
7. Name ten ways you can assist the resident who has a pressure sore. (LO 6)

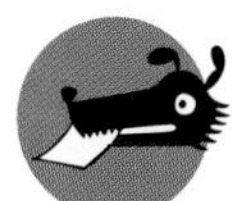

Star Student's Chapter Checklist

1. I have read my textbook chapter.
2. I have reviewed my own "Pocketful of Terms."
3. I have listened to my tutor tape.
4. I have reviewed and highlighted my class notes
5. I have read and completed any handouts from this chapter.
6. I have completed "The Finish Line."
7. Star Time! Choose your reward!

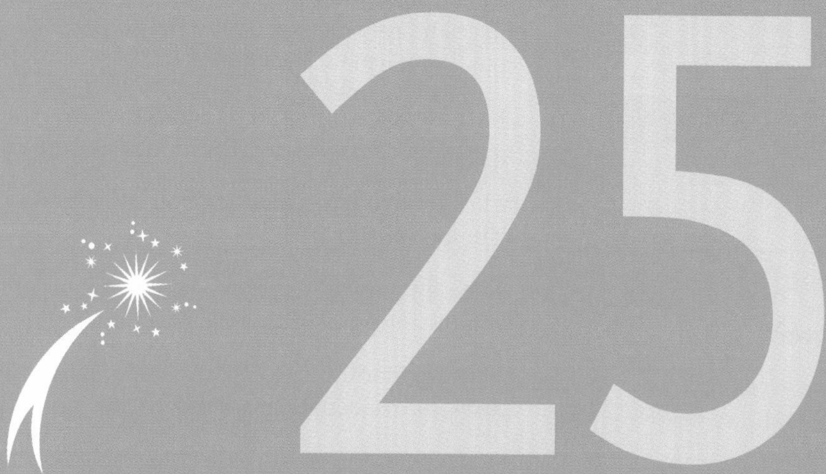

Specialized Care: The Muscular System

Look Like a Star!

Look at the Learning Objectives and The Finish Line before you begin reading this chapter.

Look at your pocket calendar.
With your pencil, put a bracket ( ) around a study period every single day.

Look at your homework for this chapter.
Plug each piece of homework into a certain time slot.

Look at the Star Student's Chapter Checklist at the end of this chapter. Check off each item as it is completed.

"In life's small things be resolute and great. To keep thy muscle trained."

James Russell Lowell 1819-1891

"And the muscular strength. . . has lasted the rest of my life."

Lewis Carroll, 1832-1898 from *Alice's Adventures in Wonderland*

Learning Objectives

1. **Spell and define all STAR words.**
2. **Identify two ways to protect your resident's muscular system.**
3. **Summarize the changes that occur in muscles during normal aging.**
4. **Name two common disorders of the muscular system.**
5. **Explain the difference between sprains and strains.**
6. **Explain guidelines for care of a muscle injury as described in the acronym "RICE."**

Successfully perform this Practical Procedure

Applying Elastic Bandages

Do muscles really create electricity?

In the 18th century, people began examining muscles and nerves and the way electrical activity affected them. Muscle contraction creates both heat and electrical activity. Luigi Galvi [1737- 1798] performed experiments using metal connected to a machine that actually caused the contraction of muscles.
Later, Carlo Malleucci [1811-1868] identified the fact that muscular contraction and electrical activity were always related. He accomplished this by performing experiments using the nerves of frogs. This enabled the development of methods to treat types of disorders.

1 Spell and define all **STAR** words.

atrophy: a wasting, weakening, or decrease in size of a muscle due to disease, injury, or lack of use.

contracture: a permanent shortening of the muscle.

elastic bandage: bandage used to compress and wrap an injured area, hold the extremity in place, and try to reduce pain and discomfort.

muscular dystrophy: hereditary disease causing destruction, wasting away, and atrophy of muscle.

RICE: acronym which stands for rest, ice, compression, and elevation.

sprain: condition in which the ligaments connecting the bones tear or stretch too much.

strain: trauma to the muscle due to stretching.

2 Identify two ways to protect your resident's muscular system.

The following guidelines can help your residents maintain a healthy muscular system and reduce the risk of injury.

Body mechanics: Teach your residents to use good body mechanics. Body mechanics is discussed in detail in Chapter 17. If you see residents reaching for something, offer to get the object for them. Reaching devices can also assist residents. If they do lift something, encourage them to bend at the knees while lifting. This reduces pressure on the lower back.

Exercise and movement: Regular exercise and movement helps prevent physical problems and disease. It improves mental state, and also increases circulation of blood, oxygen, and nutrients and improves muscle tone. Encourage movement and exercise for residents who are able.

If a resident is confined to bed, he may have range of motion exercises ordered. If you assist with these exercises, encourage the resident's participation, allowing him to do as much as possible for himself.

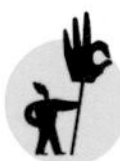

Personal Health Tip!

Have you ever "wrenched" your neck? Your neck and back are very fragile structures. People often reach without taking the time to get a sturdy stool to avoid reaching. When we reach for things, we put the muscles and nerves in our neck and back at risk. Find a stool or a sturdy chair if you need to reach for something. It only takes a minute to find a stool; it could take weeks or more to heal a neck or shoulder injury. It is also a possibility that the injury will never heal, and the person may suffer with the pain for years afterward.

3 Summarize the changes that occur in muscles during normal aging.

As people age, muscles tend to lose muscle tone and overall strength. People may also lose weight due to the loss of muscle mass in the body. Muscle weighs more than fat, so the percentage of weight lost is generally greater with a progressive loss of muscle. In addition, the person's ability to respond to circumstances diminishes. For example, an older person's ability to respond quickly to another car darting in front of his car may be reduced due to slowed muscle reflexes. This problem could be compounded by visual changes, causing poor eyesight, and hearing changes, reducing hearing ability.

Da Vinci: The REAL Father of Anatomy?

Leonardo da Vinci dissected more than 30 bodies by the light of candles in a mortuary in Rome. He spent a great deal of time studying the muscle system and came to understand each muscle's action. Had his notebooks, which simply lay gathering dust for over 200 years, actually been found earlier, they may have given HIM the title "Father of Anatomy" instead of Andreas Vesalius [1514-1563].

4 Name two common disorders of the muscular system.

1. Muscular Dystrophy

Muscular dystrophy is a hereditary disease that destroys muscle tissue. The muscles atrophy, causing various degrees of disability. Muscle **atrophy** means the muscle wastes away, decreases in size, and becomes weak. People with this disorder have muscle weakness and may be confined to a wheelchair.

CAUSE: Muscular dystrophy is a genetic disorder caused by a specific gene. Duchenne's muscular dystrophy is a disorder that is more common in males. The gene for this disorder is found on the X chromosome.

CURE/TREATMENT: At the present time, there is no cure for muscular dystrophy. Genetic breakthroughs have been made. For example, the muscular dystrophy gene that occurs on the X chromosome has now been identified. Finding the genes for these types of disorders may allow researchers to develop therapy or find a cure.

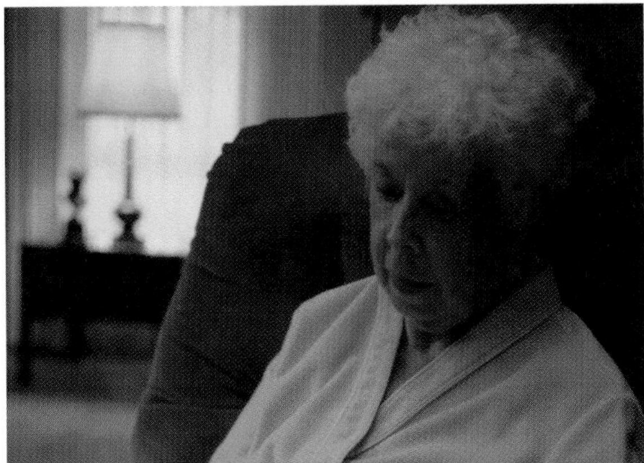

Figure 25-1. **Encouraging movement and exercise helps prevent atrophy and contractures and promotes a good mental state.**

Star K.A.R.E.

Muscular Dystrophy

KNOW your resident's care plan.
ASSIST the resident/nurse.

- *Allow enough time for the person to move about with braces or in wheelchair.*
- *Give excellent skin care.*
- *Reposition resident as ordered to help prevent pressure sores or contractures.*
- *Perform range of motion exercises as directed.*

REPORT observations
RECORD data
RECHECK resident as needed.

If the following occurs:

- *red skin, pale skin, or the start of a pressure sore*
- *the start of a contracture*
- *pain, swelling, or burning in a leg, especially the lower leg and the calf*
- *uncontrolled bleeding*
- *urinary tract infections*
- *signs of pneumonia, such as fever, chills, cough, and chest pains*

★ *"Don't Delay. Report Right Away!"*

ENCOURAGE resident's independence and progress.

- *Encourage independence with activities of daily living to the fullest extent possible so functioning muscles will not atrophy.*

2. Contractures

When a **contracture** develops, the muscle shortens, becomes inflexible, and "freezes" in position, causing permanent disability of the limb.

CAUSE: When muscles are not used, contractures develop. In addition to lack of exercise and movement, they occur as a result of improper support and positioning of joints. Contractures are very painful and contribute to skin breakdown.

CURE/TREATMENT: Preventing contractures before they happen is most important. Scheduled assistance with range of motion exercises and frequent positioning changes help prevent contractures.

5 Explain the difference between sprains and strains.

Muscle sprains and strains are fairly common injuries. A **sprain** occurs when the ligaments, which are the tissues that connect bones together, tear or stretch too much. If there is repeated extreme stretching, there is an increased risk of repeated sprains. A **strain** occurs when muscle tissue, which contracts so that bones may move, partially tears. Sprains and strains may be more painful in the long-term than broken bones.

Both of these injuries require a course of treatment and follow-up care. It is important that your residents treat these injuries promptly. Delaying treatment can cause worse damage and prevent the injury from healing as rapidly.

6 Explain guidelines for care of a muscle injury as described in the acronym "RICE."

Use the acronym "**RICE**" to help prevent further injury and support the healing process when a resident sustains a muscle injury.

RICE

Rest: Rest is vital in the healing process. Putting any weight on the injury could cause more harm.

Ice: Ice is important in the prevention and reduction of swelling. The skin should always be protected when using ice.

Compression: **Elastic bandages** are used to compress the injured area, hold the extremity in place, and try to reduce pain and discomfort. In addition, elastic bandages may decrease the tissue swelling that occurs with an injury. When using elastic bandages, it is important for you to not wrap the bandage too tightly. The person with the elastic

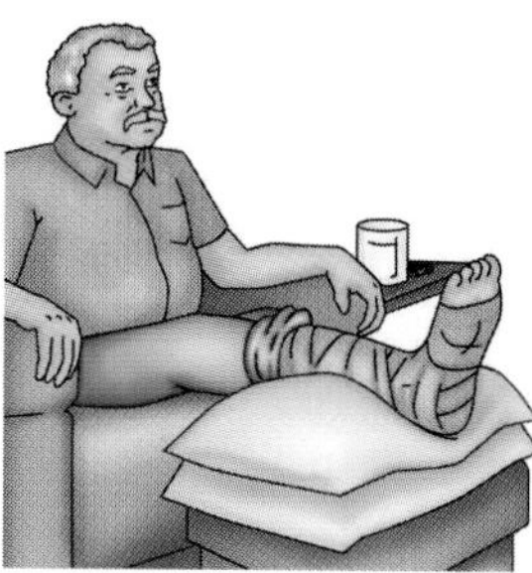
Figure 25-2.

bandage should be checked about 15 minutes after the bandage is first applied. At this time, you need to determine if the bandage needs to be re-wrapped. You must decide if the bandage is wrapped just right, or is too loose or too tight for the person's comfort.

Elevation: The extremity should be elevated, which may also help reduce or prevent swelling. When an extremity is elevated above the level of the heart, the swelling may decrease.

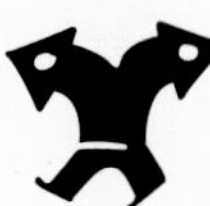
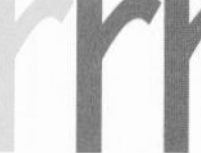

Beginning Steps

★ RESPECT
Knock first, ask and receive permission to enter a resident's room.

★ INFECTION CONTROL
Wash hands.

★ COMMUNICATION
Greet and identify the resident. Identify yourself. Explain the procedure, encouraging the resident to be as independent as possible throughout.

★ BED SAFETY
Lock bed wheels. Raise bed to safe working height. Lower one side rail if required.

★ PRIVACY
Provide for privacy by closing the door and covering the resident appropriately.

Ending Steps

★ RESIDENT SAFETY AND COMFORT
Secure the resident, lowering the bed, and raising the side rails if ordered. Check that the resident is comfortable and properly aligned.

★ PRIVACY
Remove any added privacy measures, such as a drape or a privacy screen.

★ ESSENTIALS
Place the call light, fresh beverage, and other items within reach.

★ COURTESY
Ask the resident if he or she needs anything else. Say thank you and goodbye.

★ INFECTION CONTROL
Wash hands.

r **Report** your care and any important observations to the nurse.

r **Record** your care and any important information/observations such as vital signs in the appropriate place.

r **Recheck** your resident for any changes as directed by the nurse!

Don't leave home without it!

When you travel anywhere, consider packing an elastic bandage in your first aid kit. It may be handy when going on hikes, as you never know when you will twist your ankle or sustain a fall unexpectedly.

Applying Elastic Bandages

Follow all standard and/or transmission-based precautions. Follow all rules for body mechanics.

Collect equipment:
- **elastic bandage in the correct size**
- **clip, safety pin, or tape (if using self-closing bandage, these are not needed)**

1. **Perform the "5 Stars."**

PREPARE:

2. **Assist resident to get into the supine position.**

PERFORM:

3. **Expose the part to be bandaged.**
4. **Hold the bandage with the free end down and the roll upward.**
5. **Wrap extremity beginning at the spot furthest from the heart. Circulation returns toward the heart and this allows extra fluid to flow to the heart and leave the area. (For the wrist, begin wrapping at the injured hand. For the ankle, begin at the foot.)**

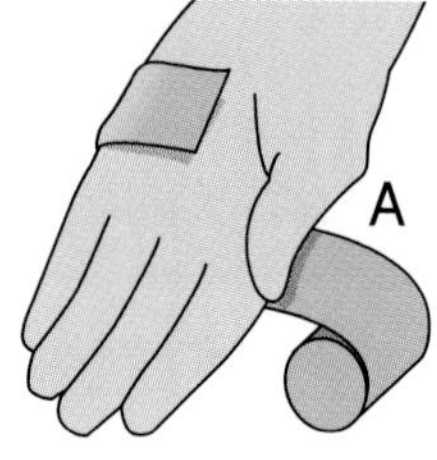

Figure 25-3.

6. **Wrap bandage once around the beginning spot and turn over the tip so that an anchor is made.**
7. **Wrap one more time around spot where anchor lies and then begin slowly wrapping.**
8. **Check for wrinkles and smooth entire bandage.**
9. **Secure bandage with self-closure, clip, safety pin, or tape. If using pin, take great care to NOT pierce the resident's skin.**

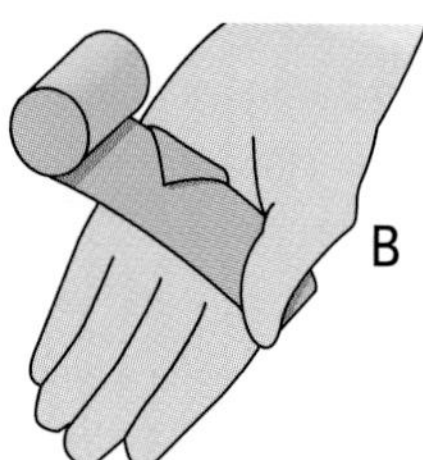

Figure 25-4.

FINISHING TOUCHES:

10. **Straighten all of the linens.**
11. **Perform the "5 Stars and 3 Rs."**

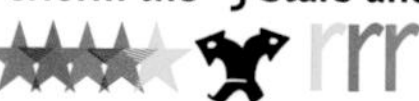

12. **Remove and re-apply bandage as directed. Wash and dry bandages as necessary.**

Summary

The function of the muscular system is to provide the body's movement. When a part of the muscular system is injured, there is usually quite a bit of pain involved. Muscle atrophy and contractures can be prevented by assisting with range of motion exercises and encouraging exercise and independence to promote muscle use. Ignored muscle injuries can worsen. Follow the plan of care closely, as well as any nurse's or doctor's orders. When an injury has been diagnosed, rest is very important in order to ensure proper healing.

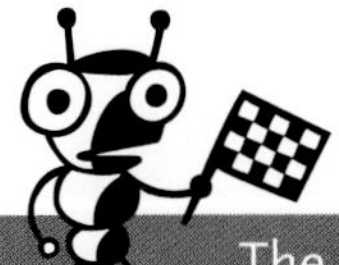

The Finish Line

What's Wrong With This Picture?

1. Look at the steps listed for Applying Elastic Bandages, shown below. Correct the incorrect step.

   Hold the bandage with the free end down and the roll upward.

   Wrap extremity, beginning at the spot closest to the heart. Circulation returns toward the heart and this allows extra fluid to flow to the heart and leave the area.

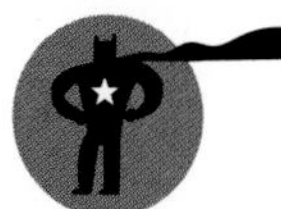

Star Student Central

1. Purchase an elastic bandage and practice wrapping it on a member of your family. This will help prepare you for the time when an injury occurs and you have to wrap an elastic bandage.
2. From the library, Internet, or your doctor's office, find more information on preventing muscle contractures and atrophy. Share this with your class.

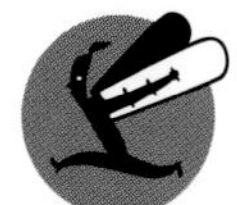

You Can Do It Corner!

1. What is the difference between a muscle sprain and a strain? (LO 5)
2. What are two ways you can protect your resident's muscular system? (LO 2)
3. What are contractures? How can they be prevented? (LO 4)
4. Identify the reason why an elastic bandage is to be wrapped in the direction of the heart. (LO 6)
5. Which weighs more, muscle or fat? (LO 3)
6. What does "RICE" stand for and when is it used? (LO 6)
7. What is muscle atrophy? (LO 3)

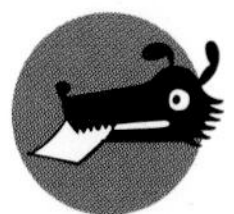

Star Student's Chapter Checklist

1. I have read my textbook chapter.
2. I have reviewed my own "Pocketful of Terms."
3. I have listened to my tutor tape.
4. I have reviewed and highlighted my class notes.
5. I have read and completed any handouts from this chapter.
6. I have completed "The Finish Line."
7. Star Time! Choose your reward!

26

Specialized Care: The Skeletal System

Look Like a Star!

Look at the Learning Objectives and The Finish Line before you begin reading this chapter.

Look at your pocket calendar.
With your pencil, put a bracket ( ) around a study period every single day.

Look at your homework for this chapter.
Plug each piece of homework into a certain time slot.

Look at the Star Student's Chapter Checklist at the end of this chapter. Check off each item as it is completed.

"Sharp misery had worn him to the bones."

William Shakespeare, 1564-1616, from *Romeo and Juliet*

"His bones ache with the day's work that earned it."

Ralph Waldo Emerson, 1803-1882

Learning Objectives

1. **Spell and define all STAR words.**
2. **Summarize the changes that occur in bones and joints during normal aging.**
3. **Name four common disorders of the skeletal system.**
4. **Describe consequences of falls and identify risk factors for falls and the nursing assistant's role in fall prevention.**
5. **Describe how to discover the extent of a bone or joint injury.**
6. **Explain the nursing assistant's role in caring for a resident in traction.**

Roentgen and The Discovery of the X-ray

On November 8, 1895, Wilhelm Konrad Roentgen (1845-1923) passed electric current through a type of tube and noted afterward that some special-coated cardboard nearby had developed a glow. He found that this glow came from the radiation coming out of the tube. He named the radiation X-rays. One of his early X-rays was of his own wife's hand. The tremendous impact of this discovery was felt over the weeks that followed throughout the entire world. An amazing method to actually see fractures and diseases of the bones had at last been found!

1 Spell and define all STAR words.

amputation: surgical or traumatic removal of an extremity.

amputee: individual who has had an extremity amputated.

estrogen: female sex hormone.

HRT: hormone replacement therapy.

ORIF: open reduction and internal fixation; type of surgery to "reduce" a fracture.

orthopedics: branch of medicine that deals with preventing or correcting disorders that occur in the parts of the body that provide motion.

osteoarthritis: chronic disorder involving the joints, usually weight-bearing.

osteoblasts: cell concerned with bone formation.

osteoporosis: disease causing a reduction of bone mass.

phantom pain: sensation that pain exists in an amputated body part.

prosthesis, prostheses: artificial replacement of amputated extremity.

rejection: destruction of transplanted material by the host.

stump: distal portion of an amputated extremity.

total hip replacement (THR): a surgical procedure involving replacement of the head of the long bone of the leg (femur) at the joint where it joins the hip.

2 Summarize the changes that occur in bones and joints during normal aging.

When people age, the bones lose calcium, causing them to become porous and brittle (easily broken). The space normally found in between the vertebrae in the spine may shrink, causing loss of height. The joints are less flexible, and may stiffen, which slows normal body movements.

It is important to know that most problems happen not because of aging itself, but because of inactivity that often occurs among the elderly. Just supporting one's own weight can help prevent the calcium loss in bones that causes osteoporosis.

3 Name four common disorders of the skeletal system.

1. Osteoporosis

Osteoporosis is a condition in which the bones lose mass. The loss of bone mass eventually leads to fractures. Something as simple as turning in bed can cause fractures in people who have osteoporosis.

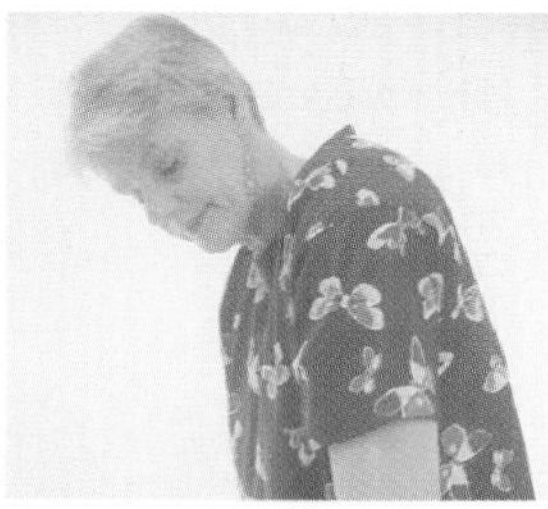

Figure 26-1. Stooped posture is a common sign of osteoporosis.

CAUSE: Osteoporosis is caused by a lack of calcium in the diet, the loss of **estrogen**, the hormone that helps bone-forming cells called **osteoblasts** form new bone, a lack of regular exercise or reduced mobility, or many other reasons.

CURE/TREATMENT: Osteoporosis is helped by attacking causes of the disorder. Taking calcium supplements, starting a doctor-approved exercise program, or taking doctor-ordered estrogen replacement (**HRT**-Hormone Replacement Therapy) may keep osteoporosis under control.

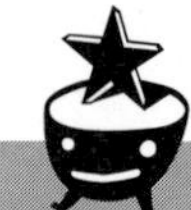

Star K.A.R.E.

Osteoporosis

KNOW your resident's care plan.
ASSIST the resident/nurse.

- *Allow enough time for the person to move about.*
- *Always move and reposition the person very carefully.*
- *Carefully follow the diet order for increased calcium.*
- *Promote the use of cane or walker if necessary.*

REPORT observations.
RECORD data.
RECHECK resident as needed.

- *If the following occurs:*
  - *medication not being taken*
  - *any decline in activity*

"Don't Delay. Report Right Away!"

ENCOURAGE resident's independence and progress.

- *Encourage ambulatory residents to walk.*

Fragile bones mean fragile residents!

When a person has osteoporosis, bones may become extremely fragile. Unfortunately, it is quite common for a bone to break with a simple movement. If you are caring for a fragile resident, it is vital that you fully understand this possibility. Movements that you take for granted, such as turning in bed, sitting down in a firm chair, or coming to a standing position can cause a fragile bone to break. If you disregard this fact with your residents and move them about carelessly, this may be considered abuse.

2. Osteoarthritis and Rheumatoid Arthritis

Osteoarthritis is a condition in which there is inflammation of the joints. The cushiony cartilage that rests between the bones and pads at the ends of the bones begins to slowly erode and disappear. Without the padding of the cartilage, the bones begin to rub together, causing inflammation and pain. If the condition worsens, the area may eventually become deformed.

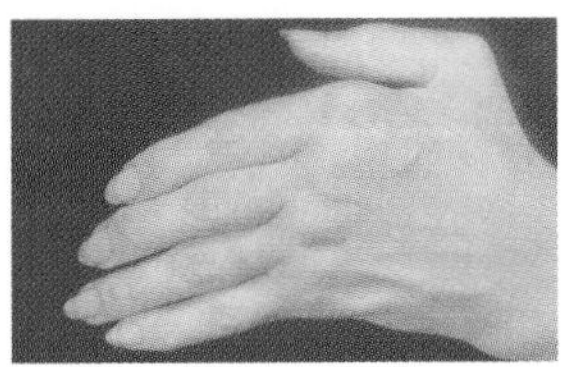

Figure 26-2. **Osteoarthritis.**

Rheumatoid arthritis is a form of arthritis that may become crippling. It usually occurs early in middle age. It affects a special membrane that lines the joint capsule, called the synovial membrane, causing stiffness and severe pain. The membrane may eventually be completely destroyed. When this occurs, the joint becomes fixed, and is unable to move.

CAUSE: Osteoarthritis is caused by the gradual erosion of the protective cartilage that normally rests between the bones at the joints. When the bones move, they scrape against each other, causing pain.

The cause of rheumatoid arthritis is not known, but it may be an autoimmune disorder. Autoimmune disorders occur when the human body makes a mistake and starts to attack itself. One theory is that a type of virus or bacteria acts as a trigger, causing the body to turn on itself.

CURE/TREATMENT: Osteoarthritis and rheumatoid arthritis are helped by a plan of care that includes rest and controlled exercise. If a problem exists with obesity, weight loss may reduce the stress on the joints. Certain types of medication reduce or relieve the pain. Heat applications are often useful in the reduction of the inflammation and pain. Ultimately, with serious deformity, joint replacement by surgery is helpful.

Star K.A.R.E.

Osteoarthritis and Rheumatoid Arthritis

KNOW your resident's care plan.
ASSIST the resident/nurse.

- *Allow enough time for the person to move about.*
- *Always move and reposition the person very carefully.*
- *Assist with exercise program as needed.*
- *Perform range of motion exercises as ordered.*
- *Let the nurse know about 30 minutes prior to exercise if pain medication is to be given beforehand.*
- *Promote the use of cane or walker if necessary.*

REPORT observations.
RECORD data.
RECHECK resident as needed.

- *If the following occurs:*
  - *pain*

★ *"Don't Delay. Report Right Away!"*

ENCOURAGE resident's independence and progress.

- *Encourage ambulatory residents to walk, even with an assistive device.*

3. Fractures

Fractures are broken bones. Many different kinds of fractures may occur in the 206 bones of the human body. The different kinds of fractures are identified below:

Closed or simple fracture: Skin is closed; bones are in proper position.
Hairline fracture: Skin is closed; bone has fine line noted on X-ray.
Open or compound fracture: Skin is open; bone may come through the skin.
Greenstick fracture: Skin is usually closed; bone has fine line noted on X-ray.
Comminuted fracture: Skin is open or closed; bone is broken in two or more places.
Spontaneous fracture: Skin is usually closed; bone breaks without trauma and may be due to osteoporosis or other condition.

CAUSE: Fractures are usually caused by some sort of trauma. Spontaneous fractures occur with diseases such as osteoporosis.

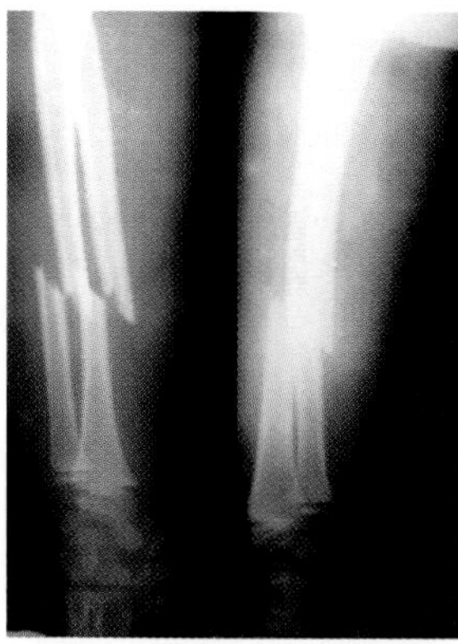

Figure 26-3. A fracture of the Ulna and Radius (forearm).

CURE/TREATMENT: Fractures are treated by specialists. The bones must be set and allowed to heal in normal alignment. Bones may take weeks or longer to heal completely. Reduction of a fractured bone, when a bone is put back in correct alignment, occurs in the doctor's office, emergency room, or urgent care facility. In other cases, special parts have to be surgically placed inside the broken bones to help them heal. These consist of plates, screws, or pins. The name of this type of surgery to "reduce" a fracture is open reduction internal fixation (**ORIF**).

Be prepared for the buzzer at the airport terminal!

If someone has a metal piece inside a bone, it is possible that the metal will trigger the buzzer at airline safety checkpoints. A special card with the location of the metal piece may be shown to the airport security personnel prior to formally going through the checkpoint, to make them aware of the situation.

Fractured Hip

Older people, especially those who have osteoporosis, will sometimes fracture a hip. This occurs because of falls or even simple movement.

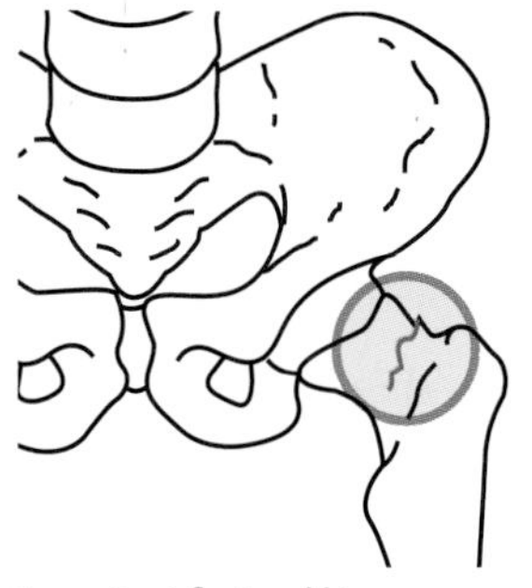

Figure 26-4. A fractured hip.

CURE/TREATMENT: The ORIF method is again used for this condition. A special pin, rod, or nail may be inserted into the bone to help keep it together and allow healing.

If a fractured hip does not heal properly or has been shattered beyond repair, surgery is performed to replace the head of the long bone of the leg (femur) at the joint where it joins the hip. This is called **total hip replacement** (THR). THR may be performed due to a fractured hip that does not heal properly, a weakened hip due to age and decreased bone strength, or a hip that is painful and stiff and no longer able to bear weight.

Once surgery has been performed, the resident will have an activity order limiting weight-bearing on that operative side. This activity order would be written as Partial weight-bearing (PWB), or Non weight-bearing (NWB). Once the person can bear weight again, the order reads: Full weight-bearing (FWB).

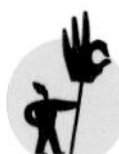

Ask for your baby's hips to be checked at birth!

If you have a baby, make sure that the healthcare provider checks the baby for congenital hip dysplasia. This occurs when the ball of the hip joint comes out of the socket too easily. It is treated with a special cast that forces the socket to become deeper so that the ball no longer comes out of the socket so easily. If this condition is missed at birth, the problem may be much more difficult to solve later in life.

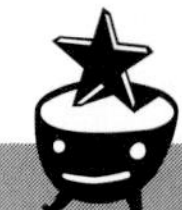

Star K.A.R.E.

Total Hip Replacement (THR)

KNOW your resident's care plan.

- *Follow the care plan exactly, even if the resident wants to do more than is ordered.*

ASSIST the resident/nurse.

- *Keep often-used items, such as medications, telephone, tissues, water, etc. within easy reach of the resident.*
- *Assist with dressing the resident, starting with the affected side first.*
- *Never rush the resident.*
- *Caution the resident not to sit with legs crossed, and not to bend the hip more than 90 degrees. Toes should not be turned inward.*
- *Never rotate hip inward towards the body (internally rotate).*
- *Use pillows in bed or chair exactly as ordered.*
- *Perform range of motion exercises only as ordered.*
- *Let the nurse know prior to exercises if pain medication is to be given beforehand.*
- *Assist with the use of cane, walker, or crutches.*

REPORT observations.
RECORD data.
RECHECK resident as needed.

- *If the following occurs:*
  - *numbness or tingling*
  - *cyanosis*
  - *increase in pain or new discomforts*
  - *changes in temperature of the skin (e.g. hot skin)*
  - *redness, drainage, bleeding, or sores of any kind*

★ *"Don't Delay. Report Right Away!"*

ENCOURAGE resident's independence and progress.

- *Use praise and encouragement often.*

4. Amputations

Amputations are the surgical removal of a limb or extremity. They are necessary when a circulatory problem becomes severe, such as with diabetes. They are also performed due to cancer or because of an accident. Traumatic amputations are due to a car accident or an accident involving some type of machinery or equipment.

There are above-the-knee amputations (AKA) and below-the-knee amputations (BKA). One problem that occurs with amputations is the condition known as **phantom pain**. A pain is felt in the missing body part, even though it is no longer attached to the body. Some people believe the pain is caused by some kind of a "memory" in the brain. This is quite real to the **amputee** and may have to be "treated" with medication.

CAUSE: Amputations are done because an extremity or a part of an extremity cannot be saved from tissue death, to remove cancer, or to treat a person who has been in a traumatic accident.

CURE/TREATMENT: Amputees—people who require amputations—may be helped by a prosthesis. A **prosthesis** is an artificial body part that is specially fitted to the **stump**, the bottom or distal part of an amputated extremity. Amazing improvements have been made to prostheses in recent years. They are much more lifelike and have greater movement and flexibility.

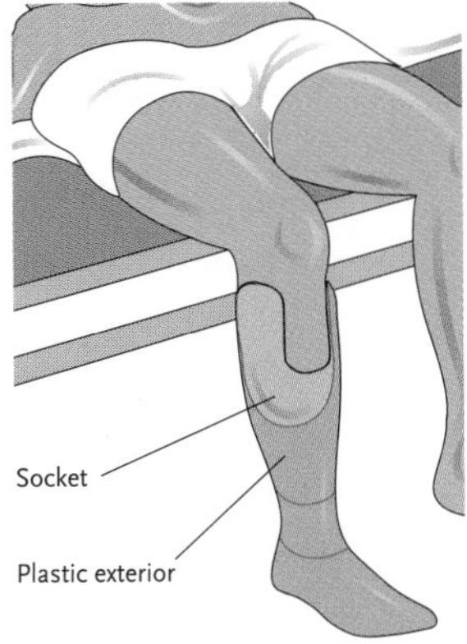

Figure 26-5. **Prostheses are specially fitted, expensive pieces of equipment.**

Transplants of certain body parts are now being done on some amputees. Hand transplants have been performed, but long-term success has not been established because the procedures are so new. **Rejection**, when the body "attacks" the surgically-attached part, is one of the most serious complications. The person must take a special medication for the rest of his life to prevent rejection of the transplanted body part.

Star K.A.R.E.

Amputations

KNOW your resident's care plan.
ASSIST the resident/nurse.

- *Allow enough time for the person to move about and adjust to changes.*
- *Follow exercise program exactly as ordered.*
- *Perform range of motion exercises only as ordered.*
- *Let the nurse know prior to exercises if pain medication is to be given beforehand.*
- *Treat phantom pain as real pain.*

REPORT observations.
RECORD data.
RECHECK resident as needed.

- *If any of the following occur:*
  - *redness or swelling of extremity*
  - *drainage, bleeding, or sores of any kind*
  - *pain or phantom pain*
  - *reduced ability to move extremity*
  - *cyanosis of any portion of the extremity*

★ *"Don't Delay. Report Right Away!"*

ENCOURAGE resident's independence and progress.

- *Provide support for anger, frustration, or grief over the loss.*
- *Provide support for phantom pain.*
- *Do not react negatively to stump or amputation site.*

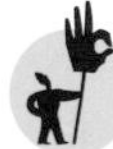

An Early Method of Amputation

Fabricus Hildanus [1560-1624] performed an early form of amputation. Hildanus used a knife that had been heated red-hot. He developed the method of cutting above the gangrene in a leg, which may have improved the survival rate for this type of patient.

4 Describe consequences of falls and identify risk factors for falls and the nursing assistant's role in fall prevention.

Residents who fall may sustain fractures. Falling, a common problem with the elderly, also contributes to many other serious physical problems, including head injuries, soft tissue injuries, and pulmonary embolisms.

It also increases the risk of problems due to physical injuries, such as immobility, dehydration, and pressure sores. It can have psychological consequences as well. Falls may trigger fear, anxiety and depression. If a resident is less confident, he may be unwilling to perform routine activities.

As the person who often spends the most time with residents, you play an important role in preventing falls. Here are some risk factors for falls and how you can help prevent them:

Risk Factors: Nursing Assistant's Role

- changes in vision: assess room and facility environment for proper lighting
- changes in hearing: encourage the use of hearing aid; clean hearing aid; reduce background noise
- changes in perception (causing balance problems): assist with balance; assist with ambulation; encourage use of assistive devices; encourage use of proper footwear; observe for environmental barriers
- dementia: assist with ambulation; give simple instructions; use bright tape to highlight stairs
- foot problems: report to nurse if there is need for a podiatrist; encourage proper footwear.

5 Describe how to discover the extent of a bone or joint injury.

When a person sustains any kind of an injury, it may be very difficult to determine the extent of the injury. Is it a sprain, strain, or fracture? No one can see inside the human body. This is a fact. No matter how well-trained a healthcare provider is, he or she is simply making a "best guess" when deciding whether an arm or leg is or is not broken. The only way to tell whether a bone is broken is to have X-rays done. If a bone is fractured and it heals in the wrong position, permanent, long-term pain may result. Bones should have plenty of time to heal correctly. This may take weeks or months.

Another problem is that sometimes X-rays do not show the fracture. This is due to the soft tissue injury around the fracture. If your resident continues to have serious pain, report it to the nurse. He may decide a second X-ray is necessary.

6 Explain the nursing assistant's role in caring for a resident in traction.

Traction is ordered for residents for a variety of reasons. It may be ordered for a person with a broken bone to keep the bone still in order for it to heal. Traction may be necessary to reduce pressure and pain due to injury or to relieve certain types of muscle spasms. When a resident is in traction, the care given has to be adjusted. Careful observation of the body is required to prevent complications.

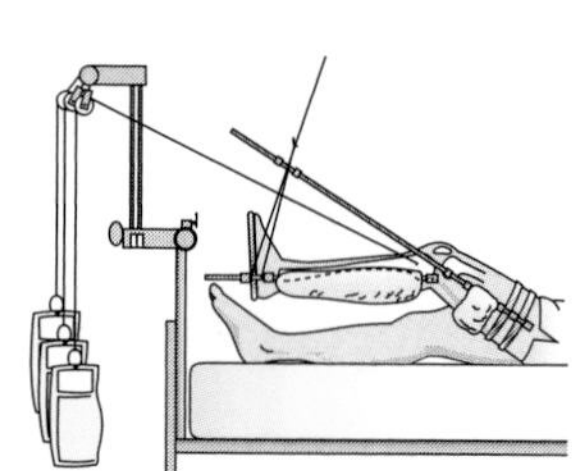

Figure 26-6. **A resident in traction may need extra care.**

Star K.A.R.E.

Traction

KNOW your resident's care plan.
ASSIST the resident/nurse.

- *Take care to protect all traction materials, such as slings or boots, from wetness or soiling.*
- *Do not allow resident to slide down in bed.*
- *Never touch the weights for any reason.*

REPORT observations.
RECORD data.
RECHECK resident as needed.

- *If any of the following occur:*
  - *numbness or tingling*
  - *cyanosis*
  - *pain, burning, pressure, swelling*
  - *changes in temperature of the skin*
  - *redness, drainage, bleeding, or sores of any kind*
  - *wetness on sling*
  - *odor around the sling or boot*
  - *sling or boot becomes loose or comes off or weights come off, touch the floor, or move*

★ *"Don't Delay. Report Right Away!"*

ENCOURAGE resident's progress.

Summary

The skeletal system contains your bones and joints. It provides the overall framework for the body. Aging causes bones to become more brittle and easily broken or fractured. When hip or other joint surgery is performed, care must focus on not harming the resident, as well as helping heal and managing pain. Falls, a major problem in long-term care, can be prevented by careful observing and reporting. X-rays are the best way to find a fracture and treat the bone properly. Improper care of skeletal disorders may result in pain, deformity, and limitation of movement for the rest of the person's life.

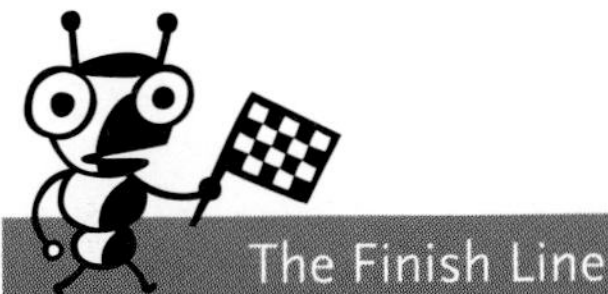

The Finish Line

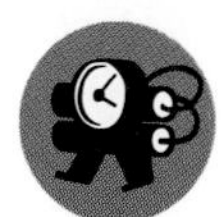

What's Wrong With This Picture?

The definitions of various fractures below are mixed up. Write the correct definition by each.

Closed or simple fracture: Skin is usually closed; bone has fine line noted on X-ray.
Hairline fracture: Skin is usually closed; bone breaks without trauma and may be due to osteoporosis or other condition.
Open or compound fracture: Skin is closed; bones are in proper position.
Greenstick fracture: Skin is open; bone may come through the skin.
Comminuted fracture: Skin is open or closed; bone is broken in two or more places.
Spontaneous fracture: Skin is closed; bone has fine line noted on X-ray.

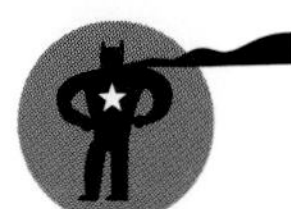

Star Student Central

1. Contact an **orthopedic** institute and ask if you can spend a couple of hours at the facility observing X-rays and casts being applied. While you are there, ask for some pamphlets about quality cast care and share them with your class.
2. Contact a local prosthesis department at a hospital or other facility. Ask for a tour and some information on some of the state-of-the art prostheses available today. Bring the information back to share with your class.

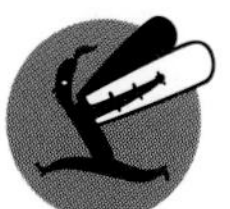

You Can Do It Corner!

1. Name one possible cause of the disorder osteoporosis. (LO 3)
2. Why do X-rays not always show a fracture? (LO 5)
3. What is one fairly common complication of an amputation? (LO 3)
4. List five risk factors for falling and two steps of prevention for each. (LO 4)
5. What causes the loss of height as we age? (LO 2)
6. What are two things you need to know to assist the resident on traction? (LO 6)
7. For a resident who has had a total hip replacement, what are six things you can do to assist the resident and/or nurse? (LO 3)

Star Student's Chapter Checklist

1. I have read my textbook chapter.
2. I have reviewed my own "Pocketful of Terms."
3. I have listened to my tutor tape.
4. I have reviewed and highlighted my class notes.
5. I have read and completed any handouts from this chapter.
6. I have completed "The Finish Line."
7. Star Time! Choose your reward!

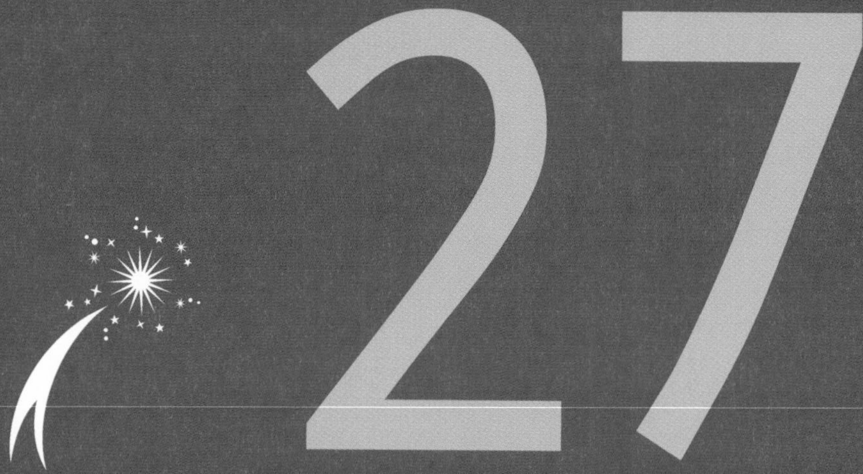

Specialized Care: The Nervous System

Look Like a Star!

Look at the Learning Objectives and The Finish Line before you begin reading this chapter.

Look at your pocket calendar.
With your pencil, put a bracket ( ) around a study period every single day.

Look at your homework for this chapter.
Plug each piece of homework into a certain time slot.

Look at the Star Student's Chapter Checklist at the end of this chapter. Check off each item as it is completed.

"Oh the nerves, the nerves; the mysteries of this machine called Man. . ."

Charles Dickens, 1812-1870

"He that wrestles with us strengthens our nerves and sharpens our skill. . ."

Edmund Burke, 1729-1797

Learning Objectives

1. **Spell and define all STAR words.**
2. **Summarize the changes that occur in the nervous system during normal aging.**
3. **Name seven common disorders of the nervous system.**
4. **Describe safety precautions to protect visually-impaired residents.**
5. **Summarize the safety precautions when caring for an artificial eye.**
6. **Describe safety precautions to protect hearing-impaired residents.**
7. **Define Alzheimer's disease and list ten warning signs.**
8. **List three possible stages of the progression of Alzheimer's disease.**
9. **Identify seven attitudes helpful in caring for residents with Alzheimer's or any dementia.**
10. **List strategies for better communication with residents who have Alzheimer's or any dementia.**
11. **Describe five guidelines for assisting the resident with Alzheimer's with personal care and activities of daily living.**
12. **List eight difficult behaviors commonly exhibited by residents with Alzheimer's and describe ways to manage each.**

Successfully perform these Practical Procedures

Care of Eyeglasses

Care of the Artificial Eye

Galen pondered, "Why did the Persian patient lose sensation only in certain fingers?"

Galen, who lived and worked in ancient Rome, treated a man from Persia who had a loss of sensation only in certain parts of his hand. Galen determined the patient had fallen on his back and that may have caused the injury. He then treated the patient with rest and the application of a type of compress to the back. He believed nerve damage actually caused the loss of sensation. Galen thought it was amazing that the man could still move his hand. To him, this meant that different nerves controlled different parts of the body. In addition, Galen thought that an injury could affect feeling, but perhaps not always movement. This was a new and exciting idea at the time!

1 Spell and define all **STAR** words.

Alzheimer's disease: a nervous system disorder that is progressive (the disease gets worse) and irreversible (the disease cannot be cured); tangled nerve fibers and protein deposits form in the brain, eventually causing dementia.

aphasia: loss of ability to speak or recognize words.

cataract: opaqueness, or lack of transparency, of the eye.

catastrophic reaction: overreaction; unreasonable reaction.

cerebrovascular accident (CVA): stroke; caused by the blockage of the blood supply to a part of the brain by a clot or ruptured blood vessel.

dementia: loss of mental abilities, such as thinking, remembering, reasoning, and communicating.

dysphagia: difficulty swallowing or the total inability to swallow.

emotional lability: inappropriate or unprovoked emotional responses including crying, laughing, and anger.

gait: manner of walking.

glaucoma: disorder of the eye caused by increased intraocular pressure.

hemiplegia: paralysis of one-half of the body.

multiple sclerosis: inflammatory disorder of the central nervous system; myelin sheath that covers the nerves, spinal cord, and white matter of the brain breaks down over time; nerves cannot conduct impulses to and from the brain in a normal way; symptoms include blurred vision, poor balance, numbness, incontinence, and difficulty walking.

one-sided neglect: lack of awareness of one side of the body.

Parkinson's disease: chronic nervous system disorder; a section of the brain degenerates (gets worse) slowly; symptoms include tremors, muscle weakness, muscle rigidity, and a shuffling gait.

prognosis: prediction of the course and end of a disease and the estimated chance of recovery.

regenerate: regrow, repair, or restore, as a tissue.

seizures: convulsions, rapid muscular contractions that last for a period of time.

spasms: involuntary movements or muscle contractions.

stroke: cerebrovascular accident (CVA); caused by the blockage of the blood supply to a part of the brain by a clot or ruptured blood vessel.

transient ischemic attack (TIA): "little stroke;" results from a temporary lack of oxygen to the brain; considered a warning sign of CVA.

vertigo: sense of moving about or having objects move about a person; room seems to be spinning.

2 Summarize the changes that occur in the nervous system during normal aging.

As people age, the number of neurons decreases. There is a diminished ability to send impulses to and from the brain. The movements we initiate, called voluntary movements, slow down, further slowing responses and reflexes.

Aging can also affect concentration and memory. Elderly people may experience memory loss of recent events.

The inner ear undergoes structural changes that can cause hearing loss. This may also affect a person's balance, which puts him at risk of falling. Weakened sense of vision, smell, taste, and touch are also common.

3 Name seven common disorders of the nervous system.

1. Stroke (Cerebrovascular Accident—CVA)

In the past, a **stroke**, or **cerebrovascular accident**, usually meant permanent disability and a difficult life from that point on. Now, the treatment of stroke patients has advanced so much that many stroke patients recover completely. The best way to accomplish this recovery is to get the person to a doctor or to the emergency room immediately.

Right-sided CVA: When a stroke occurs on the right side of the body, the blood flow to the right side of the brain has been decreased. Damage may have occurred to the right side of the brain due to this reduction in blood flow. Possible symptoms of a right-sided CVA include left-sided paralysis (hemiplegia) and a change in personality.

Left-sided CVA: If a stroke occurs on the left side of

the body, the blood flow to the left side of the brain has been decreased. Damage may have occurred to the left side of the brain due to the reduction in blood flow. Possible symptoms of a left-sided CVA include right-sided paralysis (**hemiplegia**) and **aphasia** (loss of ability to speak or recognize words).

Some conditions that are common to either right or left brain damage include the following:

- **dysphagia**: difficulty swallowing or the total inability to swallow
- **one-sided neglect**: lack of awareness of one side of the body
- **emotional lability**: inappropriate or unprovoked emotional responses, including crying, laughing, and anger

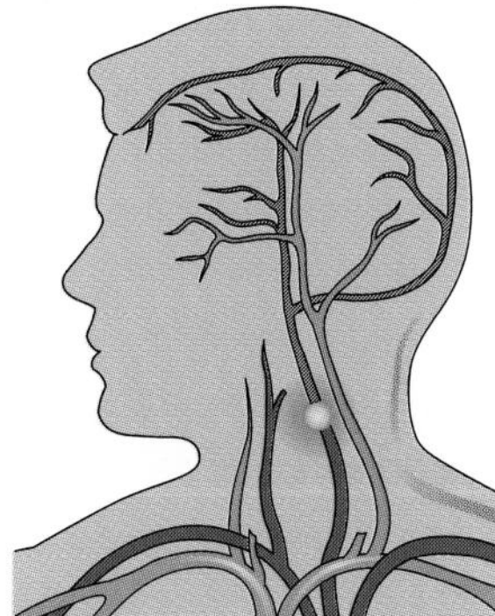

Figure 27-1. CVA, or stroke, is caused when blood supply to the brain is cut off suddenly by a clot or a ruptured blood vessel.

CAUSE: Strokes are caused by either an obstruction or the rupture of a blood vessel.

CURE/TREATMENT: When the person sees a doctor immediately, the outlook or **prognosis** may be better. When a stroke is caused by an obstructed blood vessel, sometimes doctors can dissolve the obstruction. If the cause of the stroke is a ruptured blood vessel, the prognosis is dependent upon the degree of damage inside the brain due to the bleeding.

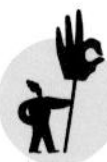

CVA: Right=Left and Left=Right

Facilities document strokes in their care plans and other forms differently. For one facility, a right-sided CVA means the person had a stroke on the right side and has left-sided paralysis. For other facilities, a right-sided CVA means that the resident is paralyzed or affected on the right side. As a caregiver, all you need to know is the side of the body that is affected by the stroke. This will determine the type of care you provide to your residents.

Transient Ischemic Attacks (TIA) — Box 27-1

A **transient ischemic attack**, or TIA, is a warning sign of a stroke. It occurs when the brain loses a portion of its blood supply. The attack is usually quite sudden, lasting from a number of minutes to a full day.

People who experience TIAs are at risk of having a full-blown stroke in the future. TIAs may occur many times before a full-blown stroke happens. A person may experience a brief blackout when he or she cannot account for a few seconds or minutes in time. Speech may be slightly slurred and dizziness may occur. Numbness or tingling may appear and then suddenly disappear.

Whether you suspect a TIA or a stroke, the key to survival with the least permanent disability is to GET HELP RIGHT AWAY.

★ *"Don't Delay. Report Right Away!"*

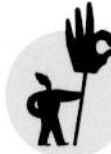

Possible Signs and Symptoms of a TIA or a CVA

If you ever notice any of the following in your residents:

- *dizziness*
- *confusion*
- *sudden loss of sight in one eye*
- *development of blurred vision*
- *sudden change in the ability to hear or speak*
- *intense headache that will not go away*
- *brief blackout when resident is unable to account for a period of time*
- *unexplained shaking or trembling*
- *numbness or tingling on one side of the body that will not go away*
- *loss of the use of one side of the body or the use of arm and/or leg on one side (e.g. you drop something and can't seem to pick it up and hold it)*
- *drooping of one side of the mouth or one eyelid*
- *pupil of one eye seems larger than the other eye*

★ *"Don't Delay. Report Right Away!"*

Star K.A.R.E.

Resident with a CVA/Stroke

KNOW your resident's care plan.
ASSIST the resident/nurse.

- *Assist with ambulation to prevent falls.*
- *Be patient with self-care and communication. Allow the resident time to do things.*
- *Give excellent skin care to prevent pressure sores.*
- *Reposition resident often to help prevent pressure sores and contractures. Position in proper alignment using special positioning devices when necessary.*
- *Assist with range of motion exercises exactly as ordered to prevent contractures and to strengthen muscles.*
- *Carefully assist with shaving, grooming, and bathing. Diminished sensation or paralysis causes lack of*

awareness about such things as water temperature and sharpness of razors. Take care so that injury does not occur.

- *Encourage fluids and proper nutrition to prevent weight loss, constipation, and dehydration.*
- *When assisting with eating, always place food in the unaffected or strong side of the mouth.*
- *Break any instructions down into short, simple sentences. Use communication boards or cards to help make communication easier.*

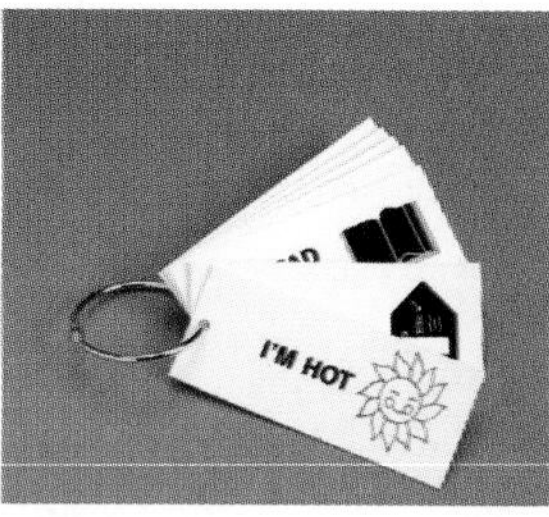

Figure 27-2. **Picture cards can help a post-CVA resident communicate.**

- *With one-sided neglect, remind resident frequently of weak side. Repeatedly orient resident when changing his or her location.*
- *With emotional lability, either distract the resident, which will often stop the emotional outburst, or redirect the resident to something else. Try asking a question or pointing out something in the room.*

REPORT observations.
RECORD data.
RECHECK resident as needed.

If the following occur:

- *red skin, pale skin, or the start of a pressure sore*
- *the start of a contracture*
- *pain, swelling, or burning in a leg, especially the lower leg and the calf*
- *uncontrolled bleeding (possibly due to blood-thinning medication)*
- *urinary tract infections*
- *constipation*
- *dehydration*
- *weight loss*

★ *"Don't Delay. Report Right Away!"*

ENCOURAGE resident's independence and progress.

- *Encourage person to remember paralyzed limbs.*
- *Prevent withdrawal and feelings of isolation. Listen to resident if he/she wants to talk.*
- *Encourage fluids every time you see resident.*
- *Praise acts of independence, no matter how small.*

Star K.A.R.E.

Aspiration Safety and the CVA Resident

(For more information on Aspiration Safety, see Chapter 22.)

KNOW your resident's care plan.
ASSIST the resident/nurse.

- *Place stroke residents in Fowler's position for eating; have resident maintain this position 30 minutes after eating and drinking.*
- *Avoid distractions.*
- *Food must be placed into the unaffected or strong side of the mouth.*
- *Feed stroke residents very slowly, cutting food into tiny pieces or offering small spoonfuls of pureed food. Be patient.*
- *Give a solid, then a liquid, then repeat.*
- *Make sure resident actually swallows food after each bite so that it is not stored in the paralyzed side of the mouth. Do not put your fingers inside the mouth; you may use swabs if needed to open the mouth.*
- *Provide mouth care after eating.*

REPORT observations.
RECORD data.
RECHECK resident as needed.

If the following occur:

- *choking*
- *shortness of breath or dyspnea*
- *signs of pneumonia*
- *chest pain or tightness*

★ *"Don't Delay. Report Right Away!"*

ENCOURAGE resident's independence and progress.

Encourage proper nutrition and offer fluids.

2. Parkinson's disease

Parkinson's disease is a disorder that usually begins after the age of 40 but can occur in younger people. The neurons in the brain that produce the special substance called dopamine begin to break down and die. This causes symptoms such as tremors or shaking that are not voluntary. Some other characteristics of the disorder are a mask-like face, pill-rolling (moving the thumb and first finger together like rolling a pill), rigid muscles, and a shuffling walk or **gait**.

CAUSE: The dopamine-producing neurons in the brain that lie in the midbrain (section of the brain that transfers impulses from the cerebrum to the cerebellum and impulses from the spinal cord upward) begin to break down and die. The basal ganglia in the brain experience a drop in dopamine, which causes the specific symptoms.

CURE/TREATMENT: Drug therapy is one way to treat this disorder. Dopamine may not be used because it is not able to pass through the area called the blood-brain barrier. The blood-brain barrier is a membrane that protects the brain from harmful substances and microorganisms. Unfortunately, the barrier sometimes also prevents good medications from passing through into the brain. Studies are being done to find new and successful methods of transferring certain medications into the brain. Another substance called L-dopa is able to get through the barrier and is used to treat the disorder. However, L-dopa sometimes loses its effectiveness over time. New medications are being tested that may prove helpful for the disease. Some people are candidates for surgery that helps the course of this disorder.

Star K.A.R.E.

Parkinson's Disease

KNOW your resident's care plan.
ASSIST the resident/nurse.

- *Assist with ambulation to prevent falls due to shuffling walk or gait.*
- *Be patient with self-care and communication. Allow the resident time to do and say things. Listen.*
- *Assist with range of motion exercises exactly as ordered to prevent contractures and to strengthen muscles.*
- *Encourage fluids and proper nutrition to prevent weight loss, constipation, and dehydration.*

REPORT observations.
RECORD data.
RECHECK resident as needed.

If the following occur:

- *severe trembling*
- *severe muscle rigidity/contractures*
- *sudden incontinence*
- *severe mood swings*
- *constipation*
- *dehydration*
- *weight loss*
- *depression*

★ *"Don't Delay. Report Right Away!"*

ENCOURAGE resident's progress.

- *Encourage self-care.*
- *Prevent depression. Listen to resident if he/she wants to talk.*
- *Encourage resident to stand as straight as possible when ambulating.*

3. Multiple Sclerosis (MS)

Multiple sclerosis is a disorder that may occur in young adults. With MS, there is a loss of myelin, the protective covering that covers the nerves and spinal cord. This loss causes a sort of "short-circuit" in the impulses, eventually preventing the impulses from being transported to and from the brain.

Symptoms include numbness and tingling, muscle weakness and fatigue (tiredness), tremors, a feeling of **vertigo** (a spinning feeling), a reduced ability to feel sensations, blurred or double vision along with jerky eye movements, poor balance, incontinence, and possibly paralysis.

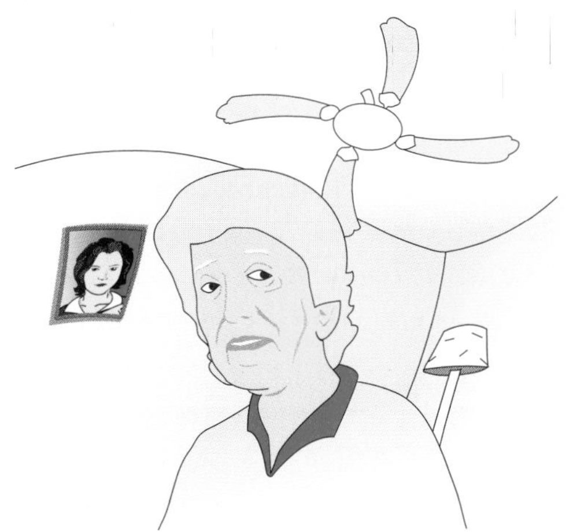

Figure 27-3. Vertigo is different from dizziness in that with vertigo, the room actually seems to spin around you.

CAUSE: The exact cause of multiple sclerosis is not known. It may be an autoimmune disorder caused by a type of virus. Autoimmune disorders occur when the human body makes a mistake and starts to attack itself. The antibodies in this case work to destroy the body's own myelin.

CURE/TREATMENT: There is no cure for this disease at this time. Interferon is a substance that has shown some promise with these patients. New therapies are being tested all the time.

Star K.A.R.E.

Multiple Sclerosis (MS)

***KNOW** your resident's care plan.*
***ASSIST** the resident/nurse.*

- *Assist with ambulation to prevent falls due to lack of coordination, fatigue, and vision impairments.*
- *Be patient with self-care and movement. Allow the resident time to do things.*
- *Offer rest periods as necessary.*
- *Give excellent skin care to prevent pressure sores.*
- *Assist with range of motion exercises exactly as ordered to prevent contractures and to strengthen muscles.*

***REPORT** observations.*
***RECORD** data.*
***RECHECK** resident as needed.*

If the following occurs:

- *red skin, pale skin, or the start of a pressure sore*
- *the start of a contracture*
- *urinary tract infections*
- *depression*

★ *"Don't Delay. Report Right Away!"*

***ENCOURAGE** resident's independence and progress.*

- *Symptoms of MS sometimes change from day to day; offer support and encouragement.*
- *Prevent depression. Listen to resident if he/she wants to talk.*

4. Spinal Cord Injuries

When a person sustains a spinal cord injury, the spinal cord is cut, partially cut, or damaged in some way. Symptoms include paralysis. Paralysis is determined by the exact area of the spinal cord that is injured.

Paraplegia is the inability to use the legs. It is caused by injuries in the thoracic or lumbar area of the spinal cord.

Quadriplegia means all extremities are paralyzed. It is caused by injuries in the cervical area of the spine.

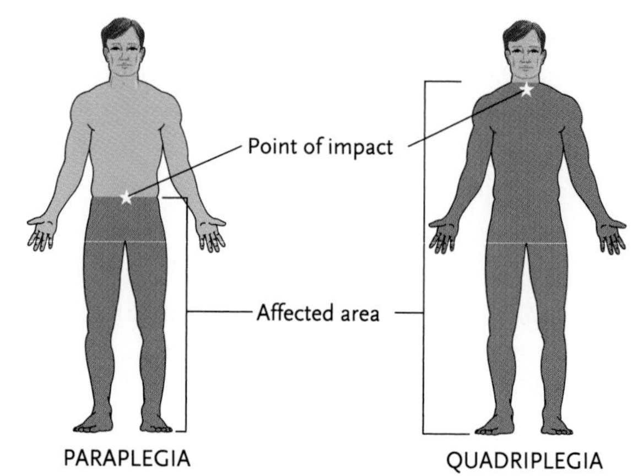

Figure 27-4.

CAUSE: Accidents, such as vehicle accidents, sporting injuries, gunshot wounds (GSW), stab wounds, or falls may cause the injury.

CURE/TREATMENT: Spinal cord injuries are treated with some success if the cord is not completely cut or severed. The results of these injuries range from **spasms**, weakness, and difficulty coordinating movements to complete paralysis. In time, with rehabilitation, some, or in certain cases all, of the former movement may be regained.

There is no current method to **regenerate** or regrow spinal cord tissue. Research is being conducted that may prove successful in the future in the treatment of spinal cord injuries.

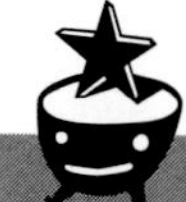

Star K.A.R.E.

Spinal Cord Injuries

***KNOW** your resident's care plan.*
***ASSIST** the resident/nurse.*

- *Be patient with all care.*

Integumentary System:

- *Give excellent skin care to prevent pressure sores. Remember that lack of sensation will prevent awareness that a pressure sore is developing.*

Muscular System:

- *Perform passive range of motion exercises exactly as*

ordered to prevent contractures and to strengthen muscles.

- *Allow as much independence as possible with ADLs.*

Skeletal System:

- *Be gentle when turning and repositioning.*

Gastrointestinal System:

- *Immobility leads to constipation. Encourage fluids and proper diet—high in fiber, if ordered.*

Urinary System:

- *Loss of control of urination leads to the need of a catheter. Urinary tract infections are common. Encourage a high intake of fluids and give extra catheter care as needed.*

Nervous System:

- *Protect residents from harm due to lack of sensation. Prevent burns from water or other sources due to the inability to feel.*

Circulatory System:

- *Lack of activity leads to poor circulation and fatigue. Use special stockings to help increase circulation as ordered.*
- *Offer rest periods as necessary.*

Respiratory System:

- *Difficulty coughing and shallow breathing can lead to pneumonia. Encourage deep breathing exercises as ordered.*

Reproductive System:

- *Male residents may have involuntary erections that have nothing to do with a deliberate reaction. Provide for privacy and be sensitive to this.*

REPORT observations.
RECORD data.
RECHECK resident as needed.

If the following occurs:

- *red skin, pale skin, or the start of a pressure sore*
- *start of a contracture*
- *urinary tract infection*
- *shortness of breath or dyspnea*
- *constipation*
- *dehydration*
- *weight loss*
- *depression*

★ *"Don't Delay. Report Right Away!"*

ENCOURAGE resident's independence and progress.

- *Encourage the resident to participate fully in her care. Listen to the resident.*

5. Seizures (Epilepsy, Convulsions)

Seizures are sometimes called convulsions. People who have seizures may have an aura prior to the start of the seizure. An aura is when a person hears a strange sound, smells something odd, or sees a flash of light. There are two primary kinds of seizures, grand-mal and petit mal.

Grand-mal seizures have these characteristics:

- generalized shaking and twitching
- loss of consciousness
- incontinence

Petit mal seizures have these characteristics:

- brief blackout period
- daydreaming
- eyes rolling back into the head for a short time

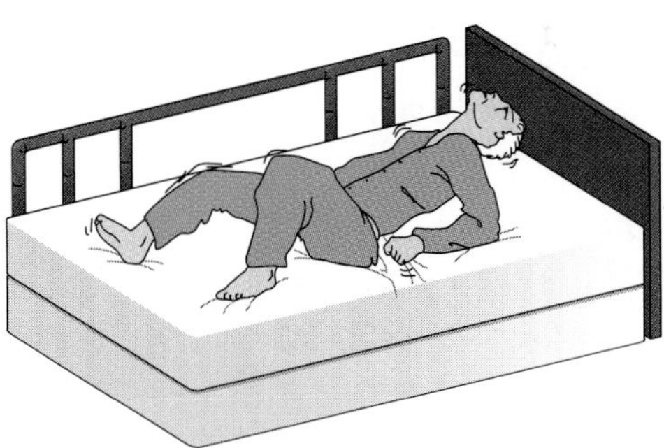

Figure 27-5. **A grand-mal seizure involves generalized shaking and twitching. Padded side rails will be raised during a seizure.**

CAUSE: Sometimes the cause of seizures is unknown. Some of the known causes of seizures are tumors, head injuries, injuries to the brain during birth, high fevers, or alcohol and drug abuse. When the cause of the seizures is not one of these things, it is called epilepsy.

CURE/TREATMENT: The cause of the seizure, if known, may be targeted by the doctor. If the cause is a tumor, it is possible to reduce or eliminate the seizures with surgical removal of the tumor. High fevers are treated with methods to reduce fever. Drug or alcohol rehabilitation helps control seizures that are caused by substance abuse. For other non-specific causes of seizures, the goal for healthcare providers is to order the right medications that will control the seizures. People with epilepsy may have to take this medication for the rest of their lives.

"Man's Best Friend" to the rescue again?

Some people have noted an interesting response from their dogs just before the start of a seizure. Some dogs are extremely sensitive to subtle changes right before a seizure begins. If you ever notice odd behavior in a dog, pay attention. The dog may be warning you about a resident's seizure.

Star K.A.R.E.

Seizures

KNOW your resident's care plan.
ASSIST the resident/nurse.

- *Become familiar with your resident's aura, if present.*
- *Cradle and protect the head during seizures.*
- *Clear other objects to protect the body.*
- *Do not try to restrain person.*
- *Loosen necktie or tight shirt or blouse.*
- *Prevent aspiration by turning head to the side.*
- *Time the exact length of the seizure.*

REPORT observations.
RECORD data.
RECHECK resident as needed.

If the following occurs:

- *stoppage of breathing, especially due to aspiration*
- *noticeable injury, bleeding, or bruising*

★ *"Don't Delay. Report Right Away!"*

ENCOURAGE resident's progress.

- *Provide support following seizure.*

Nurses may attempt to place a tongue blade inside the resident's mouth, asking her to bite down on it to prevent biting the tongue when muscles clamp down at the start of a seizure. (Note: Some states do not allow the use of tongue blades. Follow facility policy regarding tongue blades.)

Once a seizure has actually started, neither you nor anyone else should put ANYTHING inside the resident's mouth. Forcing an object inside the mouth can cause harm.

6. Cataracts

A **cataract** occurs when the lens of the eye, which is normally clear, becomes cloudy. Light has difficulty getting through, causing decreased vision. The first symptom is blurred vision. Other symptoms are glare when driving at night or a yellowing of vision.

CAUSE: In infants, cataracts may occur due to an infection or a developmental problem. Cataracts may be inherited. In adults, cataracts may be caused by diabetes or an eye injury. Cataracts may just be caused by the normal aging process.

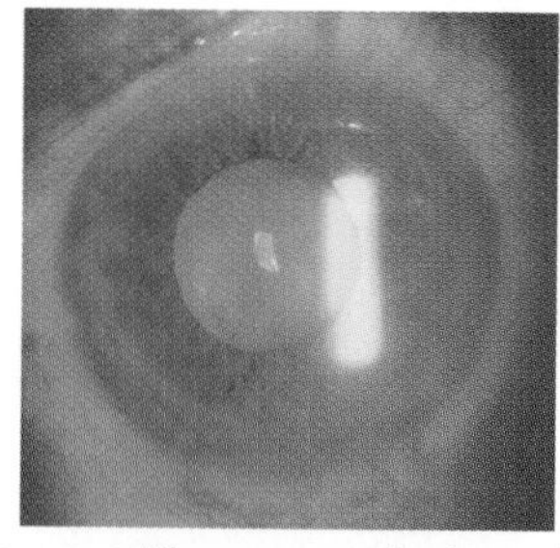

Figure 27-6. **When a cataract develops, the lens of the eye becomes cloudy, preventing light from entering the eye.**

CURE/TREATMENT: When cataracts become "mature," they become completely white. It is at this time when most eye surgeons schedule eye surgery to remove the cataract. The lens that has turned cloudy is removed and a new plastic lens implant is put in place. The eye must be carefully measured for the lens implant prior to the surgery. This lens implant is meant to be permanent. It rarely has to be removed. It is only removed when inflammation occurs or if the implant moves out of place.

7. Glaucoma

Pressure inside the eye is produced due to fluid called aqueous humor. This fluid helps keep the eye at a normal pressure by flowing into and out of an area called the anterior chamber. When the ability of this fluid to drain out of the eye is affected, the intraocular pressure may rise. This increase in pressure is the disorder known as **glaucoma**, which may ultimately cause a loss of vision.

CAUSE: There are two types of glaucoma, primary and secondary glaucoma. The majority of glaucoma found in the United States is primary, which has no known cause. However, glaucoma can be hereditary. All people with a family history of glaucoma should have their intraocular pressure checked at least once a year. Secondary glaucoma is caused by an eye injury or eye disease and makes up a small percentage of the glaucoma in this country.

CURE/TREATMENT: Normal pressure inside the eye runs between 10 and 20mmHg on a device called a tonometer. Doctors who treat glaucoma try to reduce the pressure to the normal range. They may do this by prescribing drops that, when taken as directed, work to keep the pressure as steady as possible. Other medications are available if the drops do not maintain a normal pressure. When drops and medications do not work, regular or laser surgery may be attempted to try to correct the problem. The surgery does not work on every patient.

What's your pressure?

When was the last time you had the pressure tested inside YOUR eyes? It is a test that everyone should have done during normal eye exams. Make an appointment to have an eye exam done and make sure the pressure inside your eyes is checked. This should be done no matter how young or old you may be. Glaucoma can strike at any age!

Alzheimer's disease is discussed in detail later in this chapter.

4 Describe safety precautions to protect visually-impaired residents.

There are many things you must do to protect visually-impaired or blind residents. Some guidelines are identified below:

Entering or Leaving Rooms

1. Always identify yourself as you enter the room and leave the room.
2. When you enter or leave a room, make sure you either completely open or close the door; never leave any door partly open.

New Residents

1. Walk new residents around the entire room to help orient them.
2. Walk new residents around the entire facility after they are settled.
3. Allow residents to touch your face and the faces of other staff members if they desire. This helps them perceive how you look.
4. Assist resident by helping him complete menus.

Ambulating

1. Walk a little ahead of a visually-impaired resident while he touches your arm. This allows you to guide the person and warn him of steps, curbs, etc.
2. Walk at the resident's pace, not yours.

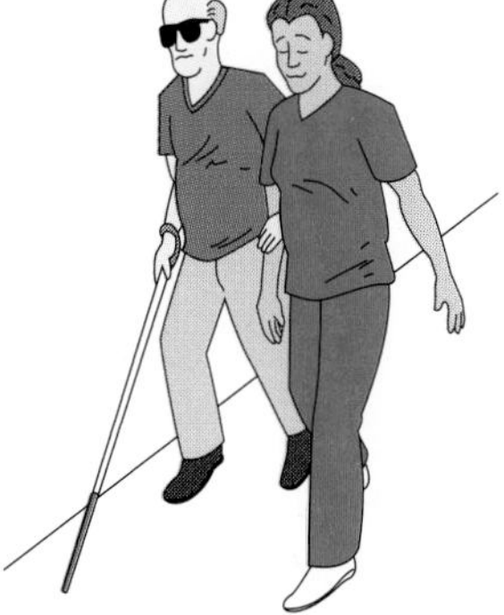

Figure 27-7.

More than three-quarters of residents will have some vision impairment. Never move furniture without telling them. Keep eyeglasses clean and in good repair. Describe procedures fully.

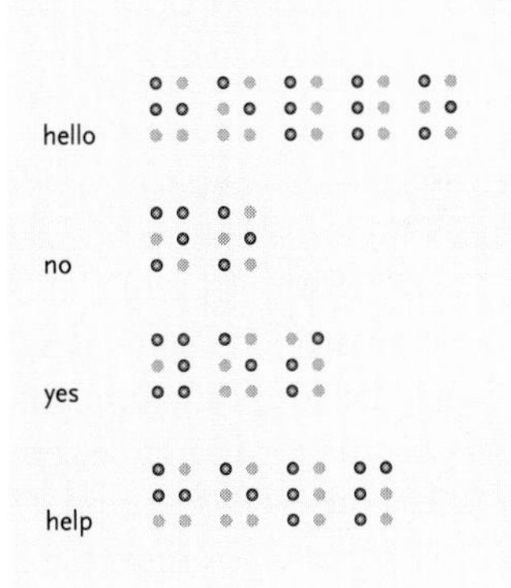

Figure 27-8. **Braille: Some examples of simple phrases.**

Wheelchairs are not rollercoasters!

When caring for visually-impaired residents, never move them too quickly in a wheelchair. It can be terrifying to be unable to see well and unable to control the speed of a rapidly-moving wheelchair. And make sure you never hit the footrests or a resident's feet against a wall or other object.

Care of Eyeglasses

Follow all standard and/or transmission-based precautions. Follow all rules for body mechanics.

Collect equipment:

- **kidney basin**
- **eyeglass cleaning equipment as needed**

1. **Perform the "5 Stars."**

PREPARE:

2. **Position resident comfortably.**

PERFORM:

3. **Carefully remove eyeglasses and place in kidney basin.**
4. **SECURE THE RESIDENT! Raise side rails, if necessary, and lower bed.**
5. **Line sink with towel.**
6. **Wash eyeglasses with lukewarm water, rinse, and place inside kidney basin. While washing, observe for loose screws or loose or broken lenses.**
7. **Dry with soft 100% cotton cloth or lens cleaning tissue. Do not dry with tissues, as they may scratch eyeglasses.**
8. **Store eyeglasses in special eyeglass case in safe place, or prepare to replace on resident.**
9. **Return to bedside.**
10. **Replacing the eyeglasses: place gently over the ears and position comfortably. Observe for proper fit.**

FINISHING TOUCHES:

11. **Perform the "5 Stars and 3 Rs."**

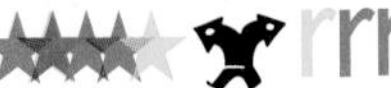

5 Summarize the safety precautions when caring for an artificial eye.

Artificial eyes are necessary for people who have lost an eye to cancer, disease, or an injury like a gunshot wound (GSW). An artificial eye is a type of prosthesis, or an artificial body part. Sometimes the artificial eye will be surgically implanted into the eye socket. This means it will not be removed daily for cleaning. It is essentially permanent. Other people have artificial eyes that are removed for cleaning and storage.

Artificial eyes made of glass are very fragile and must be treated with the utmost care. A newer type of artificial eye is made of plastic. It is very important to work very slowly and carefully with the eye. Never use any kind of cleaning agent on the artificial eye, for it may dull the shine of the eye or hurt the resident. Follow the cleaning directions exactly when cleaning the eye. When moving the eye from the bed or chair to the sink, it is very important to place the eye inside an eyecup or a basin on a piece of gauze. This may prevent you from accidentally dropping the eye. Store the eye in a covered container in the fluid the resident chooses, usually water or a type of saline solution.

The eye socket is cleaned carefully when the eye is removed. This is done with cotton balls and water or another solution. It is important not to appear uneasy when cleaning the eye socket. Always act professionally when performing this task.

Care of the Artificial Eye

Follow all standard and/or transmission-based precautions. Follow all rules for body mechanics.

Collect equipment:
- two pairs of disposable gloves • cotton balls
- kidney basin with warm water • additional gauze
- towel and washcloth • eyecup or denture cup lined with gauze and half-filled with lukewarm water

1. Perform the "5 Stars."

2. Apply gloves.

PREPARE:

3. Position resident in the supine position with a towel over the chest.
4. Position eyecup on flat surface.

PERFORM:

5. Ask resident to close both eyes and cleanse eyes with moistened cotton balls. Wipe gently from inner corner (canthus) of each eye outward. Use clean cotton ball for each eye.
6. Removing the eye:
   a. Hold hand under eye area so that eye will move out into the hand.
   b. Pull lower eyelid down with thumb and lift the upper lid gently with first finger.
   c. Eye should come out into the hand.

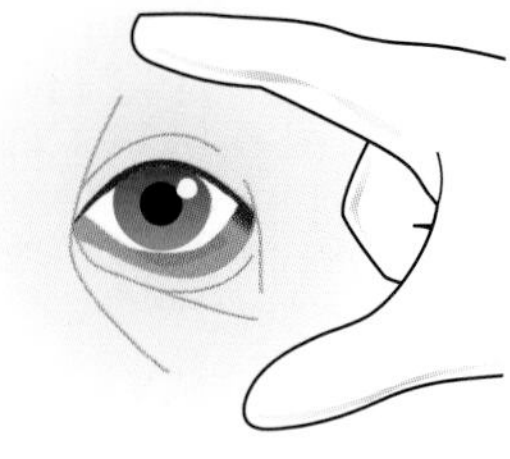

Figure 27-9.

7. Place eye carefully in eye cup on gauze.
8. SECURE THE RESIDENT.

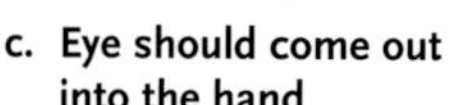

9. Bring the eyecup to bathroom and put it down on a flat surface.
10. Line sink with towel. Empty and rinse eyecup, place new gauze inside it, and replace cup on flat surface.
11. Wash eye with lukewarm water, rinse, and place on clean gauze inside eye cup. Do not dry the eye.
12. Store eye or prepare to replace inside eye socket.
13. Remove gloves and wash hands.
14. Return to bedside and put on second pair of gloves.
15. Clean eye socket, if needed, with moistened cotton balls, and dry.
16. Inserting the eye:
   a. Hold notched edge toward the nose.
   b. Lift upper lid with first finger and, using other hand, gently insert eye.
   c. Press down on the lower lid until the eye slips into its place. It is held in place by suction.

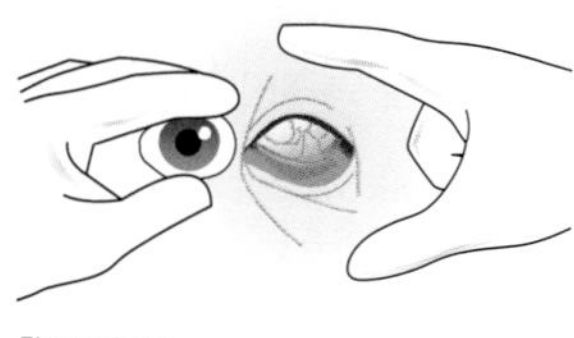

Figure 27-10.

FINISHING TOUCHES:

17. Remove gloves and wash hands.
18. Perform the "5 Stars and 3 Rs."

6 Describe safety precautions to protect hearing-impaired residents.

The deaf or hearing-impaired resident has a greater risk of injury than a resident who has no hearing impairment. Some of the safety precautions you should follow when caring for a hearing-impaired person are listed on the next page:

Entering or Leaving Rooms

1. Always lightly touch the resident as you enter the room and leave the room.

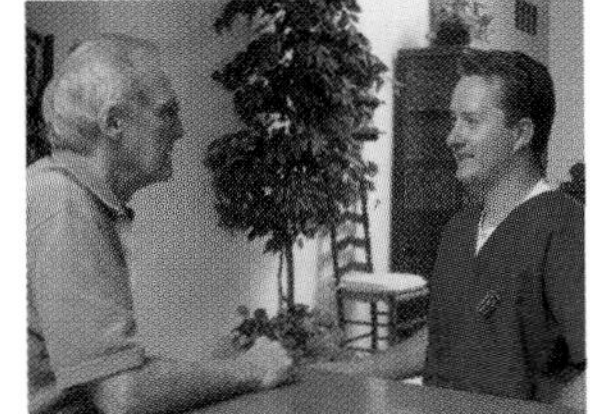

Figure 27-11. **Look directly at a hearing-impaired resident when speaking.**

2. Look directly at the person so he may see your lips as you speak. Some residents may have the ability to lip-read.
3. Communicate in good lighting.
4. Never shout at the person.
5. Speak slowly and clearly.
6. Repeat comments as necessary.

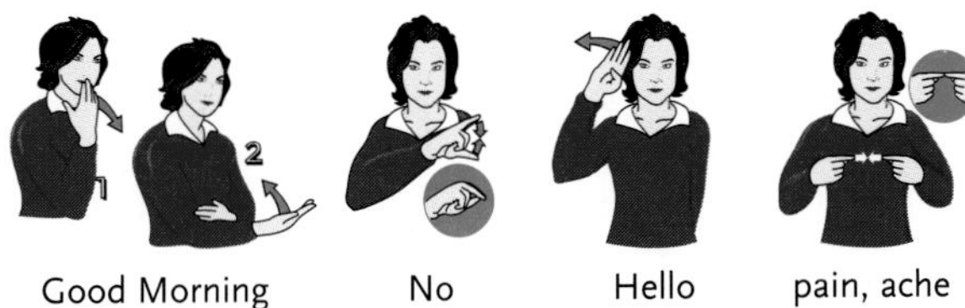

Figure 27-12. **Four Common Signs.**

New Residents

Introduce resident to other residents and staff. Have resident face each person in order to see their lips.

Ambulating

Protect hearing-impaired people from any objects they may be unable to hear coming towards them. Oncoming carts, people or pets may frighten hearing-impaired people or cause them to stumble or fall.

There are many different kinds of hearing aids. Follow the manufacturer's or your facility's directions for cleaning them. While cleaning, observe for wax buildup. Do not submerge the hearing aid or allow the section that houses the battery to get wet. Hearing aids are expensive, and you must handle them carefully. Turn it off and keep it in safe place when it is not being worn.

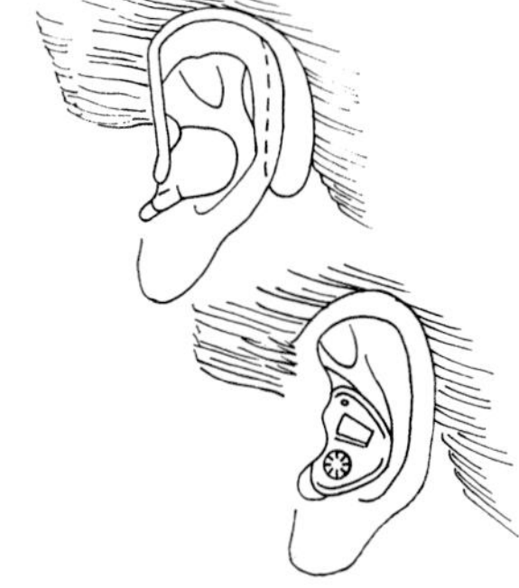

Figure 27-13. **Several types of hearing aids are available, depending on a person's needs.**

Be gentle when inserting it. Make sure it sits snugly in place before turning it on. Check that the volume is properly adjusted. If you see any sores or abrasions in the ear, report these to the nurse.

7 Define Alzheimer's disease and list ten warning signs.

Alzheimer's disease was first identified by Alois Alzheimer in 1907. The brain is affected by this disorder. Alzheimer's disease (AD) is a nervous system disorder that is both progressive (the disease gets worse) and irreversible (the disease cannot be cured). People with Alzheimer's disease may lose memory, be completely unable to care for themselves, and behave inappropriately. There is no known cause of Alzheimer's disease. Recent studies have identified alarming increases in the percentage of older people with Alzheimer's disease. Research is being conducted all over the world to unlock the key to this devastating disease.

Ten Warning Signs of Alzheimer's — Box 27-2

Alzheimer's disease is a disorder that affects all cultures and levels of society. At this time, the cause of the disease is unknown. However, certain warning signs have been identified to help diagnose a person developing the disease.

To help family members and healthcare professionals recognize warning signs of Alzheimer's disease, the Alzheimer's Association has developed a checklist of common symptoms.

1. Memory loss. One of the most common early signs of dementia is forgetting recently-learned information. While it's normal to forget appointments, names, or telephone numbers, those with dementia will forget such things more often and not remember them later.
2. Difficulty performing familiar tasks. People with dementia often find it hard to complete everyday tasks that are so familiar that we usually do not think about how to do them. A person with Alzheimer's may not know the steps for preparing a meal, using a household appliance, or participating in a lifelong hobby.
3. Problems with language. Everyone has trouble finding the right word sometimes, but a person with Alzheimer's disease often forgets simple words or substitutes unusual words, making his or her speech or writing hard to understand. If a person with Alzheimer's is unable to find his or her toothbrush, for example, the individual may ask for "that thing for my mouth."
4. Disorientation to time and place. It is normal to forget the day of the week or where you are going. But people with

Alzheimer's disease can become lost on their own street, forget where they are and how they got there, and not know how to get back home.

5. Poor or decreased judgment. No one has perfect judgment all of the time. Those with Alzheimer's may dress without regard to the weather, wearing several shirts or blouses on a warm day or very little clothing in cold weather. Individuals with dementia often show poor judgment about money, giving away large amounts of money to telemarketers or paying for home repairs or products they do not need.

6. Problems with abstract thinking. Balancing a checkbook may be hard when the task is more complicated than usual. Someone with Alzheimer's disease could forget completely what the numbers are and what needs to be done with them.

7. Misplacing things. Anyone can temporarily misplace a wallet or key. A person with Alzheimer's disease may put things in unusual places: an iron in the freezer, a wristwatch in the sugar bowl, or a sandwich under the sofa.

8. Changes in mood or behavior. Everyone can become sad or moody from time to time. Someone with Alzheimer's disease can show rapid mood swings—from calm to tears to anger—for no apparent reason.

9. Changes in personality. People's personalities ordinarily change somewhat with age. But a person with Alzheimer's disease can change a lot, becoming extremely confused, suspicious, fearful, or dependent on a family member.

10. Loss of initiative. It is normal to tire of housework, business activities, or social obligations at times. The person with Alzheimer's disease may become very passive, sitting in front of the television for hours, sleeping more than usual, or not wanting to do usual activities.

(Reproduced courtesy of the Alzheimer's Association)

8 List three possible stages of the progression of Alzheimer's disease.

A resident with Alzheimer's disease may move through three distinct stages. In each stage, the resident becomes progressively worse. He is less able to perform his ADLs, finally becoming completely dependent upon others for all of his daily care. Alzheimer's disease progresses at different rates and in different ways in different people. Remember that a resident with Alzheimer's disease is an individual and may show symptoms from two or more stages at once and may never show certain symptoms at all.

Stage I

- recent (short-term) memory loss
- disorientation to time
- lack of interest in doing things, including work, dress, recreation
- inability to concentrate
- mood swings
- irritability
- petulance: peevish, ill-humored, rude behavior
- tendency to blame others
- carelessness in personal habits
- poor judgment

Stage II

- increased memory loss, may forget family members and friends
- slurred speech
- difficulty finding right words, finishing thoughts, or following directions
- tendency to make statements that are illogical
- inability to read, write, or do math
- inability to care for self or perform ADLs without assistance
- incontinence
- dulled senses (for example, cannot distinguish between hot and cold)
- restlessness, wandering, and/or agitation (increase of these in the evening is called "sundowning")
- sleep problems
- lack of impulse control (for example, swears excessively or is sexually aggressive or rude)
- obsessive repetition of movements, behavior, or words (called perseveration)
- temper tantrums
- hallucinations or delusions

Stage III

- total disorientation to time, place, and person
- apathy
- total dependence on others for care
- total incontinence
- inability to speak or communicate, except for grunting, groaning, or screaming
- total immobility/confinement to bed
- inability to recognize family members or self
- increased sleep disturbances
- difficulty swallowing, which produces the risk of choking
- seizures
- coma
- death

9 Identify seven attitudes helpful in caring for residents with Alzheimer's or any dementia.

People with Alzheimer's disease are individuals.

- AD develops differently in different people.
- One care plan cannot serve all residents with AD.
- Take an interest in each individual. Knowing your

residents' likes and dislikes helps you manage their behavior.

- Be an expert on the residents you care for.

Work with the symptoms or behaviors you see.

- People with AD show different symptoms from day to day. Focus on the symptoms and behaviors you see, rather than on the disease.
- Notice changes in behavior, mood, and independence and report your observations.

Be understanding and compassionate.

- AD is a devastating mental and physical disorder that affects everyone who surrounds and cares for the one with AD.
- Remember that residents with AD do not always have control over their behavior. Do not take their behavior personally.
- AD can strike anyone, even you. Think about the symptoms of AD in terms of your own life. How would you want to be treated?
- Assume that residents with AD have insight and are aware of the changes in their abilities.
- Provide security and comfort.
- Provide opportunities for success and personal satisfaction.

Work as a team.

- People with AD may not distinguish between nursing assistants, nurses, or administrators, so be prepared to help when needed.
- Share insights and observations with your healthcare team.
- Part of AD care is noticing changes in behavior or physical and emotional health. Working as a team, more subtle changes will be noticed.

Take care of yourself.

- Acknowledge that caring for someone with **dementia** can be emotionally and physically demanding.
- Be good to yourself physically and emotionally.
- Be aware of your body's signals to slow down, rest, or eat better.
- Remember that your feelings are real and you have a right to them.
- Share your feelings with others, especially those experiencing similar situations.
- Do not worry about mistakes. Use them as learning experiences.

Work with family members.

- Family may know things you would have to learn by trial and error.
- Family can be of great comfort to dementia victims, helping you provide excellent care.
- Suggest environmental changes or modifications as appropriate to the person with AD.

Always remember the care program goals, including:

- Providing security and comfort.
- Maintaining dignity and self-esteem.
- Promoting independence.
- Providing assistance with appropriate care and interventions during each stage of the illness.

10 List strategies for better communication with residents who have Alzheimer's or any dementia.

Communication with residents with AD can be helped by following these guidelines:

1. If your resident is frightened or anxious:

- Move and speak slowly.
- Try to see and hear yourself as they might. Always describe what you are going to do.
- Use simple language and short sentences. If performing a procedure or assisting with self-care, simplify and list steps one at a time.
- Check your nonverbal language; are you tense or hurried?

2. If your resident forgets or shows memory loss:

- Use the same words if you need to repeat an instruction or question. However, you may be using a word the resident doesn't understand, such as "tired." Try other words like "nap" or "lie down."

3. If your resident has trouble finding words or names or substitutes sound-alike words:

- Suggest what you think the word is. If this upsets the resident, learn from it and try not to correct them. As communicating with words (written and spoken) becomes more difficult, smiling, touching, and hugging can help communicate love and concern. But remember, some residents find touch frightening or unwelcome.

4. If your resident seems not to understand basic instructions or questions:

- Ask the resident to repeat your statements. Use short words and sentences, allowing time to answer.
- Pay attention to the communication methods that are effective and use them.
- Watch for nonverbal communication as the ability to talk diminishes. Observe body language—eyes, hands, facial expressions.

- Use signs, labels or written messages.

5. If your resident repeats phrases or questions over and over:
- This is part of the disease. Answer the questions the same way each time. Even though responding over and over may frustrate you, it communicates comfort and security.

6. If your resident wants to say something but is not able:
- Encourage resident to point, gesture, or mime. If she is obviously upset but cannot explain why, just offer comfort with a hug, a smile, or distraction techniques.

7. If your resident is disoriented to time and place:
- Post reminders, such as calendars, activity boards, pictures, and signs on doors. Prior to the final stage of dementia, signs and labels can sometimes help with orientation. However, reality orientation, discussed in Chapter 7, does not help in the later stages of Alzheimer's.

8. If your resident does not remember how to perform basic tasks:
- Help by breaking each activity into simple steps. For instance, "Let's go for a walk. Stand up. Put on your sweater. First the right arm..." Always encourage residents to do what they can.

9. If your resident reminisces or lives in the past:
- Encourage reminiscing if it seems to give pleasure. It is an opportunity for you to learn more about the resident.

10. If your resident insists on doing something that is unsafe or not allowed:
- Try to limit the times you say "don't." Instead, redirect activities toward something constructive.

11. If your resident hallucinates, is paranoid, or accusing:
- Do not take it personally. Try to redirect behavior or ignore it. Because attention span is limited, this behavior often passes quickly.

12. If your resident is depressed or lonely:
- Take time, one-on-one, to ask how the resident is feeling. Really listen. Try to involve the resident in activities. Always report depression to the nurse.

13. If your resident is verbally abusive or uses bad language:
- Remember it is the dementia speaking and not the resident. Try to ignore the language or redirect attention to something else.

14. If your resident has lost most verbal skills:
- As speaking abilities decline, use nonverbal communication. People with AD will understand touch, smiles and laughter much longer than they will understand the spoken or written word.
- However, remember that some residents will not like to be touched. Approach touching slowly. Be gentle, softly touching the hand or placing your arm around the resident. A hug or a kiss can express affection and caring. A smile can say you want to help.

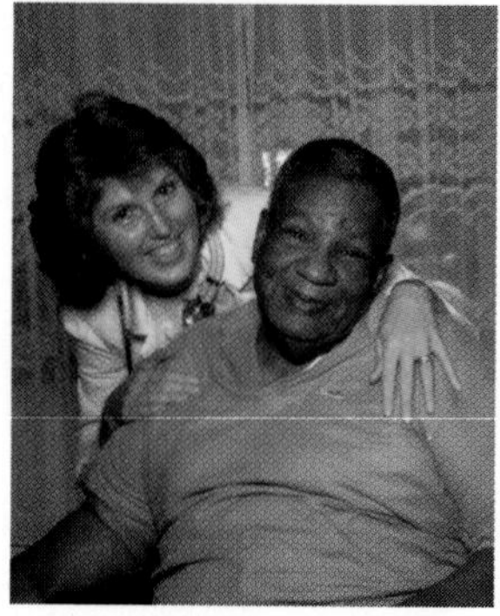
Figure 27-14. **Smiles, warm touches, and hugs can help promote positive and independent behavior in residents with Alzheimer's disease.**

- Even after verbal abilities are lost, signs, labels, and gestures can reach residents with dementia.
- Assume residents with AD can understand more than they can express. ***Never talk about them as though they were not there.***

11 Describe five guidelines for assisting the resident with Alzheimer's with personal care and activities of daily living.

The following guidelines are strategies for making resident care run more smoothly. Remember that these are general tips and may not apply to every resident. Every resident with dementia is an individual.

1. **Bathing, Grooming, and Dressing**

Ensure safety by using non-slip mats, tub seats, and hand holds. Schedule bathing when the person is least agitated. Be organized so the complete bath can be quick. Give sponge baths if a tub bath is resisted. Confusion and frustration during bathing can be reduced by always bathing at the same time, with the same steps, explaining in the same way every time. Assist with grooming. Help residents you care for to feel attractive and dignified.

Lay out clothes in the order in which they should be put on. Choose clothes that are simpler to put on, for example Velcro instead of buttons, slip-on instead of tie-up shoes, pants or skirts instead of dresses.

2. **Toileting**

Sometimes incontinence is caused by treatable medical conditions. Be certain to follow the care plan to ensure that treatment is effective. Never withhold or discourage fluids because a person is incontinent.

Though most people with AD will eventually experience incontinence, they can remain continent longer if the following tips are used:

- Set up a regular schedule for toileting and follow it.
- Mark the restroom with a sign as a reminder to use it and where it is.
- Check skin regularly for signs of irritation.
- Document bowel movements.

3. **Physical Health**

Prevent infections; they are the leading cause of death in people with Alzheimer's.

Help your residents wash their hands frequently. Observe physical health and report any potential problems. Residents with dementia may not recognize their own health problems.

4. **Nutrition**

Maintain optimal nutrition. Eating problems are common among people with AD, but can be difficult to notice. Be aware. Try to discover why a resident is not eating. Schedule meals at the same time each day and serve familiar foods. If restlessness prevents getting through an entire meal, try smaller, more frequent meals.

During meals, offer one course at a time using one utensil at a time. If your resident needs to be fed, do so slowly, offering small pieces of food. Encourage fluids. Keep nutritious snacks nearby, especially favorites. Remember to observe changes or problems in eating habits. In addition, monitor weight accurately and frequently to discover potential problems.

5. **Mental Health**

Maintain self-esteem by encouraging independence in activities of daily living. Assistance with personal grooming will increase self-esteem. Provide a daily calendar to encourage activities. Share in enjoyable activities, looking at pictures, talking, reminiscing, etc. Reward positive and independent behavior with smiles, hugs, and warm touches.

12 List eight difficult behaviors commonly exhibited by residents with Alzheimer's and describe ways to manage each.

Agitation: Dementia residents can become agitated, combative, or even violent. Feeling insecure or frustrated, encountering new people or places, and changes in routine can all trigger this behavior. Even watching television can cause extreme anxiety as people with AD lose their ability to distinguish fiction from reality. Try to recognize the triggers and eliminate them. Once behavior like this begins, your calm response and slow soothing tone can help minimize the behavior. Avoid using physical restraints; restraints can only be used with a doctor's order and should be used only to prevent injury to self or others, and then only for a limited time.

Catastrophic Reactions: When a resident with AD overreacts to something in an unreasonable way, it is called a **catastrophic reaction**. Many situations can cause these reactions, and they differ from person to person. Again, it is important to get to know the people you care for. This allows you to avoid situations that cause these reactions and to redirect them to activities you know they enjoy. As a general rule, these reactions are caused by four things:

- fatigue
- change of routine, environment, or caregiver
- overstimulation, including noise, too much activity, difficult choices or tasks
- physical pain or discomfort, including hunger or need for toileting

Pacing and Wandering: Pacing and wandering can have many causes—restlessness, hunger, disorientation, the desire to use the restroom, or even forgetting how or where to sit down. Nighttime wandering might be reduced by minimizing daytime napping. Exercise may reduce restlessness. Let residents pace and don't restrain them, but do keep an eye on them. Pacing is dangerous when it takes residents outside the safe environment. If residents attempt to leave, redirect their attention to something they enjoy.

To reduce the chance of wandering outside the home or facility:

- Create a safe place for pacing. Remove clutter and create clear paths, making certain floors are not slippery. Remove throw rugs that are not secure.
- Place stop signs or "sorry we are closed" signs on doors to remind them not to exit or have alarms on exits to indicate that the door has been opened. Locks placed either very high or very low may prevent exiting. Remember to keep a key nearby in case of emergency. Never leave a resident alone in a locked room.

Sundowning: When a resident with AD becomes

restless and agitated in the late afternoon, evening or night it is called sundowning. The best ways to reduce this restlessness are:

- Provide adequate lighting before it gets dark.
- Avoid stressful situations during this time; limit activities, appointments, trips, and visits.
- Play soft music.
- Set a bedtime routine and keep it.
- Recognize when sundowning occurs and plan a calming activity just before.
- Eliminate caffeine from the diet.
- Give a slow back massage.
- Try to redirect the behavior or distract the resident with a calm activity, like looking at a magazine.
- Maintain a daily exercise routine.

Perseveration or Repetitive Phrasing: Residents with dementia may repeat words, phrases, or questions over and over again. They may also repeat an action or task, such as tapping fingers and folding or cleaning things. Be patient with these repetitious behaviors; remember that the resident probably is unaware of what he or she is doing. If questions are asked repeatedly, respond each time with the same words.

Suspicion: As residents with AD begin to deal with their illness, they often become suspicious. Do not argue with them, as this just increases defensiveness. Instead, offer calm reassurance. Be understanding.

Hallucinations (seeing things that are not there) or delusions (thoughts believed to be true which are not): Most hallucinations and delusions are harmless and can be ignored. Respond with reassurance if residents seem agitated or worried. Disputing or challenging serves no purpose and can make matters worse. Remember that the feelings are real to the resident with AD. Again, redirecting to other activities or thoughts can be very useful. Be calm and reassure them that you are there to help.

If someone attacks you verbally or accuses you of stealing, do not take it personally. Remember, it is the disease speaking and not the resident. If someone becomes violent, stay out of the way. Block but do not hit. Stay calm and observe from a safe distance; violent behavior usually subsides quickly. Get help if necessary. Always report this behavior.

Depression: It is understandable that people who are losing independence and the ability to manage their lives become depressed. Feelings of failure and fear can cause them to become withdrawn. Be aware of these behavior and mood changes. Report depression to the nurse, as medications may help. Try to note the triggers or events that cause changes in mood. Always encourage and reward activities that improve moods and attempt to reduce situations that cause withdrawal. Find ways to help foster social relationships, such as group activities. Listen to them, as they will often share their feelings. Respect the right to feel sad; offer comfort and concern.

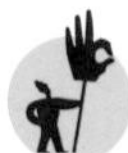

The Safe Return System

Have you ever had a knock at the door and been greeted by a person in a panic frantically searching for a missing loved one with Alzheimer's disease? The Alzheimer's Association has a Safe Return program that families can use to register their loved ones. For a small fee, the family receives an ID bracelet, labels to sew on clothing, and a special wallet card. The identification number matches the registration number with the association. It is hard for people to believe that this could happen to a loved one; however, it happens every day. If you have a relative or friend with the disease, consider protecting them with the Safe Return program. For more information about the Safe Return program, contact the Alzheimer's Association at 1- 800-272-3900 or at www.alz.org.

Summary

The function of the nervous system is to transport impulses to and from the brain in order to cause voluntary movements and other body functions. The nervous system can be injured by damaging a nerve or group of nerves. If the spinal cord is severed, the nervous system cannot function to its full capacity. Alzheimer's disease is a common disorder you will see in your residents. You will need to be able to recognize many different behaviors and techniques for dealing with them. Above all, always be patient and understanding with residents who have Alzheimer's.

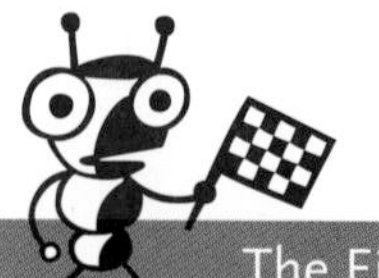

The Finish Line

What's Wrong With This Picture?

Look at the portion of the STAR KARE for aspiration safety shown below. List and correct the five errors:

Assist the resident/nurse.

- *Place stroke residents in prone position for eating. Resident should stay in prone position for about 10 minutes after eating or drinking.*

- *Feed stroke residents extremely quickly.*
- *Food must be placed into the weak or affected side of the mouth.*

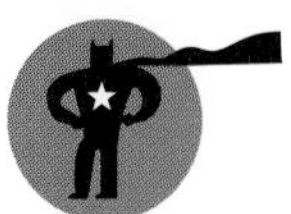

Star Student Central

1. Contact the spinal cord section of a local rehabilitation center. Ask for a tour and information regarding spinal cord injuries.
2. Contact a stroke rehabilitation center and ask if you may observe stroke patients in the rehabilitation process. Bring back any information that might be helpful for your class.

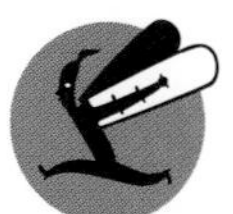

You Can Do It Corner!

1. List five things that may occur in each stage of the progression of Alzheimer's. (LO 8)
2. What is an aura? (LO 3)
3. What are five guidelines for assisting the resident with Alzheimer's disease with personal care? (LO 11)
4. What are seven attitudes that are helpful when working with Alzheimer's residents? (LO 9)
5. What are two steps you should take to try to protect a person having a seizure? (LO 3)
6. How should you enter the room of a visually impaired resident? (LO 4)
7. How should you enter the room of a hearing-impaired resident? (LO 6)
8. If your Alzheimer's resident is depressed or lonely, what can you do to help? (LO 10)
9. Why should you never use any cleaning agent on an artificial eye other than water? (LO 5)
10. A left-sided stroke may cause paralysis on which side? A right-sided CVA may cause paralysis on which side? (LO 3)
11. How can you help a resident who is experiencing sundowning? (LO 12)
12. What do the terms "irreversible" and "progressive" mean? (LO 7)
13. What are some normal changes of aging for the nervous system? (LO 2)

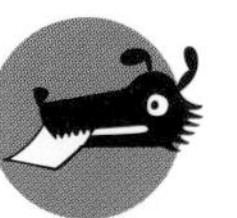

Star Student's Chapter Checklist

1. I have read my textbook chapter.
2. I have reviewed my own "Pocketful of Terms."
3. I have listened to my tutor tape.
4. I have reviewed and highlighted my class notes.
5. I have read and completed any handouts from this chapter.
6. I have completed "The Finish Line."
7. Star Time! Choose your reward!

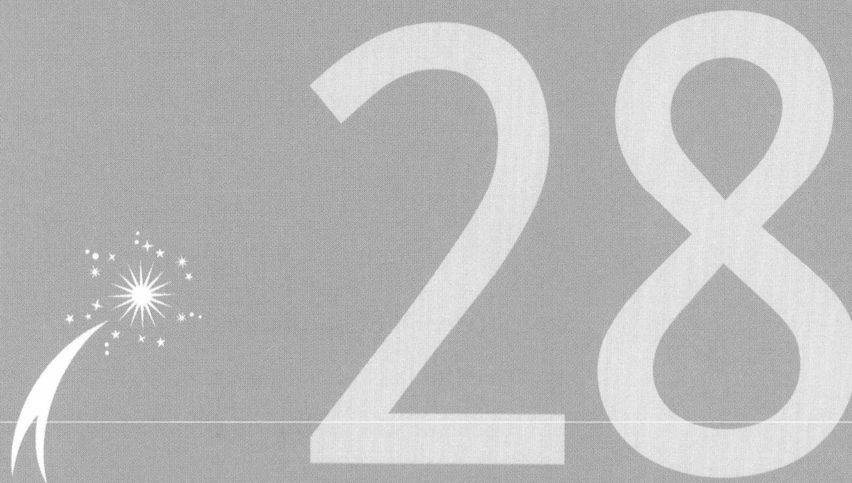

Specialized Care: The Circulatory System

Look Like a Star!

Look at the Learning Objectives and The Finish Line before you begin reading this chapter.

Look at your pocket calendar.
With your pencil, put a bracket ( ) around a study period every single day.

Look at your homework for this chapter.
Plug each piece of homework into a certain time slot.

Look at the Star Student's Chapter Checklist at the end of this chapter. Check off each item as it is completed.

"... So in my veins red life might stream again..."

John Keats, 1795-1821

"... It ennobled our hearts and enriched our blood..."

Richard Leveridge, 1670-1758

Learning Objectives

1. **Spell and define all STAR words.**
2. **Summarize the changes that occur in the circulatory system during normal aging.**
3. **Discuss five common disorders of the circulatory system.**
4. **Explain two types of circulatory stockings.**
5. **Discuss care of a resident with an intravenous line/IV and signs to observe.**

Successfully perform these Practical Procedures

Applying Anti-Embolic Stockings

Care of the Resident with Sequential Compression Therapy

The Way of the Blood in the Heart and the Vessels

William Harvey, 1578-1657, wrote *On the Movement of the Heart and Blood in Animals,* which was published in 1628. He noted the blood moves throughout the body in a closed system. He came to the conclusion that the blood actually recycles itself and moves inside the body in a single direction, not back and forth.
Harvey also identified that the heart is a pump and that it works using the force of muscle. He found the heart has two phases: systole, when the heart contracts and empties itself of blood, and diastole, when the chambers of the heart are filled with blood.

1 Spell and define all STAR words.

cardioversion: shock given to restore heart to a normal rhythm.

congestive heart failure: left or right-sided heart failure due to pumping problem with the heart.

dyspnea: difficulty breathing.

edema: swelling of the extremities, especially the ankles.

infiltration: when an intravenous line has come out of a vein, causing fluid to collect in the surrounding tissues.

orthopnea: shortness of breath when lying down that is relieved by sitting up.

2 Summarize the changes that occur in the circulatory system during normal aging.

As people age, the heart pumps less efficiently. This reduces the amount of oxygen to body cells. This can cause the elderly to tire more quickly. Blood vessels are also affected. They may become narrower due to a fatty build-up inside the arteries, usually from cholesterol. Smoking also narrows arteries.
Hypertension (high blood pressure) is also a problem for some people. When blood flow to the brain is reduced, some confusion can result.

3 Discuss five common disorders of the circulatory system.

1. Hypertension (HTN)

When blood pressure consistently measures higher than 140/90, a person is diagnosed as having hypertension. Hypertension, or high blood pressure, can develop in persons of any age. Signs and symptoms of hypertension are not always obvious, especially in the early stages of the disease. Often the illness is only discovered when a blood pressure measurement is taken by a healthcare provider. Persons with the disease may complain of headache, blurred vision, and dizziness.

Untreated hypertension may lead to a myocardial infarction (heart attack). This is often caused by one of the fatty deposits completely blocking off a coronary artery, causing damage to a part of the heart muscle from the lack of blood supply. If not treated promptly, it can also lead to a cerebrovascular accident (CVA), or stroke, due to force causing a rupture in a vessel inside the brain.

CAUSE: There are many causes of hypertension. The major cause of hypertension is a hardening and narrowing of the blood vessels. Hypertension can also result from kidney disease, tumors of the adrenal gland, complications of pregnancy, extreme stress or pain, and certain medications. Arteries may become hardened, or narrower, because of a buildup of plaque on the walls of the blood vessels, and this can cause hypertension.

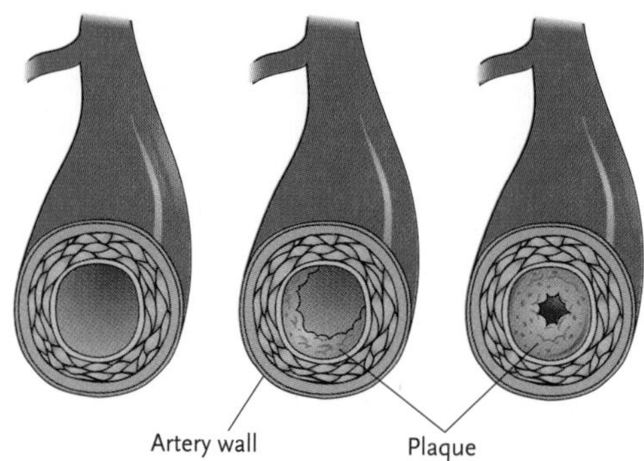

Figure 28-1. Arteries may become hardened, or narrower, because of a buildup of plaque on the walls of the blood vessels. Hardened arteries cause hypertension, or high blood pressure.

CURE/TREATMENT: High blood pressure medication is usually ordered for people with hypertension. This may keep the hypertension under control and can prevent the complications listed above. Some doctors advise their patients to seek stress management to reduce their overall stress level. Some people may have a prescribed exercise program or be on a special low-fat, low-sodium diet. Reducing the intake of sodium (salt) in the diet is ordered to reduce extra fluid in the body because of sodium. Extra fluid can increase blood volume and weight, which increases the workload on the heart. Stopping smoking can increase the size of the blood vessels, increasing the flow of blood. Nicotine constricts (closes) blood vessels.

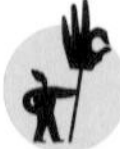

The Silent Killer

Have you noted unusual nosebleeds, eye hemorrhages (where blood shows up in the white of an eye) or symptoms like dizziness, trembling, shortness of breath, or headaches in one of your residents? Sometimes these are a sign of high blood pressure (hypertension). Hypertension may cause a serious problem, such as a stroke or a heart attack. Report to the nurse any one of these signs or symptoms. A life may depend upon it!

2. Unstable Angina (USA)

When the heart is unable to get the oxygen it needs, angina, or chest pain, occurs. Unstable angina can lead to a heart attack if untreated. People with this problem develop angina while sleeping or doing things that never caused angina before.

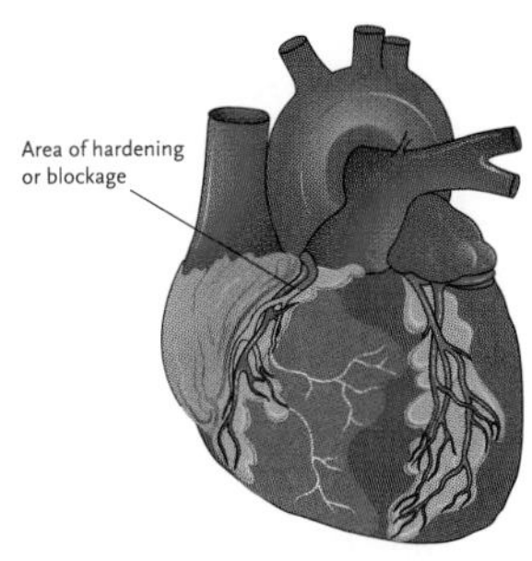

Figure 28-2. **Angina results from the heart not getting enough oxygen.**

CAUSE: A blockage in one or more of the coronary arteries, made up of fats like cholesterol, causes angina. When this blockage in a coronary artery becomes large, it sometimes tears or opens. The body tries to help heal the blockage by forming a blood clot. This clot can become so large that it blocks the flow of blood through the vessel, causing a heart attack.

CURE/TREATMENT: Blood thinners are often given to help prevent blood clots from developing. Aspirin is one of the medications ordered because it helps prevent blood clots.

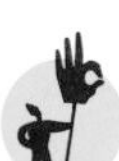

Personal Health Tip!

Commercials have discussed the positive effects of taking regular aspirin for years. They may not tell you that you should never take aspirin on a regular basis without first checking with your doctor. Aspirin may thin the blood to the extent that people develop uncontrolled bleeding after a simple injury. Ulcers can become worse with aspirin. People who are taking aspirin regularly should be under the regular care of a doctor. It is possible, for example, that a person is already on a blood thinning medication. Taking aspirin may double the blood thinning effects. If your doctor or healthcare provider tells you to take aspirin regularly, make sure you do the following:

1. *TELL YOUR DENTIST before any procedure.*
2. *TELL YOUR DOCTOR before allowing any kind of surgery.*

Quitting smoking may help unstable angina by opening the blood vessels. Taking nitroglycerin may increase the blood flow to the heart and take some of the work off the heart. A procedure called an angioplasty is an option. This procedure involves blowing up a tiny balloon inside the blood vessel to open the vessel. Coronary artery bypass surgery is a choice for people with severe blockages. The doctor grafts a piece of a vein, usually from the leg, to bypass the blocked artery inside your heart.

Myocardial Infarction (MI) or Heart Attack

Box 28-1

When the reduction in blood flow to the heart becomes more severe, the angina worsens. When the blood flow to all or part of the heart muscle is completely blocked, oxygen and important nutrients fail to reach the cells in that region. This is called a myocardial infarction or a heart attack. This means a part of the heart muscle has sustained damage and a percentage of the muscle tissue of the heart dies. A thrombus (clot) can cause a myocardial infarction by blocking the blood supply to an area of the heart. After a myocardial infarction, the area of the heart that has been damaged can no longer function and usually turns into scar tissue. The undamaged heart muscle must then compensate (take over) for the part of the heart that has died. This can increase the workload on the part of the heart that is still able to function.

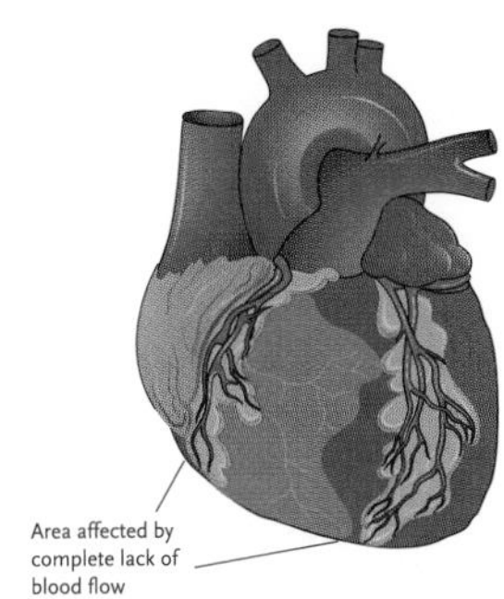

Figure 28-3. **A heart attack occurs when blood flow to the heart or a portion of the heart is cut off completely.**

Symptoms of a myocardial infarction are extreme pain in the chest, which has been likened to an elephant sitting on the person's chest. This pain may move into the left or right arm, the jaw, the neck, or the back. Nausea, diaphoresis (sweating), a change in the vital signs, especially the pulse, respiration, and blood pressure, a loss of consciousness, and a feeling of doom are other symptoms. If you observe any of these symptoms in your residents, report it to the nurse immediately.

After a myocardial infarction, a program of cardiac rehabilitation is usually ordered. Cardiac rehabilitation may continue for a period of a few months up to six months or more. This comprehensive program consists of a variety of components, including the following:

Dietary Changes: a low-cholesterol, low-fat, and low-sodium diet may be ordered. A dietician or nutritionist may plan the new diet.

Stopping Smoking: Quitting smoking will be encouraged. Even second-hand smoke may put the post-MI patient at risk. There are many new tools, both over-the-counter and prescribed, to assist people with quitting smoking.

Exercise Regimen: An exercise program done at a facility under the watchful eye of registered nurses or other healthcare professionals is ordered. The exercise program usually starts very slowly, advancing to a higher level of exercise. The person's cardiac system, including the pulse and blood pressure, will be closely watched during these exercise sessions. In some cases, the person's heart will have to be monitored during the exercise sessions.

Patient Counseling and Education: Stress management may be initiated to help reduce stress levels. Counseling about new methods to reduce possible risks during sex and other activities is an option.

3. Congestive Heart Failure (CHF)

When one or both sides of the heart stop pumping blood effectively, congestive heart failure may occur. The blood backs up during this process, causing harmful waste products to develop inside the blood. Helpful substances the body needs get "stuck" inside the blood and are unable to travel where the substance is vitally needed.

Symptoms of CHF include dizziness, fatigue, confusion, and a reduction in urination. Other symptoms may occur, depending on the side of the heart that is "congested." The different symptoms associated with congestive heart failure are listed below:

Left-sided failure: coughing, **dyspnea**, **orthopnea**, and fainting

Right-sided failure: Edema (swelling) of the extremities, especially the ankles

CAUSE: Many problems may cause congestive heart failure, including heart disease, high blood pressure, heart attacks, and heart valve problems.

CURE/TREATMENT: Congestive heart failure may be controlled through the use of certain medications and a care plan that encourages rest. Medications may help reduce the excess fluid built up inside the body, thereby reducing edema. Other medications may also help the heart contract more effectively, which increases the movement of blood through the body. Certain medications improve the flow of blood, which may reduce the workload of the heart.

Star K.A.R.E.

Congestive Heart Failure

KNOW your resident's care plan.
ASSIST the resident/nurse.

- *Carefully follow order for bedrest.*
- *Stop and have the person sit or lie down if dizziness or fainting occur.*
- *Carefully follow orders for daily weight and intake and output measurement.*
- *Carefully follow order for fluid restriction.*
- *Carefully follow a low-salt diet.*
- *Use special stockings that improve the flow of blood as ordered to reduce fluid retention (edema).*
- *Assist with range of motion exercises as ordered to improve muscle tone when activity is limited.*

REPORT observations.
RECORD data.
RECHECK resident as needed.

If any of the following occurs:

- *dizziness, confusion, or fainting*
- *increased respiratory rate, pulse, or blood pressure*
- *weight gain from fluid retention*
- *shortness of breath or dyspnea*
- *coughing*
- *chest tightness or chest pain*
- *edema (swelling)*
- *reduction in urine*

★ *"Don't Delay. Report Right Away!"*

ENCOURAGE resident's independence and progress.

- *Provide support during difficult times.*

Never ignore SOB or chest pain!

Remember, the phrase "no pain, no gain" does not belong in healthcare. If your resident is supposed to ambulate a certain number of times per day and the walking causes shortness of breath (SOB) or chest pain, stop and report this to the nurse immediately. Do not ignore if a resident has to stop periodically when walking. Do not assume the resident is just fatigued. Ask the resident if he is having any pain or difficulty getting a breath. If you ignore this, the resident may develop a more serious problem later.

4. Atrial Fibrillation

When the top chambers of the heart, known as the atria, beat in a fast, irregular manner, the person is said to have atrial fibrillation. When a person has atrial fibrillation, the atria may beat much faster than the normal 60 to 100 beats per minute. They may beat well into the hundreds per minute, and will have a tough time completely emptying of blood.

Atrial fibrillation leads to an increased risk of stroke. When the atria are unable to empty all of the blood, blood clots may form. When one of these clots or a piece of a clot begins to move, it can travel to the brain and cause a stroke. It can also travel to the heart and cause a heart attack, or to the lungs and cause a pulmonary embolism, which can be fatal. Medication may be ordered to thin the blood so that the blood clots do not form.

CAUSE: Heart disease may cause atrial fibrillation. A thyroid problem is another possible cause.

CURE/TREATMENT: A method called **cardioversion** may be used to make the heart beat normally again. This may have to be done a second or even a third time if the heartbeat becomes irregular again.

Blood thinners are ordered to thin the blood so that blood clots do not have the chance to form. This causes the person to bleed easily, so being extremely cautious will help prevent injury. Even a simple paper cut can cause uncontrolled bleeding.

5. Peripheral Vascular Disease (PVD)

The peripheral vascular system exhibits disease in different parts of the body. The blood vessels supply blood to the tips of the fingers and toes, as well as to the head. When blood supply is reduced, the oxygen supply is reduced, causing damage to tissues.

Some of the symptoms of PVD are skin that is cyanotic (slightly blue or gray-tinged), pain in the legs, especially the calves, edema of the lower extremities, feet and/or legs that feel cold to the touch, and a blue or gray tinge in the toenails.

CAUSE: Some causes for peripheral vascular disease are a reduction in cardiac output (amount of blood being pumped out of the heart) possibly due to a weakened heart, a decrease in circulation due to fatty deposits inside the blood vessels, and inflammation of the veins in the lower extremities, called phlebitis.

CURE/TREATMENT: Identifying and managing the cause of peripheral vascular disease is done to improve circulation to the peripheral blood vessels. For example, if the cause is fatty deposits, a low-cholesterol diet may be ordered to try to prevent further deposits from forming.

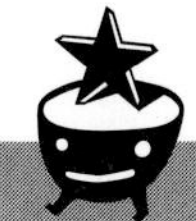

Star K.A.R.E.

Peripheral Vascular Disease

***KNOW** your resident's care plan.*
***ASSIST** the resident/nurse.*

- *Carefully check pulses and blood pressure as directed by the nurse.*
- *Carefully follow bedrest, if ordered, and any special orders for the extremities.*
- *Provide quality foot care. (Chapter 21)*
- *Carefully follow orders for daily weight and intake and output measurement.*
- *Discourage smoking.*
- *Carefully follow order for fluid restriction or low-sodium diet.*
- *Use special stockings that improve the flow of blood and reduce fluid retention (edema).*
- *Reduce overall stress as much as possible.*

***REPORT** observations.*

***RECORD** data.*

***RECHECK** resident as needed.*

If any of the following occur:

- *change in any vital sign, especially in pulse or blood pressure*
- *any complaints regarding the feet*
- *an increase in weight*
- *a change in intake or output*
- *headache or any pain in the head or neck area*
- *change in the orientation of the person, dizziness, or confusion*
- *increase in severity of edema*
- *positive Homan's sign—when the foot is dorsiflexed (toes pointed toward the head) while the rest of the leg is kept fully extended (straight), pain occurring in the back of the calf may mean a blood clot in the leg. Nursing assistants may not be able to check for Homan's sign at your facility or in your state; however, always report any pain in the calf area*
- *an increase in stress level*
- *any change noticed in the feet, legs, or arms when bathing or dressing residents*
- *any clothing items that might compromise circulation, such as tight stockings*

★ *"Don't Delay. Report Right Away!"*

- *Observe carefully when using hot or cold applications, such as hot pads, etc.*

***ENCOURAGE** resident's independence and progress.*

- *Encourage resident to do as much self-care as she is capable of doing.*
- *Help identify causes of stress and try to resolve them.*
- *Encourage following the care plan, including special diets or stopping smoking.*

4 Explain two types of circulatory stockings.

Anti-embolic stockings help people with circulatory disorders move about more comfortably. These special stockings increase the blood circulation by causing smooth, even compression of the legs so that the blood moves better through the vessels. Anti-embolic stockings are measured carefully so that the person is given the correct size. There are two styles: thigh-high and knee-high.

For thigh-high stockings, the inseam measurement and the thigh circumference are measured. To find the correct size for knee-high stockings, the calf circumference and the distance from the knee to the bottom of the foot are measured. A seamed hole

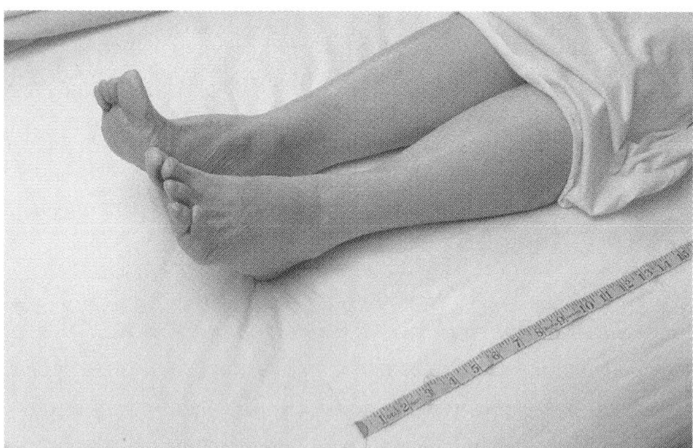

Figure 28-4. **Measuring for a knee-high stocking.**

exists in the fabric around the toe or underneath the foot. This allows the skin color of the feet and toes to be observed. Cyanosis (blue-tinged skin) can be seen without taking the stockings all the way off. Carefully observe the toes for cyanosis throughout the day.

Using anti-embolic stockings poses some risks. If this stocking is turned over at the top, the compression can double, causing the blood flow in the leg to be blocked. These stockings should be applied in the early morning hours when legs are at their smallest. It is much more difficult to apply them later on.

Sequential compression stockings are used to improve circulation and prevent blood clots. They may be used after surgery or childbirth. They are connected to a pump that normally has an on/off switch. This method of therapy is sometimes used with anti-embolic stockings. A current of air inflates and deflates throughout the wrap, which causes alternating compression of the extremities. A measurement is needed to order the correct size of sequential compression stockings.

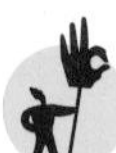

Leg and Foot Exercises

If one of your residents has leg and foot exercises ordered to improve circulation, review these steps:

1. *Exercise the toes by moving them up and down.*
2. *Make circles with the toes.*
3. *Turn the ankles in and out.*
4. *Bring each foot up and down.*
5. *Move each leg out as far as you can and bring it back to original position.*
6. *Lift the knees up and bring them down.*

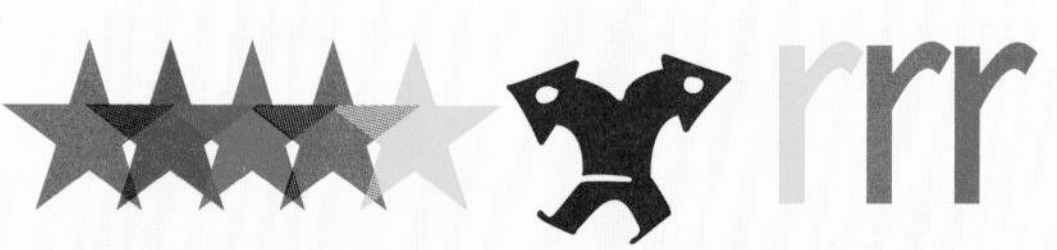

Beginning Steps

★ RESPECT
Knock first, ask and receive permission to enter a resident's room.

★ INFECTION CONTROL
Wash hands.

★ COMMUNICATION
Greet and identify the resident. Identify yourself. Explain the procedure, encouraging the resident to be as independent as possible throughout.

★ BED SAFETY
Lock bed wheels. Raise bed to safe working height. Lower one side rail if required.

★ PRIVACY
Provide for privacy by closing the door and covering the resident appropriately.

Ending Steps

★ RESIDENT SAFETY AND COMFORT
Secure the resident, lowering the bed, and raising the side rails if ordered. Check that the resident is comfortable and properly aligned.

★ PRIVACY
Remove any added privacy measures, such as a drape or a privacy screen.

★ ESSENTIALS
Place the call light, fresh beverage, and other items within reach.

★ COURTESY
Ask the resident if he or she needs anything else. Say thank you and goodbye.

★ INFECTION CONTROL
Wash hands.

r **Report** your care and any important observations to the nurse.

r **Record** your care and any important information/observations such as vital signs in the appropriate place.

r **Recheck** your resident for any changes as directed by the nurse!

Applying Anti-Embolic Stockings

Follow all standard and/or transmission-based precautions. Follow all rules for body mechanics.

Collect equipment:

- **clean stockings in the correct size**

1. **Perform the "5 Stars."**

PREPARE:

2. **Know how the stocking should be positioned, as types and brands vary.**
3. **Put resident in the supine position.**

PERFORM:

4. **Take one stocking in both hands and roll so that toe area is ready to wrap over toes of resident.**

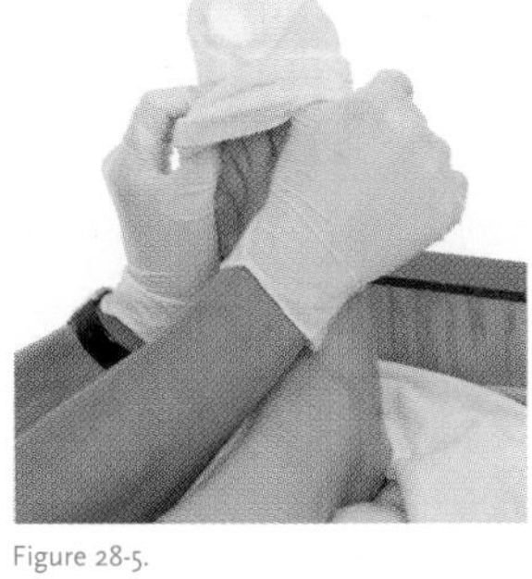

Figure 28-5.

5. **While supporting the heel, bring the stocking over the toes, then the foot and the ankle. The opening in the stocking allowing observation of skin color should be either on the top or the bottom of the toe area, depending upon the manufacturer.**
6. **Slowly bring the stocking up the leg of the resident, smoothing out any wrinkles when completely unrolled.**

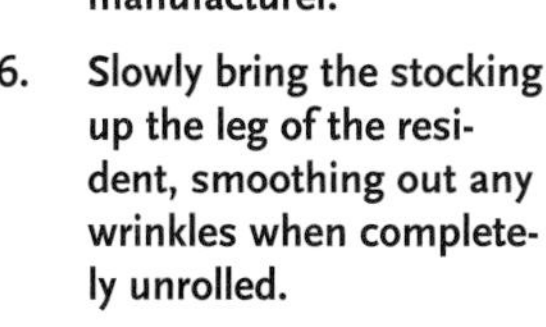

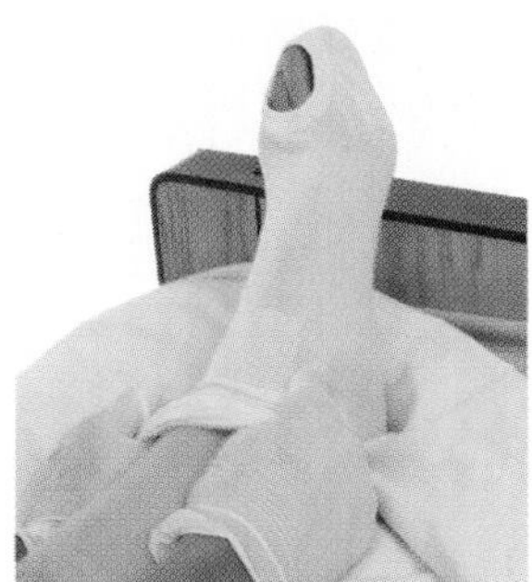

Figure 28-6.

7. **Repeat entire procedure for the other leg. Smooth out any wrinkles.**

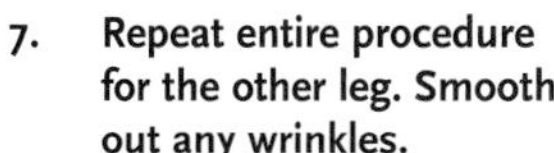

FINISHING TOUCHES:

8. **Straighten all of the linens and make sure resident is comfortable.**
9. **Perform the "5 Stars and 3 Rs."**

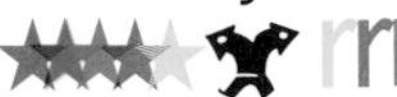

Care of the Resident with Sequential Compression Therapy

Follow all standard and/or transmission-based precautions. Follow all rules for body mechanics.

Collect equipment:

- **measuring tape • SCDs • compressor unit**

1. **Perform the "5 Stars."**

PREPARE:

2. **Position resident in the supine position.**

PERFORM:

3. **Measure upper thigh circumference according to instructions.**
4. **Look at the chart and determine size of SCDs.**
5. **SECURE THE RESIDENT.**
6. **Obtain SCDs in proper size and return to room.**
7. **Place leg on compression sleeve: back of knee over popliteal opening, and back of ankle over ankle marking.**
8. **Wrap snugly and secure with Velcro, not wrapping too tightly.**

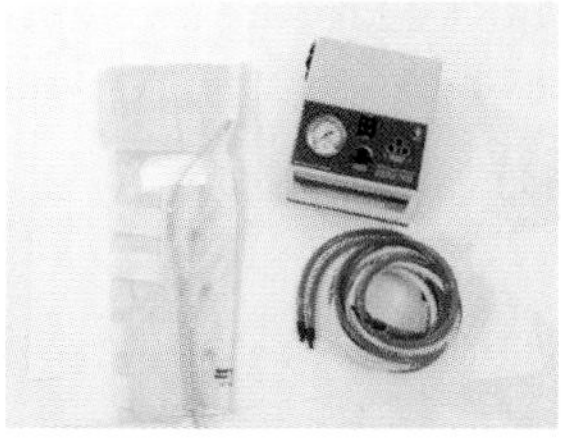

Figure 28-7.

9. **Check by inserting two to three fingers inside the sleeve.**
10. **Connect sleeves to the tubing and compressor and click into place.**
11. **Check for kinks or twists in the tubing.**
12. **Turn ON compressor unit.**
13. **Make resident comfortable. The compressor unit will remain on for long periods of time. Follow instructions from the nurse on when to turn it off.**

FINISHING TOUCHES:

14. **Perform the "5 Stars and 3 Rs."**

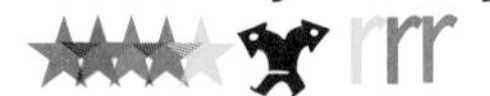

---

5 Discuss care of a resident with an intravenous line/IV and signs to observe.

A resident with an intravenous line (IV) poses many challenges for the nursing assistant trying to give the best of care. An **infiltration** means an intravenous line has come out of a vein. This happens when the resident is moved or positioned and care is not taken to support the IV tubing or catheter and tape. Be very cautious when moving residents not to tug or pull on the IV tubing. Also carefully observe the IV site for any change that may signal infiltration. Infiltration may cause tissue swelling, pain and pressure, redness, and fever. Always report these signs immediately to the nurse:

- wetness on the dressing or tape
- an arm or hand board that is coming off
- blood inside the tubing or on the dressing
- an IV pulled completely out of a vein
- air in the tubing

Summary

The circulatory system functions by moving blood through the vessels in your body. The circulatory system may be damaged when clots develop because of a decrease in blood circulation. If a blockage develops in the circulatory system, it could potentially be fatal. It is important to keep the circulatory system healthy and the blood flowing freely. Exercise and fluid intake are two things that help keep the system healthy.

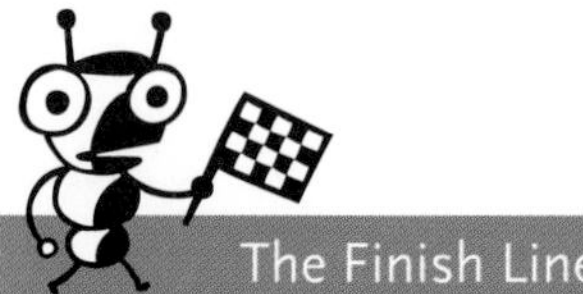

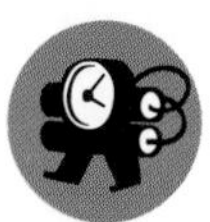

What's Wrong With This Picture?

1. Look at the portion of the STAR KARE shown below. Find and list the missing actions for assisting a CHF resident.

ASSIST the resident/nurse.

- *Carefully follow order of bedrest, if ordered.*
- *Stop and have the person sit or lie down if dizziness or fainting occur.*
- *Carefully follow order for fluid restriction.*
- *Carefully follow a low-salt diet.*
- *Assist with range of motion exercises as ordered to improve muscle tone when activity is limited.*

2. Look at the portion of STAR KARE shown below. Find and list the missing actions for assisting a resident with PVD.

ASSIST the resident/nurse.

- *Carefully check pulse and blood pressure as directed by the nurse.*
- *If a nurse asks you to feel a carotid pulse, make sure you understand the scope of practice in your state and the rules at your facility. This procedure can be very dangerous when done incorrectly.*
- *Carefully follow bedrest, if ordered, and any special orders for the extremities.*
- *Carefully follow orders for daily weight and intake and output measurement.*
- *Discourage smoking.*
- *Use special stockings that improve the flow of blood and reduce fluid retention (edema).*

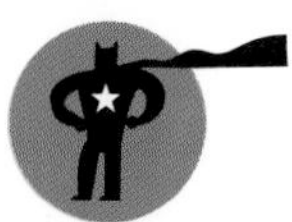

Star Student Central

1. Pick a circulatory disorder in this chapter. Research it at the library or on the Internet. If you have a family history of this disorder, find out what your risks are. Share your findings with your class.
2. Ask your doctor if you're at the right age for a stress test. This tests the stress the heart experiences during a period of supervised exercise (e.g. a treadmill). Many doctors want their patients to have a baseline stress test at a certain age.

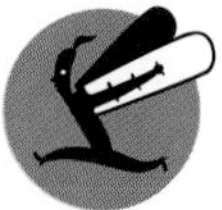

You Can Do It Corner!

1. What is the name for the problem that occurs when an IV comes out of a vein? (LO 5)
2. What is a possible complication of turning over an anti-embolic stocking and doubling up the fabric? (LO 4)
3. What are six signs of an MI? (LO 3)
4. What are five symptoms of PVD? (LO 3)
5. What is the purpose for the opening in the toes in anti-embolic stockings? (LO 4)
6. What are two changes that occur in normal aging of the circulatory system? (LO 2)
7. What are symptoms of left- and right-sided CHF? (LO 3)

Star Student's Chapter Checklist

1. I have read my textbook chapter.
2. I have reviewed my own "Pocketful of Terms."
3. I have listened to my tutor tape.
4. I have reviewed and highlighted my class notes.

5. I have read and completed any handouts from this chapter.
6. I have completed "The Finish Line."
7. Star Time! Choose your reward!

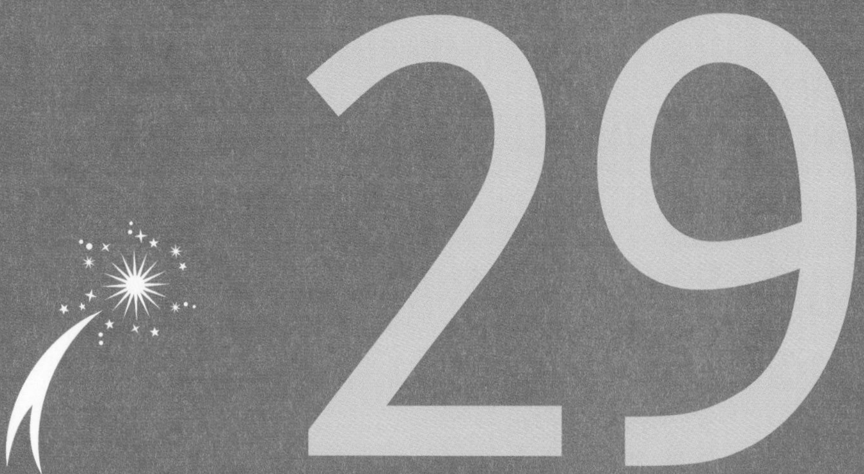

Specialized Care: The Respiratory System

Look Like a Star!

Look at the Learning Objectives and The Finish Line before you begin reading this chapter.

Look at your pocket calendar.
With your pencil, put a bracket ( ) around a study period every single day.

Look at your homework for this chapter.
Plug each piece of homework into a certain time slot.

Look at the Star Student's Chapter Checklist at the end of this chapter. Check off each item as it is completed.

"... Full of sweet dreams, and health, and quiet breathing."

John Keats, 1795-1821

"Nothing to breathe but air. Quick as a flash tis' gone. . ."

Benjamin Franklin King, Jr., 1857- 1894

Learning Objectives

1. **Spell and define all STAR words.**
2. **Summarize the changes that occur in the respiratory system during normal aging.**
3. **Discuss four common disorders of the respiratory system.**
4. **Define tuberculosis and explain how it is transmitted.**
5. **Explain care guidelines for residents with known or suspected TB.**
6. **Describe care guidelines for a resident on oxygen therapy and explain six oxygen delivery devices.**
7. **Describe safe and accurate sputum specimen collection.**
8. **Describe the benefits of deep breathing exercises.**

Successfully perform this Practical Procedure

Collecting a Sputum Specimen

Respiration and the "Vapours" of the Heart

Galen, an early physician and author of many volumes of medical knowledge, believed that the process of respiration cooled a person's heart. He thought that chest movement added air that helped get rid of certain "vapours" of the heart. Much later, William Harvey, a doctor, lecturer, researcher, and writer, developed the theory that the lungs change venous blood to arterial blood.

1 Spell and define all STAR words.

asthma: dyspnea, or difficulty breathing, from wheezing caused by bronchial spasms.

bronchitis: inflammation of mucous membrane of the bronchial tubes.

claustrophobia: fear of being confined in any space.

continuous: without break or interruption.

cyanosis: bluish or grayish discoloration of the skin due to low oxygen.

dyspnea: difficulty breathing.

emphysema: disorder where the alveoli of the lungs become filled with trapped air; usually caused by smoking.

humidifier: device used to increase the humidity content of air in the room.

intermittent: starting and stopping at intervals.

nasal cannula: oxygen delivery device that rests in the nose.

nasal catheter: oxygen delivery device that is inserted into the nasal passages.

oxygen concentrator: device that uses room air to make and deliver more pure oxygen.

oxygen tent: oxygen delivery device for the head and shoulders; an airtight enclosure to deliver oxygen in an increased amount.

pneumonia: inflammation of the lungs caused by bacteria or viruses.

sputum: substance expelled by coughing or clearing the throat.

trigger: event that initiates some other action.

tuberculosis: a disease spread by tiny germs called bacilli that float in the air; an infected person can spread the disease by coughing, breathing, singing, sneezing, or laughing; if untreated, it can be deadly.

wheeze: whistling resulting from narrowed respiratory passages.

2 Summarize the changes that occur in the respiratory system during normal aging.

As people age, the air sacs in the lungs, called the alveoli, become less elastic. This prevents the proper air exchange inside the lungs. In addition, airways can become less elastic and stiffer, preventing the adequate movement of air inside the lungs and contributing to less oxygen in the blood. This can cause elderly people to tire easily and not have enough energy to get through the day. The capacity of our lungs also may decrease. This causes more shallow breathing, which increases the risk of pneumonia.

3 Discuss four common disorders of the respiratory system.

1. Asthma

Asthma is a disorder in which **triggers**—substances or certain conditions—cause inflammation and swelling in the air passages in the lungs. These fragile air passages become very sensitive to any irritant. A person may have an "asthma attack" due to something as simple as the smell of perfume. The symptoms of asthma attacks include heavy wheezing, difficulty breathing, or **dyspnea**, and a tight feeling in the chest.

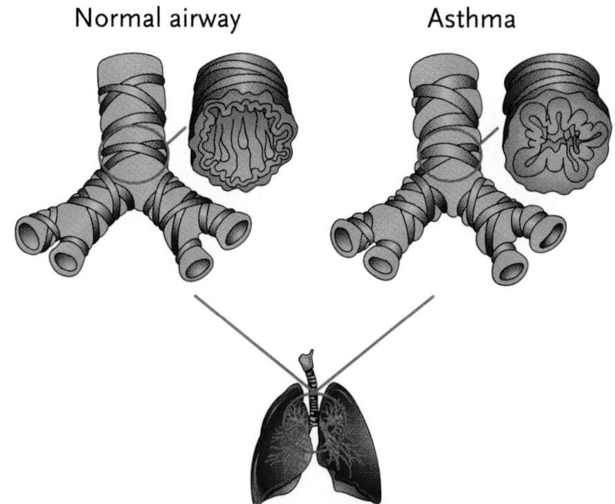

Figure 29-1. With asthma, air passages in the lungs become swollen and inflamed.

CAUSE: The cause of asthma is unknown.

CURE/TREATMENT: Asthma may go away for a time and then return, or it may disappear forever. There are some things that people can do to help decrease the chances of an asthma attack.

Taking medications correctly that have been ordered by a healthcare provider is an important step. For example, if an inhaler is ordered, asthmatics should carry the inhaler with them at all times. You may help remind that person to do this.

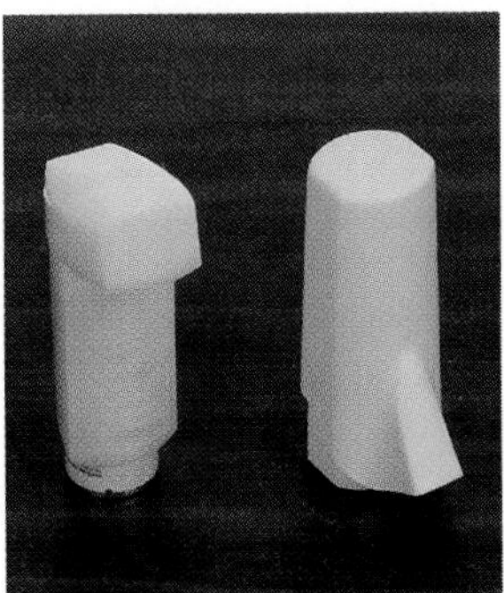

Figure 29-2. **An inhaler.**

Avoiding the triggers that cause asthma attacks is also a very important step. For example, a resident with asthma should never be put in the same room with another resident who wears heavy perfume. If someone gets asthma attacks around cats, help prevent him from being exposed to cats.

Smoking and second-hand smoke should be avoided as much as possible. Residents with asthma should not have a roommate who goes outside of the facility to smoke and then returns to the room. The smoking resident will still have smoke on her clothing and hands. This could trigger an attack.

Stress has been identified as a trigger for asthma attacks. Stress levels may be evaluated to try to find ways to reduce stress in the life of an asthmatic.

It is possible for people with allergies to improve their quality of life by going through allergy testing. This may pinpoint the trigger. Then the doctor can give allergy shots to help reduce the severity of the allergy symptoms. However, allergy testing may not help a person with serious asthma.

Star K.A.R.E.

Asthma

***KNOW** your resident's care plan.*
***ASSIST** the resident/nurse.*

- *Try to reduce stress in the resident's daily life.*
- *Never smoke around an asthmatic or allow anyone who has been smoking to come near the resident.*
- *Do not wear cologne or perfume or use any type of powder around an asthmatic.*
- *Consider replacing aerosol products with non-aerosol products.*
- *Remind asthmatics to carry their inhalers with them at all times.*

***REPORT** observations.*
***RECORD** data.*
***RECHECK** resident as needed.*

If the following occurs:

- *stressful episodes that may trigger an attack*
- *changes in vital signs, especially respiratory rate or pulse*
- ***wheezing**, shortness of breath, or dyspnea*
- ***cyanosis** (blue-tinged skin)*
- *chest pain or tightness*

★ *"Don't Delay. Report Right Away!"*

***ENCOURAGE** resident's independence and progress.*

- *Think about possible triggers and help the resident avoid them.*
- *Talking with and listening to residents may help decrease stress levels.*

2. Pneumonia

Pneumonia is an inflammation of the lungs. Symptoms of pneumonia include fatigue, fever, or pain in the chest, especially when a person inhales or coughs. Inhaling causes pain because the alveoli are filled with fluid, which prevents the air from getting inside. Pneumonia can be a serious and potentially fatal disease. If you ever note any of these symptoms in a resident, report it to the nurse as soon as possible. A delay may make a big difference in the ability of the doctors to treat the person successfully.

CAUSE: Pneumonia is caused by a virus, a bacterium, a fungus, or another organism.

CURE/TREATMENT: Antibiotics are helpful for pneumonias caused by bacteria. It is extremely important for the person to take all of the antibiotics, every single pill or dose. If the entire amount is not taken, some of the microscopic bacteria may start growing and multiplying, causing the person to become even sicker.

Taking medications correctly that have been ordered is an important step. Sometimes an inhaler is ordered for people recovering from pneumonia. It may be necessary for a resident or family member to carry the inhaler with them at all times. Help remind that person to bring the inhaler along wherever he or she goes.

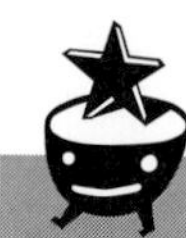

Star K.A.R.E.

Pneumonia

KNOW your resident's care plan.
ASSIST the resident/nurse.

- *Remind the person to follow the instructions regarding their antibiotics and to take all of the medication.*
- *Remind the person to follow the instructions regarding their inhalers and, if necessary, carry the inhaler with them at all times.*

REPORT observations.
RECORD data.
RECHECK resident as needed.

If the following occurs:

- *fever returns or the temperature rises*
- *confusion*
- *shortness of breath, difficulty breathing (dyspnea) or shallow breathing*
- *chest pain or tightness, especially when inhaling*

★ *"Don't Delay. Report Right Away!"*

ENCOURAGE resident's progress.

- *Provide support during pain or dyspnea.*
- *Be supportive of residents who are quitting smoking.*

3. Bronchitis

Bronchitis is an inflammation of the bronchi. There are two types of bronchitis, acute and chronic. Symptoms of bronchitis include cough, fever, and pain in the chest and perhaps the lower neck area. Symptoms of chronic bronchitis are a serious cough and **sputum** (phlegm) production. This sputum may have blood in it if the condition worsens. Bronchitis can become so severe that the person eventually develops dyspnea and has difficulty completing normal activities of daily living.

CAUSE: Acute bronchitis is a disorder that is usually caused by some type of infection. Chronic bronchitis is a condition usually caused by smoking, severe air pollution, or other irritants in the air.

CURE/TREATMENT: Antibiotics are used to treat acute bronchitis. It is extremely important for the person to take all of the antibiotics, every single pill or dose. If the entire amount is not taken, some of the microscopic bacteria may start growing and multiplying, causing the person to become even sicker.

Chronic bronchitis is a much more difficult disorder to treat. The cause of the bronchitis must be tackled. If this is smoking, the person may choose not to quit. If the cause is air pollution, it may not be possible for the person to move out of the area. Other irritants in the air may be controlled or reduced, depending on what they are.

Star K.A.R.E.

Bronchitis

KNOW your resident's care plan.
ASSIST the resident/nurse.

Remind the person to follow the instructions regarding their antibiotics and to take all of the medication.

REPORT observations.
RECORD data.
RECHECK resident as needed.

- *If the following occurs:*
  - *serious coughing episodes*
  - *fever returns or the temperature rises*
  - *confusion*
  - *shortness of breath, or dyspnea*
  - *chest pain or tightness, especially when inhaling*

★ *"Don't Delay. Report Right Away!"*

ENCOURAGE resident's progress.

- *Be supportive of residents who are quitting smoking.*

4. Emphysema

Emphysema is a condition in which the alveoli become stretched because they are "stuffed" with air and cannot perform their normal air exchange. As more alveoli are affected, breathing becomes more challenging. Symptoms of emphysema include shortness of breath and dyspnea, and eventually a "barrel-shaped" chest as more and more alveoli become "stuffed" with air.

CAUSE: Emphysema is usually caused by smoking and the chronic bronchitis that develops over time.

CURE/TREATMENT: Emphysema is a disorder that has no cure. Comfort measures are taken to try to allow the person to breathe as normally as possible. Oxygen is used, and eventually the person may need to use oxygen constantly. Smaller portable oxygen units are used in the community to help the person maintain some measure of freedom and independence. It is important for the person to stop smoking immediately to try to maximize the time he or she has left. Regular respiratory therapy and certain medications may reduce discomfort.

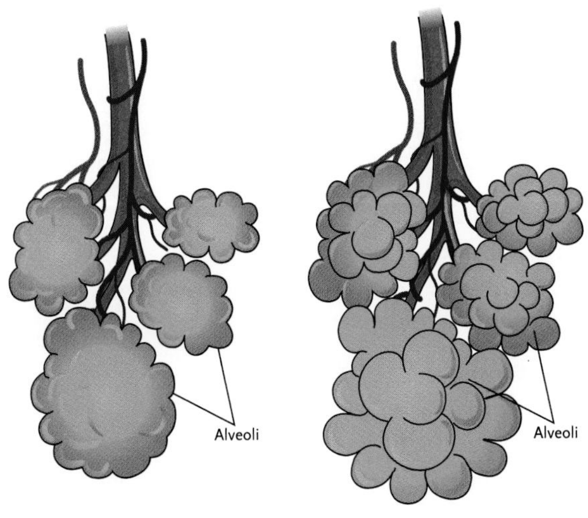

Figure 29-3. **With emphysema, the alveoli cannot perform their normal air exchange.**

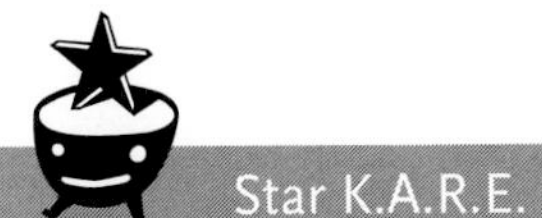
Star K.A.R.E.

Emphysema

KNOW your resident's care plan.
ASSIST the resident/nurse.

- *Use pillows to help the person breathe more comfortably at night.*
- *Allow rest periods when breathing becomes difficult.*

REPORT observations.
RECORD data.
RECHECK resident as needed.

If the following occurs:
- *shortness of breath, or dyspnea*
- *weight loss or loss of appetite*
- *excessive pain*

★ *"Don't Delay. Report Right Away!"*

ENCOURAGE resident's progress.

- *Provide support during shortness of breath or dyspnea.*

The History of the Mask

Masks were brought into use during the 1940s and 1950s. It is hard for us to believe, but many top surgeons at that time actually left the nose uncovered, wearing the mask over the mouth only. If only they had known. . .

4 Define tuberculosis and explain how it is transmitted.

Tuberculosis, or TB, is spread by tiny germs called bacilli that can float in the air. Diseases like this are called airborne diseases.

People can be exposed to TB when they spend time with a person who is infected with TB. The infected person can spread the disease by coughing, breathing, singing, sneezing, or even laughing.

TB usually infects the lungs, causing coughing, difficulty breathing, fever, and fatigue. If left untreated TB may cause death. However, TB can be cured by taking drugs that kill TB bacilli. It takes six months to a year of daily medication to wipe them out. It is very important to take all medication prescribed.

There are two types of TB: TB infection and TB disease. People with TB infection carry the disease but may not feel sick. A skin test is the only way to tell if a person has TB infection.

People with TB disease show symptoms of the disease and can spread it. Symptoms include:
- feeling weak
- losing their appetite
- losing weight
- fever
- sweating a lot at night
- coughing up blood

TB is more likely to be spread in areas with poor ventilation or small, confined spaces. People are more likely to get TB disease if they are alcoholics or injection drug users and if their immune systems are weakened by HIV/AIDS, illness, or malnutrition.

5 Explain care guidelines for residents with known or suspected TB.

It is important to follow these guidelines and any others your facility has to prevent infection from TB.

1. Follow standard precautions.
2. Wear personal protective equipment (PPE) during care. You may need to wear an N95 or HEPA respirator mask to provide care. See Chapter 11 to find more information on using one of these special masks.
3. Be especially careful when handling sputum (phlegm).
4. If in the care plan, follow isolation procedures.
5. Encourage and remind resident to take all the medication prescribed. Failure to take medication can spread TB.

6 Describe care guidelines for a resident on oxygen therapy and explain six oxygen delivery devices.

Residents who have an order for oxygen either require the oxygen use **intermittently** or **continuously**. When a resident has an order for intermittent oxygen, she may use the oxygen on a p.r.n. basis, or when needed. A continuous oxygen order means just that—the oxygen must be on at all times. The many guidelines and precautions you should follow when caring for a person on oxygen are listed below:

Guidelines for the Use of Oxygen Therapy

1. Post "No-Smoking" signs.
2. Know location of fire extinguisher.
3. Never use oxygen near electrical equipment, flammable liquids, open flames, or wool or synthetic clothing.
4. Check the following periodically:
   - equipment, for working order
   - the **humidifier** level, if in use
   - the tank level, when using tank oxygen
   - the ear, nose, mouth, or chin area for any dryness, discomfort, or soreness; adjust as needed
   - the nasal cannula, for proper fit and comfort

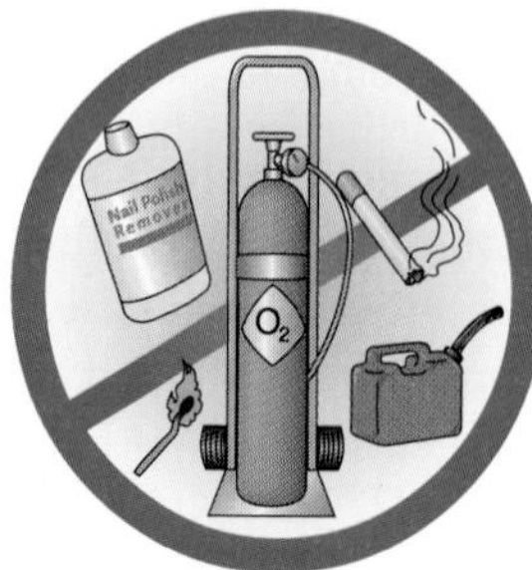

Figure 29-4.

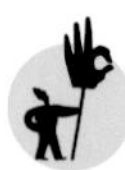

Portable Oxygen Tank Needed in Power Outages

When you are caring for anyone using an oxygen concentrator, it is important that you have a portable oxygen tank available in case of a power outage. Make sure you know how to use a portable oxygen tank. It could be dangerous for your residents if you don't know how to hook it up in an emergency.

There are six different devices for oxygen delivery available to people who need oxygen. Each device has its pros and cons. The doctor determines which device is the best for the resident or person at home.

Nasal Cannula
Pros: simple
Cons: limited to lower percent oxygen delivery

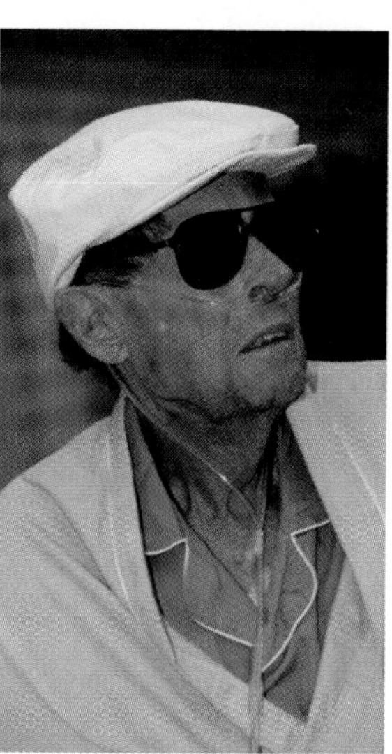
Figure 29-5. Resident with a nasal cannula.

Nasal Catheter
Pros: works better with restless residents; is disposable
Cons: irritates mucous membranes; catheter tube may kink/plug; uncomfortable

Face Mask
Pros: delivers high percent oxygen; delivers humidity; less mucous membrane irritation
Cons: irritates skin; hot; **claustrophobic**; prevents normal talking and eating

Venturi Mask
Pros: less mucous membrane irritation; delivers high humidity; always delivers exact oxygen order
Cons: irritates skin; hot; claustrophobic; prevents normal talking/eating

Oxygen Tent
Pros: delivers high humidity
Cons: claustrophobic

Oxygen Concentrator
Pros: uses room air; quiet and efficient
Cons: large and bulky; tubing may cause trips and/or falls; not usable during power outages

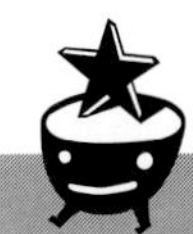

Star K.A.R.E.

Safe Oxygen Therapy

KNOW your resident's care plan.
ASSIST the resident/nurse.

- *Provide as much care as is needed to reduce dyspnea.*
- *Add pillows as needed to improve breathing.*
- *Be alert for smoking materials, flammable liquids, open flames, or wool or synthetic clothing, which can spark and cause fire.*
- *Check the tank level often.*
- *Clean areas on face where oxygen device rests, as ordered.*
- *Check for soreness or discomfort in ear, nose, mouth, or chin area.*
- *Lubricate sensitive areas on the nose and mouth.*

REPORT observations.
RECORD data.
RECHECK resident as needed.

If any of the following occur:

- *tank level drops to point where replacement is needed*
- *shortness of breath or dyspnea*
- *changes in vital signs, especially respiratory rate or pulse*
- *cyanosis (blue-tinged skin)*
- *chest pain or tightness*

★ *"Don't Delay. Report Right Away!"*

ENCOURAGE resident's independence and progress.

- *Provide support; some oxygen delivery devices can be claustrophobic and cumbersome.*
- *Encourage activity as permitted so resident does not withdraw or feel isolated.*

Continuous means constant!

When a resident has a continuous order for oxygen therapy, it means CONTINUOUS. It does not mean any person caring for the resident may remove the oxygen for their convenience. Never remove an oxygen delivery system, such as a nasal cannula, without first getting the approval of the nurse. You may cause the resident's blood oxygen level to drop, which would put him in serious danger.

7 Describe safe and accurate sputum specimen collection.

It is sometimes necessary to collect a specimen of mucus that comes from inside the respiratory system. Sputum is not the same as saliva, which comes from the salivary glands inside the mouth. Sputum, upon examination by the lab, may show evidence of various conditions, such as cancer or a bacterial pneumonia. The lab will study the sputum, looking for abnormal cells, microorganisms, or blood.

Sputum specimens are normally collected by respiratory therapy technicians or by registered or practical nurses. Some facilities allow nursing assistants to collect sputum specimens. It is very important to follow the guidelines so that you get the specimen you are supposed to collect, and not a specimen of saliva.

It is best to collect sputum specimens in the early morning. When people are flat on their backs for an entire night, mucus tends to collect inside the respiratory passages. This makes it easier to collect the sputum specimen. The resident should rinse her mouth before obtaining the sputum specimen. This removes any leftover food or any excess saliva inside the mouth. The person must never rinse with mouthwash before a sputum specimen collection. Mouthwash kills certain kinds of bacteria and other organisms that are helpful in analyzing the sputum.

Collecting a Sputum Specimen

Follow all standard and/or transmission-based precautions.
Follow all rules for body mechanics.

Collect equipment:

- **two pairs of disposable gloves • HEPA or N-95 mask**
- **face towel • cup of water • emesis basin**
- **two facial tissues • washcloth or wipes**
- **wash basin with warm water**
- **labeled specimen container • disposable plastic bag**
- **laboratory requisition slip**

1. **Perform the "5 Stars."**

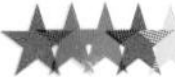

PREPARE:

2. **Apply gloves and special mask if resident has tuberculosis or an airborne or droplet disease.**

PERFORM:

3. **Help the resident to an upright position in the bed.**

4. Place towel under the resident's mouth and chin.
5. Ask resident to rinse mouth and spit water into emesis basin. Hold emesis basin carefully under mouth.

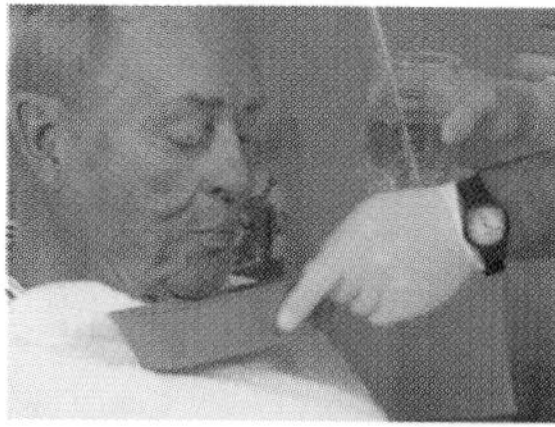
Figure 29-6.

6. Instruct resident to take three deep breaths in a row and then cough to bring up the sputum.
7. Hand the resident two tissues and tell him to hold the tissues together in front of the mouth when he coughs. This helps prevent the spread of bacteria.
8. Have the resident spit the sputum specimen into the sputum specimen container according to specific instructions.
9. Immediately cover the specimen container without touching the inside of the cover.
10. Place the specimen container inside the plastic bag, tie bag, and attach laboratory requisition slip.

FINISHING TOUCHES:

11. Remove gloves and mask.
12. Perform the "5 Stars and 3 Rs."

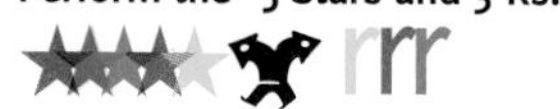

13. Bring disposable bag with specimen container inside to appropriate area.
14. Wash hands again.

8 Describe the benefits of deep breathing exercises.

Deep breathing exercises help expand the lungs, clearing them of mucus and preventing infections (such as pneumonia). Residents who are paralyzed or who have had abdominal surgery are often instructed to do deep breathing exercises to expand the lungs regularly. The care plan may include using a deep breathing device called an incentive spirometer. Incentive spirometry encourages the resident to take long, slow, deep breaths. The spirometer provides residents with visual or other positive feedback when they inhale. Usually a "goal" volume is set and they attempt at this rate for a minimum of three seconds. Regular use can increase the capacity of the lungs and strengthen the breathing muscles. It also helps clear the lungs. Do not assist with these exercises if you have not been trained.

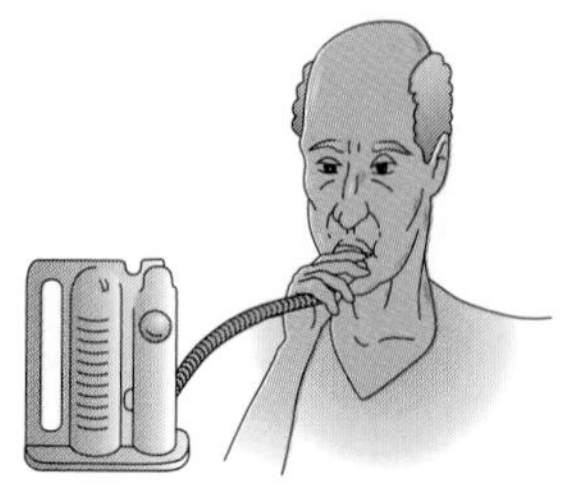
Figure 29-7. **Incentive spirometers are used for deep breathing exercises.**

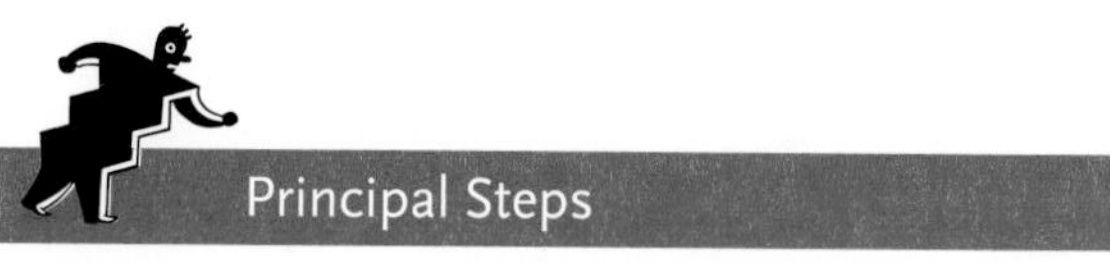

Safe Use of the Incentive Spirometer

1. *Each resident must have a separate incentive spirometer. Never borrow an incentive spirometer. The resident's name should be labeled on the spirometer.*
2. *Make sure both you and the resident wash your hands prior to using the spirometer.*

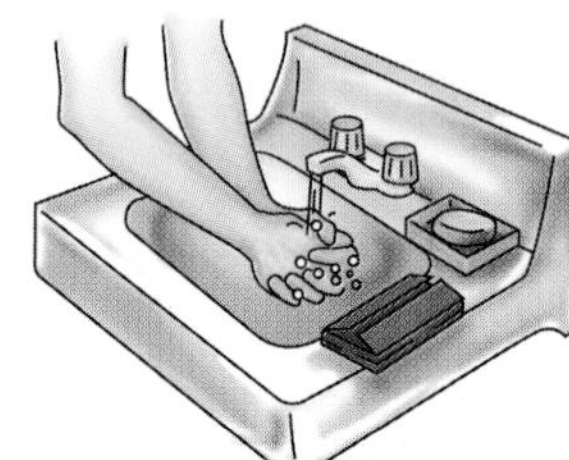
Figure 29-8. **Washing your hands is one of the most important ways to stop the spread of infection.**

3. *Residents may need encouragement from you to use this device. However, you should never "push" the resident to use one of these units. Check with the nurse to find out what is appropriate.*
4. *Depending upon the manufacturer, the spirometer's mouthpiece should be rinsed after each use. The unit may have its own storage bag. Follow the nurse's instructions regarding cleaning and storing an incentive spirometer.*

Summary

The function of the respiratory system is to take in oxygen and remove carbon dioxide from the body cells. Smoking and other toxins may cause temporary or permanent injury to the respiratory system. The act of breathing and bringing oxygen into the body cells is vital for survival. It is important to try to protect the respiratory system of your residents and your family. This will help everyone breathe easier and live longer.

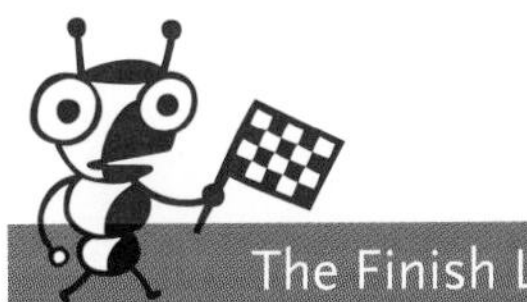

The Finish Line

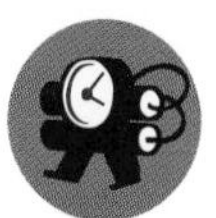

What's Wrong With This Picture?

1. Look at the guidelines for oxygen use shown below. List one missing item.

   Post "No-Smoking" signs.

   Know location of fire extinguisher.

   Never use oxygen near electrical equipment, flammable liquids, or open flames.

   Check the following periodically:
   - equipment, for working order
   - the humidifier level, if in use
   - the tank level, when using tank oxygen
   - the ear, nose, mouth, or chin area for any dryness, discomfort, or soreness and adjust as needed
   - the nasal cannula, for proper fit and comfort

2. Look at the equipment listed for the Practical Procedure: Collecting a Sputum Specimen, shown below. List the one missing piece of equipment.

Collect equipment:
- **two pairs of disposable gloves • HEPA or N-95 mask**
- **face towel • cup of water • emesis basin**
- **two facial tissues • washcloth or wipes**
- **wash basin with warm water • disposable plastic bag**
- **laboratory requisition slip**

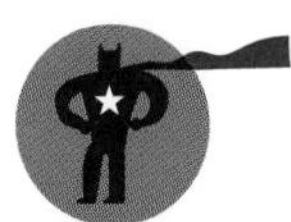

Star Student Central

1. Visit your local chapter of the American Lung Association. Ask for literature on various lung disorders. Share the information with your class.
2. Visit a respiratory therapy department at a local facility. Ask for information on what the department does. Ask for pamphlets or other information about oxygen delivery or other respiratory issues to share with your class.

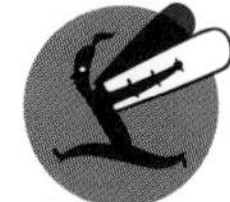

You Can Do It Corner!

1. List the ways tuberculosis can be spread. (LO 4)
2. What is one important way you can assist a resident who has pneumonia? (LO 3)
3. Why is it important for you to try to identify triggers for a resident with asthma? (LO 3)
4. What is one positive and one negative aspect of using a nasal cannula? (LO 6)
5. List three benefits of deep breathing exercises. (LO 8)
6. What is one important way you can encourage a resident who has bronchitis? (LO 3)
7. List an important reminder for a resident with TB. (LO 5)
8. At what time of day is it best to collect a sputum specimen? (LO 7)
9. What change in the respiratory system due to aging can cause an elderly person to tire more easily? (LO 2)

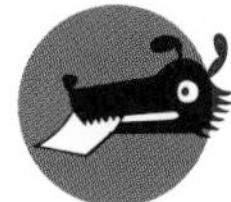

Star Student's Chapter Checklist

1. I have read my textbook chapter.
2. I have reviewed my own "Pocketful of Terms."
3. I have listened to my tutor tape.
4. I have reviewed and highlighted my class notes.
5. I have read and completed any handouts from this chapter.
6. I have completed "The Finish Line."
7. Star Time! Choose your reward!

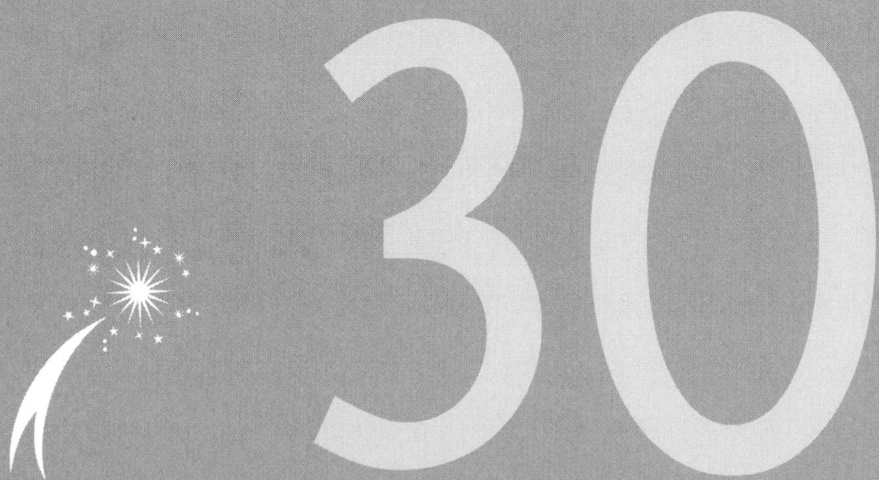

Specialized Care: The Gastrointestinal System

Look Like a Star!

Look at the Learning Objectives and The Finish Line before you begin reading this chapter.

Look at your pocket calendar.
With your pencil, put a bracket (   ) around a study period every single day.

Look at your homework for this chapter.
Plug each piece of homework into a certain time slot.

Look at the Star Student's Chapter Checklist at the end of this chapter. Check off each item as it is completed.

"... Give no more to every guest
Than he's able to digest."

Jonathan Swift, 1667-1745

"Canary birds feed on sugar and seed/Parrots have crackers to crunch/And as for the poodles, they tell me the noodles/Have chicken and cream for their lunch/But there's never a question/About my digestion—/Anything does for me! "

Charles Edward Carryl, 1842-1920

Learning Objectives

1. **Spell and define all STAR words.**
2. **Summarize the changes that occur in the gastrointestinal system during normal aging.**
3. **Discuss six common disorders of the gastrointestinal system.**
4. **List the signs of and risk factors for dehydration.**
5. **Recognize danger signs when caring for a resident with a tube feeding.**
6. **List eight signs and symptoms of a fecal impaction.**
7. **Describe the care of a resident receiving a suppository.**
8. **List ways to promote dignity for residents with ostomies.**

Successfully perform these Practical Procedures

Colostomy Care

Ileostomy Care

The moral is: Never give up on a patient!

A surgeon in the U.S. Army, William Beaumont, 1785-1853, discovered much about the study of digestion. While he was at Fort Michitimackinac on June 6,1822, he provided care for a Canadian trapper named Alexis St. Martin, who had suffered a shotgun blast to the abdomen. The doctor dressed St. Martin's large wound and then essentially waited for him to die. His patient did not die as expected, but survived with a fistula (an abnormal opening from one cavity to another). Beaumont then performed numerous experiments on his miracle patient that offered a much better understanding of the gastric process. He wrote *Experiments and Observation on the Gastric Juice and the Physiology of Digestion.* St. Martin lived with this opening into his stomach for the rest of his life.

1 Spell and define all STAR words.

biliary colic: pain caused by pressure or passing of gallstones.

cholecystectomy: the removal of the entire gallbladder.

colostomy: opening of a portion of the colon through the abdominal wall to the outside.

diverticulitis: inflammation of diverticula, causing pain and trapping feces inside the little sacs.

diverticulosis: diverticula of the colon.

enteral feeding: feeding via a tube inserted into the stomach by way of the nasal passages.

gangrene: death of tissue, usually due to absent blood supply.

gastric gavage: feeding with a tube passed through the nose into the stomach.

internal pouch: pouch usually created with the person's own intestine creating a collection area for feces instead of an external bag.

ileostomy: creation of a surgical opening through the abdominal wall into the ileum to drain feces into an external bag.

nasogastric (NG) tube: tube inserted through the nose into the stomach; used for feeding or removal of stomach contents.

ostomy: surgical removal of a portion of the intestines; end of the intestine is brought out of the body through an artificial opening in the abdomen called a stoma.

perforate: to puncture.

peritonitis: escape of contents from an internal organ into the abdominal cavity.

stoma: an artificial opening in the abdomen.

suppository: substance inserted into the rectum or vagina, usually with a medication that dissolves.

tube feeding: providing fluids and nutrition by introducing food into the stomach via a tube.

ulcers: sores that occur in the mucous membranes in the GI tract.

2 Summarize the changes that occur in the gastrointestinal system during normal aging.

As people get older, they experience changes in the gastrointestinal system. Foods do not have as strong a taste as they used to. Dental problems affect the ability to eat favorite foods and also prevent eating a balanced diet. If any difficulty swallowing develops, eating becomes a very slow and difficult process. Digestive difficulties cause discomfort as well, and can interfere with a normal day or a good night's sleep. Older people become constipated more often. They have to be very careful to prevent bowel obstructions, which are very serious complications. While inactivity requires fewer calories, it is more common for the elderly to be malnourished than overnourished.

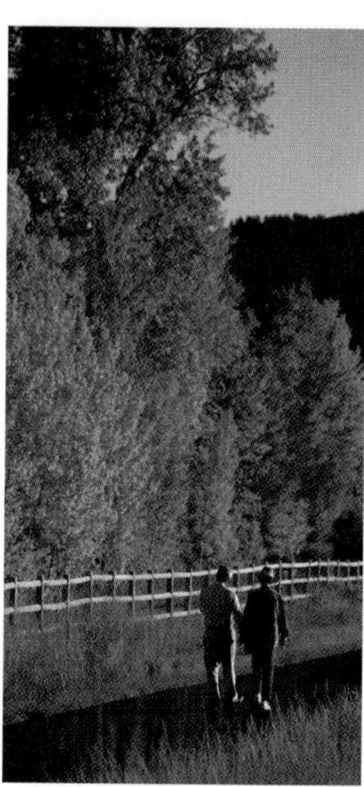

Figure 30-1. **Moderate exercise helps older adults promote a healthy gastrointestinal system.**

3 Discuss six common disorders of the gastrointestinal system.

1. Ulcers

Ulcers are sores that occur in the mucous membranes in the GI tract. These sores are usually found in the stomach (peptic or gastric ulcers) and the duodenum (duodenal ulcers). Ulcers cause a burning pain that occurs anywhere from an hour to three or more hours after eating. If ulcers become serious, they can **perforate** (puncture or make holes in) the wall of the stomach or the duodenum and lead to a life-threatening hemorrhage. Bleeding, if it does not lead to hemorrhage, may cause anemia.

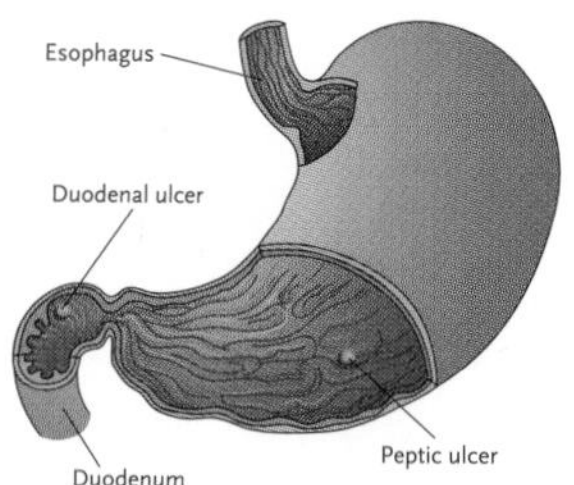

Figure 30-2. **Ulcers can occur in the stomach (peptic) or the duodenum (duodenal).**

CAUSE: Many ulcers are now thought to be caused by the bacterium Helicobacter pylori (H. pylori). These bacteria wiggle their way into the GI tract, where they work to stop the tract's lining from forming enough mucus. This mucus is needed to protect the walls of the stomach and the duodenum from the acid of the stomach. Stress and anxiety may play a part in the development or severity of ulcers.

CURE/TREATMENT: Antibiotics are used to treat ulcers thought to be caused by bacteria. Other medications that reduce the acid secretion in the stomach are also used to treat ulcers.

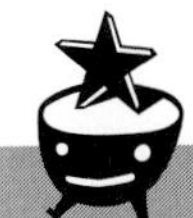

Star K.A.R.E.

Ulcers

KNOW your resident's care plan.
ASSIST the resident/nurse.

- *Reduce stressful episodes.*
- *Note foods that cause pain and discomfort.*

REPORT observations.
RECORD data.
RECHECK resident as needed.

If the following occurs:

- *vomiting, especially with blood*
- *severe pain*
- *black stools (sometimes called "tarry")*
- *unusual weakness or fatigue*
- *signs of GI bleeding*

★ *"Don't Delay. Report Right Away!"*

ENCOURAGE resident's progress.

- *Encourage maintenance of special diets.*

Certain birds helped show how food is dissolved in the stomach.

Lazzaro Spallanzani [1729-1799] studied the process of digestion. He performed experiments with birds called kites. In his studies with these birds, Spallanzani was able to determine that gastric juice works to dissolve food in the stomach.

2. Gallbladder Disorders

The gallbladder secretes bile into the duodenum in order to help digest the fat we eat. There are different problems that can occur with the gallbladder. Inflammation of the gallbladder is called cholecystitis. Gallstones (cholelithiasis) can also occur, blocking the flow of bile from the gallbladder to the duodenum. This causes extreme pain, called **biliary colic**.

CAUSE: Gallstones may be caused by the crystallization of cholesterol found in the bile inside the gallbladder. When a gallstone develops, it gets bigger and bigger, and more gallstones may form.

CURE/TREATMENT: Some people require surgical removal of gallstones. A special type of laproscopic surgery, not requiring a large incision, can remove the gallstones. A special method called lithotripsy can break apart the gallstones and make them easier to remove. In some cases, it is necessary to remove the entire gallbladder, a procedure which is called a **cholecystectomy**.

3. Diverticulosis and Diverticulitis

Diverticulosis is a disorder in which saclike pouchings of the intestinal wall of the large intestine (colon) develop in weakened areas of the wall. A small percentage of people with diverticulosis develop inflammation inside the pouchings, called diverticulitis. With **diverticulitis**, stool and bacteria become "stuck" inside the sacs, causing extreme pain and sometimes fever. If the condition worsens, the intestine can perforate, causing the stool to enter the abdominal cavity and cause **peritonitis** (when the lining of the abdominal cavity becomes inflamed due to the entrance of microorganisms).

CAUSE: One cause of diverticulitis is a low-fiber diet. The lack of fiber may cause the weakening of the intestinal wall. High-fiber diets can help improve the disorder.

CURE/TREATMENT: Diverticulitis is usually treated with rest, medications to reduce inflammation and treat infection, and a special diet. Sometimes, people with this disorder may need surgery to cut out part of the diseased colon. A **colostomy**, an opening from the colon to the outside of the abdominal wall for elimination of feces, is sometimes performed temporarily to allow the colon enough time to heal.

4. Appendicitis

Appendicitis is the inflammation of the appendix. Symptoms include an initial pain in the center of the abdomen that moves to the right lower quadrant (RLQ). The pain ranges from a dull to a severe ache.

A low-grade fever may develop as well. Other symptoms include nausea, vomiting, or decreased appetite. The infection that follows can cause **gangrene** (tissue death), and the appendix may perforate. When the appendix ruptures, the material that has gathered inside bursts out into the abdomen and causes peritonitis. If left untreated, this condition is serious and, ultimately, can be fatal.

CAUSE: Appendicitis is caused when an obstruction occurs in the appendix. This blockage may be caused by stool, a foreign body of some kind, or cancer.

CURE/TREATMENT: Immediate surgery is done to remove the appendix before it ruptures and causes peritonitis. Once peritonitis develops, the situation becomes more difficult. It is much easier and safer to remove the appendix before it bursts.

Warning signs of appendicitis include the following:
- decreased appetite
- nausea or vomiting and burping
- severe pain, especially in the RLQ
- fever
- tenderness and severe pain in the abdomen
- swollen or rigid abdomen (with peritonitis)

If you see any of these symptoms, report to the nurse immediately.

5. Colon Cancer

Colon cancer is one of the most common cancers. Symptoms include abdominal pain, gas, cramping, blood in the stool, other changes in the stool, and vomiting.

CAUSE: A family link exists in some cases of colon cancer. Other causes are being studied, such as low-fiber diets; however, no definitive causes have been identified at this time.

CURE/TREATMENT: When colon cancer is found in the early stages, surgery is performed to remove the cancer and to prevent it from spreading. Surgery can involve the creation of a colostomy, an artificial opening from the intestine to the outside of the abdomen for the elimination of feces, or an ileostomy. Advances in this type of surgery are being developed. An **internal pouch** made of the person's intestine is being studied as a possible replacement for the external bag that people currently wear. Everyone is not a good candidate for this type of internal pouch. The key to treatment is early detection. Adults over age 40 should be screened regularly for colon cancer.

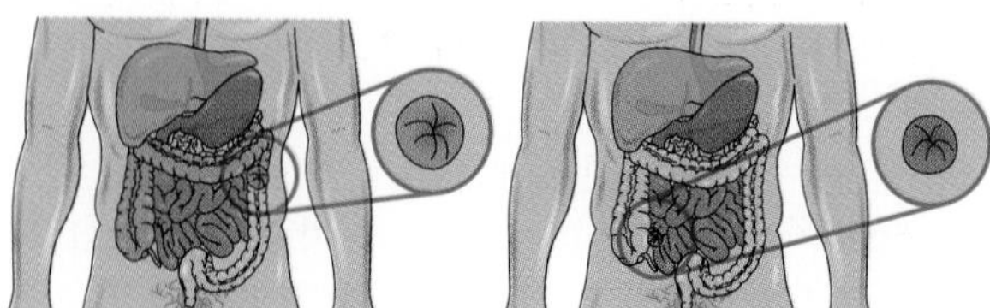

Figure 30-3. **A colostomy and an ileostomy.**

Star K.A.R.E.

Colon Cancer

KNOW your resident's care plan.
ASSIST the resident/nurse.

- *Observe residents for signs of pain or discomfort.*
- *Observe stool carefully for changes and blood.*
- *Perform Hemoccult tests exactly as ordered.*

REPORT observations.
RECORD data.
RECHECK resident as needed.

If the following occurs:
- *nausea, indigestion, or vomiting*
- *pain or discomfort*
- *gas (flatus) or cramping*
- *constipation*
- *any changes in the stool, especially blood in the stool*

★ *"Don't Delay. Report Right Away!"*

ENCOURAGE resident's independence and progress.

- *Provide support during periods of pain and post-operatively.*
- *Encourage high-fiber diets as ordered.*

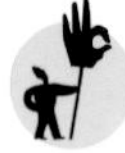

What are ulcerative colitis and Crohn's disease?

Ulcerative colitis is a disorder that causes sores to develop in the lining of the large intestine (colon). The person may have diarrhea, which becomes bloody, and abdominal pain.

Crohn's disease causes the wall of the intestines to become sore, red, and swollen. Symptoms include diarrhea, abdominal pain, fever, weight loss, and sometimes joint pain. This disorder occurs in the small or the large intestine.

Certain medications help people with these disorders. Surgery may be performed if medications do not help the disorders. An ***ileostomy****, colostomy, or an internal pouch may be created to try to help people with these disorders.*

6. Hemorrhoids

Hemorrhoids are swollen tissues that contain veins located in the wall of the rectum and anus. They can become enlarged, inflamed, bleed, or itch. Some people experience a burning sensation. Typically, bleeding occurs after a bowel movement.

CAUSE: Hemorrhoids may develop from straining during bowel movements. Constipation can make the straining worse.

CURE/TREATMENT: If hemorrhoids cause symptoms, they require treatment. Stool softeners are used to relieve constipation and straining. Sitz baths and ointments may also be used. Other procedures, such as special injections and treatments, may be ordered.

4 List the signs of and risk factors for dehydration.

Dehydration is a problem that is more and more common in long-term care facilities. It may occur due to vomiting, diarrhea, fever, diaphoresis (heavy sweating), increased urinary output, hemorrhage, and severe burns. Sadly, dehydration can also occur because fluids are not left within a resident's reach or if a resident is unable to drink without assistance. When dehydration is identified in the early stages, a full recovery is much more likely. Dehydration, if allowed to become serious, can interfere with normal heart and kidney function and ultimately, may be fatal if not treated. Chapter 22 has more information on preventing dehydration.

It is very important to recognize the signs of dehydration. Signs and risk factors of dehydration include the following: drinking less than six cups of liquids per day; needing help drinking from a cup or glass; dry mouth, cracked lips, sunken eyes, and/or dark urine; trouble swallowing liquids; frequent vomiting, diarrhea, and fever; confusion or fatigue.

When signs of dehydration are noted, immediate action must be taken. There is no time for delay. If the electrolytes in the body reach dangerously low levels, a serious complication called a heart arrhythmia may develop. This is an irregular rhythm of the heart and occurs especially when the potassium level drops to extremely low levels. Dehydration should be taken very seriously and should never be allowed to "wait until the morning."

A request for a drink must be honored!

When residents are thirsty, they may ask staff members for a glass of water, juice, coffee, tea or some other beverage. It is very important for staff members to respond promptly to a request for a drink. Ignoring a resident's request for a drink is considered abuse. The only time a request for a drink should not be answered promptly is when a resident is on a fluid restriction for some reason or NPO due to surgery or a test. In this situation, you need to explain to the resident the reasons why a drink cannot be given and report the request to the nurse.

5 Recognize danger signs when caring for a resident with a tube feeding.

A **tube feeding** (**gastric gavage**, **enteral feeding**, **nasogastric tube**) is necessary for some residents who have swallowing difficulties, a gastrointestinal upset that prevents them from eating normally, or for residents who have had a stroke or are unconscious. A tube is normally inserted through the nose, down the back of the throat into the esophagus, and finally into the stomach. Sometimes the tube is inserted directly into an opening in the stomach.

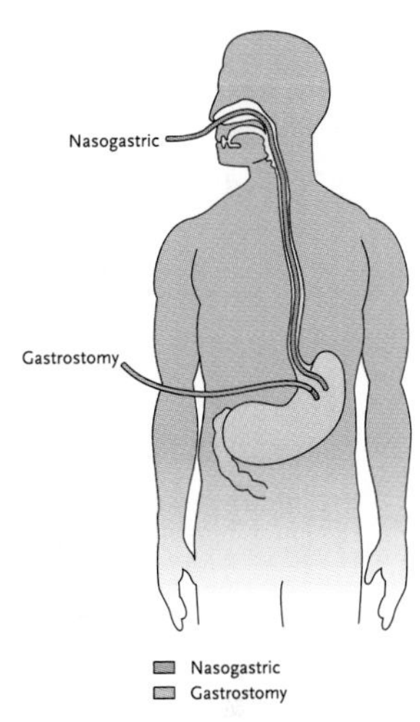

Figure 30-4.

One of the risks that residents receiving tube feedings have is aspiration of fluids (choking). It is vitally important to observe the resident carefully for any signs of aspiration during and after a tube feeding. In addition, it is important to follow all instructions from the nurse exactly regarding positioning your resident during and after tube feedings.

Immediately report choking, nausea, vomiting, cramping, pale or blue-tinged skin (cyanosis), difficulty breathing, or shortness of breath to the nurse. In addition, residents may pull on their tube, causing an increased risk of aspiration. Pulling on the tube causes the tube to move upwards out of the stomach, which causes the fluid to flow into the lungs. If your resident shows any sign of pulling on the tube, notify the nurse right away.

Star K.A.R.E.

Caring for a Resident with a Tube Feeding

KNOW your resident's care plan.
ASSIST the resident/nurse.

- *Follow fluid order.*
- *Follow orders exactly on moving and positioning.*
- *Keep HOB elevated for exact time ordered after tube feeding.*
- *Listen for feeding pump alarm.*
- *Observe for kinks in the tubing.*
- *Give excellent mouth and nose care.*

REPORT observations.
RECORD data.
RECHECK resident as needed.

If any of the following occur:

- *sores around the nose or mouth*
- *shortness of breath or dyspnea*
- *pale skin or blue-tinged skin (cyanosis)*
- *nausea, choking, vomiting, or cramping*
- *resident pulling on the tube*

★ *"Don't Delay. Report Right Away!"*

ENCOURAGE resident's progress.

- *Provide support during tube feeding; it may be uncomfortable.*
- *Help keep a social environment during feeding. Talk to resident during feeding.*

6 List eight signs and symptoms of a fecal impaction.

Many symptoms occur that warn of a possible fecal impaction. A fecal impaction is a build-up of hardened feces in the bowel that a person cannot remove naturally. Impactions can cause serious harm to residents and may require surgery if not treated promptly and successfully. When a resident has bowel movements, it is vital for the staff to document the frequency. Some facilities may not be as careful as others in the recording of regular bowel movements. When this happens, it is easier to miss the potential signs of an impaction. Older people are much more prone to impactions because they tend to get less exercise, drink less fluid, and may not eat foods that encourage regular elimination.

The embarrassment of reporting that he or she has not had a bowel movement can prevent the resident from telling anyone. You must simply get to know your residents' habits and record every time they have a bowel movement in your notes and then on the appropriate facility document. If you do not know their bowel habits, you will not notice a change in them.

Some of the signs and symptoms of a fecal impaction include abdominal or rectal pain, abdominal swelling (distention), and N,V, or D (nausea, vomiting, or diarrhea). Another sign is the seeping of stool, which can be mistaken as diarrhea. Other signs to watch for are an increase in urination or the inability to urinate, a fever or any change in the other vital signs, or confusion or disorientation. If a fecal impaction becomes serious, it can be fatal when a complete bowel obstruction occurs and it is not promptly treated. You must report any of these signs you observe to the nurse.

7 Describe the care of a resident receiving a suppository.

A **suppository** is a medication given rectally by the nurse to help the resident have a bowel movement. The nursing assistant may assist with the insertion of a suppository. The normal position is the left Sims' position. The nurse must apply gloves and lubricant and insert the suppository into the rectum until it passes over the ridge in the rectum. Once the suppository passes over the ridge, it has a better chance of staying inside the rectum and causing a bowel movement. You can also be helpful during the insertion by holding the resident's hand, if desired. After the insertion of a suppository, it is important for you to place the signal light near the resident's hand and instruct the resident to press the button when he wishes to use the bathroom or bedpan. It is vital to respond promptly to a signal light after a suppository insertion.

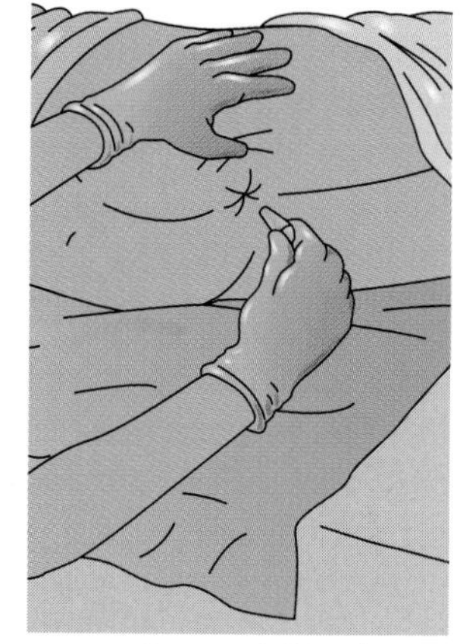

Figure 30-5. **A nurse administering a rectal suppository.**

Star K.A.R.E.

Care of a Resident Using a Suppository

KNOW your resident's care plan.
ASSIST the resident/nurse.

- *Follow nurse's instructions regarding positioning resident (i.e. Left Sims').*
- *Hold resident's hand if desired by resident.*
- *Remind resident to take deep breaths and relax.*
- *Remind resident to hold suppository in as long as possible for best results.*

REPORT observations.
RECORD data.
RECHECK resident as needed.

If any of the following occur:

- *complaints of abdominal pain or discomfort*
- *bowel movement; nurse will want to see results*

★ *"Don't Delay. Report Right Away!"*

ENCOURAGE resident's progress.

- *Provide emotional support during insertion as this may be uncomfortable or embarrassing.*

8 List ways to promote dignity for residents with ostomies.

An ostomy is created to provide an alternate method for stool to be eliminated from the body. An **ostomy** is the surgical removal of a portion of the intestines. The end of the intestine is brought out of the body through an artificial opening in the abdomen. This opening is called a **stoma**. An ostomy may be necessary due to cancer of the colon, a disease such as diverticulitis or Crohn's disease, or a stabbing or gunshot wound (GSW). An ostomy is either permanent or temporary, allowing the intestine time to heal.

Having an ostomy may be extremely embarrassing for a person, especially directly after the ostomy is created. Residents often feel they have lost control of a basic bodily function. Ostomies can cause odor, can feel uncomfortable, and can cause great fear of the ostomy bag "falling off." Many people wear an ostomy belt so that they can guard against the ostomy bag falling off.

You can do a great deal to help your residents with ostomies feel better about themselves. There are also ostomy therapists that can help residents adjust to this change. Be sensitive and supportive when working with residents with ostomies. Always provide privacy for ostomy care. Do not act uncomfortable with any aspect of ostomy care, especially the odor or the changing of the bag. Make sure when you release the ostomy appliance, or bag, that you allow a tiny bit of air out first. This decreases the risk of the bag and its contents exploding due to the build-up of the gas inside.

Check the placement of the ostomy bag before the resident goes out into the dayroom or to any activity. Make sure the bag is as secure as you can make it. Your support will really help the resident's ability to handle this big change in lifestyle.

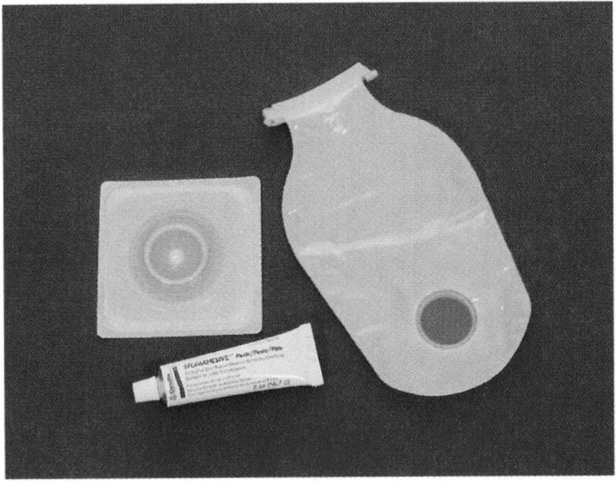

Figure 30-6. **An ostomy bag.**

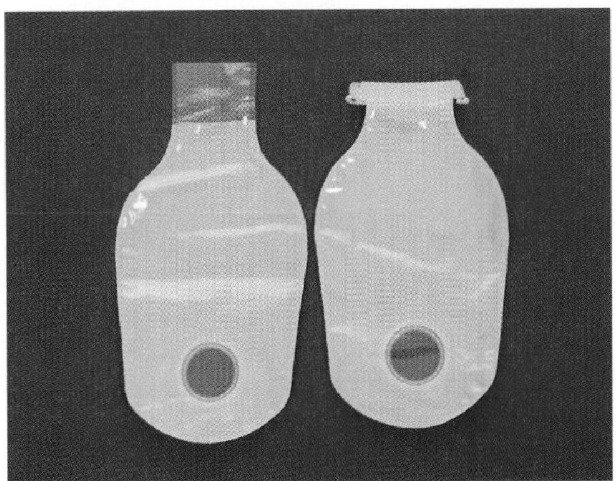

Figure 30-7. **An open and closed ostomy bag.**

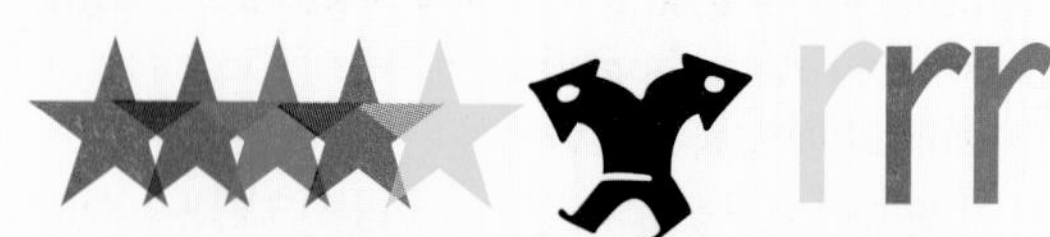

Beginning Steps

★ RESPECT
Knock first, ask and receive permission to enter a resident's room.

★ INFECTION CONTROL
Wash hands.

★ COMMUNICATION
Greet and identify the resident. Identify yourself. Explain the procedure, encouraging the resident to be as independent as possible throughout.

★ BED SAFETY
Lock bed wheels. Raise bed to safe working height. Lower one side rail if required.

★ PRIVACY
Provide for privacy by closing the door and covering the resident appropriately.

Ending Steps

★ RESIDENT SAFETY AND COMFORT
Secure the resident, lowering the bed, and raising the side rails if ordered. Check that the resident is comfortable and properly aligned.

★ PRIVACY
Remove any added privacy measures, such as a drape or a privacy screen.

★ ESSENTIALS
Place the call light, fresh beverage, and other items within reach.

★ COURTESY
Ask the resident if he or she needs anything else. Say thank you and goodbye.

★ INFECTION CONTROL
Wash hands.

r **Report** your care and any important observations to the nurse.

r **Record** your care and any important information/observations such as vital signs in the appropriate place.

r **Recheck** your resident for any changes as directed by the nurse!

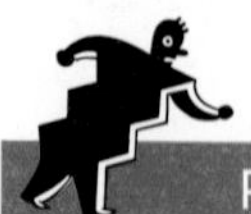

Principal Steps

Ostomy Care

1. *Follow all standard and/or transmission-based precautions, including wearing gloves, when caring for a resident with an ostomy.*
2. *Be careful to protect clothing or gown from wetness or soiling during procedure.*
3. *Never rush when providing ostomy care. If you try to remove appliances too quickly, you may remove some of the person's skin as well.*
4. *Before removing appliance, allow a tiny bit of air out of the bag to remove any built-up pressure. This can prevent the bag from exploding.*

   The consistency of colostomy and ileostomy drainage varies. Colostomy drainage ranges from formed stool to semi-formed or a liquid consistency. Ileostomy drainage is usually liquid.
5. *Use soap as directed by the nurse.*
6. *Follow directions about using skin protectors and skin creams around the stoma.*
7. *Wafer, ring, or other adhesive device should be pre-cut and pre-sized to fit the individual stoma. Make sure it fits the stoma well and is not too large or too small.*
8. *Make sure bottom of appliance/bag is securely clamped before applying it to the stoma.*
9. *Make sure bag is attached securely to the resident before allowing him to go outside of room.*
10. *Observe for any signs of skin irritation, rashes, swelling, or bleeding around stoma and report these, along with any complaints of pain or discomfort, promptly.*

Colostomy Care

Follow all standard and/or transmission-based precautions. Follow all rules for body mechanics.

Collect equipment:
- two pairs of disposable gloves • scissors
- bedpan with cover • towel • toilet tissue • paper towel
- disposable bed protector • bath blanket or drape
- wash basin with warm water • wash cloths or wipes
- wafers • gauze • clamp, if used • special paste (optional)
- ostomy appliances or bags • deodorant (optional)
- ostomy belt (optional)

1. **Perform the "5 Stars."**

PREPARE:

2. **Apply gloves.**
3. **Position the resident comfortably with disposable bed protector underneath mid-section.**

PERFORM:

4. **Lift gown or pajamas and cover with bath blanket or drape.**
5. **Carefully release a tiny bit of air from one corner of the ostomy bag before removing bag.**
6. **Remove rest of bag and place inside bedpan.**
7. **Gently clean and dry skin around stoma using soap only if directed. First use toilet tissue, then warm water and washcloth.**

8. Immediately cover opening with gauze or washcloth.
9. Wafer is often pre-cut and pre-sized to fit the individual stoma. If further sizing is necessary, notify the nurse. Wafer will have a snug fit, and there should be no skin seen around stoma.
10. Apply paste or cream to skin, if desired, and press new wafer against skin around stoma.
11. Press out all air bubbles in wafer. HOLD in place until it sticks securely.
12. Add deodorant to bag, if used. Attach appliance and make sure it snaps into place securely (Figure 30-8). Attach to ostomy belt, if used.

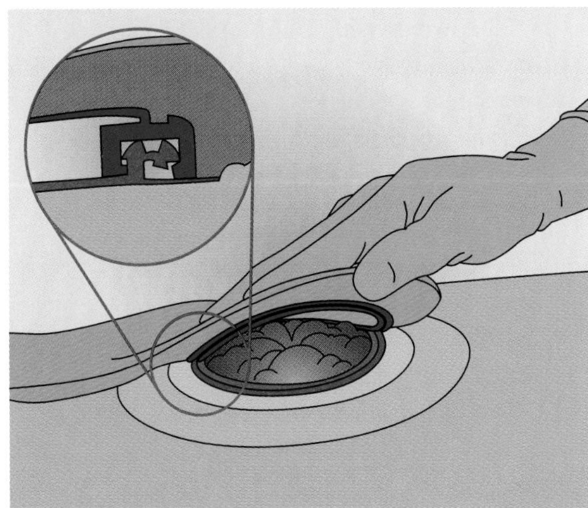

Figure 30-8.

13. If clamp is used at the bottom of the bag, make sure clamp is secure.

FINISHING TOUCHES:

14. Replace gown or clothing and SECURE THE RESIDENT.
15. Take bedpan to bathroom and measure contents of bag if on I & O.
16. Empty and dispose of old appliance according to facility policy and clean bedpan. Return bedpan to storage area.
17. Remove gloves and wash hands, and apply second pair of gloves.
18. Return to bedside and help resident wash hands. Remove and replace disposable bed protector, if needed.
19. Remove gloves.
20. Perform the "5 Stars and 3 Rs."

Ileostomy Care

Follow all standard and/or transmission-based precautions. Follow all rules for body mechanics.

Collect equipment:

• two pairs of disposable gloves • scissors
• bedpan with cover • toilet tissue • paper towel
• disposable bed protector • bath blanket or drape
• wash basin with warm water • towel
• wash cloths or wipes • gauze • special rings
• special solvent with dropper • ileostomy appliances or bags • clamp, if used • special paste or cream (optional)
• ostomy belt (optional) • deodorant (optional)

PREPARE:

1. Perform the "5 Stars."

2. Apply gloves.
3. Position the resident comfortably.
4. Lift gown or pajamas and cover with bath blanket or drape.

PERFORM:

METHOD 1: Draining and Daily Care of Ileostomy Bag

1. Place bedpan up against resident. Open clamp and allow bag to drain into bedpan. Cover bedpan. Clean inside of bag with large bulb syringe full of water.

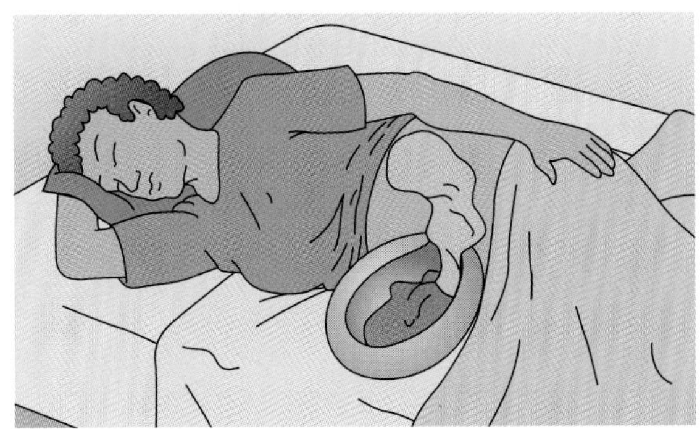

Figure 30-9.

2. Clean end of bag with toilet tissue and allow bag to rest on disposable pad. Add deodorant, if used.
3. Reclamp snugly, check that bag is securely attached to skin and belt.

FINISHING TOUCHES:

4. Replace gown or clothing and SECURE THE RESIDENT.
5. Take bedpan to bathroom and measure contents of bag if on I & O.
6. Empty and dispose of contents according to facility policy and clean bedpan. Return bedpan to storage area.
7. Remove gloves and wash hands, and apply second pair of gloves.
8. Return to bedside and help resident wash hands.
9. Remove gloves and wash hands.
10. Perform the "5 Stars and 3 Rs."

METHOD 2: Changing the Ileostomy Bag

1. Place bedpan up against resident. Open clamp and allow bag to drain into bedpan. Cover bedpan.

2. Remove belt and place on paper towel or pad.
3. Apply special solvent remover to loosen ring. After waiting to allow solvent to work, carefully release a tiny bit of air from one corner of the ileostomy bag before removing bag.
4. Remove rest of bag and place inside bedpan.
5. Gently clean and dry skin around stoma without using soap.
6. Immediately cover opening with gauze or washcloth.
7. Prepare new ring. Remove gauze and place on paper towel. Apply skin cream or paste if used. Attach ring, making sure no skin is seen around stoma and ring has a snug fit. HOLD in place until it sticks securely.
8. Attach appliance and make sure it snaps into place securely. Apply belt and attach bag to belt.
9. Make sure clamp is secure.

FINISHING TOUCHES:

10. Replace gown or clothing and SECURE THE RESIDENT.
11. Take bedpan to bathroom and measure contents of bag if on I & O.
12. Empty and dispose of old appliance according to facility policy and clean bedpan. Return bedpan to storage area.
13. Remove gloves and wash hands, and apply second pair of gloves.
14. Return to bedside and help resident wash hands.
15. Remove gloves.
16. Perform the "5 Stars and 3 Rs."

Summary

The function of the digestive system is to ingest, absorb, and remove waste products from the GI tract. When the normal functioning of the gastrointestinal system is disrupted for some reason, the ability to take in and absorb nutrition may be reduced. In addition, when the body's ability to remove solid wastes is affected, the person may be at risk of a serious complication. Staying alert for signs and symptoms of problems with the digestive tract will help keep your residents healthy.

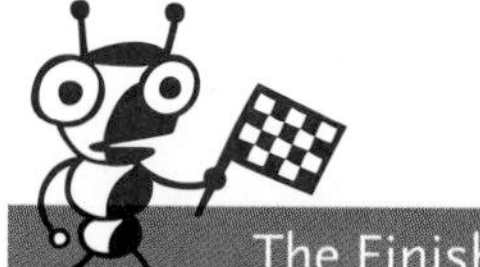

The Finish Line

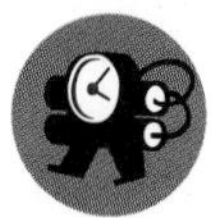

What's Wrong With This Picture?

1. Look at the STAR KARE for ulcers shown below. List the two missing symptoms to observe.
   - *vomiting, especially with blood*
   - *severe pain*
   - *unusual weakness or fatigue*

2. Look at the STAR KARE for tube feeding shown below. List the one missing step.
   - *Follow fluid order; may be NPO.*
   - *Follow orders exactly on moving and positioning.*
   - *Listen for feeding pump alarm.*
   - *Observe for kinks in the tubing.*
   - *Give excellent mouth and nose care.*

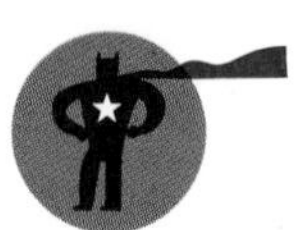

Star Student Central

1. Ask your doctor at what age you should have a colonoscopy. A colonoscopy is done to look inside the colon to try to detect a potential problem before it becomes serious or to try to identify and treat things at an early stage, such as cancer. Styles of colonscopy equipment are being used that do not require a long piece of tubing to be inserted into the colon. Some have a tiny camera on the end of the device that allows the doctor to look at the colon.
2. Visit with an Ostomy Care Therapist. Ask for pamphlets about the various types of ostomies and bring them back to share with the class.

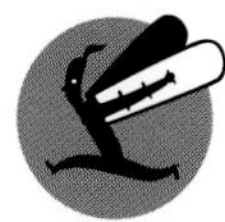

You Can Do It Corner!

1. What should you do immediately after the insertion of a suppository? (LO 7)
2. What is the key to treating colon cancer? (LO 3)
3. Identify six risk factors for and symptoms of dehydration. (LO 4)
4. Are the elderly more at risk f or being over- or undernourished? (LO 2)
5. Why is peritonitis an emergency situation? (LO 3)
6. Identify five signs of aspiration with a tube feeding resident that must be reported to the nurse. (LO 5)
7. What are three signs that a resident may have a fecal impaction? (LO 6)
8. Why might residents feel embarrassed or uncomfortable if they have an ostomy? (LO 8)
9. What important step should be taken before removing the ostomy bag? (LO 8)

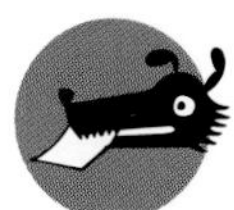

Star Student's Chapter Checklist

1. I have read my textbook chapter.
2. I have reviewed my own "Pocketful of Terms."
3. I have listened to my tutor tape.
4. I have reviewed and highlighted my class notes.
5. I have read and completed any handouts from this chapter.
6. I have completed "The Finish Line."
7. Star Time! Choose your reward!

Specialized Care: The Urinary System

Look Like a Star!

Look at the Learning Objectives and The Finish Line before you begin reading this chapter.

Look at your pocket calendar.
With your pencil, put a bracket ( ) around a study period every single day.

Look at your homework for this chapter.
Plug each piece of homework into a certain time slot.

Look at the Star Student's Chapter Checklist at the end of this chapter. Check off each item as it is completed.

"A human being: an ingenious assembly of portable plumbing."

Christopher Morley, 1890-1957

"Now is this golden crown like a deep well
That owes two buckets filling one another;
The emptier dancing in the air,
The other down, unseen and full of water"

William Shakespeare, from *Richard II*

Learning Objectives

1. **Spell and define all STAR words.**
2. **Summarize the changes that occur in the urinary system during normal aging.**
3. **Discuss four common disorders of the urinary system.**
4. **Describe the process of "weaning" a resident from a catheter.**
5. **Review the safety guidelines for a resident with a urinary catheter and discuss the reasons a supra-pubic catheter is used.**
6. **Describe continuous bladder irrigation (CBI) and list reasons why it is ordered.**
7. **Explain the specific gravity test and list one reason it is ordered.**

Successfully perform these Practical Procedures

Urine Straining

Performing Specific Gravity Test

Watching the Kidneys

Galen, 130-200 A.D., wrote a 17-book set entitled *On the Uses of the Parts of the Body of Man*. One portion of the work dealt with the function of the kidneys. To help determine how the kidneys produced urine, Galen tied up the ureters and watched the kidneys swell up with urine!

1 Spell and define all STAR words.

calculi: kidney stones; also called renal calculi.

continuous bladder irrigation (CBI): irrigation used to flush the bladder and the catheter system of clots and other materials.

crystallize: to cause to form crystals.

cystitis: infection of the bladder.

Foley Clamp and Drain: a program that involves clamping and unclamping the catheter tubing in order to "wean" a resident from a urinary catheter.

Kegel exercises: exercises done to strengthen the muscles that control urination and defecation.

kidney stones: stones made of mineral salts that accumulate inside the kidneys.

lithotripsy: use of sound waves to crush kidney stones.

nephritis: inflammation of the kidneys.

patency: the state of being open.

specific gravity: the comparison of the weight of a liquid (such as urine) with the weight of water; a number is assigned to show that relationship.

2 Summarize the changes that occur in the urinary system during normal aging.

As people age, the urinary system is affected in many ways. The bladder is not able to hold the same amount of urine as it used to. Older people may need to urinate more frequently. The ability of the kidneys to filter the blood decreases. Older people are more prone to dehydration due to inadequate fluids. This may decrease the kidneys' ability to flush the poisons out of the blood. Because the kidneys are less efficient, medications also have greater effect, positive or negative.

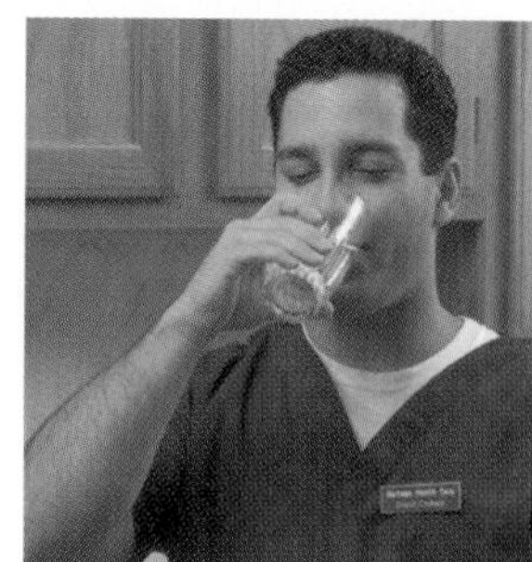

Figure 31-1. Drinking plenty of water is good for you and your residents!

Don't wait; urinate!

Do your residents wait to go to the bathroom? This is unhealthy for their urinary systems. Residents should be taken to the bathroom as soon as they need to urinate. They should never have to wait to go to the bathroom. Accidents are not the only problem with waiting; it is also dangerous to the person's health. Poisons may gather inside the bodies of people who routinely have to wait to go to the bathroom.

3 Discuss four common disorders of the urinary system.

1. Cystitis

Cystitis is an infection of the bladder. Symptoms include pain with urination, blood in the urine, and frequency and urgency of urination. Urine is often cloudy.

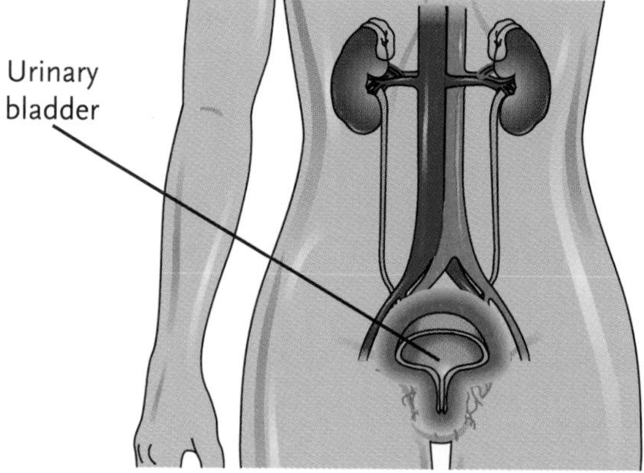

Figure 31-2. The most common cause of cystitis is the E-coli bacteria moving from the colon into the urinary tract.

CAUSE: There are many possible causes of cystitis; however, the most common is the E-coli bacteria. It moves from the colon into the urinary tract very easily, causing cystitis. Women often develop bladder infections after having sex.

CURE/TREATMENT: Drinking plenty of water and other fluids may help prevent mild bladder infections. Antibiotics are often prescribed for cystitis. The physician may evaluate risk factors of repeat cystitis attacks and can offer helpful suggestions on how to decrease the risk of a repeat episode.

Cystitis can often be prevented by following these instructions:

- wiping from front to back after going to the bathroom, which prevents E-coli from traveling from the colon to the urinary tract
- drinking plenty of water and other fluids to provide enough fluid for the kidneys to cleanse the blood of impurities; fruit juices high in vitamin C are encouraged to keep the urinary tract acidic
- urinating immediately after sex

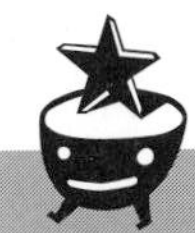

Star K.A.R.E.

Cystitis

KNOW your resident's care plan.
ASSIST the resident/nurse.

- *Encourage rest.*
- *Encourage fluids as ordered.*
- *Ensure that all prescribed antibiotics are taken.*

REPORT observations.
RECORD data.
RECHECK resident as needed.

If the following occurs:

- *pain or discomfort*
- *change in urination*
- *bleeding*
- *cloudy urine*

★ *"Don't Delay. Report Right Away!"*

ENCOURAGE resident's progress.

- *Provide support during painful episodes.*

Personal Health Tip!

After sex, it is important for women to urinate immediately. It is a good idea for men to urinate after sex too. This is important because during and after sex, bacteria can enter the urethra. The female urethra is shorter than the male's, so the bacteria do not have very far to travel to reach the bladder. This can cause what many healthcare providers have called "Honeymoon Cystitis." Cystitis is a bladder infection caused by bacteria that can lead to more serious kidney trouble if the bacteria are able to "crawl" up the ureters into the kidneys. If you ever have symptoms of cystitis, such as bloody, dark amber, or rust-colored urine, pain with urination, frequency, and urgency, seek help from your healthcare provider right away. If a resident ever shows these signs and symptoms, report it immediately.

2. Nephritis

Nephritis is an inflammation of the kidneys. It is also called pyelonephritis. Nephritis may occur when cystitis is not treated. Symptoms include fever, high blood pressure, and pain around the kidney area. Other symptoms include blood and/or protein in the urine along with swelling in the extremities (edema).

CAUSE: Nephritis may be caused by cystitis that has not been treated or a bacterial infection that has become systemic and spread throughout the body.

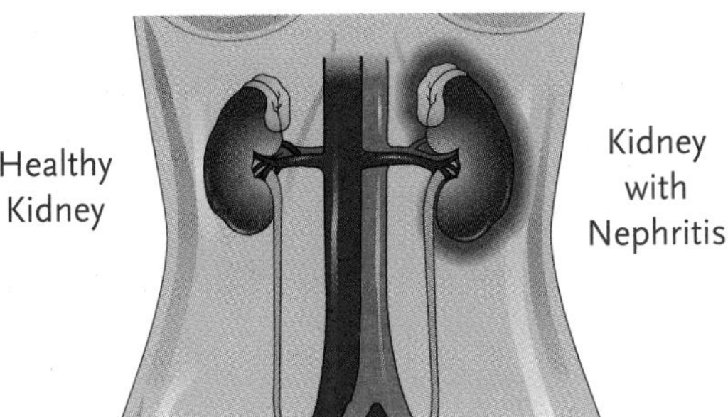

Figure 31-3. **Untreated cystitis may turn into nephritis.**

CURE/TREATMENT: Dialysis may be necessary if the nephritis affects both kidneys. This is done at home or at a hospital or dialysis facility. A kidney transplant may be available for the resident if a match is found. Drugs must be taken to prevent rejection of the transplanted kidney, and the patient must follow the instructions of healthcare providers carefully, including dietary restriction of sodium.

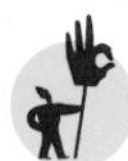

The Bladder: Exposed

In 1879, Nitze and Leiter developed the first cystoscope, an instrument used to examine the inside of the bladder and the ureters. The electric light bulb had not been invented at the time, so they used an exposed platinum wire lit by an electric current for light. By the 1920s, an IV technique for looking at the urological tract was created. This method ultimately became the modern technique known as angiography, which uses a special dye injected into the bloodstream in order to view and examine our blood vessels.

3. Calculi

Calculi or renal calculi are also called **kidney stones**. People may experience no pain or mild to extreme pain with kidney stones.

CAUSE: Stones also occur inside other areas of the body, such as the gallbladder. Kidney stones may be very large or very tiny. They are made up of one of the salts that normally exist in the urine. When the amount of one of these salts increases, a kidney stone forms. This can be caused by a number of problems, such as the parathyroid gland releasing too much calcium. This causes the excess calcium to **crystallize**, or come together inside the kidney. Other causes include a decreased fluid intake or an increase of a type of mineral supplement, such as calcium supplements. Many healthcare providers believe calcium supplements are very important, especially for women. It is possible that vitamin C causes kidney stones, so it is also important to drink enough water and other fluids while taking vitamin C supplements.

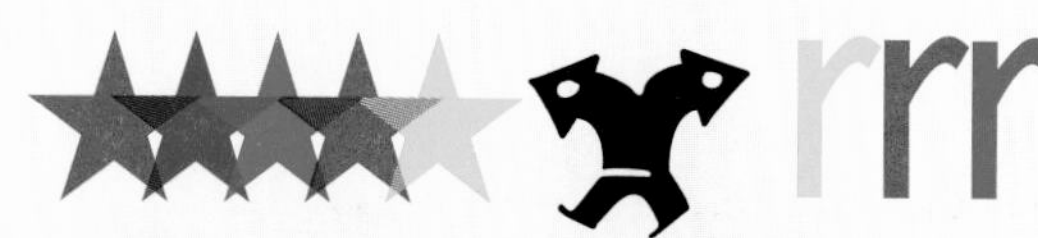

Beginning Steps

★ RESPECT
Knock first, ask and receive permission to enter a resident's room.

★ INFECTION CONTROL
Wash hands.

★ COMMUNICATION
Greet and identify the resident. Identify yourself. Explain the procedure, encouraging the resident to be as independent as possible throughout.

★ BED SAFETY
Lock bed wheels. Raise bed to safe working height. Lower one side rail if required.

★ PRIVACY
Provide for privacy by closing the door and covering the resident appropriately.

Ending Steps

★ RESIDENT SAFETY AND COMFORT
Secure the resident, lowering the bed, and raising the side rails if ordered. Check that the resident is comfortable and properly aligned.

★ PRIVACY
Remove any added privacy measures, such as a drape or a privacy screen.

★ ESSENTIALS
Place the call light, fresh beverage, and other items within reach.

★ COURTESY
Ask the resident if he or she needs anything else. Say thank you and goodbye.

★ INFECTION CONTROL
Wash hands.

r **Report** your care and any important observations to the nurse.

r **Record** your care and any important information/observations such as vital signs in the appropriate place.

r **Recheck** your resident for any changes as directed by the nurse!

CURE/TREATMENT: Stones may simply pass through the system by themselves, causing mild to very serious pain for the resident. Surgery may also be done to remove the stone. Another option is **lithotripsy**, which prevents the need for surgery. This method uses sound waves to crush the kidney stones into small enough pieces that they may pass through the urinary tract on their own.

Urine straining is done when renal calculi exist. Urine straining is the process of pouring all urine discharged from the body through a fine filter of some kind in order to catch particles that are too large to run through the filter. Caregivers are asked to observe and monitor urine from certain residents to watch for these stones or pieces of stones. The type of urine strainer is chosen by the facility and used for that resident until the stones are all passed or removed by surgery or another special procedure. Special plastic strainers may be chosen, or a coffee-filter-like strainer may be used.

4. Nocturia

Nocturia is frequent urination during the night.

CAUSE: Nocturia may be caused by a urinary tract infection; high fluid intake, especially of fluids that may encourage diuresis, such as tea or coffee; diabetes mellitus; kidney disease; or a disorder of the prostate. Nocturia can also be caused by a weakened urinary sphincter, which occurs more often in the elderly and women who have had children.

CURE/TREATMENT: Limiting fluids after a certain time of the day can be helpful. Also, taking the person to the bathroom immediately before going to bed and while providing care during the night is a good idea.

Urine Straining

Follow all standard and/or transmission-based precautions. Follow all rules for body mechanics.

Collect equipment:

- two pairs of disposable gloves • bedpan and cover
- toilet tissue • bed protector • specimen container
- special filter for straining • laboratory requisition slip
- disposable plastic bag

1. Perform the "5 Stars."

2. Apply gloves.

PREPARE:

3. Help the resident onto the bedpan (or onto the commode or to the bathroom). Ask resident to urinate.
4. Ask resident not to place toilet tissue into the container.
5. Use toilet tissue to clean perineal area and place tissue on bed protector or directly in toilet.
6. Cover and SECURE the resident.

PERFORM:

7. Bring bedpan to bathroom and pour urine through the filter into the specimen container.
8. Place the filter in the disposable plastic bag.

FINISHING TOUCHES:

9. Dispose of the urine in the toilet.
10. Clean bedpan and remove gloves. Replace bedpan in storage area.

11. Perform the "5 Stars and 3 Rs."

12. Bring disposable bag with specimen container inside and take lab slip to appropriate area.

4 Describe the process of "weaning" a resident from a catheter.

Residents who have been catheterized for a long period may require "weaning" from the catheter and retraining in urination. This is sometimes called a "**Foley Clamp and Drain**" program and is ordered by the doctor. If one of your residents is on this program, make sure you are familiar with your responsibilities. Ask the nurse to clarify anything you do not understand.

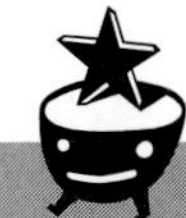

Star K.A.R.E.

"Foley Clamp and Drain" Order

KNOW your resident's care plan.
ASSIST the resident/nurse.

- *Post schedules if approved by supervisors.*
- *Follow schedules developed in the care plan. Communicate schedule to resident and to staff.*
- *Note if the resident is unable to maintain the clamping at any time.*
- *If nursing assistants are allowed to do this at your facility, clamp and unclamp catheter at times ordered. NEVER FORGET THE CATHETER IS CLAMPED! SET A TIMER, if needed.*

REPORT observations.
RECORD data.

- *Make charts of each daily clamping process.*

RECHECK resident as needed.

If the following occurs:

- *pain or discomfort*
- *the tubing becomes disconnected*

★ *"Don't Delay. Report Right Away!"*

ENCOURAGE resident's independence and progress.

- *Be consistent with the daily schedule.*
- *Provide plenty of encouragement and praise during this treatment method.*

Make your Kegel muscles work for you!

As women get older, especially after having children, they may experience the onset of dribbling or leaking of urine. This can occur at any time and may cause embarrassment. In the past, women had to wear sanitary napkins, but today special types of incontinence pads are available.

There is an exercise that women can perform to help reduce the amount of dribbling and leaking of urine. This involves exercising the Kegel muscles. These muscles control the starting and stopping of urine.

Follow these guidelines for **Kegel exercises**:

1. *When urinating, stop the flow of urine once or twice during urination. This will help you recognize your Kegel muscles and the way it feels when you squeeze them.*
2. *Squeeze your Kegel muscles and try to keep them squeezed for at least five to ten seconds.*
3. *Relax the muscles and repeat the exercise at least five times.*
4. *Set a goal of performing Kegel exercises at least three to four times at set times every day. Continue until you notice a decrease in dribbling or leaking of urine. If you do not note improvement after three to four weeks, contact your healthcare provider for professional advice.*

5 Review the safety guidelines for a resident with a urinary catheter and discuss the reasons a supra-pubic catheter is used.

Residents with urinary catheters are at increased risk of infection. When caring for catheterized residents, make sure you follow these guidelines:

Drainage Bags

- Never allow the catheter bag to touch the floor.
- Never allow the tip of the catheter drainage spout to touch the graduate when draining the catheter bag.
- When ambulating a resident, make sure the bag is always carried below the level of the resident's bladder.
- When returning to a resident's room, the catheter bag should never be placed on the bed.
- The drainage bag must hang from the bed frame, not from the side rail.

Tubing

- Never allow the tubing to touch the floor.
- Never re-attach a catheter tube that has disconnected for any reason.
- Make sure there are no kinks or twists in the catheter tubing.
- Make sure the resident is not lying on top of the tubing.

Catheter Care

- Provide catheter care with caution, carefully following facility guidelines.

- Always wear clean gloves when performing catheter care.
- Never tug on the catheter when performing care or moving the resident.
- When cleaning the urinary meatus, clean from front to back and then down, one motion at a time. Start the cleaning motion at the opening into the body and move downward from there.

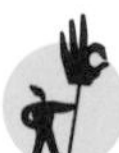

When catheter tubing separates:

★ *"Don't Delay. Report Right Away!"*

When a resident has a urinary catheter, the tubing may separate. This is a serious situation and must be handled by the nurse. Nursing assistants do not reattach the catheter tubing. Bacteria may enter the tubing and travel to the urinary tract causing a very serious infection. So, if a resident's catheter tubing separates:

★ *"Don't Delay. Report Right Away!"*

A supra-pubic catheter is inserted directly into the bladder in order to drain urine out of the bladder without having it drain through the urethra. This is done for a variety of reasons, such as urethral blockage, some types of trauma, problems with the neurological system that affect the ability to urinate normally, or after certain types of surgery. This type of catheter may be inserted temporarily or long-term.

A supra-pubic catheter is secured at the insertion site with sutures or a special type of seal. The catheter site is considered sterile, and sterile dressing changes are done by the nurse. The drainage system must remain closed. Blockages, kinks, and tugging of the tubing should be avoided. If you observe any pain, redness, or drainage, report it immediately to the nurse.

6 Describe continuous bladder irrigation (CBI) and list reasons why it is ordered.

Some residents with a Foley catheter have an order written for a **continuous bladder irrigation** (CBI). This occurs after surgery on the urinary tract, which may cause blood clots or bits of tissue to gather inside the tract. It may also be needed when a resident has had a catheter for some time and needs a flushing of the system periodically to clear out any debris. The goal of this procedure is to maintain the **patency**, which means the state of being open, of the catheter system.

When a CBI is ordered, a special type of catheter tubing is needed. This tubing has a 3-in-1 style:
- Tube 1 drains the urine.
- Tube 2 allows fluid to be injected to blow up the tiny balloon inside the bladder.
- Tube 3 allows the irrigation fluid to flow inside the bladder to flush out the system.

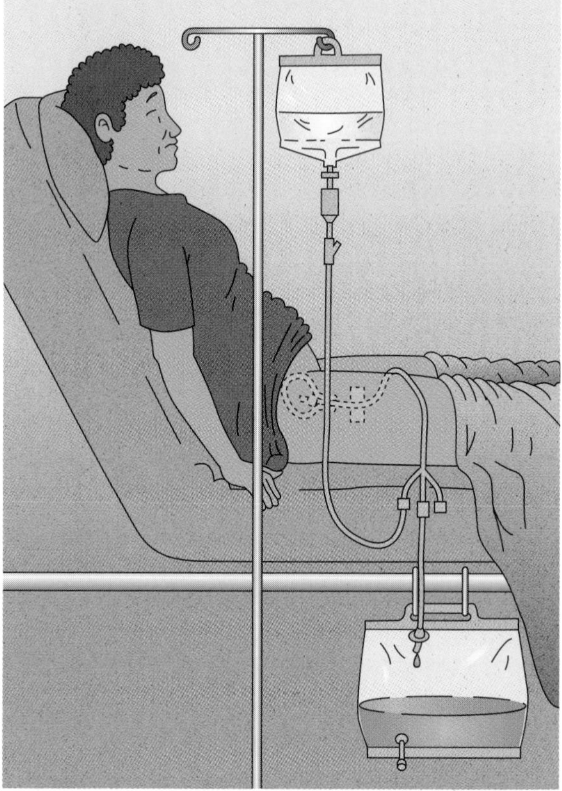

Figure 31-4. **Bladder irrigation using a three way catheter.**

When a resident has this order, the nurse performs the irrigation procedure. Be careful to follow the nurse's instructions when caring for this resident. When determining urine output on a resident with a CBI in place, follow this example:

Irrigation fluid used during shift: 750 cc

Fluid output in the catheter drainage bag when emptied: 1250 cc

1250 cc
-750 cc

---

500 cc urine output total
750 cc irrigation fluid total

Star K.A.R.E.

Continuous Bladder Irrigation

KNOW your resident's care plan.
ASSIST the resident/nurse.

- *Provide fluids as ordered to maintain urine output.*
- *Make sure drainage tubing stays clear.*
- *Make sure tubing does not disconnect or leak.*
- *Empty catheter drainage bag when asked to do so.*

REPORT observations.
RECORD data.
RECHECK resident as needed.

Watch urine output regularly during your shift.

If the following occurs:

- *pain*
- *redness*
- *drainage*

★ *"Don't Delay. Report Right Away!"*

ENCOURAGE resident's progress.

- *Provide encouragement and praise.*

7 Explain the specific gravity test and list one reason it is ordered.

A **specific gravity** test is performed on a resident's urine to determine the density of the urine. It can be ordered to make sure the kidneys are functioning properly. Density means how much the substance weighs compared to another substance, which in this case is water. Urine can be very dilute, or close to water. It can also be very dense, or concentrated. This test is done to see how the urine compares to water.

For example, if a person drinks a lot of water, her urine's specific gravity will decrease (be more diluted and closer to water).If a person is dehydrated, his urine's specific gravity will increase (be more concentrated). Urine can have a different specific gravity at various times of the day.

Different facilities use different methods to test urine. Your facility may use a special dip strip, interpreted by the caregiver, that can test for things like specific gravity, pH level, and glucose. Based upon the specific gravity, a resident may need further tests and medication or treatment.

Performing Specific Gravity Test

Follow all standard and/or transmission-based precautions. Follow all rules for body mechanics.

Collect equipment:

- **two pairs of disposable gloves • bedpan and cover**
- **toilet tissue • bed protector • specimen container**
- **specific gravity glass tube • test tube**
- **disposable plastic bag (if lab specimen ordered)**

1. **Perform the "5 Stars."**

2. **Apply gloves.**

PREPARE:

3. **Help the resident onto the bedpan (or onto the commode or to the bathroom). Ask resident to urinate.**
4. **Ask the resident not to place toilet tissue into container.**
5. **Use toilet tissue to clean perineal area and place tissue on bed protector or directly in toilet.**
6. **Cover and SECURE the resident.**

PERFORM:

7. **Bring bedpan to bathroom and pour urine into the special test tube until about three-fourths full.**
8. **Set the test tube down on a flat surface at eye level.**
9. **Place the specific gravity glass tube inside the test tube and "twirl."**
10. **Wait until the tube stops twirling. Read the number at the level the specific gravity tube meets the level of the urine. Note the results.**

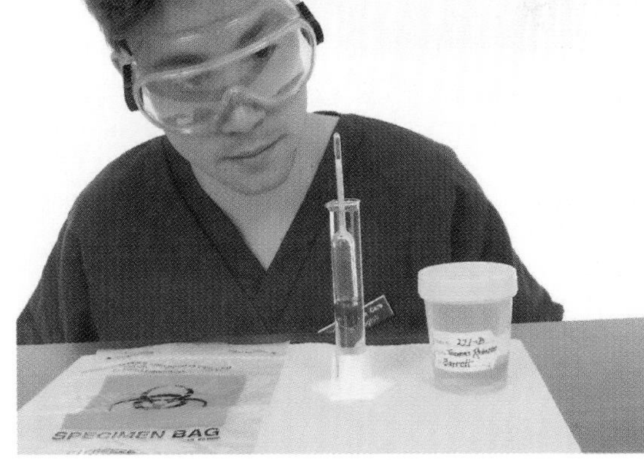

Figure 31-5.

FINISHING TOUCHES:

11. **Dispose of the urine in the toilet.**
12. **Clean bedpan and remove gloves. Replace bedpan in storage area.**
13. **Perform the "5 Stars and 3 Rs."**

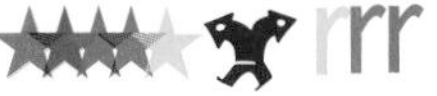

14. **If lab specimen is ordered, bring disposable bag with specimen container inside and take lab slip to appropriate area.**

Summary

The function of the urinary system is to remove liquid waste products from the body. When the urinary system is damaged in any way, the body's ability to eliminate waste products is reduced. Dangerous toxins can increase in the blood. It is vital that you be constantly on the lookout for any sign or symptom that may indicate a urinary tract problem. Urinary problems can rapidly become serious if not treated promptly.

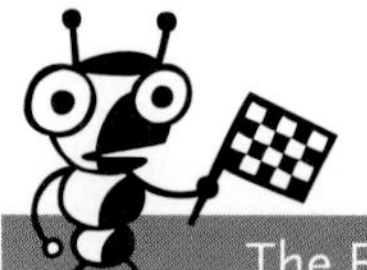

The Finish Line

What's Wrong With This Picture?

1. Look at the steps shown below for recording output after a continuous bladder irrigation. There are two errors listed. Find the errors and fix them.

   Irrigation Fluid Used During Shift: 525 cc

   Fluid output in the catheter drainage bag when emptied: 975 cc

   975 cc
   -525 cc
   ______
   425 cc urine output total
   575 cc irrigation fluid total

2. Look at the guidelines below. Find the two errors and fix them.

Drainage Bags

- Never allow the catheter bag to touch the floor.
- Never allow the tip of the catheter drainage spout to touch the graduate when draining the catheter bag.
- When ambulating a resident, make sure the bag is always carried above the level of the resident's bladder.
- When returning to a resident's room, the catheter bag should never be placed on the bed for any length of time.
- The drainage bag must hang from the side rail, not from the bed frame.

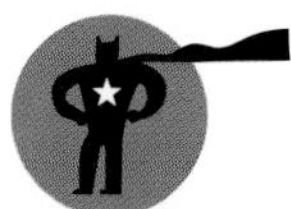

Star Student Central

1. Contact a local dialysis center and ask for a tour. Gather pamphlets about kidney disease and the process of dialysis to share with your class.
2. Find out the location of your local organ donor network association. Go to the office and ask for literature and donor cards to share with your class, family, and friends. Remember that organ donation is a personal decision.

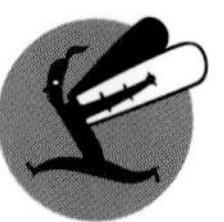

You Can Do It Corner!

1. Why is it important for women to urinate after sexual intercourse? (LO 3)
2. List one reasons why medication has more of an effect on the elderly. (LO 2)
3. Why would a specific gravity test be ordered for a resident? (LO 7)
4. What is another name for kidney stones? (LO 3)
5. Identify one cause of cystitis. (LO 3)
6. Why would a separation of catheter tubing be such an emergency? What would your first step be if this occurred? (LO 5)
7. What is the purpose of a Continuous Bladder Irrigation (CBI)? (LO 6)
8. List four ways you can assist the resident and nurse with a Foley Clamp and Drain order. (LO 4)

Star Student's Chapter Checklist

1. I have read my textbook chapter.
2. I have reviewed my own "Pocketful of Terms."
3. I have listened to my tutor tape.
4. I have reviewed and highlighted my class notes.

5. I have read and completed any handouts from this chapter.
6. I have completed "The Finish Line."
7. Star Time! Choose your reward!

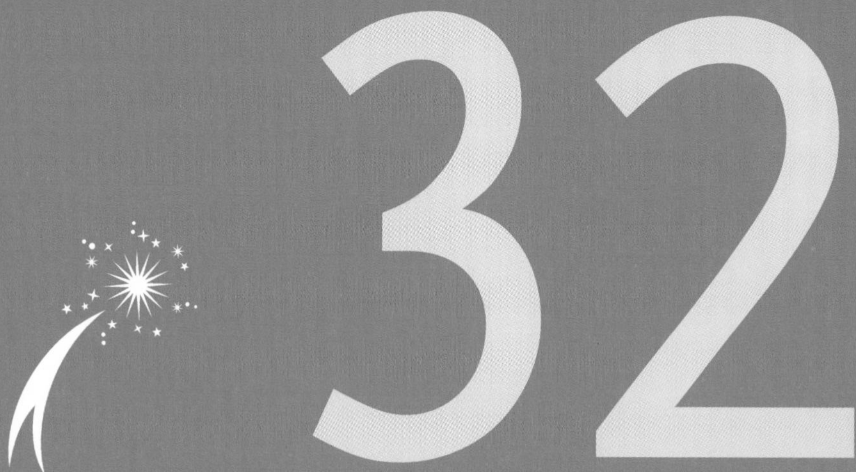

Specialized Care: The Reproductive System

Look Like a Star!

Look at the Learning Objectives and The Finish Line before you begin reading this chapter.

Look at your pocket calendar.
With your pencil, put a bracket (   ) around a study period every single day.

Look at your homework for this chapter.
Plug each piece of homework into a certain time slot.

Look at the Star Student's Chapter Checklist at the end of this chapter. Check off each item as it is completed.

"When I was born, I drew in the common air, and fell upon the earth, which is of like nature, and the first voice which I uttered was crying, as all others do."

Wisdom of Solomon 7:3

"In the dark womb where I began/My mother's life made me. . . Through all the months of human birth/Her beauty fed my common earth."

John Masefield, 1878-1967

Learning Objectives

1. **Spell and define all STAR words.**
2. **Summarize the changes that occur in the reproductive system during normal aging.**
3. **Describe sexual needs of the elderly and explain how nursing assistants can help promote dignity and respect.**
4. **Discuss seven common disorders of the reproductive system.**
5. **Describe vaginal irrigation.**
6. **Successfully provide accurate breast self-examination instruction to another person.**
7. **Successfully provide accurate testicular self-examination instruction to another person.**
8. **Discuss the six most common sexually transmitted diseases.**
9. **Describe the importance of privacy during a gynecological exam.**

Successfully perform this Practical Procedure

Assisting the Nurse with a Vaginal Irrigation

An Amazing Recovery!

Ephraim McDowell, 1771-1830, a doctor of the Kentucky frontier, was visited in 1809 by a patient with a large ovarian cyst. He asked her to consider traveling 60 miles to his office for an operation which she would probably not survive. She decided to travel the distance on horseback. The physician opened her abdomen without anesthesia while she read from the Bible and cut out an ovary weighing nearly 20 pounds. She left the area and returned home after a 25- day recovery. The woman lived another 31 years. McDowell gained international fame for his removal of cysts.

1 Spell and define all **STAR** words.

breast cancer: cancer of one or both female or male breasts.

cervical cancer: cancer in a female's cervix.

chlamydia: sexually transmitted disease (STD) that can cause infertility if not treated.

digital rectal exam: an examination of the rectum to check for lumps or an enlarged prostate.

erectile dysfunction (E.D.): the inability of a male to get or keep an erection in order to satisfy himself and/or his partner.

genital herpes: STD causing itching, burning, and blister-like sores.

gonorrhea: STD caused by bacteria; symptoms include painful urination and discharge.

HPV: STD causing wart-like spots on the genitals.

ovarian cancer: cancer in one or both ovaries.

ovarian cysts: cysts found on one or both ovaries.

sexually transmitted disease (STD): also called venereal disease; passed through sexual contact with an infected person.

syphilis: STD causing sores on the genitals; fatal if not treated.

testicular cancer: cancer in one or both testicles.

uterine cancer: cancer in the uterus.

vaginal irrigation: introduction of fluid into the vagina for treatment or cleansing; may or may not have doctor-ordered additive, such as vinegar or Betadine; also called a douche.

2 Summarize the changes that occur in the reproductive system during normal aging.

As we age, many changes occur within the male and female reproductive systems. Menopause occurs within the female reproductive system when the menstrual period ends. This happens anywhere from age 35 to 55. The production of estrogen and progesterone drops and other symptoms occur, such as hot flashes, night sweats, and mood swings. Vaginal walls become drier and thinner.

In men, testosterone production drops; this can cause a decreased interest in sex. Sperm also decrease in number, and the sperm's ability to successfully fertilize an egg, also known as viability, decreases. The prostate gland becomes larger and can cause difficulty in urination.

3 Describe sexual needs of the elderly and explain how nursing assistants can help promote dignity and respect.

While interest in sex may decline in the elderly, it does not go away. The elderly are no less inclined to desire intimate relationships than younger adults. The ability to engage in sexual activities, such as intercourse and masturbation, continues unless a disease or injury occurs. You can help by providing privacy whenever necessary for sexual activity and respecting your residents' sexual needs.

Some things that can affect sexual activity in the elderly include:

- illness reducing or affecting the ability of men and women to perform sexually
- erectile dysfunction in males
- vaginal atrophy, pain and dryness in females
- fear of inadequate sexual performance
- depression
- a lack of privacy
- medications

Remember that older adults are sexual like all humans, and they have the right to choose how they express their sexuality. In all age groups, there is a wide variety of sexual behavior. This is also true of your residents. An attitude that any expression of sexuality by the elderly is either disgusting or cute deprives your residents of their right to dignity and respect. All of your residents have a right to be treated with dignity and have their privacy respected.

What is a Bundling Bag?

Bundling bags were used at the time of the American Revolution when an unmarried gentleman visited a home. The matron (or woman) of the house or another woman inside the home would literally sew a bag completely around the man so that they could all be assured he would not creep into the bed of any unmarried female in the home.

4 Discuss seven common disorders of the reproductive system.

Female

1. Breast Cancer

Breast cancer is a leading cause of death in women. Women may be at a greater risk of getting breast cancer if they have a family history, have never had children, or had a first child after age 30.

CAUSE: No one knows for sure what causes breast cancer. Researchers have found a gene in some individuals that is involved in the development of breast cancer.

CURE/TREATMENT: Breast cancer has a much higher cure rate when caught in the very early stages. Performing a monthly breast self-exam helps to detect potential problems. Mammograms are thought to be able to find tiny lumps as much as two years before a person might feel the lumps.

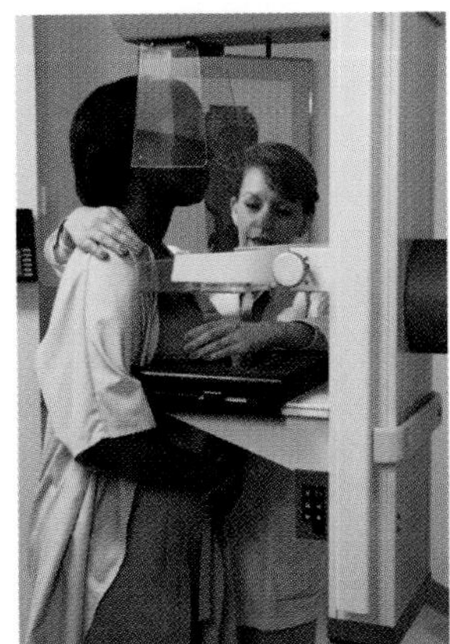

Figure 32-1. Mammograms can help prevent breast cancer.

A Different Kind of Gift

What do you give yourself for Christmas, Hanukkah, or a special holiday you celebrate? My gift to myself is a mammogram. Think about how important this gift might be to you and your loved ones. It could truly be the gift of life!

2. Ovarian Cysts

Ovarian cysts are growths that develop on the ovaries, the female sex glands. These organs produce the eggs that are fertilized by the sperm and create a fetus. Cysts are common in women in their reproductive years. Symptoms of an ovarian cyst include backaches, abdominal pain, pressure inside the abdomen, or pain during sex. Other symptoms are spotting between periods, irregular periods, stoppage of periods, or very painful periods. Abdominal distention can also occur, which is swelling of the abdomen. Some women experience no symptoms.

CAUSE: The process of ovulation causes normal cysts to form. Abnormal cysts may be formed due to an imbalance in the female hormones.

CURE/TREATMENT: Treatment depends upon the age of the woman. It also depends upon the severity and size of the cyst(s). In some cases, medications are used and in others, surgery, such as a hysterectomy (removal of the uterus), may be performed.

3. Uterine, Cervical, and Ovarian Cancer

Cervical cancer is almost 100% curable if caught and treated in the early stages. It can occur at any age and is occurring at younger ages. One reason for this increase in younger women may be the increase in the number of sex partners a woman might have.

Uterine cancer affects more women who are obese, who are taking estrogen supplements, who have a family history of uterine cancer, and who have infertility problems.

Ovarian cancer is a hidden and quiet cancer that may strike at any age. There may be few symptoms, or the person may have a mild persistent backache or other mild symptoms.

CAUSE: No one knows for sure what causes uterine, cervical, or ovarian cancer. Researchers believe women who have sexual intercourse at an early age, who have many sex partners, or who are infected with a certain virus called the HPV—Human Papilloma Virus—are at a greater risk for cervical cancer. Women who are at higher risk for cancer of the uterus include women taking estrogen, obese women, those with a family history of cancer, and women suffering from infertility.

CURE/TREATMENT: The best way to prevent cervical cancer and uterine cancer is to have an annual exam with a Pap smear. An annual pelvic and **digital rectal exam** is very important for women because this may detect problems in the early stages while they are still curable. This is done by a doctor or healthcare provider skilled in this procedure.

There is a test called the CA-125 blood test that may help a doctor diagnose ovarian cancer.

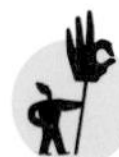

Personal Health Tip!

Sometimes when a woman asks for a certain test, a healthcare provider feels the test is unnecessary. You may have to be persistent and ask for the test directly. If you are having any symptoms that make you think you have a reproductive cancer, ask for a Pap smear, pelvic exam, possibly an abdominal pelvic ultrasound, and a CA-125 blood test. If your regular doctor will not order them for you, get a second opinion!

Male

1. Prostate Cancer

Prostate cancer is the most common cancer found in males, especially in older men; it can occur in younger men as well. There may be few symptoms or there may be pain during urination or difficulty urinating.

CAUSE: The cause of prostate cancer is unknown.

CURE/TREATMENT: The best way to prevent prostate cancer is to have an annual physical exam that includes a digital rectal exam. The doctor can sometimes feel an enlargement of the prostate during this part of the exam. An annual digital rectal exam is very important for men because this may detect problems in the early stages while they are still curable. This is done by a doctor or healthcare provider skilled in this procedure.

There is a test called the PSA blood test that may help a doctor diagnose prostate cancer.

2. Testicular Cancer

Testicular cancer is a cancer of the male reproductive glands. It is most common in young men from about the mid-teen years to the mid-30's. A symptom is a slight enlargement of one or both testes. Pain may or may not be a symptom, but there may be a kind of pressure in the abdomen or the groin area. The person may feel a sort of "dragging" or heaviness in this area, as well.

CAUSE: No one knows for sure what causes testicular cancer. One thing that may increase a man's chances of getting this disorder is if he ever had an undescended or partially undescended testicle.

CURE/TREATMENT: Testicular cancer has a much higher cure rate when caught in the very early stages. Surgery is the usual treatment, and it may be combined with radiation and possibly chemotherapy.

Cancer care is covered in Chapter 35.

3. Erectile Dysfunction (E.D.)

Erectile Dysfunction (E.D.) is a disorder in which a man is unable to get or keep an erection in order to satisfy himself and/or his partner. Impotence is another term used to identify this disorder.

CAUSE: There are many physical and psychological causes of this problem. Some physical causes are diabetes mellitus, multiple sclerosis, spinal cord injuries, and trauma or surgery that affects the nerves in the male genital area. Examples of psychological causes include life stressors and fear related to the ability to achieve an erection. Medications, especially anti-hypertensive drugs (drugs to treat high blood pressure) can also have a negative affect on male erectile ability.

CURE/TREATMENT: Counseling, drug therapy, or special surgical implants placed in the penis may be utilized.

4. Benign Prostatic Hypertrophy (BPH)

Benign prostatic hypertrophy is a disorder that is quite common in men over the age of 60. There are estimates that one-third to one-half of all men over this age show signs of this disorder.

CAUSE: The cause of BPH is still unclear. It rarely affects men under 40 years of age, with symptoms generally beginning between 60 to 65 years of age. The prostate gland enlarges due to unknown causes, and this change in size causes a narrowing of the urethra. The urethra passes through the center of the prostate gland. When the urethra becomes compressed, the discharge of urine becomes more difficult. Urinary retention may occur due to this situation, causing discomfort. Prostate enlargement is not a cancerous condition.

CURE/TREATMENT: A prostatectomy may be performed which removes part of or all of the prostate gland. Partial or total erectile dysfunction (E.D., impotence) can result from this surgery. State-of-the art, nerve-sparing surgery is utilized in some cases where a great concern about E.D. exists. One abbreviation you may see used to identify one of these surgeries is TURP, Transurethral Prostatectomy, where a specific part of the prostate gland is removed in order to re-open the urethra and try to eliminate the urinary retention. In some cases, non-surgical treatment is used to attempt to reduce or eliminate the prostatic enlargement. There are many non-surgical treatments used to treat this disorder, such as a variety of medications and radiation therapy.

5 Describe vaginal irrigation.

Vaginal irrigations are performed in order to cleanse the vaginal tract prior to surgical procedures or due to vaginal drainage. They are also performed to introduce medication into the vagina to reduce discomfort such as itching or redness, along with pain or vaginal drainage.

Many facilities do not allow nursing assistants to perform this procedure; however, you may be asked to assist the nurse in performing it. Generally, doctors and healthcare providers do not believe regular irrigations are needed without evidence of a problem of some kind.

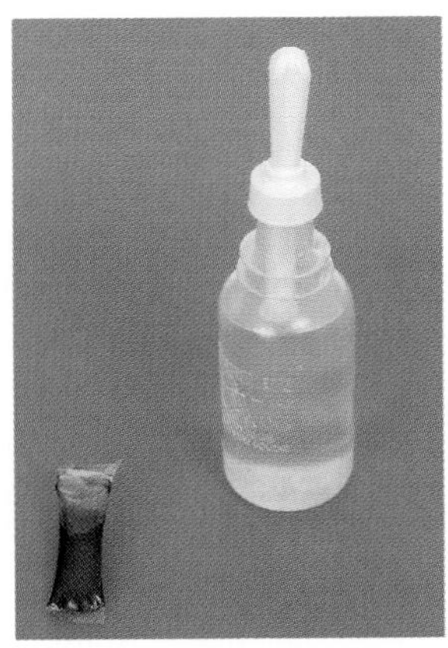

Figure 32-2. Betadine and a ready-to-use douche.

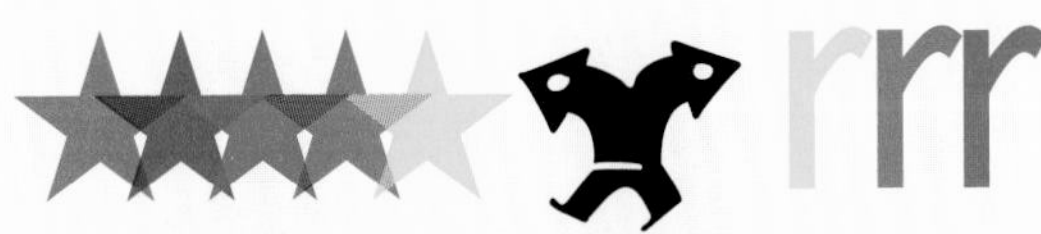

Beginning Steps

★ **RESPECT**
Knock first, ask and receive permission to enter a resident's room.

★ **INFECTION CONTROL**
Wash hands.

★ **COMMUNICATION**
Greet and identify the resident. Identify yourself. Explain the procedure, encouraging the resident to be as independent as possible throughout.

★ **BED SAFETY**
Lock bed wheels. Raise bed to safe working height. Lower one side rail if required.

★ **PRIVACY**
Provide for privacy by closing the door and covering the resident appropriately.

Ending Steps

★ **RESIDENT SAFETY AND COMFORT**
Secure the resident, lowering the bed, and raising the side rails if ordered. Check that the resident is comfortable and properly aligned.

★ **PRIVACY**
Remove any added privacy measures, such as a drape or a privacy screen.

★ **ESSENTIALS**
Place the call light, fresh beverage, and other items within reach.

★ **COURTESY**
Ask the resident if he or she needs anything else. Say thank you and goodbye.

★ **INFECTION CONTROL**
Wash hands.

r **Report** your care and any important observations to the nurse.

r **Record** your care and any important information/observations such as vital signs in the appropriate place.

r **Recheck** your resident for any changes as directed by the nurse!

Assisting the Nurse with a Vaginal Irrigation

Follow all standard and/or transmission-based precautions. Follow all rules for body mechanics.

Collect equipment:

- 2 pairs of disposable gloves • bedpan and cover
- toilet tissue • bed protector
- disposable douche or prepared vaginal irrigation bag
- drape or bath blanket • plastic bag

1. Perform the "5 Stars."

2. Apply gloves. Assist resident to urinate.

PREPARE:

3. Hang prepared vaginal irrigation bag on IV pole and lower pole so that bag is 12 inches above resident's perineal area.

PERFORM:

4. Place disposable bed protector.
5. Help the resident onto the bedpan (or onto the commode or to the bathroom) and place in dorsal recumbent position. (Figure 32-3)

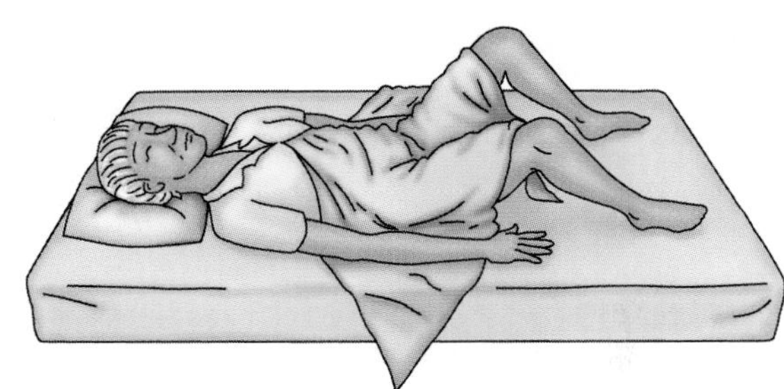

Figure 32-3.

6. Drape resident.
7. Release air from the tubing into the bedpan.

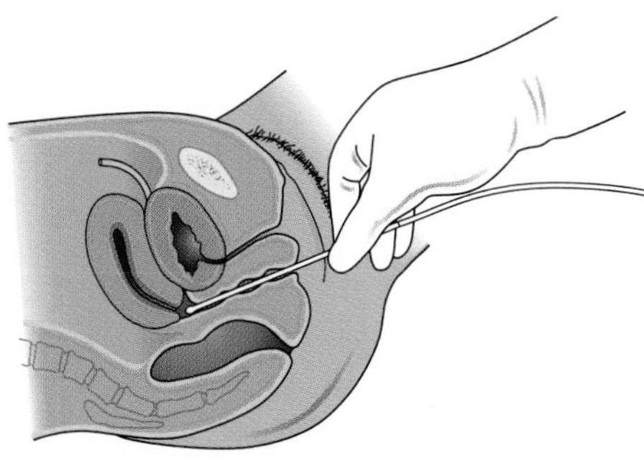

Figure 32-4.

8. Insert nozzle very slowly and gently into vagina about two to three inches. (Figure 32-4)
9. Begin slow flow of water or fluid by releasing clamp. Before vaginal irrigation bag is empty, clamp tubing.
10. Remove tubing slowly and gently and place tubing tip inside top of bag.

11. **Position resident in Fowler's position on the bedpan so that solution can drain.**

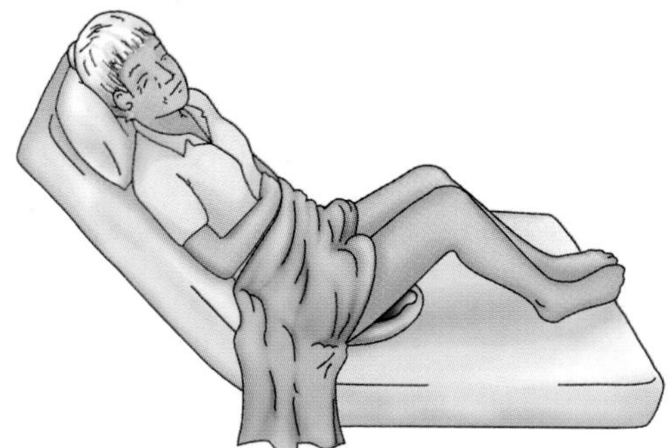

Figure 32-5.

12. **Dry perineal area and buttocks and replace clothing or gown.**
13. **Remove disposable bed protector and replace if needed.**
14. **SECURE THE RESIDENT.**
15. **Bring covered bedpan to bathroom, observe contents for anything unusual and pour contents into the toilet.**

FINISHING TOUCHES:

16. **Remove gloves and wash hands.**
17. **Perform the "5 Stars and 3 Rs."**

6 Successfully provide accurate breast self-examination instruction to another person.

Breast cancer has one of the highest fatality rates among cancers in women. By the time the cancer becomes painful, it may be quite advanced. A breast self-exam, in which the person searches for lumps or anything unusual, should be done every month on the same day. Always report any lumps to a physician. Figure 32-6 shows the correct way to do a breast self-examination.

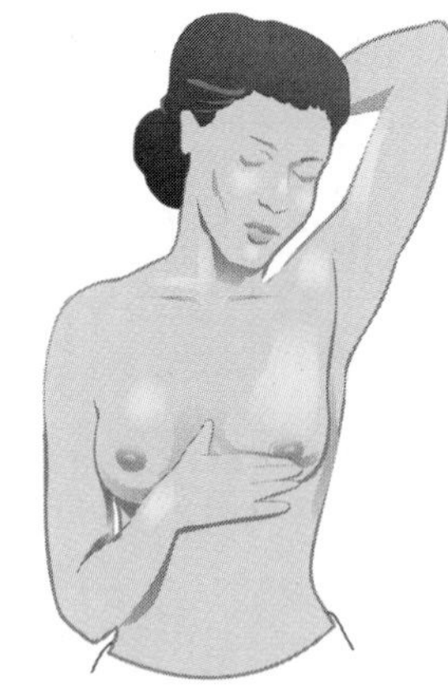

Figure 32-6. **Breast self-examination.**

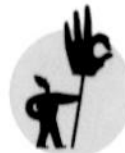

BSE: Write it on your calendar!

Write BSE on your calendar in big letters on the first of every month. Also, add BSE to your calendar book, if you carry one. This way, you will never forget to do your own exam each month.

7 Successfully provide accurate testicular self-examination instruction to another person.

Men of all ages should develop a habit of doing a monthly examination of their testicles, in which the person searches for lumps or anything unusual. Testicular cancer is more common in young men than in older men. Any man can do this exam himself or with the help of another person. It should be done every month on the same day. Figure 32-7 shows the correct method to perform a testicular self-examination.

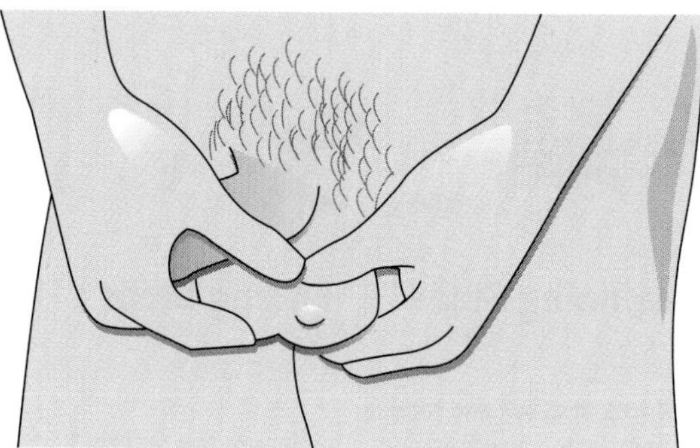

Figure 32-7. **Testicular self-examination.**

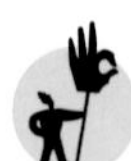

TSE: Write it on your calendar!

Write TSE on your calendar in big letters on the first of every month. Also, add TSE to your calendar book, if you carry one. This way, you will never forget to do your own exam each month.

8 Discuss the six most common sexually transmitted diseases.

AIDS, which can be transmitted through sex, is discussed in Chapter 34 (the lymphatic system).

1. Chlamydia

CAUSE: Microorganisms

SYMPTOMS: urethritis, an inflammation of the urethra; pain and discomfort with urination and/or sex.

Men: discharge from the penis and swelling of the testes.

Women: no symptoms or symptoms include vaginal discharge and low back pain.

TREATMENT: antibiotics; may cause infertility if left untreated.

2. Genital Herpes

CAUSE: virus called Herpes Simplex Type II

SYMPTOMS: itching, burning sensation, and blisters that look like cold sores on the genitals and possibly other parts of the body. These may appear quickly after the sexual contact.

TREATMENT: It is a virus and cannot be treated with antibiotics. Once infected, a person cannot be cured and may suffer repeated outbreaks of the disease for the rest of his life.

3. HPV (Genital Warts)

CAUSE: virus called human papilloma virus

SYMPTOMS: tiny wart-like growths on the genitals

TREATMENT: There is no cure; freezing, burning, and laser surgery may help. HPV may cause an increased risk of cervical and other cancers.

4. Gonorrhea

CAUSE: bacteria

SYMPTOMS:

Men: No symptoms, or painful urination, a cloudy pus-like discharge from the penis, and swelling of the testes.

Women: No symptoms, or a cloudy vaginal discharge, or burning with urination.

TREATMENT: antibiotics

5. Syphilis

CAUSE: bacteria

SYMPTOMS: small, painless sore at the point of infection; this stage (primary) passes in one to five weeks.

In second stage, rashes occur on the skin, in the genital area, and the mouth. A headache, fever, and joint and muscle aches are common. Syphilis can be fatal. Once it reaches the late stage, it can spread to vital organs and the nervous system and cause death.

TREATMENT: antibiotics

6. Trichomoniasis

CAUSE: protozoa

SYMPTOMS:

Men: may be a carrier without symptoms; lives in the urethra

Women: severe burning and itching of the vulva area and a heavy, white, frothy vaginal discharge

TREATMENT: anti-infective medications

The Scourge of Syphilis

The first epidemic of syphilis affected the sailors who returned from Columbus' first voyage to the New World. It was first called Naples Disease and the French Disease.

Paul Ehrlich, 1854-1915, developed a substance called salvarsan in 1910. He then used it to treat patients with syphilis. It was found after experimenting with hundreds of substances. Persistence pays off!

9 Describe the importance of privacy during a gynecological exam.

The gynecological examination may occur in the resident's room or in a special examination room. It can also occur in an emergency room or an urgent care center, and you may be asked to go there with a resident. It is important to be sensitive to the concerns of the resident who is in this position. Gynecological examinations may be very embarrassing or frightening for many residents. Nursing assistants and other staff need to be very careful to ensure the privacy of each resident. Privacy must never be compromised. This means that you should never allow yourself to relax your standards.

Star K.A.R.E.

Assisting with a Gynecologic Procedure

KNOW your resident's care plan.
ASSIST the resident/nurse.

- *Assist resident to empty bladder before procedure.*
- *Position resident appropriately.*
- *Help feet into stirrups, if needed.*
- *Drape resident for privacy.*
- *Hand doctor instruments as needed.*
- *Provide doctor with lubricant as needed.*
- *Hold slide for doctor as needed.*
- *Provide tissues to resident for clean-up after exam.*

REPORT observations.
RECORD data.
RECHECK resident as needed.

If any of the following occur after the procedure:

- *bleeding or discharge*
- *pain or discomfort*
- *dizziness*
- *change in vital signs*

★ *"Don't Delay. Report Right Away!"*

ENCOURAGE resident's progress.

- *Provide support during gynecological procedures because they can cause discomfort and fear.*

Knock first, then listen for the magic words!

At some point in your life, you may have had a healthcare provider or doctor knock on the door to an examination room and not wait to hear you say "come in." If so, you may have felt uncomfortable. With a resident, when you do not wait those few seconds, you may expose him or her not only to you, but also to people walking through the hallways. This is potentially embarrassing to all involved, but most importantly, to the resident. Ensure your residents' dignity; wait to hear "come in."

Summary

Remember that your residents are sexual human beings. Their ability to engage in sexual activity may be affected by a wide range of factors. There is a wide variety of sexual behavior in older people, just as there is in younger people. You must promote their privacy and their right to express themselves sexually. Always be respectful.

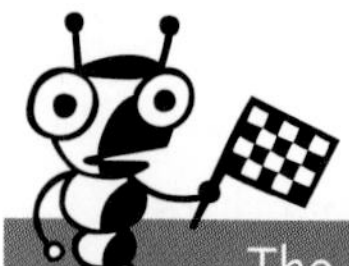

The Finish Line

What's Wrong With This Picture?

Look at the following sexually transmitted diseases. Change the symptoms for each to make them correct.

Chlamydia: tiny, wart-like growths on the genitals.
Trichomoniasis: small, painless sore in the primary stage.
HPV (Genital warts): urethritis, pain and discomfort with urination.
Syphilis: cloudy discharge.
Gonorrhea: lives in the urethra of males; males may be carriers without symptoms.

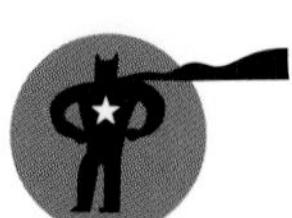

Star Student Central

1. Go to your local health department and gather pamphlets on all of the STDs to share with your class.
2. Visit your local American Cancer Society and gather pamphlets on the various cancers of the reproductive system to share with your family and your class.

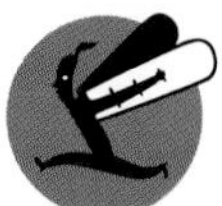

You Can Do It Corner!

1. How often should a breast self-exam (BSE) be done? (LO 6)
2. Why is it important to provide privacy during a gynecological exam? (LO 9)
3. List two changes of aging for men and women in the reproductive system. (LO 2)
4. Why are vaginal irrigations performed? (LO 5)
5. List six STDs and treatment for each. (LO 8)
6. What is the most common reproductive cancer? List for males and females. (LO 4)
7. What are men looking for when they perform a testicular self-exam? (LO 7)
8. How can a nursing assistant promote dignity with the sexual needs of residents? (LO 3)

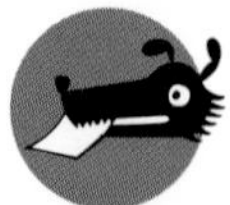

Star Student's Chapter Checklist

1. I have read my textbook chapter.

2. I have reviewed my own "Pocketful of Terms."
3. I have listened to my tutor tape.
4. I have reviewed and highlighted my class notes.
5. I have read and completed any handouts from this chapter.
6. I have completed "The Finish Line."
7. Star Time! Choose your reward!

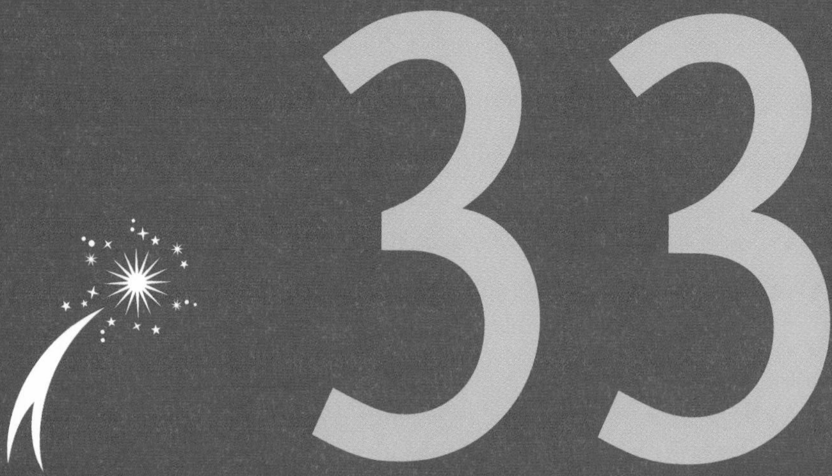

Specialized Care: The Endocrine System

Look Like a Star!

Look at the Learning Objectives and The Finish Line before you begin reading this chapter.

Look at your pocket calendar.
With your pencil, put a bracket (   ) around a study period every single day.

Look at your homework for this chapter.
Plug each piece of homework into a certain time slot.

Look at the Star Student's Chapter Checklist at the end of this chapter. Check off each item as it is completed.

"... Who dodges life's stress and its strains..."

Donald Robert Perry, 1878-1937

"...Complaints is many and various/And my feet are cold..."

Robert Graves, 1895-1985

Learning Objectives

1. Spell and define all STAR words.
2. Summarize the changes that occur in the endocrine system during normal aging.
3. Discuss two common disorders of the endocrine system.
4. Identify three "Ps" of diabetes mellitus.
5. Describe nutrition for a diabetic resident and discuss guidelines of insulin therapy.
6. Describe a diabetic's test for glucose levels to determine how much insulin to take.
7. Discuss the importance of safe foot care with the diabetic resident.
8. Describe the body's physical response to stress.
9. Describe ways to cope with stress.
10. Describe ways to decrease stress in your residents' lives.

Successfully perform this Practical Procedure

Ketone Testing

Early Work with Hormones

Thophile de Bordeau, 1722-1776, developed the idea that certain organs like the brain discharged a type of substance. He believed this substance moved into the blood. If there was a sufficient quantity of the substance inside the blood, it actually helped keep people healthy.

1 Spell and define all STAR words.

hyperglycemia: increase in the blood sugar; signs and symptoms include the 3 Ps (polydipsia, polyphagia, and polyuria), nausea or vomiting, aches and pains, sweet or fruity breath smell.

hypoglycemia: deficiency of sugar inside the blood; signs and symptoms may include sweating, faintness, dizziness, headache, nervousness, shaking, rapid heartbeat, anxiety, hunger, visual problems, weakness, irritability.

nocturia: tendency to urinate frequently during the night.

podiatrist: physician who diagnoses, treats, and cares for conditions of the human feet.

polydipsia: excessive thirst.

polyphagia: excessive hunger.

polyuria: discharge of large amounts of urine.

stressor: anything that causes stress.

Type 1 diabetes: formerly called juvenile diabetes or insulin-dependent diabetes; begins at a younger age; insulin injections required for rest of life.

Type 2 diabetes: formerly called adult-onset diabetes or non-insulin-dependent; person may take oral medication or insulin injections.

2 Summarize the changes that occur in the endocrine system during normal aging.

As we age, our levels of hormones decrease. This can affect the day-to-day functioning of the organs that the hormones control. The functioning of the male and female sex organs usually decreases, which lessens the sex drive. The pancreas may not produce enough insulin, and this causes the body to build up sugar in the blood. Enough blood may not be released for energy when the body does not produce enough insulin. This causes the body to start showing signs and symptoms of diabetes mellitus.

3 Discuss two common disorders of the endocrine system.

1. Type 1 Diabetes

Type 1 Diabetes usually occurs before the mid-30s. Prior names for this disorder were juvenile diabetes and insulin-dependent diabetes mellitus (IDDM). With this disorder, the body does not produce any insulin.

CAUSE: Some think the reason for this lack of insulin is a problem with the immune system. There may also be a genetic link.

CURE/TREATMENT: People will require daily injections of insulin for the rest of their lives. These injections do not always prevent the many complications that occur with this disorder. Special diets help treat this disorder and must be followed exactly.

2. Type 2 Diabetes

Type 2 Diabetes can occur in adults. Prior names for this disorder were adult-onset diabetes or non-insulin-dependent diabetes mellitus (NIDDM).

CAUSE: The body either does not make enough insulin or it becomes unable to use insulin for some reason.

CURE/TREATMENT: Treatment for type 2 diabetes is either oral medication or injections of insulin. Special diets help treat this disorder.

Brown-Sequard: The Father of Endocrinology?

Although others did much research in the field, Charles Eduoard Brown-Sequard [1817-1894] is considered by some to be the "Father of Endocrinology." He was the son of an American sea captain and a French mother, and he traveled and lectured widely. Brown-Sequard noted that organs like the thyroid, liver, spleen, and kidneys secreted substances that traveled into the blood. These substances were ultimately called hormones.

4 Identify three "Ps" of diabetes mellitus.

Diabetes mellitus is a disease that can affect people of virtually any age. Approximately four out of five people over 65 have some form of diabetes.

This disorder is due to the pancreas not manufacturing the hormone insulin or not making enough insulin. Diabetes prevents the sugar taken in from food from moving into the cells and being changed into much-needed energy. Sugar then builds up inside the blood, causing **hyperglycemia**, or high blood sugar. Because the body is unable to get energy in the usual way, from the sugar in the blood, the body has to find energy in another manner. Usually the energy is obtained by burning fat.

Insulin acts like a key because it "unlocks" the door to the blood and allows the sugar to come out, be transferred into the cells, and turn into energy. Figure 33-1 outlines this process.

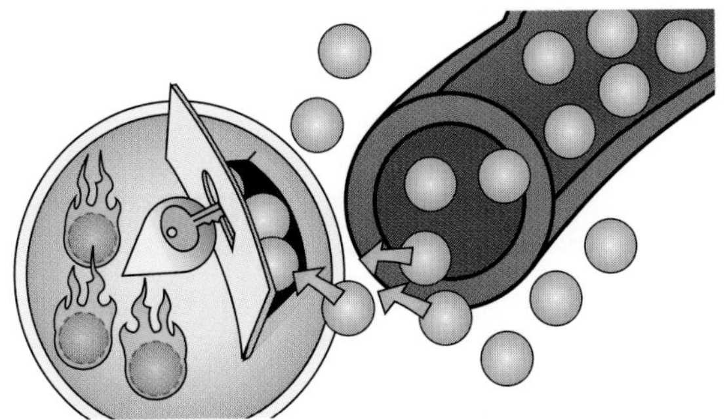

Figure 33-1. Insulin acts as a key, unlocking the cells to let the glucose enter.

Many signs and symptoms occur in a person who develops diabetes. There is a trio of symptoms that alerts a person or a doctor to the development of diabetes. That person should immediately be tested. This group of symptoms is outlined below:

The 3 Ps

- **Polydipsia**: excessive thirst
- **Polyphagia**: excessive hunger
- **Polyuria**: excessive urination

Polyuria may show up as a tendency to urinate frequently during the night, known as **nocturia**. This occurs in a person who, prior to this, rarely got up in the night to urinate. Nocturia can be one of the first signs of the disorder.

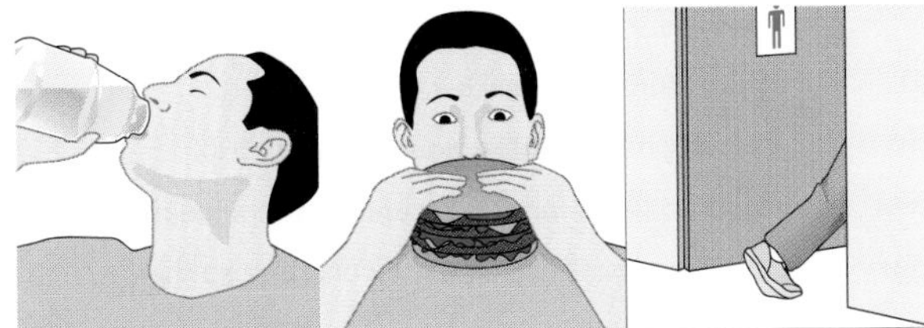

Figure 33-2. Excessive thirst, excessive hunger, and excessive urination make up the three Ps.

What is your risk for diabetes?

The American Diabetes Association (ADA) has developed a test to see whether or not you may be at risk for diabetes. You may want to take the test and share it with members of your family.

The ADA has lowered the at-risk blood sugar level to 126, down from 140. This means that people with a fasting blood sugar level of 126 are considered diabetic. Fasting blood sugar refers to the level of sugar in the blood when a person has not taken in food or fluids, except for water. Normal fasting blood sugar levels are from 70 to 110.

Star K.A.R.E.

Resident with Diabetes

KNOW your resident's care plan.
ASSIST the resident/nurse.

- *Carefully monitor vital signs.*
- *Watch for signs of low or high blood sugar.*

SKIN:

- *Observe skin for complications, such as sores, blisters, cuts, or nail problems on the hands or feet.*
- *Give good oral hygiene and observe for mouth sores.*
- *Watch for signs of dehydration.*
- *Give excellent skin care.*

SKELETAL and MUSCULAR:

- *Ambulate with care.*
- *Give range of motion exercises.*
- *Change position every two hours.*

CIRCULATORY:

- *Be alert for signs of blood clots, such as pain in the legs, especially the calves.*
- *Monitor pulse, including pedal pulse, and blood pressure.*
- *Watch for signs of faintness, dizziness, or headache.*
- *Discourage smoking.*

RESPIRATORY:

- *Monitor respiratory rate.*

GASTROINTESTINAL:

- *Watch for nausea, vomiting, or complaints of thirst.*
- *Watch for signs of dehydration or weight loss.*
- *Follow fluid order carefully.*
- *Measure intake carefully.*
- *Weigh resident as ordered.*

URINARY:

- *Follow fluid order carefully.*
- *Measure output carefully.*
- *Observe for signs of urinary problems, such as burning or difficulty urinating, which could lead to infection.*

NERVOUS:

- *Watch for signs of nervousness, shaking, or trembling.*
- *Observe for signs of visual or hearing problems.*
- *Watch for numbness or tingling in arms or legs, especially the feet and hands.*
- *Be alert for irritability or confusion.*

REPORT observations.
RECORD data.
RECHECK resident as needed.

If any of the following occur:

- *changes in vital signs*
- *signs of hypoglycemia: sweating, faintness, dizziness, headache, nervousness, shaking, rapid heartbeat, anxiety, hunger, visual problems, irritability*
- *signs of hyperglycemia: 3 Ps (polydipsia, polyphagia, and polyuria), nausea, or vomiting, aches and pains, sweet or fruity breath smell*

SKIN:

- *signs of pressure sores*
- *redness or blood around any injection site*

SKELETAL:

- *ambulating difficulty, change in gait*

MUSCULAR:

- *muscle weakness*

CIRCULATORY:

- *chest pain or tightness*
- *tachycardia or palpitations*
- *signs of blood clots in the legs*

RESPIRATORY:

- *shortness of breath or dyspnea*

GASTROINTESTINAL:

- *signs of dehydration or weight loss*
- *hunger or thirst*
- *increased or decreased intake of food or drink*
- *nausea or vomiting or abdominal pain*
- *flatus, diarrhea, or constipation*
- *fruity breath odor*

URINARY:

- *change in output*
- *frequency of urination or incontinence*
- *signs of urinary tract infection, such as burning or dysuria*

IMMUNE:

- *fever or other signs of infection*

NERVOUS:

- *visual difficulties such as blurred vision*
- *any numbness or tingling anywhere on the body*
- *irritability or confusion*

★ *"Don't Delay. Report Right Away!"*

ENCOURAGE resident's independence and progress.

- *Encourage taking prescribed medication.*
- *Encourage following proper diet.*
- *Encourage exercise and movement as allowed.*

Ketones are formed when the body breaks down fat. Uncontrolled diabetes can produce ketones in the urine. When the ketone buildup is excessive, the body is unable to excrete these substances safely. They can reach dangerous levels. Ketones in the urine can be detected by test strips. Your facility may ask you to perform this kind of urine testing.

Ketone Testing

Follow all standard and/or transmission-based precautions. Follow all rules for body mechanics.

Collect equipment:

• two pairs disposable gloves • bedpan and cover
• toilet tissue • bed protector • specimen container
• ketone test strips • plastic bag
• laboratory requisition slip • paper towel

1. **Perform the "5 Stars."**

2. **Apply gloves.**

PREPARE:

3. **Help the resident onto the bedpan (or onto the commode or to the bathroom).**
4. **Ask the resident to urinate in container and not to place toilet tissue into container.**
5. **Use toilet tissue to clean perineal area and place tissue in plastic bag.**
6. **Remove gloves and place in disposable bag.**
7. **Cover and SECURE THE RESIDENT.**

PERFORM:

8. **Apply second pair of gloves. Bring urine to bathroom. If necessary, pour urine into urine cup.**
9. **Place urine cup on paper towel.**
10. **Open testing bottle and remove one test strip.**
11. **Dip strip into urine for one second and remove right away.**
12. **Tap the strip onto the side of the container so that excess urine falls off.**
13. **Follow the instructions on the container regarding the wait time for the test.**
14. **Holding the strip in one gloved hand and container in the other, compare the color of the strip with the color chart. If the color has changed, match the color with the closest color in the chart. Do not touch bottle with strip.**

FINISHING TOUCHES:

15. **If necessary, clean and replace bedpan in storage area.**
16. **Perform the "5 Stars and 3 Rs."**

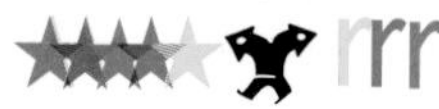

17. **Bring disposable plastic bag to biohazard area.**
18. **Wash hands again.**

5 Describe nutrition for a diabetic resident and discuss guidelines for insulin therapy.

People with diabetes must be very careful about what they eat. It is very important for a diabetic to eat meals at about the same time each day. This helps control the diabetes. The sugar or glucose in the blood must stay balanced and not become too high, which causes hyperglycemia, or too low, which causes **hypoglycemia**. When a resident is taking regular insulin, all staff members must play a part in this careful balance of blood sugar.

When the doctor orders insulin, the amount is carefully matched to the exact amount of food the resident eats throughout the normal day. Residents must never eat more food than ordered for them because it would upset the delicate balance of blood sugar. When diabetics eat too much, it causes their blood sugar to be too high. People with diabetes are usually taught by a dietitian to follow meal plans and use exchange lists. A sample meal plan and partial exchange list is shown in Box 33-1.

Sample Meal Plan and Exchange List Box 33-1

The following is a sample meal plan and a partial exchange list a person with diabetes might use. Keep in mind that this is only an example. A resident's diet may also be under other restrictions, and the diet will vary according to the resident's daily calorie needs. Exchange lists contain many more choices than the sample below.

Sample Meal Plan

Breakfast (to be eaten between 7:30 and 8:30 a.m.): two starches, one milk, one fruit, one fat

Snack (to be eaten between 10 and 11 a.m.): one milk

Lunch (12:30 to 1:30 p.m.): one meat, one milk, two starches, one vegetable, one fruit

Snack (3:00 to 4:00 p.m.): one vegetable, one milk

Dinner (5:30 to 6:30 p.m.): three meats, one starch, two vegetables, one milk, two fats

Snack (7:30 to 8:30 p.m.): one milk, one starch

Following the meal plan for what types of food and how many servings to eat, the person chooses specific foods and determines serving size using the exchange lists.

Exchange List Sample Items

Starch list: 1 slice of bread, one-half bagel, one-half cup cereal, one-half cup pasta, one-half cup rice, 1 baked potato, 3 cups popcorn, 15-20 fat-free potato chips

Milk list: 1 cup milk (skim, 1%, 2%, or whole, depending on other dietary guidelines), three-fourths cup yogurt

Fruit list: one-half cup unsweetened applesauce, 1 small banana, one-half cup orange juice, 2 tablespoons raisins, 1 small orange, one-half cup canned pears

Vegetable list: one-half cup cooked vegetables or vegetable juice, 1 cup raw vegetables (not included are corn, potatoes, and peas, which are on the starch exchange list instead)

Meat list: 1 oz. meat, fish, poultry, or cheese, 1 egg, or one-half cup dried beans

Fat list: 1 teaspoon margarine or butter, 2 teaspoons peanut butter, 2 tablespoons sour cream, 1 tsp mayonnaise, 10 peanuts

---

Low or high blood sugar occurs for a variety of reasons. Closely monitoring your diabetic residents throughout the day prevents complications of insulin therapy. It is especially important for you to know a diabetic's habits well so you can recognize any change.

Five Questions to Protect Residents on Insulin

1. What type of insulin are your residents receiving? There are fast-acting and slow-acting insulins.
2. What time are the insulin injections given? Does the resident have any tests due today?
3. Has the resident finished each meal and snack during your shift?
4. Has the resident received any snacks or treats from other residents or visitors?
5. Does the resident seem to be acting like him- or herself?

Be watchful for any signs that a resident on insulin has high or low blood sugar. Observe intake of food and drink carefully. If you notice any problems, report them immediately to the nurse.

6 Describe a diabetic's test for glucose levels to determine how much insulin to take.

As a nursing assistant, you may assist a nurse with blood glucose monitoring equipment or be trained in its use. This type of monitoring equipment measures the level of glucose inside the blood throughout the day. Normal blood glucose is from 70 to 110 mg.

When assisting with this procedure, make sure the strips are not discolored in any way. In addition, make sure the strips have not expired. Discolored or expired strips may not be accurate. The strips will be in a container with an expiration date marked. Check the date before you go to the resident's room.

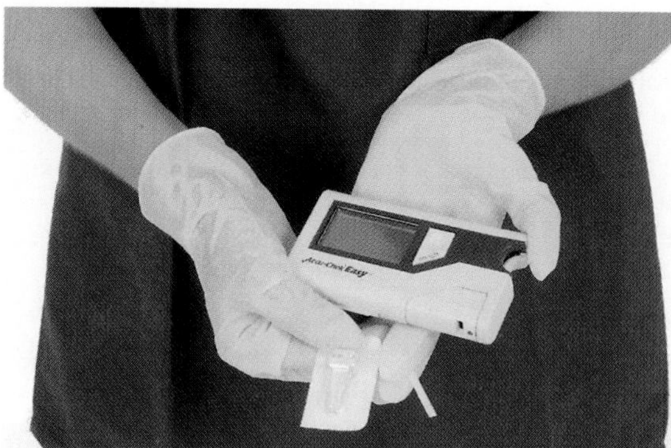

Figure 33-3. **Blood glucose monitoring equipment.**

Star K.A.R.E.

Blood Glucose Monitoring

KNOW your resident's care plan.
ASSIST the resident/nurse.

- *Wear gloves if you are assisting the nurse with this procedure.*
- *Look at the strip for any sign of discoloration.*
- *Check expiration date on the strips.*
- *Be careful handling any sharps.*
- *Dispose of equipment properly.*

REPORT observations.
RECORD data.
RECHECK resident as needed.

If any of the following occur:

- *signs of hypoglycemia: sweating, faintness, dizziness, shaking, rapid heartbeat, anxiety, hunger, visual problems, weakness, irritability*
- *signs of hyperglycemia: 3 Ps (polydipsia, polyphagia, polyuria) extreme thirst, extreme hunger, frequent urination, nausea, or vomiting, aches and pains, sweet or fruity breath smell*
- *redness or blood around any insulin injection site*

★ *"Don't Delay. Report Right Away!"*

ENCOURAGE resident's progress.

7 Discuss the importance of safe foot care with the diabetic resident.

Diabetes may cause potentially serious problems with the feet. One of the most common foot problems in diabetics is the risk of foot infection. Diabetes weakens the immune system, which reduces resistance to infections. Poor circulation due to the narrowing of the blood vessels also increases chances of infection. When foot infections are noted in the early stages, there is a good chance of a full recovery. However, when this kind of an infection is allowed to remain unchecked, a diabetic may ultimately need to have a toe, foot, or leg amputated due to spread of the infection. Sixty-four percent of diabetes-related amputations are in people 65 and older.

Common problems that a healthy person would recover from easily may have a different effect on a person with diabetes. You must be very careful when handling a diabetic's feet. Box 33-2 outlines some common problems to observe and report.

Common Diabetic Foot Problems Box 33-2

Problems with toenails: an ingrown toenail may cause a serious infection; there can be fungus around the toenails; they may be yellow in color.

Problems with rashes: any kind of a rash on the feet, such as athlete's foot, should be reported promptly and treated.

Problems with corns, calluses, or warts: infections can easily occur in these areas; they should be watched closely and treated immediately.

Problems with poor-fitting shoes: complaints of shoes being too tight or uncomfortable should be reported immediately; pressure caused by a shoe could cause an ulcer, which can lead to infection.

It is extremely important for all diabetic residents to see a **podiatrist** regularly. Many facilities have this type of doctor visit twice a month or more to provide care for residents' feet. Nursing assistants may have the responsibility of signing up their residents for a visit to the podiatrist. Always err on the side of safety; if in doubt, sign the resident up. If you need help with this decision, ask the nurse.

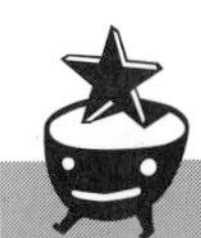

Star K.A.R.E.

Safe Diabetic Foot Care

KNOW your resident's care plan.
ASSIST the resident/nurse.

- *Inspect resident's feet every day during daily bath, making sure to check between the toes for rashes, cuts, sores, blisters, bruises, or fungus.*
- *Give excellent skin care, especially to the feet.*
- *Avoid harsh soaps and hot water when bathing feet.*
- *Always dry feet thoroughly, especially between toes.*
- *Never cut toenails, corns, or calluses for any reason.*
- *Never use any object to try to remove dirt from a toenail, like a nail stick.*
- *Use a doctor-recommended cream or lotion on the feet, but avoid the area between the toes.*
- *Avoid hot water bottles or hot packs near the feet.*
- *Check shoes for tiny rocks or other objects prior to resident putting them on.*
- *Remind the resident not to walk around barefoot.*
- *Encourage high-quality shoes, such as leather shoes. Make sure shoes fit properly.*
- *Discourage high heels or sandals.*
- *Wash and change socks daily. Keep socks dry and free of bumps or lumps.*
- *Avoid socks that are too tight.*

REPORT observations.
RECORD data.
RECHECK resident as needed.

If any of the following occur:

- *redness, cut, scrape, sore, bruise, or blister anywhere on the body*
- *rash or fungus*
- *corn or callus*
- *problems with toenails*
- *blood on the feet or toes*
- *pain or burning in the feet*
- *wetness, such as a discharge around the feet*
- *poorly-fitting shoes*
- *other injuries on or around the feet*
- *pain in the feet or legs, especially the calves*

★ *"Don't Delay. Report Right Away!"*

ENCOURAGE resident's progress.

8 Describe the body's physical response to stress.

Stress is the state of being frightened, excited, confused, in danger, or irritated. We think of stress as being a purely emotional or mental state. Why would we include information on stress and stress management in a chapter on the endocrine system? Because stress produces physical changes in your body, largely regulated by the endocrine system.

While the physical response to stress is quite complicated, here are a few examples of what happens. The hypothalamus begins our response. First a "fight or flight response" begins. This releases adrenaline and readies the body for physical action. This brings huge amounts of glucose and oxygen to the brain, skeletal muscles, and the heart. To achieve this, the pulse races. Blood vessels in our skin and other organs contract to get the extra blood to our skeletal muscles, heart and brain. The spleen contracts, releasing stored blood into our system. The liver releases glucose to feed the cells, which increases temperature and causes sweating. Respiratory passageways expand and breathing becomes faster. Our digestive system slows to save energy. Our adrenal glands release hormones, including epinephrine, to maintain this stress response. And all this is just the beginning!

The endocrine system continues to release hormones that see us through the **stressor** after the initial response ends. If the stressor is great enough, the effect on organs can actually cause death.

We do not know the exact relationship between stress and disease. We do know that stress is linked to many diseases, including hypertension, depression, ulcers, migraines, and rheumatoid arthritis. It also increases the risk of developing other chronic diseases and is linked to dying prematurely.

9 Describe ways to cope with stress.

The most obvious way to deal with stress is to remove or avoid stressors. Research shows that being asked to do things for which you are not trained causes great stress. Sadly, sometimes this stress is turned toward residents in the form of abuse and neglect. This, of course, is unacceptable. As care providers, you must always seek help in dealing with difficult situations. For example, having to deal with a combative resident or an angry family member can cause great stress. By recognizing the signs of stress, you will have a signal that you may need assistance dealing with a stressful situation. Only you can ask for this help.

When stressors cannot be avoided, which is often the case, try to undo the effects of stress. Some immediate responses you can attempt are listed below:

Abdominal Breathing
- Stop and breathe.
- Hold your hands on your abdomen and close your eyes.
- Breathe slowly and regularly, pushing your hands out with each breath.
- Do this a few times until you feel yourself begin to relax.
- A feeling of peace should begin moving over your entire body.

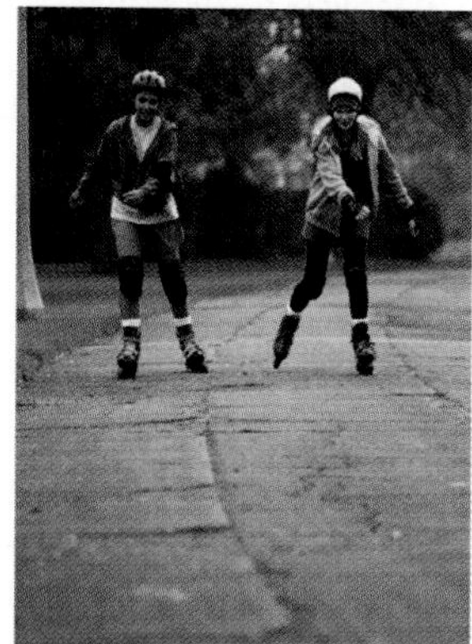

Figure 33-4. **Exercising by yourself or with a friend can help decrease stress.**

Muscle Relaxation
- Starting with your head and jaw, relax as many muscles as you can.
- Do this one muscle at a time, from top to bottom, until you reach the muscles of your feet and toes.

Leave your stress at home!

When you experience a great deal of stress, sometimes it takes a superhuman effort not to show it on the job. When we bring stress to the workplace, we may take out our stress on our residents. This is very unfair to them and should never be done. If you become angry or impatient with a resident because you are upset with someone else or stressed about something, it is abuse. Remember to always try to leave your stress and anger at home. If you feel that you cannot do this, contact your supervisor. He or she may be able to give you more resources to help manage your stress.

10 Describe ways to decrease stress in your residents' lives.

Many people forget that residents feel stress, too. There are many possible causes for the stress your residents may have. Here are some to consider:

- moving into a long-term care facility
- a family member or friend who is ill
- uncertainty about their health
- a family member or friend who has moved away
- illness of a beloved pet
- a loved one who has not visited for quite awhile
- the facility has announced financial difficulties; residents might have to move
- increasing dependence on staff
- frequent change in caregivers
- incontinence

When residents feel stress, it can affect all of the people at the facility. Other residents may feel bad; staff members can get upset, and the whole morale of the unit can suffer. Here are some ways to combat a resident's stress:

1. Determine the reason for the stress as best you can. This may be done by listening carefully to them and possibly talking to the nurses about it. Spending time with residents can also have a calming effect.

2. Find out if anything can be done to change the situation. For example, perhaps a family member can be contacted to determine the reason he has not visited for some time.

3. If nothing can be done to fix the stressor, try to find a way to improve the situation.

4. Try to involve the resident in an activity. Encourage an activity the resident has not participated in before.

Summary

The endocrine system functions by producing the substances called hormones in sufficient quantity to keep the body healthy. Hormones control many body functions. When the level of a certain hormone goes up or down, the normal functioning of the body can be affected. If you are caring for diabetic residents, remember to encourage proper diet and taking prescribed medication. Also, take care to protect a diabetic's toes and feet. If you are experiencing high levels of stress, you may need to seek resources to help you manage the stress.

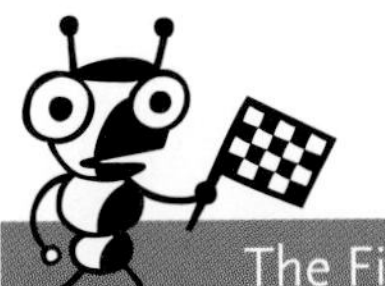

The Finish Line

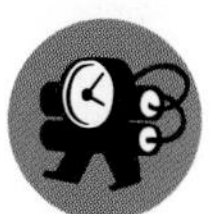

What's Wrong With This Picture?

Look at the STAR KARE on safe diabetic foot care listed below. List the two missing observations.

If any of the following occur:

- *redness, cut, scrape, sore, bruise, or blister anywhere on the body*
- *corn or callus*
- *blood on the feet or toes*
- *pain or burning in the feet*
- *wetness, such as a discharge around the feet*
- *poorly-fitting shoes*
- *other injuries on or around the feet*
- *pain in the feet or legs, especially the calves*

★ *"Don't Delay. Report Right Away!"*

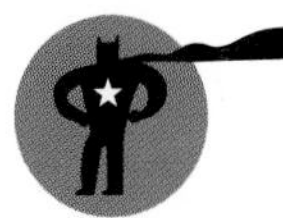

Star Student Central

1. Visit the American Diabetic Association and pick up pamphlets for your class.
2. Take a copy of the ADA diabetic quiz home with you and give to friends and family. Provide any help needed in completing the quiz. If anyone shows a risk of diabetes, encourage an immediate check-up.

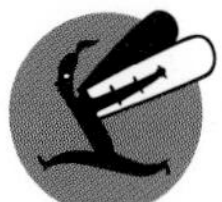

You Can Do It Corner!

1. What can happen when a foot infection is not noted in the early stages? (LO 7)
2. List two ways to cope with stress. (LO 9)
3. Describe the two types of diabetes. (LO 3)
4. Identify the 3 Ps of diabetes. (LO 4)
5. What are some reasons why your residents could be stressed? (LO 10)
6. What is a normal level of blood glucose? (LO 6)
7. What happens when the pancreas does not produce enough insulin? (LO 2)
8. Why do diabetic residents need to eat the exact amount of food on their diets? (LO 5)
9. List some of the body's physical responses to stress. (LO 8)

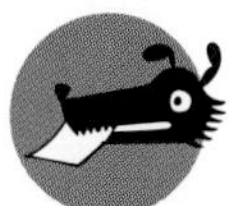

Star Student's Chapter Checklist

1. I have read my textbook chapter.
2. I have reviewed my own "Pocketful of Terms."
3. I have listened to my tutor tape.
4. I have reviewed and highlighted my class notes.
5. I have read and completed any handouts from this chapter.
6. I have completed "The Finish Line."
7. Star Time! Choose your reward!

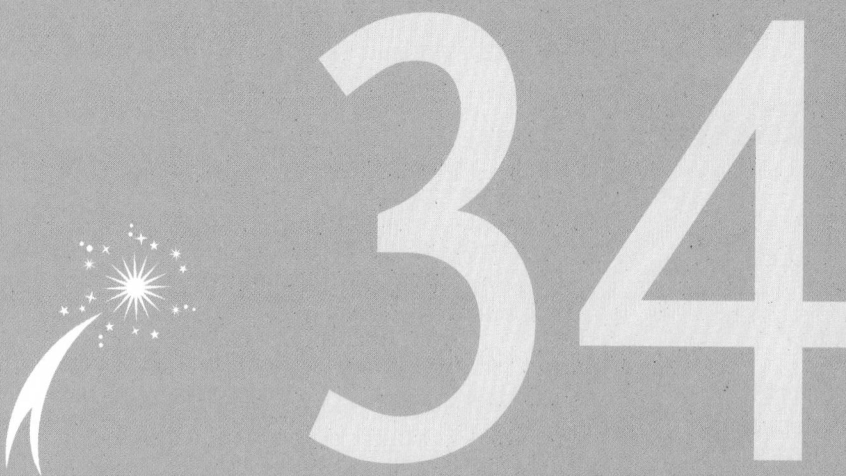

34

Specialized Care: The Lymphatic System and Immunity

Look Like a Star!

Look at the Learning Objectives and The Finish Line before you begin reading this chapter.

Look at your pocket calendar.
With your pencil, put a bracket ( ) around a study period every single day.

Look at your homework for this chapter.
Plug each piece of homework into a certain time slot.

Look at the Star Student's Chapter Checklist at the end of this chapter. Check off each item as it is completed.

"Healing is a matter of time, but it is sometimes also a matter of opportunity."

Hippocrates, 460-377 B.C.

"Extreme remedies are very appropriate for extreme diseases."

Hippocrates, 460-377 B.C.

Learning Objectives

1. **Spell and define all STAR words.**
2. **Summarize the changes that occur in the immune system during normal aging.**
3. **Discuss four common disorders of the immune system.**
4. **Discuss ways to provide emotional support to the resident with AIDS.**
5. **Identify community resources and services available to the resident with HIV/AIDS.**
6. **Explain the precautions you should take when caring for people with AIDS.**
7. **Demonstrate knowledge of the legal aspects of AIDS, including testing.**

Amazing Cells that Gobble up Bacteria

Elie Melchnekoff, 1845-1916, identified that bacteria could be destroyed by certain cells that seemed to "gobble them up." This process was eventually called "phagocytosis." He won the Nobel Prize in 1908.

1 Spell and define all STAR words.

AIDS: acquired immunodeficiency syndrome; an illness caused by human immunodeficiency virus, or HIV.

HIV: human immunodeficiency virus; the virus that causes AIDS.

Hodgkin's disease: disease producing enlarged lymph tissue, usually curable when caught in early stages.

homophobia: a fear of homosexuality.

lymphoma: general term used to describe diseases of the lymph system; includes Hodgkin's disease.

pneumovax: the vaccine given to older people that provides protection from many types of pneumonia.

Systemic Lupus Erythematosis (SLE): disorder of the immune system that causes an inflammation of the connective tissue.

T-cells: vital T-lymphocytes that help fight infection.

2 Summarize the changes that occur in the immune system during normal aging.

As we age, the ability of our immune system to function may decrease. When this happens, there is usually an increase in the number of infections or illnesses per year. The response of the antibodies may also slow down, which can cause more infection. The very important T-lymphocytes may decrease in number, reducing the number of helper T cells available to fight infection.

The body can have a reduced response to certain vaccines as it ages. This decreases the person's ability to prevent a certain disease despite the fact that he or she had the vaccine.

Personal Health Tip!

Be up-to-date on all vaccinations, and consider getting a flu shot. Vaccinations are important to protect you and your residents from serious diseases. Outbreaks of certain diseases still occur, especially in cities with large populations.

Flu shots are not an absolute protection against the flu, but they can make a flu episode less serious. Some facilities encourage employees to get flu shots.

*The **pneumovax** vaccine is a one-time vaccine that may help protect older people against different types of pneumonia. Doctors can give more information about this vaccine and help people make an informed decision about it.*

3 Discuss four common disorders of the immune system.

1. Allergies

Allergies occur in people who are hypersensitive to a foreign substance called an allergen. Examples of allergens include pollen, dust, colognes, and certain foods. The immune system responds to the allergen by releasing histamine and other substances that cause the characteristic runny nose and watery eyes. These substances may trigger a life-threatening response in some people to certain allergens. This is called an anaphylactic reaction or anaphylactic shock. If help is not obtained immediately, the person can die due to the shortness of breath, dyspnea, and wheezing that develops.

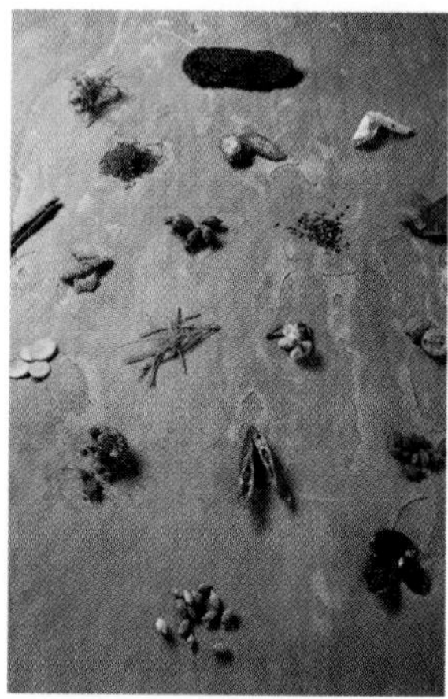

Figure 34-1. There are many possible allergens.

CAUSE: There may be a genetic link to allergies that people suffer.

CURE/TREATMENT: People who have severe allergies can see a specialist called an allergist. Allergists first try to determine the things the people are allergic to and then attempt to decrease their sensitivity to the allergens. They do this by giving them tiny amounts of the allergens. This amount is not enough to cause a serious reaction, but is enough to de-sensitize them from the allergen. This process may take a very long time, and there is no guarantee of success.

Star K.A.R.E.

Allergies

KNOW your resident's care plan.
ASSIST the resident/nurse.

- *Closely observe resident for any allergic reaction.*

- *Keep known allergens out of resident's room (flowers, perfumes, cosmetics).*
- *Keep resident away from others who have known allergens nearby.*

REPORT observations.
RECORD data.
RECHECK resident as needed.

If any of the following occur:
- *watery eyes, runny nose, or sneezing attacks*
- *hives or any skin rash*
- *difficulty breathing or shortness of breath*

★ *"Don't Delay. Report Right Away!"*

ENCOURAGE resident's progress and independence.
- *Provide support during allergy attacks.*
- *Residents who are careful to avoid allergens and who take any prescribed medication will feel better and be more active.*

2. The Lymphomas: Hodgkin's Disease

The lymphomas are cancers of the lymphatic system. There are different kinds of **lymphoma**. One of the most common is **Hodgkin's disease**. The first symptom is a painless enlargement of one of the lymph nodes. Some of the other symptoms are fever, weight loss, night sweats, and fatigue.

CAUSE: No absolute cause is known, although there may be a genetic link. It may also be caused by a problem with the immune system.

CURE/TREATMENT: Hodgkin's disease is known as a "curable cancer" when discovered and treated in its early stages. Chemotherapy may be effective with or without radiation therapy. In some cases, bone marrow transplants are performed.

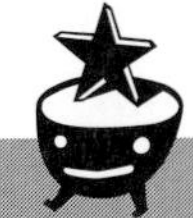

Star K.A.R.E.

Hodgkin's Disease

KNOW your resident's care plan.
ASSIST the resident/nurse.

If on radiation therapy or chemotherapy:
- *Follow any special skin care orders exactly (for example: no hot or cold packs, no soap or other cosmetics, no garters or tight stockings).*
- *Take great care when moving and positioning to reduce bruising.*
- *Take great care when brushing teeth; soft brushes or special swabs should be used.*
- *Test stool as ordered for hidden (occult) blood.*

REPORT observations.
RECORD data.
RECHECK resident as needed.

If any of the following occur:
- *nausea, vomiting, or diarrhea*
- *stomatitis (inflammation of the mouth)*
- *bleeding from gums or any other bleeding*
- *bruising of the skin*
- *cracks, breaks, or sores anywhere on the skin*
- *blood in the stool*
- *changes in vital signs, especially fever*

★ *"Don't Delay. Report Right Away!"*

ENCOURAGE resident's progress.
- *Provide support during difficult times.*

The Discovery of Hodgkin's Disease

Thomas Hodgkin [1798-1866] was one of a few great men who became known for their work at the world-renowned Guy's Hospital in London. He was a pathologist who, in 1832, examined specimens of Hodgkin's disease without using a microscope. Samuel Wilks coined the term "Hodgkin's Disease" in 1865.

3. Systemic Lupus Erythematosis (SLE)

Systemic lupus erythematosis (lupus) is a disorder of the immune system that causes an inflammation of connective tissue. It is most common in young women. Symptoms may include joint pain, fever, fatigue, mouth ulcers, and the characteristic "butterfly rash" across the nose and cheeks. Many organs may be affected, including the spleen, kidneys, nervous system, lungs, heart, and the liver. Serious cases can lead to death.

CAUSE: We do not know what causes SLE, although there may be a genetic link. For example, researchers seem to find other connective tissue disorders in relatives of SLE patients, such as rheumatoid arthritis.

CURE/TREATMENT: Some cases are mild and may be treated with anti-inflammatory medications. In severe cases, more powerful medications may be used. There is no cure.

4. Acquired Immunodeficiency Syndrome (AIDS)

AIDS is an illness caused by the human immunodeficiency virus (**HIV**). The syndrome was noted by the CDC (Centers for Disease Control) in 1981, but the virus itself was not discovered until 1983. The virus has actually been found in samples of blood from 1959 that have been tested.

HIV attacks the body's immune system and gradually disables it. AIDS may begin with a mild, flu-like sickness when the body is making antibodies to the HIV virus. People can test positive for these HIV antibodies but not yet have AIDS. Without medication, the HIV-infected person's weakened resistance to other infections will lead to AIDS and eventually to death.

Some of the symptoms that may be seen with AIDS are weight loss, fever, night sweats, cough, swollen lymph nodes, mouth sores, white patches inside the mouth, rashes, nausea and vomiting, and diarrhea. During a period of years, the HIV virus destroys the **T-cells**. People then begin developing the diseases that are commonly seen in AIDS patients. The types of disorders seen are pneumocystis pneumonia, a lung infection, and Kaposi's sarcoma, a skin cancer.

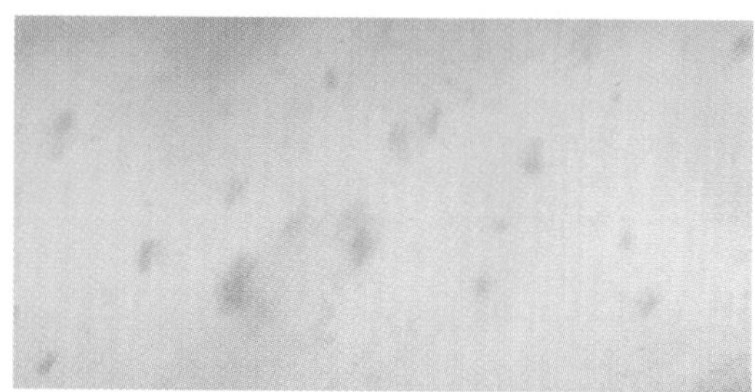

Figure 34-2. **A purple or red skin lesion called Kaposi's sarcoma can be a sign of AIDS.**

At its worse, AIDS so weakens the immune system that many infections can make one very, very ill, including an attack on the nervous system that causes dementia.

CAUSE: AIDS is caused by acquiring the HIV virus through an exchange of blood or body fluid from an infected person. The most common transmission is through unprotected or poorly-protected sex with an infected person. However, transmission may also occur through:

- sharing needles
- accidents, such as being stuck by a needle that was used on a person with HIV
- blood transfusions from infected blood (this occurred before 1985 when transfused blood began being tested)
- from an infected mother who passes the virus to her newborn during pregnancy, delivery, or breastfeeding
- receiving tattoos or any body piercing from a facility not using proper infection control methods

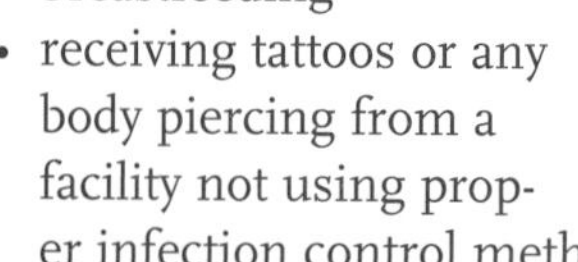

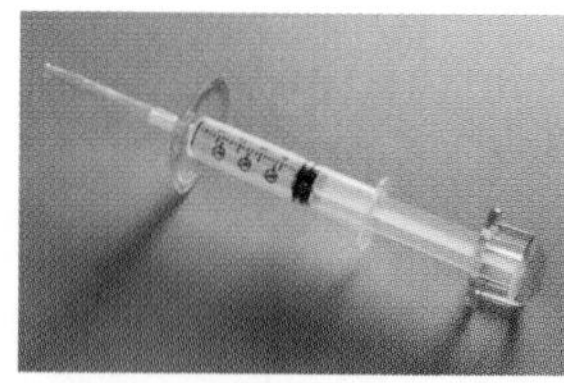

Figure 34-3. **Sharing needles greatly increases the risks of bloodborne diseases.**

CURE/TREATMENT: There is no cure for this disease. There is no vaccine to prevent the disease.

Many people are living longer with HIV by taking "cocktails" of certain drugs every day. In the past decade these drugs have slowed the huge number of AIDS-related deaths in the developed world. However, these treatments must be taken at precise times throughout the day. They are very expensive. They produce many unpleasant side effects. While we know they "hold off" many symptoms of AIDS, we do not know how long these drugs stay effective.

Star K.A.R.E.

Resident with AIDS

KNOW your resident's care plan.
ASSIST the resident/nurse.

- *Protect the person from people having known contagious diseases, even the common cold.*
- *Consider getting a flu shot to help protect the person with AIDS.*
- *Never feed the person raw or undercooked eggs.*
- *Cook meat and poultry all the way through.*
- *Use proper precautions when cooking, such as washing hands frequently and cleaning kitchen often.*
- *Follow diet order carefully (for example, a soft diet may be needed; spicy foods may cause discomfort; high fiber may aggravate diarrhea).*
- *Give fluids as ordered.*
- *Take great care when cleaning the mouth and brushing teeth; use soft toothbrushes or special swabs.*
- *Take great care when moving and positioning to reduce bruising.*
- *Take great care to follow special skin care orders exactly (for example, you may not use soap on some AIDS residents).*
- *Carefully measure weight and intake and output.*

REPORT observations.
RECORD data.
RECHECK resident as needed.

If any of the following occur:

- *loss of appetite, nausea, vomiting, or diarrhea*
- *weight loss*
- *reduced intake of fluids*
- *mouth sores or discomfort*
- *dysphagia (difficulty swallowing)*
- *bleeding from anywhere on the body*
- *bruising of the skin*
- *cracks, breaks, rashes, lumps, or sores anywhere on the skin*
- *blood in the stool*
- *changes in vital signs, especially fever*
- *nervousness, withdrawal, severe mood swings, or depression*
- *any behavior that puts themselves or others at risk*

★ *"Don't Delay. Report Right Away!"*

ENCOURAGE resident's progress and independence.

- *Encourage involvement in activities.*
- *Spend time listening if the resident wants to talk.*
- *Arrange for visits from family and friends.*

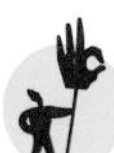

High-risk behaviors can spread HIV/AIDS!

Behaviors that put people at high risk for HIV/AIDS include:

sharing used drug needles

having unprotected sex

having sexual contact with multiple partners or with a partner who has had many sexual partners

Ways to protect against the spread of HIV/AIDS:

Never share needles for injections of any type of drug.

Do not have unprotected sex. Use condoms if you have sex.

Stay in a monogamous relationship. Monogamous means having only one sexual partner. You and your partner can be tested for bloodborne diseases like AIDS and hepatitis before sleeping together.

Practice abstinence. Abstinence means not having sexual contact with anyone.

AIDS and the T-cells

You may have heard of a link between the AIDS virus and the helpful T-cell. The AIDS virus infects T-cells, which reduces the number of cells available to fight common infections. This reduces the body's ability to ward off these infections, making the person more susceptible to illness.

4 Discuss ways to provide emotional support to the resident with AIDS.

Residents who have HIV/AIDS may be experiencing many difficulties. They may have been abandoned by family or friends due to the fear of the disease itself. Another real problem associated with HIV and AIDS is **homophobia**, or a fear of homosexuality. Some emotions he or she may be experiencing include anxiety, fear, guilt, sadness, depression, and loneliness. It is important to treat your residents with respect and help provide the emotional support they need.

Residents with AIDS will benefit from a set schedule and as much independence as possible. It is important for you not to avoid a resident who has AIDS. Spending quality time with a resident may mean sitting and listening quietly to their concerns. If the person likes to read, make sure he has enough reading material available. Any activities that the residents wants to participate in should be encouraged.

Residents with HIV/AIDS need support from others. Arrange for family and friends to visit whenever possible. Take whatever precautions you need when arranging for visitors, such as making sure the visitors are not suffering from a contagious illness.

If the AIDS diagnosis is known, other residents may be hesitant about being close to the resident. You cannot insist that anyone pay attention to the person with AIDS. It is possible once they are educated about the ways AIDS is transmitted, people will feel safer and change their minds.

If AIDS-related dementia is present, the person may have to be protected from harm. She may lose her mental alertness, become forgetful, and have slowed reflexes and thinking processes. This puts the person at very high risk of injury. She can also have mood swings that may frighten other residents and visitors.

Don't be stingy with your handshakes and hugs!

People need to educate themselves about HIV/AIDS and take care not to ignore or feel afraid of the person who has this disease. It is very important to understand that a handshake or a hug cannot spread the AIDS virus.

Current facts tell us the disease CANNOT be transmitted by telephones, door knobs, tables, chairs, toilets, mosquitoes, or by breathing the same air as an infected person.

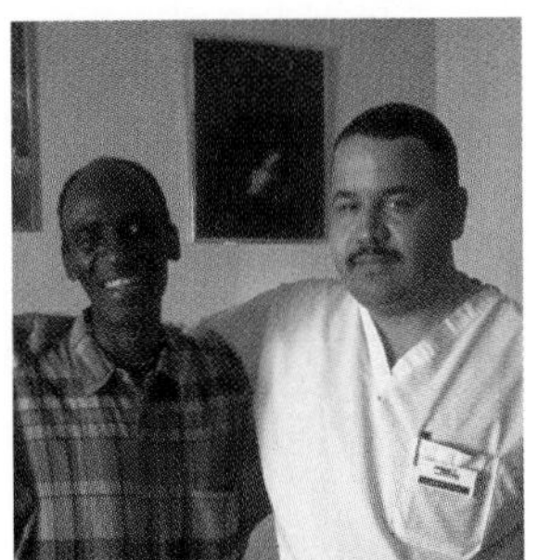

Figure 34-4. **Hugs and touches cannot spread the AIDS virus.**

5 Identify community resources and services available to the resident with HIV/AIDS.

Depending on your community, many resources and services may be available for people with HIV/AIDS. These include counseling, meal services, access to experimental drugs and any number of other services. Look in the phone book for resources available in your area, or speak to your supervisor if you feel a resident with HIV/AIDS needs more help. A social worker or another member of the care team may be able to coordinate services for residents with HIV/AIDS.

6 Explain the precautions you should take when caring for people with AIDS.

If you are practicing standard and transmission-based precautions correctly, there should be no difference in your care for a known AIDS resident and other residents.

1. It is worth saying again: the reason to always follow standard and transmission-based precautions is that you cannot tell by looking at people if they carry a bloodborne disease or not.
2. If you have any cuts, sores, or breaks in the skin, report these to your supervisor BEFORE you begin your care. Your supervisor may either assign the resident to someone else, or might ask you to double-glove.
3. Never leave out any razors or toothbrushes of a resident with AIDS that could be accidentally used by a roommate.
4. If you are pregnant, ask your supervisor if you should care for the person with AIDS. People with AIDS sometimes have a virus called CMV (cytomegalovirus) which may be passed from an infected mother to her baby.

If in doubt about what to do in any situation, check with your supervisor first.

7 Demonstrate knowledge of the legal aspects of AIDS, including testing.

The right to confidentiality is especially important to people with HIV/AIDS, because others may pass judgment on people with this disease. A person with HIV/AIDS cannot be fired from a job because of the disease; however, a healthcare worker with HIV/AIDS may be reassigned to job duties with a lower risk of transmitting the disease.

HIV testing requires consent. That means no one can force you to be tested for HIV unless you agree. HIV test results are confidential and should not be shared with a person's family, friends, or employer without his or her consent. If you are HIV-positive, you might want to confide in your supervisor so your assignments can be adjusted to avoid putting you at high risk for exposure to other infections. Everyone has a right to privacy regarding their health status. Never discuss a resident's status with anyone.

Summary

The immune system functions by attacking toxins and invading cells. When the immune system is damaged, the body's ability to defend itself may be reduced. Education about high-risk behaviors is one of the best ways to prevent the spread of HIV/AIDS. Informing yourself and others about how AIDS is transmitted is important and will help you give the best care to your residents.

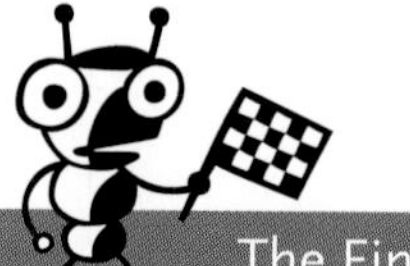

The Finish Line

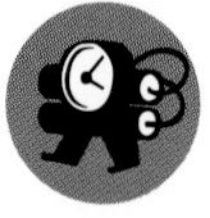

What's Wrong With This Picture?

Look at the list of precautions and guidelines for caring for residents with AIDS. Correct the errors in each of the statements.

1. Practice standard and transmission-based precautions only on residents you think have a bloodborne disease. It is relatively easy to tell if a resident has a bloodborne disease just by looking at him.
2. If you have any cuts, sores, or breaks in the skin, you usually do not have to wear gloves.
3. It is fine for a resident with AIDS to share a razor with another resident. It is not okay for a resident with AIDS to hug another person.

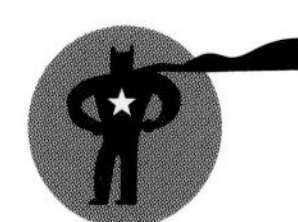

Star Student Central

1. Ask yourself if you have any risk factors for HIV/AIDS and think about getting tested. There are usually places in the community to get a free test. All testing is confidential.
2. Research the Internet to learn more about the typical drug schedule for an HIV-infected person. Share any information with your class.

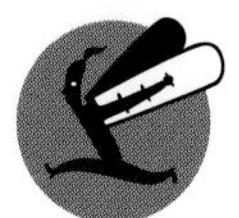

You Can Do It Corner!

1. Name four ways to reduce your risk of acquiring HIV/AIDS. (LO 3)
2. What are two reasons a resident with AIDS may need emotional support? (LO 4)
3. What happens when the response of antibodies slows? (LO 2)
4. What are five ways AIDS can be transmitted? (LO 3)
5. What are some ways communities can help people with AIDS? (LO 5)
6. Why is it especially important to maintain confidentiality of a diagnosis of AIDS? (LO 7)
7. Identify one way allergies can be treated. (LO 3)
8. How should you practice standard precautions differently with a resident with AIDS? (LO 6)

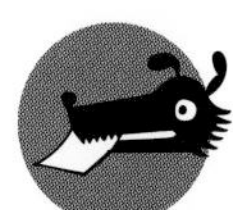

Star Student's Chapter Checklist

1. I have read my textbook chapter.
2. I have reviewed my own "Pocketful of Terms."
3. I have listened to my tutor tape.
4. I have reviewed and highlighted my class notes.
5. I have read and completed any handouts from this chapter.
6. I have completed "The Finish Line."
7. Star Time! Choose your reward!

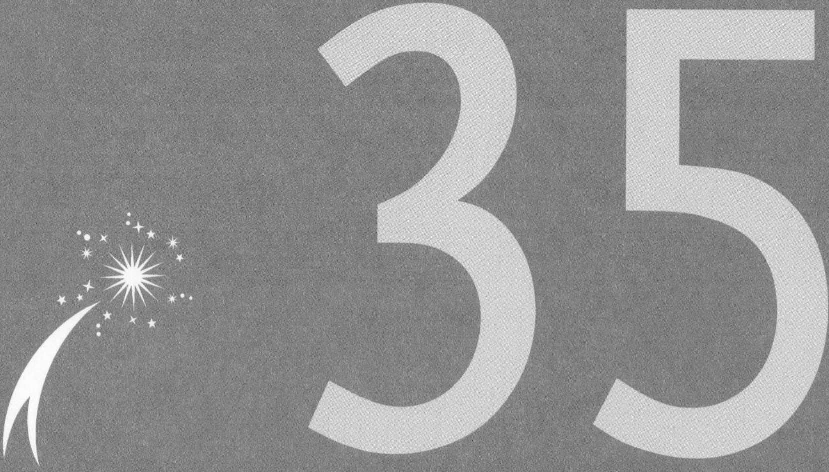

An Expanded View: Subacute Care and Oncology

Look Like a Star!

Look at the Learning Objectives and The Finish Line before you begin reading this chapter.

Look at your pocket calendar.
With your pencil, put a bracket ( ) around a study period every single day.

Look at your homework for this chapter.
Plug each piece of homework into a certain time slot.

Look at the Star Student's Chapter Checklist at the end of this chapter. Check off each item as it is completed.

"And in this harsh world draw thy breath in pain......"

William Shakespeare, 1564-1616, from *Hamlet*

"There are some remedies worse than the disease."

Publilius Syrus, circa 42 B.C.

Learning Objectives

1. **Spell and define all STAR words.**
2. **Discuss the types of residents you will see in a subacute care setting.**
3. **Describe the type of resident requiring pulse oximetry and list guidelines for care.**
4. **Describe telemetry and related care.**
5. **List a nursing assistant's responsibilities with residents on ventilators.**
6. **Describe residents who require frequent suctioning and list signs of respiratory distress.**
7. **Discuss the care of the resident with a tracheostomy.**
8. **Discuss the need for a central intravenous line and total parenteral nutrition (TPN).**
9. **Explain the nursing assistant's role in the observation of a resident requiring a blood transfusion.**
10. **Describe a gastrostomy and related care.**
11. **Describe physical and emotional care of the resident with cancer and list seven warning signs of cancer.**
12. **Explain chemotherapy and radiation therapy and related care.**

The Ventilator in its Infancy

Robert Hooke, 1635-1703, developed one of the earliest forms of ventilators. He attached a bellows to the trachea of a dog and discovered that the dog could be kept alive without any lung or chest motion. This meant that an artificial means of breathing might actually be used to keep a human body alive.

1 Spell and define all STAR words.

chemotherapy: treatment with chemical agents that have a toxic effect on disease.

dialysis: a process that cleanses the body of waste products usually due to kidney failure.

intubation: insertion of a tube into the trachea for the entrance of air.

oncology: branch of medicine dealing with the study of tumors.

oxygen saturation (oxygen sat): oxygen content of the blood expressed in a percentage.

pallor: extreme or unnatural paleness of skin.

patient-controlled analgesia (PCA): drug administration method used for pain control that allows the person to control the delivery of the pain medication.

pulse oximeter: clip-on device that measures a person's blood oxygen level along with the pulse.

radiation therapy: branch of medicine utilizing radiation in the treatment of malignant tumors.

subacute care: level of care for people who no longer require hospitalization but need a higher level of care than typical nursing home residents require.

tracheostomy: surgical creation of an opening in the trachea that performs as an airway.

ventilator: a mechanical device used for artificial ventilation of the lungs.

2 Discuss the types of residents you will see in a subacute care setting.

A subacute setting is a unit or facility that accepts people who need more care for a period of time than a typical long-term care facility can provide. **Subacute care** can be found in both hospital-based skilled care facilities and free-standing nursing homes. The subacute resident needs a higher level of care than many long-term care residents. This resident will require the most direct care and close observation by staff.

Rehabilitation, perhaps from a stroke or some type of serious injury, may be a goal with the subacute resident. The resident may have recently had surgery or may have a chronic illness, such as AIDS or cancer, that creates a need for ongoing care. The cost for subacute care is usually less than care received in an acute care setting such as a hospital. However, it is more expensive than normal long-term care.

Others who require subacute care are those with serious burns or people with kidney problems who require dialysis. **Dialysis** cleanses the body of waste products that the kidneys are unable to remove due to kidney failure. People in subacute units may also be on a mechanical **ventilator**, a machine that literally "breathes" for the person.

3 Describe the type of resident requiring pulse oximetry and list guidelines for care.

One device that may be used in subacute care is a **pulse oximeter**. When residents are on oxygen, going to or coming from surgery, or experiencing bleeding or some other problem, a pulse oximeter may be attached to the resident. A pulse oximeter measures a person's blood oxygen level, as well as measuring pulse rate. Blood oxygen is the oxygen level inside the arteries and is sometimes called **oxygen saturation**. A sensor is clipped on a resident's finger, ear lobe or toe. It is so sensitive that it warns of a low blood oxygen level before any noticeable signs or symptoms develop. It works by moving two kinds of light, red and infrared light, through the skin and then measuring the amount of each type of light absorbed by the hemoglobin inside the blood. Blood with oxygen absorbs more of the infrared light while blood without oxygen absorbs more red light.

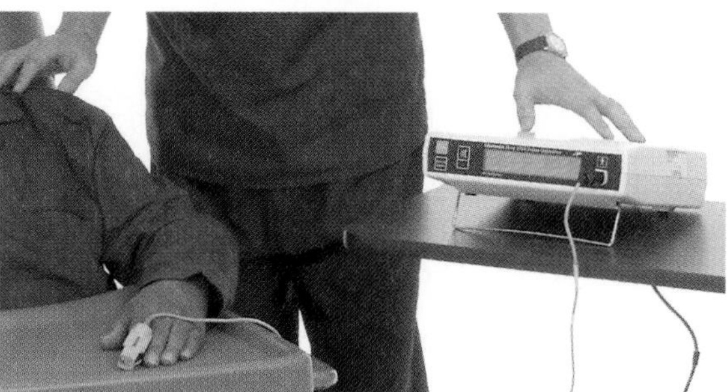

Figure 35-1. **A pulse oximeter.**

A normal blood oxygen level is usually measured between about 95% and 100%. The danger zone for blood oxygen is approximately 70%.

A resident requiring pulse oximetry will need to be observed for any change in the blood oxygen level. If the alarm on the device sounds, it is important that you notify the nurse right away. A very low blood oxygen level may eventually cause death if not treated immediately.

Star K.A.R.E.

Resident Requiring a Pulse Oximeter

KNOW your resident's care plan.
ASSIST the resident/nurse.

- *Remove nail polish if requested by nurse prior to oximeter placement.*
- *Take great care when moving and positioning to prevent oximeter from coming off or moving.*
- *Observe skin carefully for* ***pallor*** *or cyanosis.*
- *Watch skin for signs of skin breakdown due to device.*
- *Carefully monitor all vital signs.*

REPORT observations.
RECORD data.
RECHECK resident as needed.

If any of the following occur:

- *alarm sounds*
- *cracks, breaks, rashes, or sores on the skin around or under the oximeter*
- *changes in vital signs*

★ *"Don't Delay. Report Right Away!"*

ENCOURAGE resident's progress.

- *Provide support during difficulty breathing or shortness of breath.*

4 Describe telemetry and related care.

Telemetry is the application of a cardiac monitoring device which transmits data about the heart rhythm and heart rate for assessment by a skilled staff member. The data is sent to an area within a facility watched constantly by a specialist trained to read these monitoring screens.

Caring for a resident on telemetry requires some additional skills. You must be aware of the proper care of the telemetry unit or device. You must also know which circumstances require the assistance of a nurse. The unit attaches to a resident's chest and is carried in a pack that allows for movement. The resident may have to be reminded not to leave the central monitoring area during ambulation.

There are different methods of connecting the device to the person's chest. One type uses sponge-like adhesive pads or patches (also called leads or electrodes) that stick to different parts of the person's chest. The pad attaches to a wire that is connected to the telemetry pack. Do not get the unit, wires, or pads wet during bathing. If any rash or irritation occurs, ask the nurse for a hypoallergenic pad/patch.

Star K.A.R.E.

Resident on Telemetry

KNOW your resident's care plan.
ASSIST the resident/nurse.

- *Listen for the alarm.*
- *Carefully monitor all vital signs.*
- *Never get unit, wires, pads/patches, or electrodes/leads wet.*
- *Observe all pads/patches (electrodes, leads) for loosening.*
- *Remind residents the alarm may trigger with their movement, a disconnected lead, or a low battery.*

REPORT observations.
RECORD data.
RECHECK resident as needed.

If any of the following occur:

- *alarm sounds*
- *change in vital signs*
- *resident needs to leave unit area*
- *chest pain or discomfort, tachycardia, sweating, SOB, dyspnea, or dizziness*
- *leads become loose or unit or leads become wet*
- *rash or irritation under or around pad/patch*
- *low battery*

★ *"Don't Delay. Report Right Away!"*

ENCOURAGE resident's progress.

- *Provide support during periods of chest pain, shortness of breath, or anxiety.*

5 List a nursing assistant's responsibilities with residents on ventilators.

People in a subacute unit may be on a ventilator. A ventilator performs the mechanism of breathing for a person who is unable to breathe on her own. Many problems cause a person to require a mechanical ventilator. Injuries that affect the ability to breathe or diseases such as cancer are examples.

When a person is on a ventilator, she must have an **intubation** performed. When a person is intubated, a special tube called an endotracheal tube is inserted into the mouth or the nose and then into the trachea. A special scope is used to insert the tube. Sometimes a person will have a tracheostomy tube instead. This is inserted into a **tracheostomy**, which is an artificial opening into the trachea (windpipe).

While a person is on a ventilator, usually she will not be able to speak. This is because air will no longer reach the larynx (vocal cords). She will need a lot of support during the time she is connected to the ventilator. Clipboards, pads of paper, or special communication boards with common questions or pictures are used to communicate with this person.

If a resident on a ventilator is unconscious, remember to act as though he is able to understand everything going on around him.

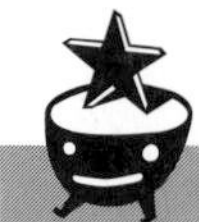

Star K.A.R.E.

Resident on a Ventilator

KNOW your resident's care plan.
ASSIST the resident/nurse.

- *Listen carefully for the sound of the alarm.*
- *Watch for kinks or disconnected tubing.*
- *Answer the call light promptly.*
- *Take great care when cleaning the mouth to prevent aspiration; special swabs should be used.*
- *Reposition at least every two hours. Follow instructions carefully when moving and positioning. Always get enough help and have nurse check resident after a move.*
- *Give excellent skin care to prevent pressure sores.*
- *Provide frequent oral care.*
- *Carefully monitor vital signs, if not measured by machine.*
- *Do not tire resident when performing care.*

REPORT observations.
RECORD data.
RECHECK resident as needed.

If any of the following occur:

- *the alarm goes off*
- *the pressure gauge on the ventilator looks like it is going down*
- *mouth sores or discomfort*
- *cracks, breaks, or sores anywhere on the skin, especially at site of intubation*
- *change in vital signs*
- *nervousness*
- *depression*

★ *"Don't Delay. Report Right Away!"*

ENCOURAGE resident's progress and independence.

- *Be patient during communication with the resident. Offer communication aids to assist.*
- *Provide for quality rest time.*
- *Provide support during difficult times. Being dependent can create feelings of despair.*

6 Describe residents who require frequent suctioning and list signs of respiratory distress.

Subacute care units include residents who require frequent suctioning by the nurses. Suctioning is necessary when a resident has collected secretions in the upper respiratory system. A person may need suctioning with or without a tracheostomy.

Suctioning comes from a wall hook-up or a portable pump at the bedside. A bottle is provided that collects the suctioned material from the airway. The nurse or the respiratory therapist will suction the resident. Water is normally used to rinse the suction catheter in between suctioning.

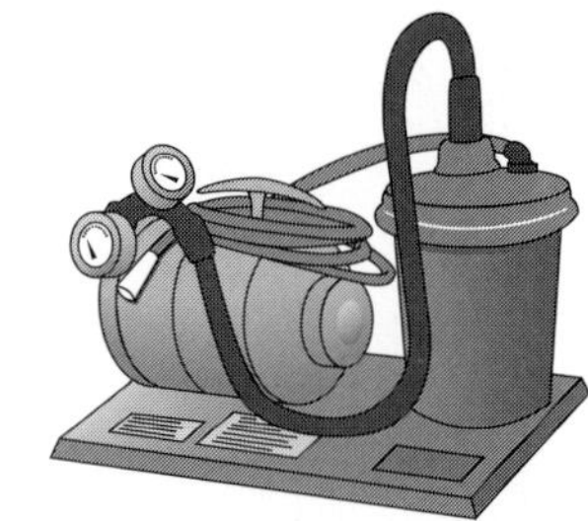

Figure 35-2. **Although nursing assistants do not perform suctioning, they can help by notifying the nurse immediately if there is any sign of respiratory distress.**

A resident who has frequent suctioning may show signs of respiratory distress. Signs of respiratory distress include gurgling, an elevated respiratory rate, shortness of breath, dyspnea, pallor, or cyanosis.

The resident requiring suctioning must have the call light answered promptly. When a nursing assistant sees a resident in respiratory distress, it is vital for the nursing assistant to report the problem right away. The inability to breathe freely causes great anxiety. Allowing a resident to stay in respiratory distress for a lengthy period of time is very dangerous.

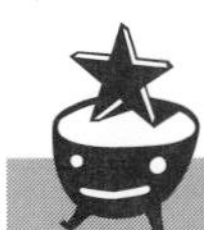

Star K.A.R.E.

Resident Requiring Suctioning

KNOW your resident's care plan.
ASSIST the resident/nurse.

- *Watch for signs that a resident needs suctioning.*
- *Observe skin carefully for pallor or cyanosis.*
- *Monitor vital signs closely, especially respiratory rate.*
- *Put on gloves, gown, mask, or goggles as directed by the nurse.*
- *Place resident in position as directed by nurse, normally semi-Fowler's or lateral.*
- *Place pad or towel under the chin; have wet washcloth ready.*
- *Hold person's hand, if appropriate.*
- *Perform oral hygiene after suctioning as directed by the nurse.*

REPORT observations.
RECORD data.
RECHECK resident as needed.

If any of the following occur:

- *change in vital signs, especially respiratory rate*
- *gurgling sounds during breathing*
- *difficulty breathing (dyspnea) or shortness of breath*
- *pale skin or cyanosis*
- *nervousness*

★ *"Don't Delay. Report Right Away!"*

ENCOURAGE resident's progress.

- *Provide support during difficulty breathing.*

7 Discuss the care of the resident with a tracheostomy.

A tracheostomy is a surgically-created opening into the person's trachea or windpipe. This is performed when there is a need for an airway other than the normal airway through the nose and mouth. A tube called a tracheostomy tube is inserted into this opening to provide the new airway. This tube is normally held in place by a cuff that attaches to the end of the device in the trachea. The cuff prevents the accidental aspiration of food or fluids.

During the time the tracheostomy is in place, the resident may be unable to speak. This can cause fear and anxiety because the resident is unable to call for help from the staff. A great deal of careful observation and support is needed when caring for the person with a tracheostomy.

General tracheostomy care includes keeping the skin around the opening or stoma clean, assisting with dressing changes as necessary, and assisting with the cleansing of the inner part of the device. Suctioning may be needed frequently with this type of resident.

Star K.A.R.E.

Resident with a Tracheostomy

KNOW your resident's care plan.
ASSIST the resident/nurse.

- *Listen for the sound of the alarm on the ventilator.*
- *Answer the call light promptly.*
- *Provide resident with another method of communicating, such as a board or notepad.*
- *Watch for signs that resident needs suctioning.*
- *Do not get tracheostomy dressing wet.*
- *Do not cover opening.*
- *Inspect tape or ties often.*
- *Watch for kinks or disconnected tubing.*
- *Take great care when cleaning the mouth to prevent aspiration; special swabs should be used. Perform oral hygiene every two hours.*
- *Watch for mouth sores, cracks, breaks, or sores anywhere on the skin.*
- *Carefully follow orders when moving and positioning; always get enough help.*
- *Observe skin carefully for pallor or cyanosis.*
- *Carefully monitor vital signs, if not measured by machine.*

REPORT observations.
RECORD data.
RECHECK resident as needed.

If any of the following occur:

- *alarm sounds on ventilator*
- *mouth sores or discomfort*
- *cracks, breaks, or sores anywhere on the skin*
- *gurgling sounds during breathing, a sign that suctioning is needed*

- *difficulty breathing (dyspnea) or shortness of breath*
- *change in vital signs, especially respiratory rate*

★ *"Don't Delay. Report Right Away!"*

ENCOURAGE resident's progress.

- *Provide support during difficult times.*
- *Do not tire resident when performing care.*

It is important to note that residents on TPN may find it difficult to be on a restricted diet. Provide emotional support. Family and friends may try to bring restricted food in to the resident. You may need to remind them about the medical reasons that TPN is needed. Report any failure to follow the diet to the nurse.

If a resident attempts to remove or removes the tube, notify the nurse immediately.

8 Discuss the need for a central intravenous line and total parenteral nutrition (TPN).

Residents frequently need intravenous lines for the administration of fluids, nutrition, or blood products. When this need is expected to continue, a central line is often inserted. One type of central line is called a PICC, or a Peripherally Inserted Central Catheter. The tip is inserted into the superior vena cava, the largest vein in the human body. This procedure is done in a surgical or non-surgical setting.

Nursing assistants must be very cautious when caring for a resident with any type of central line in place. Some of the priorities for this care include:

- never get the dressing site wet
- make sure the tubing is not kinked or tangled
- allow slack in the tubing so insertion site does not pull
- observe and report swelling, redness, bleeding, or leaking at the insertion site

Sometimes a resident cannot eat or drink in a normal fashion. Total parenteral nutrition (TPN) or hyperalimentation (HYPER-AL) may be ordered until he or she is able to consume food and drink orally again. TPN may be necessary because of significant weight loss, the inability to eat due to surgery or complications from surgery or swallowing problems due to stroke, coma, and depression.

This solution provides all the nutrients the resident needs in a 24-hour period. This is based upon the resident's height, weight, and nutritional needs, taking into account any illness. When caring for a resident on TPN, watch for any signs of allergic reaction to the solution, such as fever or headache. Observe and report swelling, redness, bleeding or leaking at the insertion site. Carefully follow the nurse's directions regarding the use of TPN. Report any change in condition or anything unusual immediately.

9 Explain the nursing assistant's role in the observation of a resident requiring a blood transfusion.

A blood transfusion is the transfer of blood or a blood component from one person to another. Transfusions are given to increase the blood's ability to carry oxygen, restore the body's blood volume, improve immunity, and to correct clotting problems.

The resident who requires a blood transfusion may be anxious and frightened of this procedure. He may benefit from you staying with him during the transfusion. The nurse will direct you to perform frequent vital signs on this resident before, during, and after the transfusion. This helps warn staff promptly of a possible transfusion reaction. Transfusion reactions occur when the blood the resident is receiving is not compatible with the resident's blood.

Most people do not have a transfusion reaction. However, the few that do may be in a life-threatening situation. When any sign of a transfusion reaction occurs, the nurse will stop the blood from flowing and take immediate steps to prevent serious complications from occurring. When a person receives incompatible blood, blood may start to clump or slow down and stick together because of the new blood. This situation requires an IV of a solution of normal saline and oxygen to be administered. A special urine specimen collection or a 24-hour urine collection to check for poisons in the bloodstream may be performed. Careful monitoring of the resident is required after the episode.

An Early Form of the Blood Transfusion

Richard Lower, 1631-1691, became the first person to transfuse blood between animals.In 1669, he placed venous blood into an animal's lungs and noted it changed from dark to bright red. Blood transfusions were done from animals into men around the late 17th century. They ended after a negative public response.

Resident Receiving a Blood Transfusion

KNOW* *your resident's care plan.
ASSIST* *the resident/nurse.

- *Carefully take a set of baseline vital signs.*
- *Monitor resident closely, as directed, and watch for signs of transfusion reaction.*
- *Take repeat vital signs as directed.*

REPORT* *observations.
RECORD* *data.
RECHECK* *resident as needed.

If any of the following occur:

- *change in vital signs, especially fever, low or high B/P, or elevated pulse*
- *signs of transfusion reaction:*
  fever, chills, headache, backache, muscle aches, wheezing, dyspnea, cough, elevated respiratory rate, low or high blood pressure, tachycardia, cyanosis, flushing, anxiety, hives, rash, itching, nausea, vomiting, or diarrhea

★ *"Don't Delay. Report Right Away!"*

ENCOURAGE* *resident's progress.

- *Provide support during blood transfusions.*

"The Gift of Life"

Have you ever considered giving blood to help others? The process takes only a short while and you can actually save one or more lives. Think about calling the local Red Cross or other agency and offering "The Gift of Life." You'll be glad you did.

Blood Types Box 35-1

Type	Percentage of Population
O+	38 percent
O-	7 percent
A+	34 percent
A-	6 percent
B+	9 percent
B-	2 percent
AB+	3 percent
AB-	1 percent

10 Describe a gastrostomy and related care.

A gastrostomy is a surgically-placed tube that brings nutrition into the stomach by way of the abdomen. This is done for people who are unable to eat normally. Problems like swallowing difficulties, tumors of the throat, the tendency to choke on food or fluids, or a resident who is comatose or unconscious can require the insertion of a gastrostomy. The doctor or the nurse will insert a gastrostomy tube.

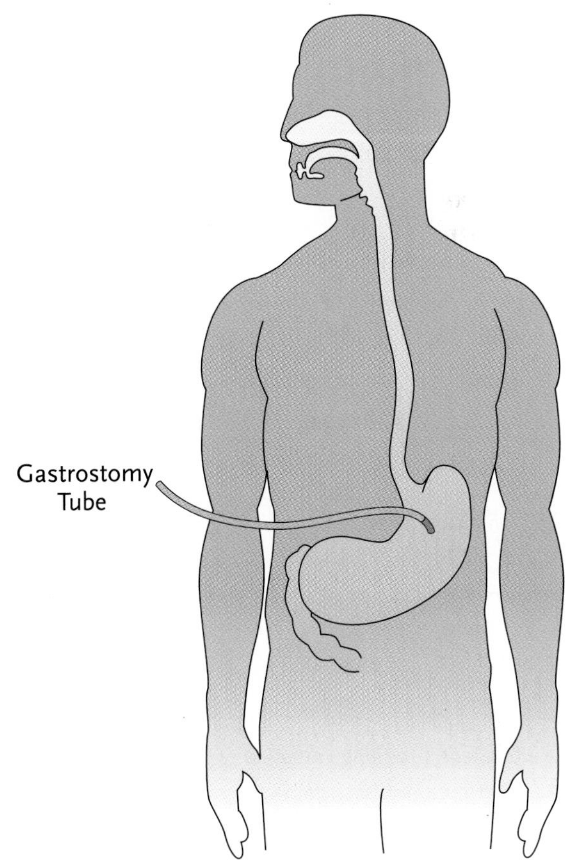

Figure 35-3. **A gastrostomy tube delivers nutrition to the stomach through the abdomen.**

When caring for a person with a gastrostomy, there are certain important steps to take to prevent complications with this device. After any feeding, follow post-feeding directions regarding the length of time to keep the resident upright or in the Hi-Fowler's position. Usually, a period of about 30 to 45 minutes in the upright position is required. The head of the bed will be elevated throughout the feeding time and for the time directed after the feeding. If the tubing becomes loose or disconnected, you must notify the nurse right away.

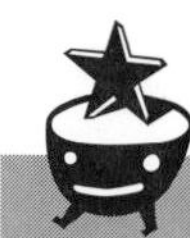

Star K.A.R.E.

Resident with a Gastrostomy

KNOW your resident's care plan.

ASSIST the resident/nurse.

- *Listen carefully for the sound of the alarm.*
- *Answer the call light promptly.*
- *Carefully monitor all vital signs, especially temperature and blood pressure.*
- *Be alert for signs of aspiration or choking.*
- *Give oral hygiene as needed.*
- *Position as directed during feedings.*
- *Carefully follow post-feeding positioning order; may require sitting upright or on right side for at least 30 minutes after feeding is completed.*
- *Follow skin care instructions around insertion site.*
- *Apply special lubricant to skin area around site as directed.*
- *Never pull, tug, or twist tubing.*
- *Inspect dressing and tape often.*
- *Take great care not to get dressing wet during care.*

REPORT observations.

RECORD data.

RECHECK resident as needed.

If any of the following occur:

- *alarm sounds*
- *signs of choking or aspiration*
- *difficulty breathing (dyspnea) or shortness of breath*
- *chest pain or discomfort*
- *diarrhea or signs of fecal impaction*
- *skin around dressing changes, such as swelling, pain, redness, warmth*
- *change in vital signs, especially fever or respiratory rate*
- *dressing becomes wet or tape comes off*
- *kinked, cracked, broken, or disconnected tubing*
- *empty bag or container*

★ *"Don't Delay. Report Right Away!"*

ENCOURAGE resident's progress.

- *Provide support during difficult times.*

11 Describe physical and emotional care of the resident with cancer and list seven warning signs of cancer.

The resident with cancer will require a great deal of your care. People with cancer may be depressed and can experience frequent mood shifts. They will benefit from staff members spending as much time as possible sitting and listening to them. Encouraging involvement in activities, depending on the abilities of the person, will help to improve mental and emotional well-being. Visitors from both inside and outside the facility can help the resident cope.

Physical care of the resident with cancer is geared toward observation for any complications and prevention of pain and discomfort. In addition, the prevention of complications, such as pressure sores or mouth sores, is a top priority. People with cancer are sometimes in great physical pain. They may be on a special pump that allows the person to press a button and obtain pain medication. This is called a PCA pump, or **patient-controlled analgesia**. There is a "lockout" period of time when the pain medication will not be available to the person. This is usually a pre-set number of minutes. You may need to explain the lock-out time to the resident. Side effects of this pump include mouth sores. Caring for a resident on a PCA pump is similar to IV care. Excellent oral hygiene and skin care should be performed. Observe and report redness, swelling, and warmth around the insertion site.

A resident who has cancer may experience difficulty eating and have special orders for more frequent meals or special orders regarding fluids.

It is important to note that many cancers can be treated and/or cured. **Oncology** is the branch of medicine dealing with the study of tumors. A discussion of specific cancers is also included in various body system chapters.

Take care not to ignore the resident with cancer!

There are some caregivers who are uncomfortable with the diagnosis of cancer. Cancer is not contagious, and people who think it is must be educated. Cancer is frightening to some people. Nursing assistants must be careful not to avoid a person with cancer. This resident deserves just as much, if not more, of your time. Make sure you try to spend as much time as is possible with all residents who have cancer. It is the loving, caring, and right thing to do.

The Seven Warning Signs of Cancer

If you notice any of these signs in your residents, report them to the nurse immediately:

- **C**hange in bowel or bladder habits
- **A** sore that does not heal
- **U**nusual bleeding or discharge
- **T**hickening or lump in breast or other part of the body
- **I**ndigestion or difficulty in swallowing
- **O**bvious change in wart or mole
- **N**agging cough or hoarseness

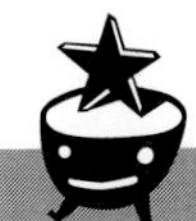

Star K.A.R.E.

Resident with Cancer

KNOW your resident's care plan.
ASSIST the resident/nurse.

SKIN:

- *Give good oral hygiene as often as needed.*
- *Give excellent skin care, keeping skin clean and dry. Try to prevent odors that often accompany cancer.*
- *Monitor temperature.*

SKELETAL/MUSCULAR:

- *Ambulate with great care.*
- *Allow time to perform ADLs.*
- *Change position every two hours.*
- *Give gentle backrubs as needed.*

CIRCULATORY:

- *Monitor pulse and blood pressure.*

RESPIRATORY:

- *Monitor respiratory rate.*

GASTROINTESTINAL:

- *Follow fluid order carefully.*
- *Provide small, frequent meals to prevent weight loss.*
- *Measure intake carefully.*
- *Weigh resident as ordered.*

URINARY:

- *Follow fluid order carefully.*
- *Give excellent catheter care.*
- *Measure output carefully.*

NERVOUS:

- *Be alert for signs of pain.*
- *Be alert for signs of depression.*

REPORT observations.
RECORD data.
RECHECK resident as needed.

If the following occur:

SKIN:

- *signs of any sores on the skin*
- *new bumps or lumps*
- *any rash*

SKELETAL/MUSCULAR:

- *ambulating difficulty*
- *muscle weakness*

CIRCULATORY:

- *chest pain or tightness*

RESPIRATORY:

- *SOB or dyspnea*

GASTROINTESTINAL:

- *weight loss*
- *difficulty swallowing*
- *nausea or vomiting*
- *flatus, diarrhea, or constipation*
- *blood in the stool*

URINARY:

- *change in output (O)*
- *any change or blood in the urine*
- *urinary tract infection*

IMMUNE:

- *fever*

NERVOUS:

- *confusion*
- *signs of depression*

★ *"Don't Delay. Report Right Away!"*

ENCOURAGE resident's progress.

- *Provide support during painful episodes and difficult times.*

12 Explain chemotherapy and radiation therapy and related care.

Radiation therapy for the treatment of cancer uses radiation to attempt to destroy cancer cells. **Chemotherapy** involves certain powerful drugs being administered, usually intravenously, in order to kill cancer cells. Sometimes this type of therapy also kills normal cells.

Both of these therapies can cause severe side effects.

Side effects include:
- fatigue
- loss of appetite/malnutrition
- nausea and vomiting
- rashes, irritation or reddened or broken areas on the skin
- dry, sore mouth
- difficulty swallowing and chewing
- hair loss
- feelings of depression, fear, and anger

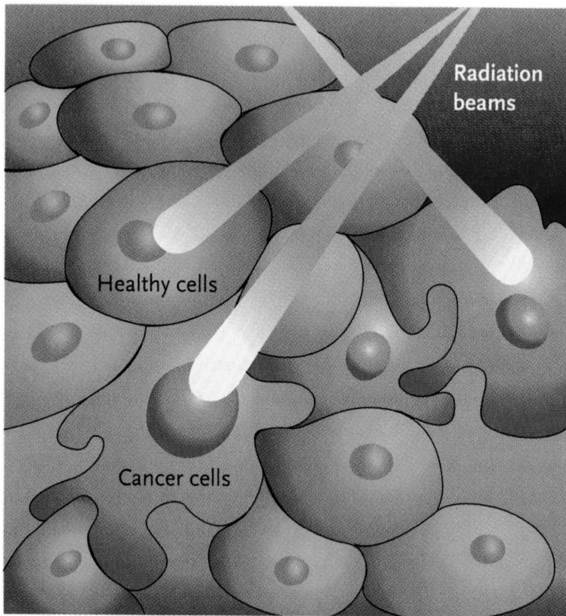

Figure 35-4. **Radiation is targeted at cancer cells, but it also destroys some healthy cells in its path.**

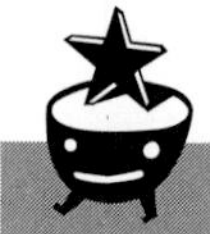

Star K.A.R.E.

Resident on Chemotherapy or Radiation Therapy

KNOW your resident's care plan.
ASSIST the resident/nurse.

- *Allow enough rest and recognize limitations.*
- *Provide food whenever hunger occurs. Keep nutritious snacks available. Provide cold food substitutes if hot foods increase nausea.*
- *During bathing, do not remove any markings that are used as a guide for the therapy.*
- *Keep skin clean and avoid irritation, pressure or injury. Follow any special skin care orders exactly (for example: no hot or cold packs, no soap or other cosmetics, no garters or tight stockings).*
- *Cut food into small pieces if necessary.*
- *Take great care when brushing teeth; soft brushes or special swabs should be used.*
- *Encourage fluids.*
- *Assist in selecting a hair covering such as a wig, scarf, or hat if resident desires.*
- *Be sensitive to emotional needs. Allow resident to express feelings.*
- *Take great care when moving and positioning to reduce bruising.*
- *Test stool as ordered for hidden (occult) blood.*

REPORT observations.
RECORD data.
RECHECK resident as needed.

If any of the following occurs:
- *severe nausea, vomiting, constipation, or diarrhea*
- *sudden weight loss or gain*
- *stomatitis, inflammation of the mouth*
- *bleeding from gums or any other bleeding*
- *bruising of the skin*
- *cracks, breaks, peeling, or sores anywhere on the skin*
- *blood in the stool*
- *changes in vital signs, especially fever*

★ *"Don't Delay. Report Right Away!"*

ENCOURAGE resident's independence and progress.
- *Help resident understand why he may feel so tired.*
- *Listen and talk with resident as often as possible.*
- *Remind resident that there can still be good days and special times ahead.*

Summary

Residents who are in subacute care will require a highly-skilled staff to care for their needs. If you decide to work in this area, extra training may be provided. It is very rewarding to care for residents who have special needs. Your skills will also be more marketable with this type of training. Subacute residents will need more of your listening time. Make sure you organize your day so that you can spend quality time with subacute residents and their families and friends.

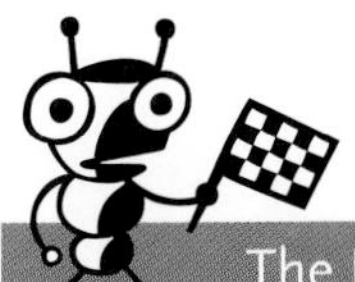

The Finish Line

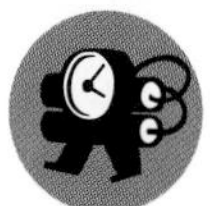

What's Wrong With This Picture?

Correct the following incorrect statements:

1. Normal blood oxygen level is usually between 75 and 85 percent.
2. A resident on a ventilator will be able to communicate normally.
3. A nursing assistant is the only person who will perform suctioning on a resident.
4. A telemetry unit, along with wires and pads, should be submerged in water when bathing a resident.
5. TPN is necessary if a resident does not feel like going to the dining room to eat.
6. An increased appetite and energy level are two side effects of chemotherapy.
7. Cancer is always incurable.

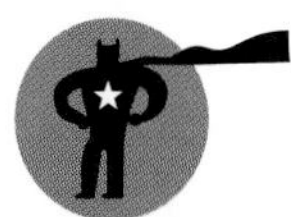

Star Student Central

1. Visit a subacute unit and ask for a tour. Take notes on any equipment you are unfamiliar with and share this information with your class.
2. Gather information, such as risk factors, recovery rate, and treatment options, on a specific type of cancer and share it with the class.

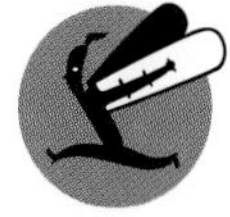

You Can Do It Corner!

1. What should a nursing assistant report immediately when caring for a resident with a pulse oximeter? (LO 3)
2. Why is monitoring vital signs with blood transfusions so important? (LO 9)
3. What are some communication aids that can help a resident on a ventilator? (LO 5)
4. List tips on caring for residents on chemotherapy or radiation therapy who are experiencing fatigue, loss of appetite, skin effects, mouth effects, hair loss, and emotional effects. (LO 12)
5. Name three reasons a resident may require subacute care. (LO 2)
6. List six signs of respiratory distress. (LO 6)
7. What is a tracheostomy? (LO 7)
8. What are four reasons for the insertion of a gastrostomy? (LO 10)
9. List what telemetry monitors. (LO 4)
10. Why is a central intravenous line inserted? (LO 8)
11. What is the name of the special pump residents with extreme pain may use to give themselves pain medication? What does a lock-out period mean? (LO 11)

Star Student's Chapter Checklist

1. I have read my textbook chapter.
2. I have reviewed my own "Pocketful of Terms."
3. I have listened to my tutor tape.
4. I have reviewed and highlighted my class notes.
5. I have read and completed any handouts from this chapter.
6. I have completed "The Finish Line."
7. Star Time! Choose your reward!

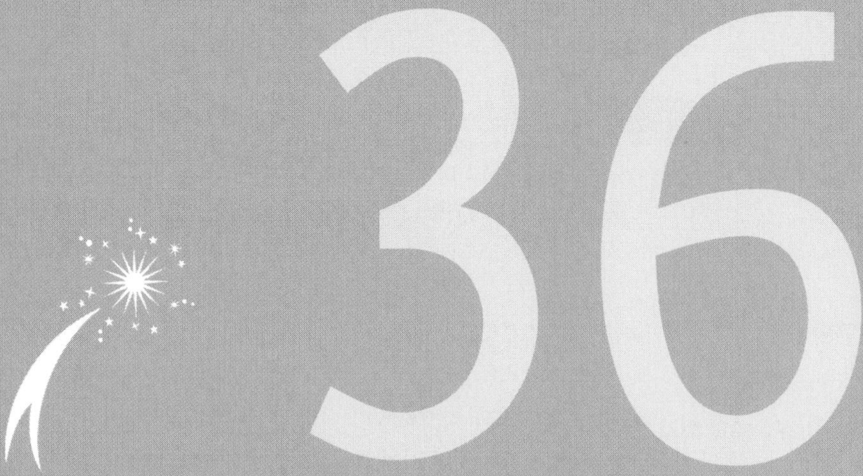

36

End-of-Life Care: Your Role in Death and Dying

Look Like a Star!

Look at the Learning Objectives and The Finish Line before you begin reading this chapter.

Look at your pocket calendar.
With your pencil, put a bracket ( ) around a study period every single day.

Look at your homework for this chapter.
Plug each piece of homework into a certain time slot.

Look at the Star Student's Chapter Checklist at the end of this chapter. Check off each item as it is completed.

"As a well-spent day brings happy sleep, so life well used brings happy death."

Leonardo Da Vinci, 1452-1519

"Men fear death as children fear to go in the dark; and as that natural fear in children is increased with tales, so is the other."

Publilius Syrus, circa 42 B.C.

Learning Objectives

1. **Spell and define all STAR words.**
2. **Define "advance directives" and list two examples.**
3. **Identify and describe the five stages of death and dying.**
4. **Describe ways to meet the psychosocial and spiritual needs of a dying resident.**
5. **Identify common signs of approaching death.**
6. **Explain the care of a dying resident.**
7. **Define "hospice" and list seven of its goals.**
8. **Discuss the changes you will see in the human body after death.**
9. **Identify ways to help the resident's family and friends deal with a resident's death.**
10. **Describe ways you can help residents and staff members cope with death.**
11. **Describe postmortem care.**

Successfully perform this Practical Procedure

Postmortem Care

The Ancient Egyptian Art of Embalming the Dead

Life in ancient Egypt was simply a preparation for the afterlife. The hope was that the afterlife would be a joyful paradise. The art of embalming dead bodies was common in ancient Egypt, especially for people of high birth. Embalming consisted of removing and preserving organs, such as the liver and the lungs. They were placed inside jars and then covered. Various cavities were washed out with spices and then the body was soaked for a period of 70 days with a substance called natron. Natron was made of clay mixed with certain salts. The body was then coated with various gums and wrapped with pieces of fine linen. People of that time who were of lower birth were destined to be buried in the sand without any of the above special preparation.

1 Spell and define all STAR words.

acceptance: the last stage of death and dying; person is able to accept death and prepare for it.

advance directive: a document that allows people to choose what kind of medical care they wish to have in the event they are unable to make those decisions themselves; an advance directive can also designate or name someone else to make medical decisions for a person if that person is disabled.

anger: the second stage of death and dying; person asks, "Why me?"

bargaining: third stage of death and dying; person says, "Yes me, but. . ."

Cheyne-Stokes breathing: method of breathing commonly seen in the dying; slow breathing with periods of no breathing at all.

denial: the first stage of death and dying; person feels disbelief: "No. Not me."

depression: the fourth stage of death and dying; the person may become deeply sad or depressed.

fixed and dilated: having pupils that do not respond to light; this occurs when there is no blood flow inside the brain; pupils may be fixed and dilated when a person is pronounced dead.

mottling: appearance of bruises on some parts of the body; can occur after death.

palliative care: care or treatment to relieve or lessen pain or other uncomfortable symptoms, not to cure.

postmortem care: care of the body after death.

shroud: a large, usually white piece of material used for covering the body after death.

2 Define "advance directives" and list two examples.

Advance directives are written documents that allow people to designate what kind of medical care they wish to have in the event they are unable to make those decisions themselves. An advance directive can also designate someone else to make medical decisions for a person if that person is disabled. Advance directives also include oral statements.

Two common types of advance directives include a Living Will and a Durable Power of Attorney for Health Care.

A Living Will is a written document that states the medical care a person wants, or does not want, in case he or she becomes unable to make those decisions him- or herself. It is called a Living Will because it takes effect while the person is still living.

A Durable Power of Attorney for Health Care is a signed, dated, and witnessed paper that appoints someone else to make the medical decisions for a person in the event he or she becomes disabled. This can include instructions about medical treatment the person wants to avoid. Because the term "power of attorney" indicates legal issues, many individuals think this means that someone can take control of a person's money, property, etc. This document, however, deals only with medical issues.

Either document may specify healthcare instructions such as a DNR (Do Not Resuscitate) order. A DNR order tells medical professionals not to perform CPR. Other healthcare instructions may include specifications on organ donation and life support.

Both types of advance directives may be used together, or a person may elect to use one or none at all. Having an advance directive is not legally required. However, it is a good way to make sure a person's wishes regarding medical treatment are known and honored.

An advance directive can be changed or canceled at any time, either in writing, or verbally, or both.

3 Identify and describe the five stages of death and dying.

Dr. Elisabeth Kubler-Ross wrote the book *On Death and Dying* in 1970. She developed the theory that dying people may experience five different emotional stages before death. The dying individual may not reach all of the stages. Some may stay in one stage until death occurs. It is also possible for people to move back and forth between stages during the process.

Stage 1. **Denial:** No. Not Me.

People in the denial stage may refuse to believe they are dying. They often believe a mistake has been made. They may demand lab work be done a second time or that a special scan be repeated. The person may not be able to talk about death throughout this stage and may simply act like it is not happening.

Stage 2. **Anger:** Why me?

When people start to face the possibility of death, they may be angry that they are the ones who are dying. They may be angry because they believe they are too young or because they have always been "good" or taken care of themselves. A dying person may express anger at anyone or anything. For example, a resident may become upset with a cold dinner or a problem with the television. Anger may be directed at staff, visitors, roommates, family, or friends. This can be very upsetting to people, especially to family members. It is important that you do not take the anger personally.

Stage 3. **Bargaining:** Yes, me, but...

Once people have begun to believe that they really are dying, they may start a bargaining process with God in hopes of recovery. It is also possible for the person to try to bargain for the ability to attend an important function, such as a bar mitzvah or first communion.

Stage 4. **Depression:** Sadness

As dying people become weaker and the symptoms of the progressing illness become more pronounced, they may become deeply sad or depressed. They may cry or become withdrawn. It is possible the person will want to talk during this stage. It is important for you to listen and be understanding.

Stage 5. **Acceptance:** Peace

Some people who are dying are eventually able to accept death and prepare for it. They may ask to see an attorney or accountant or make arrangements with loved ones for the care of important people or belongings. They may request the help of clergy to prepare for a religious ceremony before or after death, or both.

These stages of death and dying may not be possible for someone who dies suddenly, unexpectedly, or in a very short period of time. When a person goes through all of the stages, he or she may reach the point of death at greater peace. You cannot force anyone to move from stage to stage. You can only listen, and be ready to offer any help the person needs.

4 Describe ways to meet the psychosocial and spiritual needs of a dying resident.

When people deal with impending death, they bring all of their life experiences with them. Each person's life experiences are very different. You cannot expect your feelings to be the same as others. When dealing with a resident who will die soon, listening is often one of the most important things you'll do. Do not underestimate the benefit of listening to the fears and concerns of your dying residents. Some people seem to have no actual fear of death itself, but have great concerns about the situation they are leaving behind. Perhaps they have concerns over the safety and financial security of their family or other loved ones. They may not have made arrangements for the care of much-loved pets. Others are worried about their beloved plants. They have concerns over the family business or the location of all of the family assets.

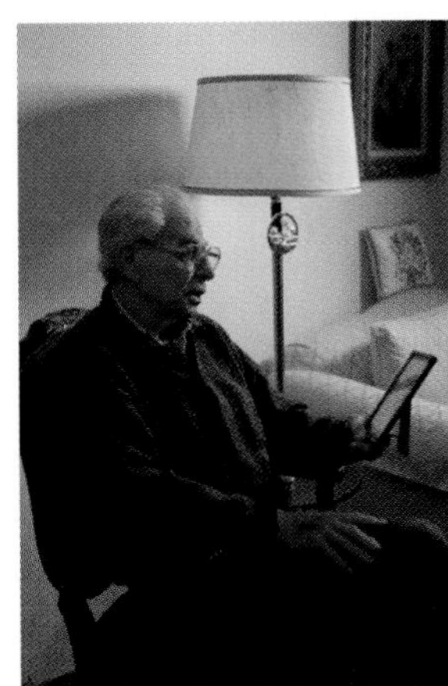

Figure 36-1. A dying resident may have many concerns. It is important to listen to him if he wants to talk.

You can take notes when listening to a resident who is expected to die soon. If he or she says anything of importance, it can be relayed to family or friends. Give any notes you take to the nurse so that he may take care of notifying the family.

Feelings and attitudes about death are influenced by many factors. These factors include the person's previous experience with death, personality type, religious beliefs, and cultural background.

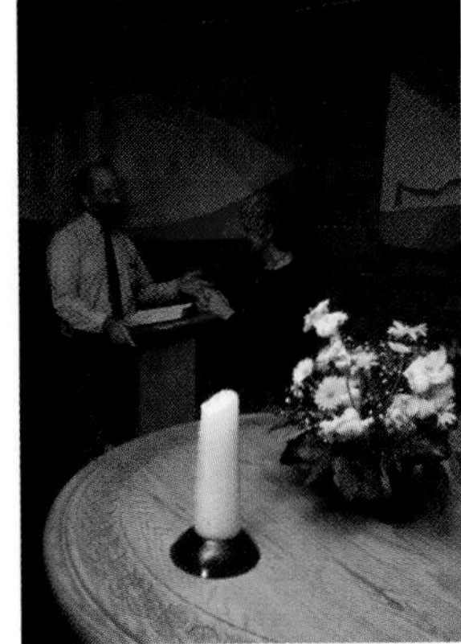

Figure 36-2. Religious beliefs influence a person's feelings about death.

A resident may request that a personal clergyperson come into the facility and spend time with the dying resident. If the clergyperson cannot be reached, you can spend some time with the resident.

When people are afraid of death, it is possible that talking about their fears may make them come to terms with the impending death. Drawing out a person's fears is sometimes a difficult process. There are some general guidelines to follow when dealing with residents who are dying soon and wish to talk.

Guidelines for Caring for a Resident Facing Death (Box 36-1)

1. Do not avoid the dying resident.
2. Never bring your religious beliefs into the conversation.
3. Never judge anything the person tells you about his or her past.
4. Listen more; talk less.
5. Notify the nurse immediately if resident requests a clergy person.
6. Provide the person with privacy for family or clergy visits.
7. Never share anything private that is said to you by the resident with anyone other than the nurse. For example, the resident says: "Please tell my cousin I have always loved him." This should be shared with the nurse first. The nurse will then share this information, if she determines it is appropriate, at the right time. There are some things that may be said that might cause pain for a loved one and the nurse should make the decision whether or not to share any information.
8. Never share anything about the resident, whether it be conversation, appearance, or anything else about the dying person, with any other person. This includes other staff members, volunteers, your own family and friends, or the newspapers or the media.

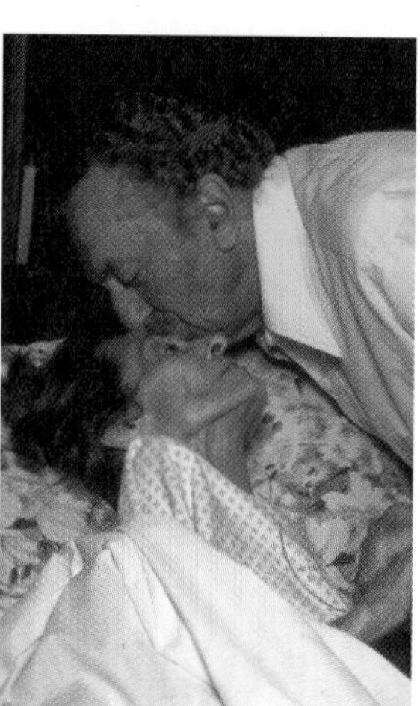

Figure 36-3. As much as possible, give your resident and his or her visitors the privacy they need.

5 Identify common signs of approaching death.

When a resident is approaching death, signs occur in many of the body systems. The common signs of impending death follow:

Signs of Impending Death (Box 36-2)

Integumentary System

Skin may:

- become cyanotic or paler than normal color
- be cold to the touch
- look bruised; called **mottling**
- perspire heavily (diaphoresis)
- be feverish

Muscular System

- loss of muscle tone, beginning with the legs and feet
- fallen jaw, causing the mouth to stay open

Nervous System

- decreased sense of touch
- loss of feeling beginning in the legs and feet
- loss of vision
- pupils dilate and eyes may stare
- loss of ability to speak
- confusion

Circulatory System

- lower blood pressure
- increased pulse

Respiratory System

- slow and irregular respirations, called **Cheyne-Stokes breathing**
- gurgling and noisy respirations

Gastrointestinal System

- dysphagia (difficulty swallowing)
- decreased appetite
- thirst
- nausea, vomiting, and diarrhea
- incontinence of stool

Urinary System

- decreased urinary output
- incontinence of urine

Hippocrates' Description of Impending Death

The "facies Hippocratica," was a very grave situation, one of impending death. The patient would be seen with "nose peaked, eyes sunken, temples hollow, ears cold and contracted with lobes turned outwards, sweat clammy, yellowish hue. . ."

6 Explain the care of a dying resident.

Integumentary System: It is important for you to perform excellent skin care for a dying person. When the resident is perspiring heavily, change gowns and sheets often for comfort. Fever may cause chills, and the resident should be protected by providing extra bedcovers to keep him warm. Remove heavier bedclothes if the resident is perspiring. If the resident is incontinent, it is very important to clean him promptly and make him comfortable. This is done not only for comfort and proper hygiene, but also to prevent pressure sores.

Oral care should be done frequently. It is needed more frequently because secretions gather inside and outside the mouth and form crusts. Also, the mouth and nose area can become dry and cracked. Lubrication applied lightly to the nose may be helpful to protect these mucous membranes.

Muscular System: Frequent turning and repositioning is important so that pressure sores do not develop. Extra assistance may be necessary to help the person move because of the decrease in muscle strength.

Nervous System: The resident may be in severe pain or may not suffer any pain at all. If the person is in pain, it is vital that the nurse be notified. The resident may be connected to a device called PCA (Patient Controlled Analgesia) that she can operate independently. This allows the resident to press a button in order to give herself a dose of pain medication. Sometimes residents cannot communicate that they are in pain. Observe your residents for signs of pain and report them promptly.

Vision may begin to fail as death nears. The person may demand that the light stay on at all times. Keep the room softly lighted without glare.

Speaking may become difficult for the dying resident. You will have to be creative to understand the resident's requests. Special picture boards can be used if vision is still adequate, or ask family for assistance if you are unable to understand a request.

It is very important to understand that the sense of hearing is usually the last sense to leave a dying person. This means you must always behave professionally when caring for a dying person. Treat this person in the same way you would any resident—explaining procedures and talking to the person normally.

Remember that hearing is the last sense to disappear!

Remember to never say anything inappropriate around a dying resident or the resident's family. The sense of hearing is the last sense to leave a person. Never act like the resident is not there or is not fully capable of understanding you.

Circulatory System: Report any change in the pulse and blood pressure to the nurse immediately. It is vital that the nurse be notified so that any necessary measures may be taken. The nurse might need to notify family members if it appears that death is near.

Respiratory System: If the dying resident experiences dyspnea (difficulty breathing), it can be very frightening to the resident and any family, friends, or roommates. The resident may also experience gurgling or rattling in breathing. This is caused by secretions building up in the throat. Notify the nurse if either of these conditions occurs. The nurse may ask you to elevate the bed or change the position of the resident to help ease the problems with breathing.

Gastrointestinal System: Feeding should be done slowly to help prevent choking and aspiration. Never force the resident to eat or drink. If the resident is thirsty, and fluids are allowed, provide them as necessary. If the resident is experiencing nausea, vomiting, or diarrhea, inform the nurse.

Urinary System: When residents are incontinent, you must clean and dry them immediately. Always behave professionally and empathize—put yourself in the resident's place.

7 Define "hospice" and list seven of its goals.

Hospice is a compassionate method of caring for people with a terminal illness and their families. Hospice care uses a holistic approach. Holistic care means treating the "whole person," including his or her physical, emotional, spiritual and social needs. Hospice care can be provided seven days a week, 24 hours a day. There is always a nurse on call to answer questions, make an additional visit, or assist with solving a problem. Hospice care is available with a physician's order.

Hospice goals include the following:

1. Offer compassionate care for a person with a terminal illness.

2. Focus on the resident and family as a unit of care.
3. Offer medically-directed/team-managed care.
4. Focus on **palliative** (relieving or soothing pain) **care** rather than trying to cure.
5. Emphasize pain and symptom control.
6. Emphasize holistic approach—address physical, spiritual, emotional and social needs.
7. Provide an alternative to traditional hospital care.

It is important to understand that palliative care is not curative. Palliative care focuses on pain and symptom control, psychosocial support, and the involvement of family and friends.

Hospice strives to help meet all possible needs of the dying resident. Both family and friends, as well the resident, are directly involved in making decisions for care. The resident is also encouraged to participate in the family life and decisions as much as possible, including choices about medical care in the event that the resident becomes disabled.

Hospice helps with pain management by monitoring the administration and effectiveness of medicine, which is prescribed by the physician. These observations are related to the physician.

Hospice encourages the involvement of the resident's own religious leader if the resident has one. A list of volunteers can be provided for a resident who wants religious support but has no specific religious leader.

Hospice also supports both the family and dying resident in continuing involvement in social activities such as reading, listening to music, going out if possible, and learning new skills.

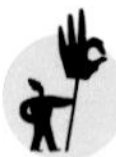

Hospice cares.

According to the National Hospice Organization, of the 115,000 people providing hospice care in America, 95,000 are volunteers. Volunteers give more than five million hours of their time each year to help people who are dying. Hospice volunteers go through a training program to prepare them for hospice work.

8 Discuss the changes you will see in the human body after death.

When death occurs, you may hear the nurse or doctor identify the exact time. She may announce the

I HAVE THE RIGHT TO:

be treated as a living human being until I die.

maintain a sense of hopefulness, however changing its focus may be.

be cared for by those who can maintain a sense of hopefulness, however changing this might be.

express my feelings and emotions about my approaching death in my own way.

participate in decisions concerning my care.

expect continuing medical and nursing attentions even though "cure" goals must be changed to "comfort" goals.

die alone.

be free from pain.

have my questions answered honestly.

not be deceived.

have help from and for my family in accepting my death.

die in peace and dignity.

retain my individuality and not be judged for my decisions which may be contrary to beliefs of others.

discuss and enlarge my religious and/or spiritual experiences, whatever these may mean to others.

expect that the sanctity of the human body will be respected after death.

be cared for by caring, sensitive, knowledgeable people who will attempt to understand my needs and will be able to gain some satisfaction in helping me face my death.

Figure 36-4. **The Dying Person's Bill of Rights.**

fact that the pupils are **fixed and dilated**. If the pupils are fixed and dilated, it means there is no blood flow inside the brain. There will be no heartbeat, pulse, respiration, or blood pressure. Other physical signs you may see include the following:

- the jaw dropping, which causes the mouth to stay open
- eyelids partially open with eyes in a fixed stare, until they are closed by the nurse
- incontinent of both urine and stool

9 Identify ways to help the resident's family and friends deal with a resident's death.

The family or friends, if present, may be quite upset at the point of death of their loved one. They may cry or scream, faint, become very nervous, or become very quiet. Everyone has an individual way of dealing with the death of a loved one. Some family members comfort other family members. Others need the help of staff or pastoral care. If a person requests pastoral care, inform the nurse immediately.

Unfortunately, it is also possible for family to become upset with staff members. They may initially say things that make it sound like they are blaming staff for the death of their loved one. This anger is usually not really directed at the staff. It can be due to the fact that they are upset with a decision they may have made concerning their loved one. Sometimes, the family may be upset with staff because of a specific problem that they feel was not addressed. In any case, refer any family complaints to the nurse. Do not try to calm a family member or friend who is upset with staff.

Your facility will have a policy for handling residents' personal items after death, such as jewelry, pictures, and even dentures. Make sure you follow your facility's policy.

10 Describe ways you can help residents and staff members cope with death.

Staff members and other residents may be extremely upset with the death of a beloved resident. It is important to understand the depth of grief you may experience for a resident who has died. Do not underestimate your feelings, and never be ashamed because you feel grief about a resident's death. This grief is a testament to the kind of person you are and the kind of person your resident was. Grieve at your own pace. Also, allow other staff and residents to grieve at their own pace. Listen and provide emotional support when appropriate. Increasingly, facilities are allowing caregivers and residents to participate in memorial or religious services following a death. Some services are held in the facility.

11 Describe postmortem care.

The care of the body after death is called **postmortem care**. Nurses may assist you with this care or ask that you do the care yourself. Try to perform postmortem care with others to provide support for each other.

Be sensitive to the needs of family and friends after death occurs. They may wish to stay with the body for a while. Allow them time to do so. Be aware of religious and cultural practices that the family wants to observe.

Ask the nurse for instructions before beginning postmortem care. A **shroud** kit containing a large white piece of material for covering the body is sometimes used by facilities. It may also include special pads and ID tags.

Do not be afraid of unexpected sounds or movements from a body after death.

There are times after death when a body makes sounds or movements unexpectedly. These movements or sounds can frighten residents, staff, family, and visitors. Things heard and seen include respiratory sounds when air moves out of the lungs during movement, muscular movements as hands or legs move, eyes opening again, jaws opening, and bouts of incontinence. Try not to be frightened when one of these situations occurs. It is common for this to happen, and it is one of the reasons that two or more people should perform postmortem care and transport the resident to the morgue together.

An Early Autopsy

An examination of a dead body was performed in 1302 when the nobleman Azzolini died under suspicious circumstances. A doctor named Bartolomeo da Varignana was called in to examine the body and determine whether or not the death had been caused by poisoning. He skillfully performed the autopsy, compiling records that showed his understanding of anatomy.

Postmortem Care

Follow all standard and/or transmission-based precautions. Follow all rules for body mechanics.

Collect equipment:
- **three pairs of gloves • disposable bed protector**
- **shroud kit or sheets • toilet tissue • washcloth or wipes**
- **wash basin of warm water • towel • cotton balls**
- **plastic bags for clothing and belongings**

PREPARE:

1. **Wash hands and provide for privacy.**
2. **Apply gloves.**
3. **Place bed in flat position.**

PERFORM:

4. **Only remove tubes if specifically directed to do so by the nurse. Most facilities leave tubes in the resident.**
5. **Turn off any oxygen, suction, or other equipment if directed by the nurse.**
6. **Gently close eyes without pressure.**
7. **Place body in good alignment.**
8. **Place chin strap or rolled towel under the chin.**
9. **Gently bathe the body. Be careful to avoid bruising. Replace any dressings if directed to do so. Otherwise, leave dressings in place.**

10. Comb or brush hair very carefully without tugging.
11. Put a clean gown on the body and place disposable pads under the buttocks.
12. Cover body to just over the shoulders with sheet. Never cover face or head.
13. Tidy room so family may visit.
14. Remove all used supplies and linen.
15. Follow your facility's policy for handling or removing personal items.
16. Remove gloves, discard, and wash hands.
17. Turn lights down and allow family to enter and spend private time with resident.
18. Return after family departs and apply clean gloves.
19. Place shroud on resident and carefully complete all ID tags.

    ID Tags:

    1-usually placed around the big toe

    2-attached to the valuables or belongings

    3-may be third tag for morgue
20. Remove gloves, discard, and wash hands.
21. Transport body to the morgue (Follow Principal Steps below).

FINISHING TOUCHES:

22. Return to room. Apply gloves. Strip bed and remove all linen and trash. If facility policy, remake room for new resident. See Chapter 15 for information on unit cleaning.
23. Remove gloves, discard, and wash hands.
24. Report and record observations.

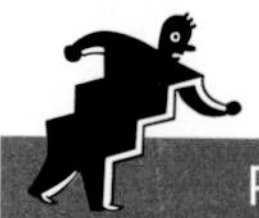

Principal Steps

Transport to the Morgue

1. *Transfer resident to stretcher with assistance.*
2. *Carefully cover with a sheet or shroud.*
3. *Carefully transport in appropriate manner, since bumping any body part can cause bruising.*
4. *Choose appropriate elevator for transfer.*
5. *Behave in professional manner during transport.*
6. *Always use two staff members to transport to the morgue.*

Summary

Death is a part of life. There is no way to avoid it. In order to care for the dying, family members, friends, staff, and other residents, it is important to thoroughly understand the process of dying. It is a good idea to examine your own feelings about death and dying before beginning your employment at a long-term care facility. People in long-term care facilities are usually at an advanced age, and more than one death may occur in a very short period of time. Being in touch with your feelings may help you cope with the possible difficulties surrounding death.

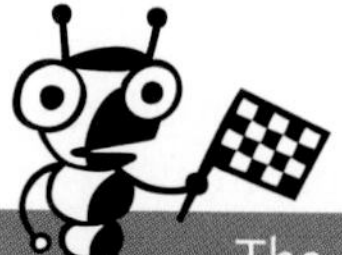

The Finish Line

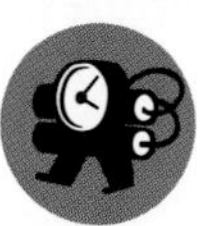

What's Wrong With This Picture?

1. Look at the equipment for the procedure on postmortem care. List the one missing piece of equipment.

Collect equipment:
- **three pairs of gloves • shroud kit or sheets**
- **toilet tissue • washcloth or wipes • cotton balls**
- **wash basin of warm water • towel**
- **plastic bags for clothing and belongings**

2. Look at the Principal Steps on transporting to the morgue. List and correct the two errors.
   1. *Transfer resident to stretcher with assistance.*
   2. *Carefully cover with a sheet or shroud.*
   3. *Carefully transport in appropriate manner, since bumping any body part can cause bruising.*
   4. *Choose busy, public elevator for transfer.*
   5. *Behave in professional manner during transport.*
   6. *Always transport to the morgue by yourself.*

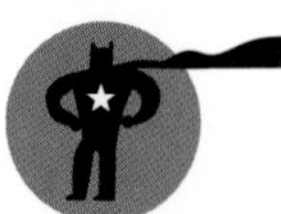

Star Student Central

1. Gather information about the following in your state:
   - DNR order
   - Living Will
   - Durable Power of Attorney for Health Care

2. What would you like your legacy to be? Legacy is defined as something left behind by a person. One way to be remembered in a positive way is by volunteering your time. A place that usually greatly appreciates volunteers is a hospice center. Volunteering is a noble thing. Consider volunteering even a couple of hours a month at a special place in need. You will be very glad you did.

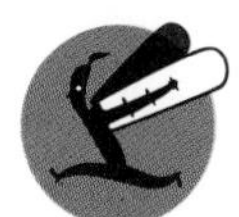

You Can Do It Corner!

1. List an advance directive and its purpose. (LO 2)
2. Define palliative care. (LO 7)
3. List possible wishes of family and friends you need to consider before performing postmortem care. (LO 11)
4. Why might clergy be called in to help staff cope with death? (LO 10)
5. What is often one of the most important things you can do for a resident who is dying? (LO 4)
6. List three changes you may see in a resident's body after death. (LO 8)
7. Identify the five stages of death and dying a resident may go through. (LO 3)
8. List one common sign of approaching death for seven different body systems. (LO 5)
9. If a family member becomes angry with you after a resident dies, what should you do? (LO 9)
10. List one care measure for a dying resident for seven different body systems. (LO 6)

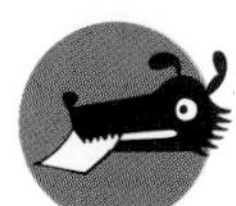

Star Student's Chapter Checklist

1. I have read my textbook chapter.
2. I have reviewed my own "Pocketful of Terms."
3. I have listened to my tutor tape.
4. I have reviewed and highlighted my class notes.
5. I have read and completed any handouts from this chapter.
6. I have completed "The Finish Line."
7. Star Time! Choose your reward!

37

Your Position: The Star Employee

Look Like a Star!

Look at the Learning Objectives and The Finish Line before you begin reading this chapter.

Look at your pocket calendar.
With your pencil, put a bracket (   ) around a study period every single day.

Look at your homework for this chapter.
Plug each piece of homework into a certain time slot.

Look at the Star Student's Chapter Checklist at the end of this chapter. Check off each item as it is completed.

"When men are employed, they are best contented; for on the days they worked they were good-natured and cheerful, and, with the consciousness of having done a good day's work, they spent the evening jollily."

Benjamin Franklin, 1706-1790

"Do not turn back when you are just at the goal."

Maxim 580

Learning Objectives

1. **Spell and define all STAR words.**
2. **Describe the components of a STAR resumé and cover letter.**
3. **Summarize the information you need to complete a STAR job application.**
4. **List eleven steps for dressing successfully for a job interview.**
5. **List the "Five Secret Techniques for Successful Interviewing."**
6. **Describe a standard job description.**
7. **Describe the competencies, or skills, necessary to succeed in the workplace as outlined by the SCANS report of 1992.**
8. **Identify four additional requirements for securing a job.**
9. **Identify the guidelines for obtaining your nursing assistant certification and keeping your certification current.**
10. **Identify the number of hours of continuing education required by federal and state law.**
11. **Discuss the annual in-services required by state and federal law.**
12. **Explain the policy for a TB skin test or chest x-ray and a hepatitis vaccine.**
13. **Discuss the process of evaluating employee performances.**

The Origins of "Nursing Attendants"

Rules for nursing assistants in the late 1700s were very different than they are today. Some of the old rules seem pretty funny and outdated by today's standards. They included rules such as outlawing bones and dirt being thrown from the windows! Some places changed the patients' bed linens only once every two weeks and washed patients' underclothing as little as once a week. "Attendants" who got drunk or argued with men were immediately fired!

1 Spell and define all **STAR** words.

certification: legal document prepared by an official body that indicates a person has met certain standards or completed a course of instruction.

competency: having necessary skills or qualities.

constructive criticism: suggestions given to help an employee improve job performance.

continuing education: formal education for adults after completion of original training.

cover letter: a letter of introduction to an employer.

Department of Health Services: department handling organization's health issues and services.

font: in printing, a set of type of particular size and appearance.

Human Resources Department: department handling all personnel issues.

in-service: an adult training session.

job description: a list of tasks for a specific job.

OBRA: Omnibus Budget Reconciliation Act.

personal reference: a reference written by a good friend or non-employer.

probationary: a trial period of employment.

performance appraisal: evaluation of an employee's work.

professional reference: a reference written by a former employer.

registry: a formal list.

resumé: a summary of experience and education.

scope of practice: a set of tasks that a state or federal agency allows certain individuals to perform.

template: a model to follow; a pattern.

title: name identifying an office or position.

2 Describe the components of a STAR resumé and cover letter.

The most important thing about getting your first position as a nursing assistant will be how well you have prepared for the job search. The first step in any job search is preparing a quality **resumé**. This is a summary of your education and experience. You will need to gather information on the following topics when preparing a resumé:

Objective: Identify your primary goal in this exciting field.

Education: List schools or G.E.D. courses completed, starting from high school and including any college courses.

Experience: Identify the jobs you have held to this point, placing your current job first and moving backward in time. A general rule of thumb is to list positions you have held for more than six months. If you have held many jobs in, say, the fast-food industry, these positions can be grouped together in one section to save space.

Volunteer Work: Describe all volunteer work, stressing work closely related to the healthcare field.

Skills Acquired: List all of your special skills, including things like typing, computer skills, speaking other languages, etc.

References: Simply identify the fact that references are available upon request.

The following general rules should apply when writing a resumé:

1. Limit your resumé to one page. Use short, precise sentences.
2. Do not add borders or color of any kind. Use quality, white paper.
3. Use a basic, size 12, plain **font**. Boldface your name and address at the top of the page and place this in the center of the page.
4. If using a computer, do not rely on a spell-check program. Use it, then check spelling yourself. Then have a friend check the spelling. Finally, read the resumé out loud to make sure you have not made an error in grammar.
5. Do not staple anything to your resumé.

An example of a well-written nursing assistant resumé is shown in Figure 37-1. A resumé should be perfect in every way. One small mistake can cost you the job you desire. Take the extra time to make it the best it can be.

The **cover letter** is a letter that will be included with a resumé during the application process. A sample cover letter is shown in Figure 37-2. It is best to have a **template** of a cover letter saved on a computer or a sample cover letter saved that you have already typed on a typewriter. This letter should be brief and serves as your introduction to the interviewer.

Sarah Louise Harris
1234 Sandia Court
Albuquerque, NM 87126
505-555-4211

OBJECTIVE:	To secure an entry-level nursing assistant job in a long-term care facility.
EDUCATION:	Hobbs High School, Hobbs, NM, Diploma 1990 Pima Medical Institute, Albuquerque, NM 1994 Certified Nursing Assistant
EXPERIENCE:	Sunnyvale Nursing Home 1995 - present Hobbs, NM **Nursing Assistant** - Performed personal care duties and assisted with ADLs. - Worked mostly with residents with dementia. - Helped plan activities for residents. Happy Home Nursing Center 1991-1993 Austin, Texas **Receptionist** - Managed multi-line phone system. - Made appointments for staff. - Visited residents and read to them. - Made arrangements for resident activities out of the facility.
SKILLS:	Microsoft Word, Microsoft Excel, Adobe Acrobat, and ACT database on a PC.
VOLUNTEER WORK	National Diabetes Foundation, Hospice Foundation
REFERENCES:	Available upon request.

Figure 37-1. **A sample resumé.**

Sarah Louise Harris
1234 Sandia Court
Albuquerque, NM 87126
505-555-4211

Mr. David Pomazal
Human Resources Manager
Rolling Meadows Nursing Home
P.O. Box 555
Albuquerque, NM 87102

Dear Mr. Pomazal:

Please consider this letter and the enclosed resume and application for the NA position advertised in last Sunday's edition of the *Albuquerque Journal.*

I am an energetic, detail-oriented person who has strong organizational skills, experience, and the ability to work well with people from all walks of life. In addition, I have held positions of responsibility in four community organizations over the last eight years and was chosen the 2000 National Diabetes Foundation Volunteer of the Year.

As you can see from my resume, I thrive in a busy atmosphere that involves many different tasks, and enjoy the opportunity to work with residents and the chance to excel. I would appreciate an interview to discuss the possibility of my joining your staff. I will call you next week to request an appointment, or you may call me at your convenience at (505) 555-4211.

Thank you for your consideration of my application. I look forward to meeting you soon.

Sincerely,

Sarah Louise Harris
Enclosure

Figure 37-2. **A sample cover letter.**

3 Summarize the information you need to complete a STAR job application.

Completing a job application can be stressful at best. If you are not prepared for this experience, you may not present yourself well. This mistake could also cost you a position. A few simple steps can help you feel ready for this task. Before filling out the application, make sure you have completed the following checklist:

1. Make a new copy of your resumé and place it in a folder to carry it safely to the facility.
2. Gather information that you may need from your home. If the **Human Resources Department** will agree to send the application to your home ahead of time, ask them to do so. The information includes the following:
   - salary information from your past and present positions
   - former and present supervisors' names, **titles**, and phone numbers
   - exact dates of employment and your reasons for leaving each of your former jobs
   - complete names, addresses, and telephone numbers of **personal references** and **professional references**.
   - names of other people you know who may work at the facility
   - certification numbers and expiration dates from Nursing Assistant **Certification** card, CPR cards, first aid cards, and any other identification you may need
3. If you must fill out the application at the facility, write out everything neatly on a yellow pad, or simply enter it into your computer, print the file, and take it with you. Put it in outline form, if possible, so that you can scan the page quickly while filling out the application.
4. Before arriving at the facility, think about any potential problems the employer may find in the job application. For example, if you have a gap in employment, a time when you did not work at all, an interviewer may ask the reason for the gap. If you took care of your second child at home for a year, be prepared to give that answer. Imagine being the interviewer and consider the questions you might ask yourself.

When you actually fill out the job application, here are a few steps that can make the process run smoothly:

1. Print neatly using ink. If you are at home, use a dictionary to check spelling.
2. Tell the truth. Never lie on a job application. If there is a criminal record section, be honest if you have a record. Remember, this employer will do a complete background check. Federal and state laws require a criminal background check before hiring a nursing assistant. The best way to handle this is to allow for no surprises. Write a complete explanation in the appropriate section so that they will have your side of the story.
3. Do not leave anything blank in the application. You may write N/A (not applicable) if the question does not apply to you.

Employment Application

Personal Information	
Name: Rosie Ferguson	Date: 1/15/02
Social Security Number: 555-99-9999	
Home Address: 8529-A Indian School Rd. NE	
City, State Zip: Albuquerque, NM 87112	
Home Phone: 505-291-1274	Business Phone: N/A
US Citizen? yes	If Not Give Visa No. & expiration:

Position Applying For	
Title Nursing Assistant	Salary Desired: $8.50/hr.
Referred By: Ms. Pendergras Instructor, NA Training Center	Date Available: 1/15/02

Education	
High School (Name, City, State): Laguna Senior High School Albuquerque, NM	
Graduation Date: December 2001	
Technical or Undergraduate School: NA Training Center Albuquerque, NM	
Dates Attended: July - Dec. 2001	Degree, Major:

References
Mr. Robert Castro, Instructor NA Training Center, 505-291-1284
Ms. Scott, Health Occupations, Laguna HS 505-555-0255
Kate Crawford, Instructor, NA Training Center, 505-291-1284

Figure 37-3. **A sample job application.**

4 List eleven steps for dressing successfully for a job interview.

In another chapter, we identified the importance our appearance plays in our daily lives. This information can be used to your advantage when dressing for an important job interview.

You must plan your outfit carefully when preparing for a job interview. First impressions are very important when you apply for a position. General guidelines on dress for interviewing follow:

1. Bathe and use deodorant.
2. Wear a nice pair of slacks, a skirt, or a dress. Make sure the skirt or dress has no wrinkles and is no shorter than knee-length. Do not wear jeans or shorts.
3. Wear a minimum of jewelry.
4. Do not overdo your makeup.
5. Wash your hands and clean and file your nails. Nails should be medium length or shorter. Females may wear clear nail polish.
6. Wear your hair in a simple manner.
7. Males should shave right before the interview.
8. Make sure your shoes are polished. Do not wear sneakers or sandals.
9. Brush your teeth. Look at your teeth right before the interview begins.
10. Do not smoke. You will smell like smoke during the interview.
11. Do not wear perfume or cologne. Many people are offended by or allergic to scents, and this alone could end up costing you the job.

5 List the "Five Secret Techniques for Successful Interviewing."

Interviewing well is truly an "art." When you learn to interview successfully, it will help you in many other new situations. Here are the five secrets to a successful interview:

1. **Practice** for the interview with a trusted friend or family member. Find a book at the library with common questions asked at interviews. Have your trusted friend or family member ask you the questions so you may practice your answers.
2. **Tests** of some kind may be given during the interview to see how skilled you are for the job. Ask if there will be a test, then study your course material while you are at home to help you feel better prepared.
3. **Map** your way to the interview site. If you are taking the bus, **get bus fare.** If you are driving, **get gas.** Make sure your car is in working order. Arrive **early** at the facility to fill out all of the paperwork. Ask the person in human resources the best time to arrive.

4. **Eye contact** is important. Do not look up or down or left or right during the interview. To some people, this means you are not telling the truth or are not interested in the conversation. Maintain eye contact during the interview.

5. **Relax.** You have worked hard to get this far. You understand the work and what is expected of you. You look great. They are going to see it!

Make sure you smile often and offer to shake hands when you arrive. Your handshake should be firm and confident.

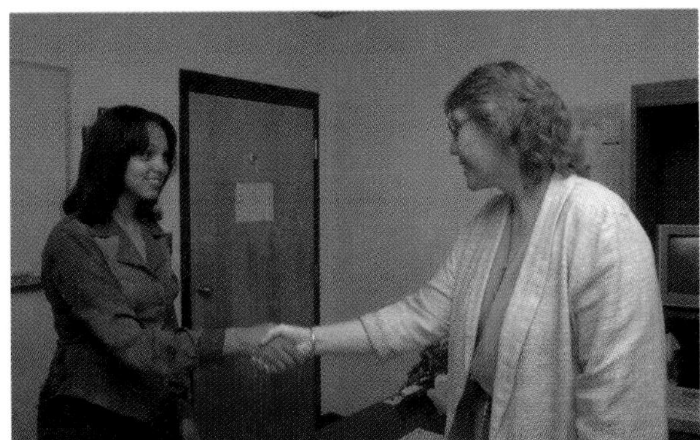

Figure 37-4. **Smile and shake hands confidently when you arrive at a job interview.**

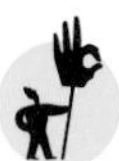

Tuition Reimbursement: Is it in your future?

When you apply for a position as a nursing assistant, request information regarding tuition reimbursement. Many nursing assistants decide to return to school to further their education in the healthcare field. Compare the tuition reimbursement offered by each facility and take this into account when accepting a nursing assistant position.

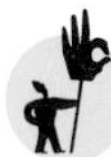

It pays to say thank you!

Always write a thank-you note following every job interview. Keeping your name in front of an interviewer can cause the employer to think of you first the next time the facility is in need of new staff members. Also, so few people do this, you are sure to stand out.

6 Describe a standard job description.

A **job description** is an outline of what you will be expected to do in your job. It can be a long, complex form and it is always best to read through any form before you sign it. An example of a job description is shown in Figure 37-5. Nursing assistants, along with other members of the healthcare team, have what is identified as a "**scope of practice**." This is a listing of skills determined by the federal and state government that includes everything nursing assistants may legally do in their position. Follow these tips when deciding whether or not to do something:

1. Do **NOT** perform the procedure if the procedure or skill is not listed in your job description. Being polite and doing things that are beyond your scope of practice could injure a resident, you, or another staff member.

2. Do **NOT** perform the procedure if you have not been trained to do the procedure.

3. Do **NOT** perform the procedure if you have forgotten how to do something you were trained to do. Ask your immediate supervisor for a reminder on how to perform the procedure before you do it.

4. If you have been trained to perform a procedure that is within your scope of practice, but you believe it may not be appropriate for a specific resident, ask a supervisor!

SERVICES FOR THE AGING

Job Title: Nursing Assistant — Department: Nursing
Responsible to: Nurse Manager/Charge Nurse — Date: November 1999

DEFINITION:

Under the supervision of a registered nurse, the nursing assistant is a recognized member of the health care team and performs nursing functions commensurate with his/her training and/or competencies. The nursing assistant is a trained and/or experienced individual who assists the nurse with the care of residents by performing appropriate nursing procedures.

JOB DUTIES:

1. Provides for the mental, emotional and physical comfort and safety of residents.

2. Observes, records and reports to the appropriate persons the general and specific physical and mental conditions of residents, and signs and symptoms which may be indicative of changes; i.e. hyperglycemia, hypoglycemia and depression.

3. Assists with rehabilitation of residents, according to Care Plans.

4. Performs the duties in connection with resident care as may be assigned from time to time.

Approved: ____________________
Director-Nursing

Figure 37-5. **A sample job description.**

7 Describe the competencies, or skills, necessary to succeed in the workplace as outlined by the SCANS report of 1992.

In 1992, the U.S. Department of Labor developed and issued a report called the SCANS, or the

Secretary's Commission on Achieving Necessary Skills. This report was updated in 2000. It outlines all of the skills needed to be a successful employee. Box 37-1 highlights the skills identified in the SCANS report.

SCANS COMPETENCIES Box 37-1

SCANS report of 1992

PART 1: WORKPLACE COMPETENCIES

RESOURCES: Identifies, organizes, plans, and allocates resources

Manages Time: Selects relevant, goal-oriented activities; ranks them in order of importance; allocates time to activities; understands, prepares, and follows schedules

Manages Money: Uses budgets, keeps records, and makes adjustments to meet objectives

Manages Material and Facilities: Acquires, stores, allocates, and uses materials or space efficiently

Manages Human Resources: Assesses skills and distributes work accordingly, evaluates performance and provides feedback

INTERPERSONAL: Works well with others

Participates as Team Member: Contributes to group effort

Teaches Others New Skills

Serves Clients/Customers: Works to satisfy customers' expectations

Exercises Leadership: Communicates ideas to justify position, persuades/convinces

Negotiates Decisions: Works toward agreements involving exchange of resources, resolves divergent interests

Works with Cultural Diversity: Works well with people from diverse backgrounds

INFORMATION: Acquires and uses information

Acquires/Evaluates Information

Organizes/Maintains Information

Interprets/Communicates Information

Uses Computers to Process Information

SYSTEMS: Understands complex social, organizational, and technological systems and interrelationships

Understands Systems: Knows how social, organizational, and technological systems work and operates effectively with them

Monitors/Corrects Performance: Distinguishes trends, predicts impacts on system operations, diagnoses deviations in systems' performance, and corrects malfunctions

Improves/Designs Systems: Suggests modifications to existing systems and develops new or alternative systems to improve performance

TECHNOLOGY: Works with a variety of technologies

Selects Technology: Chooses procedures, tools, or equipment, including computers and related technologies

Applies Technology to Tasks: Understands overall intent and proper procedures for setup and operation of equipment

Maintains/Troubleshoots Technology: Prevents, identifies, or solves problems with equipment, including computers and other technologies

PART 2: FOUNDATION SKILLS AND PERSONAL QUALITIES

BASIC SKILLS: Reads, writes, performs arithmetic/mathematical operations, listens, and speaks

Reading: locates, understands, and interprets written information, including material in documents such as manuals, graphs, and schedules

Writing: communicates thoughts, ideas, information, and messages in writing; creates documents such as letters, directions, manuals, reports, graphs, and flow charts

Arithmetic/Mathematics: Performs basic computations, approaches practical problems by choosing appropriately from a variety of mathematical techniques

Listening: Receives, attends to, interprets, and responds to verbal messages and other cues

Speaking: Organizes ideas and communicates orally

THINKING SKILLS: Thinks creatively, makes decisions, solves problems, visualizes, knows how to learn, and reasons

Creative Thinking: Generates new ideas

Decision Making: Specifies goals and constraints, generates alternatives, considers risks, and evaluates and chooses best alternative

Problem Solving: Recognizes problems and devises and implements plan of action

Knowing How to Learn: Uses efficient learning techniques to acquire and apply new knowledge and skills

Reasoning: Discovers a rule or principle underlying the relationship between two or more objects and applies it when solving a problem

PERSONAL QUALITIES: Displays responsibility, self-esteem, sociability, self-management, integrity, and honesty

Responsibility: Exerts a high level of effort, perseveres towards goal attainment

Self-Esteem: Believes in own self-worth, maintains a positive view of self

Sociability: Demonstrates understanding, friendliness, adaptability, empathy, and politeness

Self-Management: Assesses self accurately, sets personal goals, monitors progress, and exhibits self-control

Integrity/Honesty: Chooses ethical courses of action

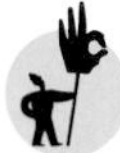

Organize your days!

When you start a new job, you will want to feel as organized as possible during your work day. You can purchase an inexpensive nylon or vinyl pocket organizer. These can be found at uniform stores as well as in many uniform catalogs. These are available ready-to-fill or as a package complete with bandage scissors, penlight, pen, and small notebook. Some organizers even have room for a stethoscope!

8 Identify four additional requirements for securing a job.

When you apply for a job as a nursing assistant, there are some additional things an employer may require you to do before you are hired. They include:

1. A complete physical. This is a good opportunity for you to have a physical, especially if you have not had an examination for a while.
2. A pre-employment drug screen. This is becoming more common in many states. Be careful not to eat food with poppy seeds beforehand.
3. Criminal background check. Criminal background checks are required by federal law. You may be asked to obtain a complete set of fingerprints and answer questions truthfully. The form may need to be notarized by a notary public. A notary public signs important documents that require verification of identity. He or she notarizes wills or other legal forms. In order to use notary services, you must produce a picture ID, pay a small fee, and sign or complete a document in front of the notary. Do not sign or fill out the form at home. A record of the transaction is kept. Banks and other agencies may have a notary public on staff.
4. A credit check. If you are unsure of your credit record, here are the addresses of the three main credit bureaus:

- **Experian**
  PO Box 2002
  Allen TX 75013
  888-397-3742
- **Trans Union**
  PO Box 1000
  Chester PA 19022
  800-888-4213
- **Equifax**
  PO Box 105873
  Atlanta GA 30348
  800-405-0081

Order a copy of your credit report before you apply for a position and check it carefully for any errors. If you find an error, follow the instructions in the report to fix it as soon as possible.

9 Identify the guidelines for obtaining your nursing assistant certification and keeping your certification current.

In 1987, the Omnibus Budget Reconciliation Act (**OBRA**), passed by the federal government, put nursing assistant requirements and education under federal regulation. In order to meet the OBRA requirements, several organizations, including the National Council of State Boards of Nursing, created **competency** evaluation programs. These programs serve as a guide for each state to follow when developing its individual nursing assistant testing program. The federal OBRA law identifies 75 hours as the minimum number of hours of training required to take the tests to become a certified nursing assistant. Today, many states' requirements exceed the minimum 75 hours.

After completing the required number of hours of training for a particular state, the nursing assistant is then eligible to take the manual and written test in that state. A fee may be required. Once the nursing assistant has passed both the written and manual skills test, a certificate is sent out. A few of the guidelines on obtaining and keeping your nursing assistant certification are listed below:

1. A nursing assistant has a certain amount of time from the date he or she is employed to take the state test. Your employer will supply you with that information the day you are hired. Pay close attention to the time frame. If you do not take

the test during this time period, you will not be able to work as a nursing assistant at that facility until you have taken and passed the written and manual tests.

2. A nursing assistant must take the state test within 24 months of training or he or she will have to start over and complete a new training course and state examination to become certified.

3. A nursing assistant must work for pay during a 24-month period. If the nursing assistant does not work during 24 months, a new training program and examination must be completed.

4. In most states, a nursing assistant has three chances to pass the state test.

5. A nursing assistant must keep his or her certification current if the state requires certification. Be sure to file a change-of-address with your state agency to make sure you receive your certification renewal.

Your employer may require that you show proof of renewal of your certificate each time it expires, as required by state law or regulation. When this is requested, you must show proof that you renewed your certificate on a timely basis. Do not allow your certificate to lapse. It is best to respond immediately to your state's request that you renew your certification. There may be a renewal fee.

The state agency in your state will keep a nursing assistant **registry**. This registry will keep track of each nursing assistant working in that particular state. Examples of the information kept in this registry include the following:

- full name along with any other names a nursing assistant may have used
- home address and other information, such as date of birth or social security number
- date that the nursing assistant was placed in the registry along with the state test scores
- expiration dates of nursing assistants' certificates
- information about investigations and hearings regarding abuse, neglect, or theft, which becomes a part of a nursing assistant's permanent record

A nursing assistant may ask that a personal written statement be added to the file. This includes information explaining the situation in the nursing assistant's own words. A nursing assistant has the right to correct any errors in a registry file.

10 Identify the number of hours of continuing education required by federal and state law.

As a team member working in the healthcare field, you will need to keep up-to-date on all aspects of your resident care. The federal government identified 12 hours per year as a minimum number of hours of **continuing education** a nursing assistant must have in order to keep certification current.

Your facility is required to provide and document this continuing education, sometimes called **in-services**, on every nursing assistant on their staff.

Some states have a requirement for more than the federal minimum of 12 hours of continuing education. Many facilities have increased the minimum requirement for continuing education. You must become familiar with both the rules in your state and your facility policy regarding continuing education.

11 Discuss the annual in-services required by state and federal law.

The federal government requires that certain continuing education training classes be provided each year. Some of the subjects are outlined below:

- Residents' rights
- Fire safety
- Safety
- CPR
- Infection control
- Confidentiality
- Bloodborne pathogens
- Tuberculosis

Many states have increased the number of required in-services. Become familiar with your state's policy and make sure you attend all of the required formal in-services. In facilities that provide computerized sessions, make sure that you attend any mandatory in-services in person when required to do so.

12 Explain the policy for a TB skin test or chest x-ray and a hepatitis vaccine.

Each year facilities are required to test all employees for exposure to dangerous diseases like tuberculosis, a disease usually affecting the respiratory system. You will receive an annual notice when it is time to have an annual TB skin test. At this time, it is your responsibility to go to the designated department to obtain the TB skin test. Once this is completed, the health services individual will ask that you return within a certain amount of time, usually 48 hours, to receive the test results.

In some cases, a person will not be able to have a TB skin test. These people must then have a chest x-ray to make sure they do not have TB. The **Department of Health Services** will notify staff members when a chest x-ray is due.

As you have learned, hepatitis refers to swelling of the liver caused by infection. Liver function can be permanently damaged by hepatitis, which can lead to other chronic, life-long illnesses. Several different viruses can cause hepatitis; the most common are hepatitis A, B, and C. Hepatitis B and C are blood-borne diseases that can cause death. Many people have hepatitis B (HBV), and it poses a serious threat to healthcare workers. Your employer must offer you a free vaccine to protect you from hepatitis B. This will usually occur when you begin your new job. Currently, there is no vaccine for hepatitis C.

13 Discuss the process of evaluating employee performances.

An annual evaluation, sometimes called a **performance appraisal** or review, is used to evaluate the performance of each employee and to give **constructive criticism**.

Some of the things you will be evaluated on are overall knowledge, conflict resolution, and team effort. Flexibility, friendliness, trustworthiness, and customer service are other qualities considered in an evaluation. A performance review or appraisal may be done after a three-month **probationary** period and then annually afterward. When you show professionalism, excellent customer service, dependability, and high ethical standards, you will usually receive a satisfactory evaluation. It is important for an employee to try each year to improve his or her performance appraisal score. Performance reviews are frequently the basis for salary increases. In addition, a satisfactory review can put a nursing assistant in a good position to advance within the facility. These evaluations almost always include ways in which you can improve your work. Be open to these suggestions as they will help you grow and be more successful in your work. Ask for and keep a copy of your probationary evaluation and each annual evaluation.

QUALITY PERFORMANCE REVIEW

EMPLOYEE NAME:____________ DATE:______ ❑90 DAY ❑ANNUAL ❑OTHER________

PERSON COMPLETING:(CIRCLE) SELF SUPERVISOR PEER CUSTOMER OTHER________

	S	NI
FOCUSED ON CUSTOMER NEEDS		
Listens to understand customer's point of view	❑	❑
Follows up with customer to ensure needs have been met	❑	❑
Reliable/dependable in completing tasks and commitments to customers	❑	❑
FRIENDLY		
Courteous, pleasant	❑	❑
Is positive when interacting with others		
Shows care and concern for others	❑	❑
FLEXIBLE		
Handles multiple assignments	❑	❑
Adjusts to changing situations and needs	❑	❑
Seeks win/win in meeting customer needs	❑	❑
FAST		
Is timely meeting customer needs	❑	❑
Corrects mistakes quickly	❑	❑
Provides accurate, appropriate service the first time	❑	❑
DEMONSTRATES HIGH ETHICAL STANDARDS		
Exhibits honesty in actions and decision making	❑	❑
Displays fairness in dealing with others	❑	❑
Is truthful in interactions	❑	❑
TRUSTWORTHY		
Makes and keeps promises	❑	❑
Refrains from speaking negatively about others	❑	❑
Apologizes when appropriate	❑	❑
MATURITY		
Is honest and forthright	❑	❑
Displays maturity in interactions and decision-making	❑	❑
Accepts constructive criticism	❑	❑
Assumes responsibility for self-improvement	❑	❑
PROFESSIONAL EFFECTIVENESS		
Seeks out and participates in learning opportunities	❑	❑
Shares job knowledge readily with others	❑	❑
Strives to balance personal and professional goals	❑	❑
LEADERSHIP EFFECTIVENESS		
Regularly provides others with constructive feedback and contributes to others' development	❑	❑
Takes time to coach and mentor others	❑	❑

	S	NI
ACHIEVING MUTUAL GOALS		
Works together with teammates to accomplish desired outcomes	❑	❑
Demonstrates commitment to team goals; holds self accountable for team effectiveness	❑	❑
contributes as an equal member of the team	❑	❑
COLLABORATION		
Seeks out others' points of view	❑	❑
Demonstrates support of teammates' accomplishments	❑	❑
Avoids placing blame on others	❑	❑
WIN/ WIN		
When dealing with conflict, strives to find solution that benefits all	❑	❑
When dealing with conflict, confronts the issue directly with the individual involved	❑	❑
Respects every individual in every interaction	❑	❑
CONTIGUOUS IMPROVEMENT OF PROCESSES		
Suggests ideas for improving the way a job gets done	❑	❑
Openly accepts suggestions for individual improvement from others	❑	❑
QUALITY/COST BALANCE		
Continually strives to improve timeliness, accuracy, and quality of outcome	❑	❑
Shares ideas for cost savings	❑	❑
INNOVATION		
Suggests ideas for new/enhanced products/services to satisfy customers	❑	❑
Displays imagination, creativity, and resourcefulness in providing cost-effective customer satisfaction	❑	❑
ACHIEVEMENT		
Continually accomplishes objectives and takes on extra tasks as necessary	❑	❑
Accepts full accountability in accomplishing tasks/projects	❑	❑
Takes pride in work	❑	❑
KNOWLEDGE/SUPPORT OF ORGANIZATIONAL GOALS		
Demonstrates understanding and support of facility's culture, purpose, and values	❑	❑
Understands how individual duties support facility's mission	❑	❑

List facts to be shared with the employee to substantiate the feedback above. (Attach additional sheets if necessary.)

BASIC JOB RESPONSIBILITIES	S	NI
1. ________	❑	❑
2. ________	❑	❑
3. ________	❑	❑
4. ________	❑	❑

GOALS	MEASURES OF SUCCESS
________	________

EMPLOYEE COMMENTS:

EMPLOYEE SIGNATURE ____________ DATE______

REVIEWER SIGNATURE ____________ DATE______

SUPERVISOR SIGNATURE ____________ DATE______

DEFINITIONS

S– Satisfactory–Has Successfully achieved performance competencies. In a few instances may have exceeded some competencies and missed others, but on balance has performed the duties of the job. Demonstrates the motivation to improve performance.

NI–Needs Improvement–Has adequately performed most responsibilities. Has completely or consistently met all competencies. Has not completely reached agreed upon standards of quantity and/or quality for these competencies. Needs to improve skills to fully qualify for position. Likely that performance will improve within the next year.

Customer Satisfaction–focused, friendly, flexible, and fast

Integrity–demonstrates high ethical standards, trustworthy, displaying character and maturity

Teamwork–achieves mutual goals, collaborating, and seeking win/win

People (skill)–professional, personal, and leadership effectiveness

Process–continuous process improvement, value, and innovation

Outcome–achievement, leadership, knowledge and support of organizational goals

Figure 37-6. **A sample performance appraisal.**

Summary

In this chapter, we have learned about the best methods of obtaining employment and keeping your position as a nursing assistant. It is best to periodically review this information in order to make sure you stay current with all of the annual requirements. You must also keep up-to-date regarding policy changes at your facility, along with any changes that may occur at the state level. You must treat your position with the respect and care it deserves. Remember, you worked very hard to get where you are!

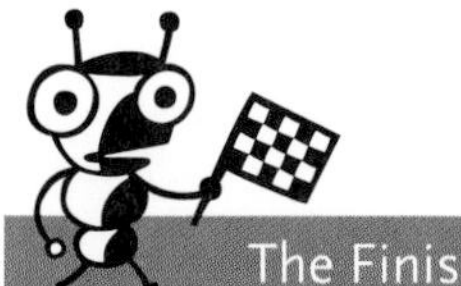

The Finish Line

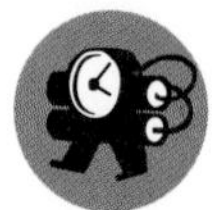

What's Wrong With This Picture?

Find all of the errors in the pictures below of people "ready" for an interview.

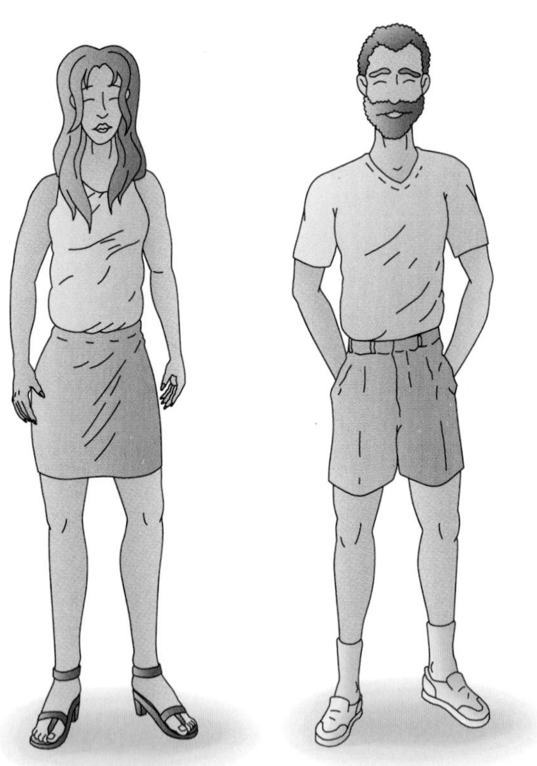

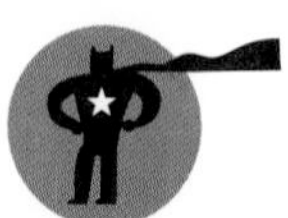

Star Student Central

1. Ask a friend, fellow student, or a family member to help you by pretending to be a potential employer. Make a short list of possible questions an employer might ask and practice going through an entire interview from start to finish. This kind of a "dry run" can help you feel more comfortable during the real interview.
2. Write a resumé and sample cover letter. Have a fellow student review it and offer suggestions.

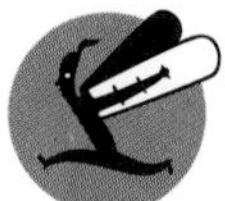

You Can Do It Corner!

1. List five necessary personal qualities in the SCANS report and what they mean. (LO 7)
2. What steps should you take when dressing for a job interview? (LO 4)
3. How and when do you receive a hepatitis B vaccine (HBV)? (LO 12)
4. List six categories found on a resumé. (LO 2)
5. Why should you be open to suggestions and constructive criticism on your job performance appraisal? (LO 13)
6. List four other requirements you may have to meet in order to secure a job. (LO 8)
7. What information do you need to bring from home to complete a job application? (LO 3)
8. Why is eye contact so important during a job interview? (LO 5)
9. List eight topics that may be required in annual in-services. (LO 11)
10. Describe five examples of information kept in a nursing assistant registry. (LO 9)
11. What are four important things to remember about scope of practice? (LO 6)
12. What is the minimum number of hours of required continuing education identified by federal law? (LO 10)

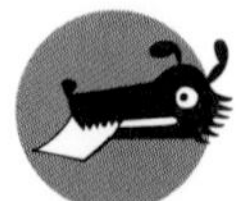

Star Student's Chapter Checklist

1. I have read my textbook chapter.
2. I have reviewed my own "Pocketful of Terms."

3. I have listened to my tutor tape.
4. I have reviewed and highlighted my class notes.
5. I have read and completed any handouts from this chapter.
6. I have completed "The Finish Line."
7. Star Time! Choose your reward!

Index